Cover design by Laura Palese
Cover photos © Leslie Klenke
Author photos © Janée Meadows
Cover copyright © 2021 by Hachette Book Group, Inc.

Grand Central Publishing
Hachette Book Group
1290 Avenue of the Americas, New York, NY 10104
grandcentralpublishing.com
twitter.com/grandcentralpub

First Edition: March 2021

Grand Central Publishing is a division of Hachette Book Group, Inc. The Grand Central Publishing name and logo is a trademark of Hachette Book Group, Inc.

The publisher is not responsible for websites (or their content) that are not owned by the publisher.

The Hachette Speakers Bureau provides a wide range of authors for speaking events. To find out more, go to www.hachettespeakersbureau.com or call (866) 376-6591. [delete if author doesn't participate]

The Carnivore Scores chart on page 62 © Dr. Paul Saladino

The Perfect Health Food Plate figure on page 59 © 2013 PerfectHealthDiet.com

Figures on pages xviii, 4, 12, 63, 68, 81, 82, 86, 121, and 126 are by Caroline DeVita

Library of Congress Control Number: 2020951069

ISBNs: 978-1-5387-3695-1 (hardcover); 978-1-5387-3694-4 (ebook)

Printed in the United States of America

LSC-C

Printing 1, 2021

Contents

Introduction

I used to run almost entirely on carbs, chowing down three or four robust grain-based meals every day. I kept a reliable supply of packaged processed energy bars and other snacks in my home, car, office, and travel bag. As soon as I finished breakfast, I would start thinking about lunch. A couple of hours after my typically huge dinners, I would wander into the kitchen to nibble on something while relaxing in the evening. Because I burned so much energy with extreme endurance workouts, I never got fat—unlike sedentary people with similar eating patterns. Yet even with my impressive physique and no obvious adverse health consequences, my hunger, appetite, and meal planning ran my life. I did not realize the culprits at the time, but gluten and other dietary toxins were destroying my intestinal tract to such an extent that I had to structure my running routes around bathroom locations.

Nearly two decades ago, I switched to an ancestral-style diet free from processed sugar, grains, and industrial seed oils and experienced a health awakening beyond my wildest dreams. In addition to healing my lifelong digestive dysfunction, my new eating habits meant that I was no longer dependent on food to stabilize my energy, mood, and cognitive functioning. By ditching high-carbohydrate, high-insulin-stimulating foods, I was able to access and burn stored body fat around the clock. I was almost never hungry and required far fewer calories to attain total satisfaction at every meal. It felt like an incredible gift to escape from the prison of carb dependency and transition into a new existence, one in line with our human genetic expectations for health that were honed through 2.5 million years of evolution. Contrary to modern marketing hype and the flawed science that's likely been programmed into your brain, we humans can do just fine without stuffing our faces morning, noon, and night and snacking incessantly to maintain energy between these round-the-clock feedings.

Essentially, my life's work has boiled down to this: helping others escape lifelong carbohydrate dependency driven by the Standard American Diet (SAD) and become what I affectionately call a *fat-burning beast*. This is the default human metabolic state that has been hardwired into our genes but has been egregiously compromised by the overconsumption of high-carbohydrate processed foods and toxic industrial seed oils (e.g., canola, sesame, soybean, and sunflower oils), which destroy our natural ability to burn stored energy. While it may take some sustained and devoted effort to reprogram your genes away from reliance on carbs, depending on the severity of your metabolic damage, the beast within you is ready to emerge when you choose the most nutritious and satiating foods, reduce meal frequency, and unlock the amazing healing powers of fasting.

Welcome to *Two Meals a Day*, a simple, sustainable, highly effective strategy to help you lose excess body fat; increase energy and focus; minimize your risk of diabetes, cancer, heart disease, and cognitive decline; and enjoy your maximum *healthspan*—a long, healthy, happy, high-energy life lived all the way to the end. *Two Meals a Day* offers a refreshing solution to the incredible frustration of carrying excess body fat. It transcends almost all the controversy and confusion over what constitutes the most healthful diet and finally does away with the pain, suffering, and sacrifice we've come to associate with dieting. I'm pretty fired up as we begin this journey together, because misguided health gurus, manipulative corporate marketing techniques, and so-called experts in government, in academia, and on the all-powerful internet are perpetuating the ridiculousness and the suffering of dieting with horrible advice and a fundamental misunderstanding and misrepresentation of human genetics and evolutionary biology. In case you haven't heard, here's the issue at hand: *We eat too much of the wrong foods too often. It's making us fat, tired, sick, and it's slowly but surely killing us.*

Recent science has made the surprising discovery that it's not laziness or lack of willpower that has made modern humans unwell but rather the *hormone dysregulation* caused by a daily pattern of high-carbohydrate breakfasts, lunches, and dinners along with frequent snacking and ingestion of toxic industrial oils. This pattern of eating has violently disrupted our magnificent evolutionary ability to burn stored body fat around the clock as a steady and reliable source of energy. Instead, we have become dependent on regular doses of ingested calories to fuel our busy days. The common phenomenon of feeling "hangry" after skipping even a single meal—a ridiculous notion from an evolutionary perspective—blatantly exposes this hormone dysregulation.

Even many enlightened folks who know to stay away from processed sugars, sweetened beverages, refined grain-based foods (wheat, corn, rice, pasta, cereal), and industrial seed oils remain unhealthy and overweight because they eat and snack too much. Consider the ketogenic diet, which has risen to popularity in recent years. While many who followed a well-formulated ketogenic diet have shed fat and improved their health, the plan has also been widely misappropriated as an opportunity to stuff one's face with "keto-approved" high-fat meals and snacks in a misguided attempt to trigger ketone production in the liver. We've forgotten keto's roots as an evolution-honed survival mechanism. Ketone production occurs in the liver to supply a steady source of fuel for the brain in times of starvation or in the absence of dietary carbohydrates. In reality, you access the main benefits of keto through fasting, not feasting on high-fat foods.

It's time to reframe our flawed and dated belief systems and behavior patterns relating to food and meals. It's as simple as this: if you want optimum health, body composition, and longevity, you have to do two things:

1. Ditch processed foods in favor of wholesome foods
2. Eat less frequently

Two Meals a Day will help you develop one of the most important health attributes imaginable: *metabolic flexibility*. This genetically preprogrammed superpower is the ability to burn a variety of fuel sources, especially stored fat, based on your body's needs at any given time. Paradoxically, you were born with robust metabolic flexibility, but it began to atrophy as soon as you were fed all manner of crunchy and mushy carbs as an infant. The good news is that you can quickly reclaim your genetic fat-burning abilities. Metabolic flexibility allows you to feel great all day long, with stable mood, energy, cognitive functioning, and appetite, *whether or not you eat regular meals*. I believe that reigniting your metabolic flexibility is the holy grail of all health pursuits. With it, you can naturally derive energy from a range of sources: the fat on your plate of food or the fat on your butt, belly, or thighs; the carbohydrates in your meal, the glucose in your bloodstream, or the glycogen in your muscles; and even from ketones, the superfuel that your liver makes when you're fasting or restricting dietary carbs. The best part is that your body doesn't care where those calories came from, because your source of calories to burn will move seamlessly from one substrate (fuel source) to another depending on your immediate energy needs.

Metabolic flexibility allows you to cruise through life not having to think about how many calories or grams of carbs you "earned" because you ran on the treadmill or how much protein you'll need to consume after your weight-lifting session to avoid muscle breakdown. Most important, metabolic flexibility will free you from the tyranny of hunger, appetite, and cravings, because your body will always be primed to get energy from body fat, glycogen (the stored form of carbohydrate in the liver and muscle tissue), and ready-made ketones. Ultimately, you'll stop living at the edge of "how much food can I stuff down my face and not get fat" and get to the point where you might want to explore how *little* food you can eat and still remain completely satisfied and energized every single day for the rest of your life.

If metabolic flexibility describes the ability to skip meals and burn fat, *metabolic efficiency* describes the result: the life-changing, life-extending ability to thrive on fewer calories.

I'm not suggesting you must starve yourself or live as an ascetic to be healthy. What I'm talking about is enjoying your life to the fullest and eating delicious and highly satisfying foods to your heart's content. I enjoy lavish meals as much as anyone, and I never deprive myself when I'm hungry. That said, I also believe that one fabulous plate of fresh sashimi or a grass-fed rib eye cooked to perfection can be more pleasurable (and ultimately more healthful) than all-you-can-eat fish and steak! I'm also not inclined to tarnish the lingering taste sensations and satisfaction of a gourmet meal by stuffing some sugar down at the end, just because dessert is a cultural mainstay.

Unfortunately, when you are locked into a carbohydrate-dependent eating pattern, you are compelled to eat an excessive amount of calories every day because your fat-burning factory is shut down and your appetite and satiety hormones are out of whack. The classic potato-chip ad campaigns of decades past are excellent examples. "Betcha can't eat just one" was the slogan for Lay's potato chips, and "Once you pop you can't stop" encouraged eating Pringles. These ads revealed the disturbing reality that nutrient-deficient foods trick your brain into eating more in a futile attempt to obtain nourishment.

The idea here is that when you can burn body fat and make ketones at any time, and your appetite and satiety hormones are optimized, you simply don't need as much food—even in pursuit of peak performance and maximum pleasure. I like to envision my metabolism as a carefully constructed closed-loop system that can operate perfectly well for days, if need be, without any visits to the fuel pump (i.e., without ingesting calories). A closed-loop metabolism ensures that you don't lose energy, muscle mass, strength, or your happy disposition. This honors our evolutionary imperative to not waste energy. In an effort to achieve widespread adoption of this empowering new strategy, I hereby declare a revision to global dietary lexicon: the popular term *intermittent fasting* is changed to the more apropos term (and mindset!) *intermittent eating*!

It's All About Insulin

Insulin is the key metabolic hormone that presides over all manner of cellular and homeostatic functions in the body. Insulin's primary role is to transport nutrients such as glucose, amino acids, and fatty acids from the bloodstream into cells. Today, we overburden our extremely delicate hormonal mechanisms in the pancreas (where insulin is manufactured) and the liver (which regulates glucose levels in the bloodstream) by consuming too many carbohydrates. Most dietary carbohydrates are converted into glucose upon ingestion. A small amount of this energy is burned right away, while the excess is quickly removed from the bloodstream and rerouted by insulin. Insulin transports the extra glucose to the muscle cells and the liver, where it is either converted into glycogen (the stored form of glucose) or triglycerides (the stored form of fat). Excess blood glucose is highly toxic—this is why a diabetic might pass out without a timely insulin injection. If you are not burning up lots of glycogen with an ambitious workout regimen, your extra calories will end up in fat-storage depots throughout your body.

When modern humans slam down high-carbohydrate breakfasts, lunches, and dinners, suck down sweetened beverages, and indulge in sugary snacks and treats, insulin must be continually pumped out to deal with the glucose burden created by these foods. Because insulin is a storage hormone, SAD eating patterns lock us into fat-storage mode around the clock. By contrast, low insulin levels allow the counterregulatory hormone glucagon to pull nutrients from storage into the bloodstream, where they're burned for energy. Three squares a day is a wholly modern construct and completely foreign to our evolutionary experience as rough-and-tumble hunter-gatherers who evolved to be fat burners in a feast-or-famine pattern.

The *Two Meals a Day* approach gets you back into the feast-or-famine rhythm that aligns with your genetic predisposition for maintaining health. This dietary modification can save your life, because when you overproduce insulin for too long—a condition known as *hyperinsulinemia*—you eventually develop the disease state known as *insulin resistance*. This happens over time as your cells become desensitized to the signals given off by insulin (because of chronic overproduction) and don't accept the package of nutrients insulin delivers to their doorstep. The NO VACANCY sign at the cell motel results in too much glucose remaining in the bloodstream. This is the start of big trouble. The liver cannot detect your blood glucose levels, instead relying on insulin signaling to decide when to release more glucose into the bloodstream. Sensing elevated blood insulin levels, the liver is deceived into releasing more glucose in a futile attempt to get you back to homeostasis. Instead, too much insulin *and* too much glucose in the bloodstream send you spiraling into decades-long disease patterns. Many medical experts believe insulin resistance is the number one health crisis facing modern-day humans across the globe.

Insulin resistance causes oxidative damage (a.k.a. free-radical damage), system-wide chronic inflammation, and *glycation*—the binding of excess glucose molecules to important structural proteins in organs throughout the body. This causes widespread dysfunction and disease patterns that affect important organs and systems. It's sobering to realize that just as the sugar in cotton candy sticks to your fingers, the sticky composition of glucose molecules tends to adhere to the delicate endothelial cell lining on the walls of your arteries and gets you started on the road to heart disease. It also sticks in the retinal microvascular endothelium to mess with your eyesight and attaches to collagen and elastin to wrinkle your skin.

Oxidation, inflammation, and glycation are the driving factors in heart disease, cancer, and accelerated aging. The direct association between atherosclerosis and a high-carbohydrate, high-insulin-producing diet is finally becoming a matter of consensus. This science replaces the flawed and dated lipid hypothesis of heart disease, which erroneously blames dietary cholesterol and saturated fat for causing heart disease. As you will learn in detail shortly, reducing excess body fat and avoiding chronic disease patterns can be achieved through minimizing insulin production rather than by restricting caloric intake and increasing caloric expenditure.

Honoring Our Ancestors

I've covered food choices extensively in other books such as *The Primal Blueprint* and *The Keto Reset Diet*. In this book, I'm going to suggest that you draw on your favorites from the surprisingly simple list of "ancestral" foods that fueled human evolution. Examining human health in an evolutionary context is without a doubt the most profound and exacting scientific study of all time. The legendary geneticist and evolutionary biologist Theodosius Dobzhansky reinforced this point in a highly acclaimed 1973 essay titled "Nothing in Biology Makes Sense Except in the Light of Evolution."

Following is a list of the ancestral foods that have made us human for the past two million years: meat, fish, fowl, eggs, vegetables, fruits, nuts, and seeds. I left off insects so you'll continue reading, but of course they are technically included in the evolutionary list and are still enjoyed today in many cuisines and indigenous populations. I also make concessions to allow for the inclusion of healthful modern foods such as organic high-fat dairy products and high-cacao-percentage dark chocolate. Noticeably absent are today's heavily processed, nutrient-deficient sugars, grains, and industrial seed oils. Bestselling author Michael Pollan memorably and accurately called today's packaged, processed fare "edible foodlike substances." Sadly, these substances make up a huge percentage of our total caloric intake today, in the process crowding out the opportunity to enjoy truly nutritious and satisfying foods. Dr. Loren Cordain, author of *The Paleo Diet* and one of the forefathers of the Paleo diet, cites a statistic: 71 percent of the calories in the grain-based Standard American Diet come from foods that were wholly absent during Paleolithic times.

You can enjoy a *Two Meals a Day* lifestyle whether you follow a vegan, vegetarian, Paleo, keto, carnivore, or any other eating strategy. It is important to remember, however, that skipping meals doesn't give you license to be indiscriminate when it's time to eat. You absolutely must ditch toxic processed foods and emphasize wholesome, nutrient-dense, ancestral-style foods in order to succeed. You cannot achieve metabolic flexibility while engaging in the wildly excessive intake of processed carbs and industrial oils in the SAD. That said, I think it's time to back off a bit from some of the dogma and intense scrutiny over food choices that's so prevalent these days in order to honor some big-picture objectives:

- Eat nutrient-dense foods of your personal preference—within ancestral guidelines, of course.
- Ditch the alarmingly destructive habit of snacking or eating frequent small meals. Snacking disrupts fat burning, increases insulin swings during the day, and increases overall daily caloric intake.
- Honor your hunger and satiety signals at all times.

Two Meals a Day is a great place to start, but as you build momentum on this journey, this guideline will likely become your *maximum* meal frequency rather than a minimum or an average. I actually thought for a moment about calling this book *The 1.5 Diet*! However, I want you to feel confident and comfortable that you "got this" when it comes to escaping the cultural norm of regimented meals and quickly being able to thrive on a haphazard and spontaneous eating pattern in which you rarely eat more than two full meals a day and occasionally less than that. You will do everything by choice, not because you are trying to adhere to a regimented program in pursuit of a short-term goal. You will get to the point where eating fewer meals and not snacking feels comfortable, easy, and intuitively correct.

If you love to eat, and recoil at the thought of passing up a dining opportunity, please understand that I support your enjoyment of life and consumption of indulgent meals to your heart's content. Take it from me: I've gone from being a young guy who ate more food more often than anyone I knew to someone who eats only when I'm truly hungry and savors every bite that goes into my mouth. If a gourmet offering is not at hand, I simply won't eat. This sometimes happens when I'm traveling and away from good choices or am engrossed in work or play. I don't consciously strive to skip meals, but I often simply forget to eat. When you regulate your appetite and metabolic hormones with the strategies presented in this book, you'll discover a remarkable ability to naturally stabilize hunger, mood, energy, and satiety by eating fewer meals and consuming fewer calories. Metabolic efficiency drives longevity, while caloric excess is one of the most prominent drivers of accelerated aging and disease.

When you develop metabolic flexibility and metabolic efficiency, you will be able to go with the flow and not worry about adhering to regimented meal patterns to keep your energy level steady. You'll be free from the prison of food obsession. When you reclaim your human genetic birthright as a fat-burning beast, dropping excess body fat will be as easy as putting your hand on a dial and turning it to the desired setting. Lower your insulin production, and you lower your body fat—it's (almost) as simple as that! Metabolic flexibility allows you to take control of your life and your daily schedule and sustain peak cognitive and physical performance without needing to eat regular meals or snacks. While losing some inches and getting new clothes is certainly a rewarding manifestation of success, the wide-ranging sense of freedom and empowerment you experience with metabolic flexibility is perhaps the richest reward of all.

SISSON'S SIMPLE SUGGESTIONS

My *Two Meals a Day* lifestyle looks like this: with rare exceptions, I eat only during the hours between 1:00 p.m. and 7:00 p.m., which means that I fast for eighteen hours every day. I usually break my fast with my world-famous Sisson Bigass Salad (see page 229), then enjoy an evening out with my wife, Carrie, at one of the many fabulous restaurants near my home in Miami Beach. Many days, I'm too busy to prepare my centerpiece salad, so I might have what amounts to half a meal (either a smoothie, a few squares of dark chocolate smothered in nut butter, a healthful meat-and-veggie frozen meal, or a small bowl of leftover steak) before enjoying a celebratory dinner later. On other days, my midday masterpiece is so satisfying that I'm really not hungry in the evening for anything more than a small serving of the previous evening's fish or steak main course.

When I'm traveling, my time-tested strategy for beating jet lag is to fast on the day of the flight (this protects against the extra oxidative stress of passing through time zones in the confinement of a jet's cabin), arrive at my destination, and stay active until bedtime (I do not eat), then eat my first meal the following morning. This quickly calibrates my digestive and circadian rhythms to the new time zone. It's an advanced strategy, but it works incredibly well once your body adapts to extended fasting. This means that there are plenty of days on my calendar when I either don't eat or have only one proper meal, paired with my typical routine at home, in which I'll eat two or maybe one and a half meals.

Excelling in the Essentials

We are going to proceed slowly and methodically on this journey together, because I want to make sure you don't struggle or feel intimidated by any part of the process. You don't have to stress about counting calories, painstakingly track macronutrient ratios, or traffic in the dogma and rigidity of many niche diets. Instead, you are going to focus on the big-picture essentials of metabolic flexibility, as follows:

- *Eliminate nutrient-deficient processed foods.* Sugars, sweetened beverages, grains (wheat, rice, corn, pasta, cereal), and refined industrial seed oils (canola, corn, cottonseed, peanut, safflower, soybean, sunflower) are insidious killers—they are directly associated with both immediate health disturbances (inflammatory and autoimmune reactions) and an elevated risk of diabetes, cancer, heart disease, and cognitive decline over the long run. In this book, you will bust out of the gate with a total elimination of these foods for twenty-one days in order to escape carbohydrate dependency and set yourself up for success with fasting, round-the-clock fat burning, and a long-term two-meals-a-day rhythm.
- *Emphasize nutrient-dense ancestral foods.* Humans evolved to thrive on an array of wholesome, colorful, nutrient-dense plant and animal foods. Once you ditch toxic modern foods, you can custom-design a dietary strategy guided by personal

preference. Cut through the hype and controversy and choose to include whatever foods on the aforementioned ancestral list make you feel happy, energetic, and well nourished.

■ *Embrace intermittent eating.* Our bodies operate most effectively in a fasted state. Fasting taps into our genetically hardwired regenerative and renewal pathways, boosting immune, cognitive, metabolic, and anti-inflammatory functions better than any superfood. However, you must first kick carb addiction before you can unlock the powers of fasting. If you can't burn fat well, fasting will be too stressful to your carb-addicted body. You'll trigger the fight-or-flight response and end up in burnout mode instead of beast mode.

■ *Reduce meal frequency and snacking.* Snacking may provide a deserved break from the intensity of the workday, but so does a walk around the block or a set of deep squats! Dr. Cate Shanahan, author of *The Fatburn Fix* and *Deep Nutrition*, reminds us that whenever you eat anything, even the "fat bombs" (homemade high-fat snack foods) favored by the keto community, burning stored body fat (along with the manufacturing of ketones in the liver) ceases abruptly while you process the ingested calories. A grazing pattern of eating throughout the day is directly associated with hyperinsulinemia, especially when you consider that most snacks are made with refined carbohydrates. Humans operate much better in a feast-or-famine pattern.

■ *Form an empowering mindset.* It's no secret that many well-meaning health enthusiasts fail miserably and repeatedly with diet and body transformation goals because of the destructive influence of self-limiting beliefs and behavior patterns and the subconscious programming that sabotages good intentions. You will learn how to gracefully live in alignment with your stated goals and make empowering, conscious choices with full accountability.

An empowering mindset starts with feeling comfortable that you have all the knowledge you need to succeed. The next steps are to forgive yourself for past mistakes and failures with extreme compassion and identify flawed subconscious thoughts, beliefs, and behaviors, such as harboring a negative body image and snacking mindlessly. Then you will awaken your amazing potential for transformation and be able to describe your goals and dreams with specificity.

Next, you'll create a winning environment and an action plan for success, including establishing some firm rules and guidelines that will help you stay

strong against the constant temptation of indulgence and excess. Finally, you'll
use repetition and endurance to create automatic habits that don't drain the
fragile and easily depleted resource of willpower (you'll be guided through this
sequence in chapter 4 and during the 12-Day Turbocharge). After this hard
internal work, you'll emerge with your natural hunger and satiety signals running the show—no more emotional or absentminded eating. You will no longer
be tethered to the "three squares a day plus snacks" clock.

- *Get your lifestyle dialed in.* Your exercise, sleep, and stress management habits are
going to make or break your dietary transformation efforts. If you are sedentary,
sleep deficient, or harried and hyperconnected, you'll sabotage your dietary transformation efforts and drift back toward carbohydrate dependency. Hectic days
can trigger carbohydrate cravings in association with fight-or-flight sympathetic
nervous system dominance. Conversely, fat burning is associated with parasympathetic "rest and digest" dominance.

The lifestyle essentials include increasing all forms of general everyday movement (especially frequent breaks from prolonged periods of stillness), following a
sensible exercise program (including brief, high-intensity efforts), implementing
superb sleep habits (which helps lower stress hormones and regulate appetite and
satiety hormones), and setting aside time every day to unwind and unplug from
hyperconnectivity.

Replacing Flawed and Dated Conventional Stupidity with Empowering New Truths

There is an enormous amount of conventional wisdom about diet and eating that is
flawed, dated, and straight-up nonsense—what Australian peak-performance coach Andre
Obradovic calls "conventional stupidity." We are going to destroy flawed and dated conventional stupidity (FDCS) and replace it with empowering new truths (ENTs). These
new truths may be contrary to what you've heard and believed your whole life, and they
may be difficult to embrace right way. However, once you put these empowering new
insights and possibilities into action, you will experience a transformation of both body
and mindset.

FDCS: Fasting will slow down your metabolism, make you feel weak and sluggish, and cause you to overeat later.

ENT: Your body operates most efficiently in a fasted state. In general, the more time you can spend in a fasted state, the healthier you'll be—provided that you possess metabolic flexibility.

FDCS: Breakfast is the most important meal of the day. It helps keep your metabolism and energy levels steady for hours.

ENT: An early morning smorgasbord is not necessarily the most important meal of the day, nor is it even necessary. Consuming a high-carbohydrate meal in the morning can put you on a blood sugar roller coaster for the rest of the day. The best time to "break-fast" is when you experience true sensations of hunger.

FDCS: Eating three square meals a day (or six small meals, as is commonly recommended for serious athletes) is the key to maintaining steady energy, mood, and focus all day and will boost your metabolism.

ENT: Eating frequently increases total caloric intake and promotes excess body fat and disease patterns associated with hyperinsulinemia, especially type 2 diabetes, heart disease, and many cancers. Departing from regimented breakfasts, lunches, and dinners to eat in a haphazard, intuitive manner is actually healthful! It will develop metabolic flexibility and efficiency and likely trigger breakthroughs in fat loss, boost cognitive and physical performance, and minimize disease risk factors.

FDCS: Whole grains are the staff of life and should be the centerpiece of your diet (as they are on the USDA's Food Guide Pyramid and MyPlate imagery).

ENT: There is no requirement for dietary carbohydrates in human biology. Humans can survive and thrive on extremely low carbohydrate intake in comparison to today's egregious excess. Grains have minimal nutritional value and contain plant toxins such as gluten and many others that can be problematic for many people. Moreover, the "healthful fiber" argument for grains has been scientifically invalidated. A high carbohydrate, grain-based diet can easily result in excess fiber intake, which is counterproductive to weight loss and health.

FDCS: Carbohydrates are essential fuel for working muscles. Athletes must fuel up before workouts (carbo-load) and reload on carbs immediately after workouts. Otherwise, they will break down hard-earned muscle mass.

ENT: Muscles can efficiently burn fatty acids as well as carbs for fuel. Even high-calorie-burning athletes can transition to fat-adapted training and racing and thrive on minimal carbohydrate intake. Fat and ketones burn more cleanly than glucose in the brain and body, promoting improved performance, less inflammation, and faster recovery from workouts.

FDCS: Dietary fat and cholesterol are the driving causes of obesity, cancer, and heart disease.

ENT: The true cause of today's epidemic diet-related disease patterns is excess consumption of refined carbohydrates and industrial seed oils, which drives hyperinsulinemia and triggers oxidation and inflammation, which are the root causes of virtually all disease. Natural, nutritious sources of fat—including high-cholesterol foods—can help support healthy hormone and metabolic functioning.

How Did We Get into This Mess?

Let's take a quick stroll through the timeline of human evolution to get some perspective on the incredible mess we have landed in today: carbohydrate-addicted humans suffering from a global epidemic of obesity, cancer, heart disease, and cognitive decline. These conditions are being increasingly tied to a grain-based, high-insulin-producing diet. *Homo erectus* and his descendants existed for more than two million years as hunter-gatherers. Our ancestors prevailed through the brutal life-or-death selection pressures of starvation and predator danger by gaining access to nutrient-dense animal foods, especially omega-3 fatty acids from marine life and land animals. Our success as hunter-gatherers enabled us to branch off from our plant-chomping ape cousins, grow incredibly large and complex brains, and rise to the top of the food chain.

The advent of agriculture and the ensuing dawn of civilized life across the globe, starting ten thousand years ago, was in some ways the most health-destructive event in the history of humanity. Granted, cultivating grains and livestock allowed us to live close together in permanent settlements, specialize labor, store cheap calories for reliable long-term access, produce more offspring, and accelerate the technological progress and affluence that continues today. Sadly, human health took a huge hit when we transitioned from hunter-gatherers, eating the planet's most bountiful foods, to carbohydrate addicts. The brain and body size of humans declined significantly with the dawn of civilization,

Human Evolution Dietary Timeline

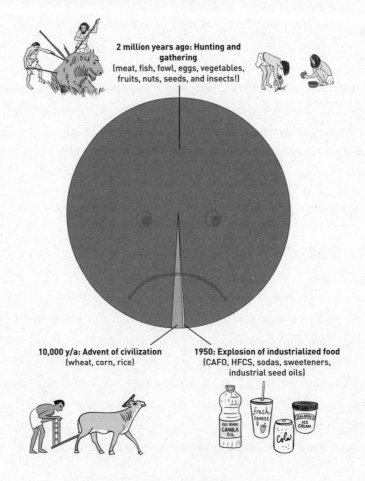

2 million years ago: Hunting and gathering
(meat, fish, fowl, eggs, vegetables, fruits, nuts, seeds, and insects!)

10,000 y/a: Advent of civilization
(wheat, corn, rice)

1950: Explosion of industrialized food
(CAFO, HFCS, sodas, sweeteners, industrial seed oils)

and conditions such as malnutrition and diet-related diseases arose for the first time. The industrialization of food over the past century—especially the increasing consumption of refined sugar, grains, and seed oils in processed and fast foods—has resulted in the fattest, least fit, most diseased population in the history of humanity.

Buying whole-grain crackers, nonfat Greek yogurt, or a freshly squeezed vegetable-and-fruit smoothie may seem like healthful and virtuous choices, but even the most health-conscious eaters can suffer from carbohydrate addiction and metabolic disease patterns by eating too frequently and drifting too far from the *Homo sapiens* evolutionary diet that was (compared to the SAD) extremely low in carbohydrates, high in natural, nutritious fats, and entirely absent of toxic processed foods. The *Two Meals a Day* journey starts with ditching nutrient-deficient processed foods and replacing them with your favorite wholesome, nutrient-dense plant and animal foods. This switch will lower insulin production and give you a fighting chance at attaining metabolic flexibility. From there, you will focus on reducing meal frequency and eliminating snacking, which will help you unlock the amazing health benefits of fasting.

Alas, making good choices for your two daily meals isn't enough: sufficient attention must also be devoted to the lifestyle and mindset factors that can make or break your success. Overly strenuous exercise routines, insufficient sleep, self-limiting beliefs and behavior patterns, and too much general stress are all associated with carbohydrate cravings, overeating, and excess insulin production.

The Magic of Hormone Optimization

It's time to reject the deeply flawed and misinterpreted "calories in, calories out" mentality of portion control and exhaustive workouts that we've been socialized to believe is the singular path to staying lean and healthy. I want you to take comfort right now in the fact that you will never have to struggle and suffer again in the name of fat loss or dietary transformation, because you are finally adopting the correct approach—one aligned with your human genetic requirements for health. You can eat when you're hungry, enjoy incredibly delicious and satiating meals (just breeze through the titles in the recipe section of this book and you'll see what I mean), and experience the bliss of *hormone optimization*—perhaps for the first time since you were a kid with boundless energy. No more counting calories or obsessing about macronutrient ratios ever again. You will embrace a new ethos of intermittent eating and get into a rhythm of intuitive eating decisions instead of thinking of food as the fuel necessary to survive a busy day without passing out.

If you possess a decent level of health, body composition, and metabolic flexibility right now—evidenced by healthful body-fat levels (males under 18 percent; females under 25 percent) or being able to skip a meal and still function smoothly for a few more hours before eating again—you can experience dramatic results in as little as three weeks. Many intermittent-eating practitioners can lose ten pounds or more in twenty-one days. This total is not just body fat but also a reduction in water retention and inflammation throughout the body—a reduction caused by eliminating toxic foods. If you are starting this journey with a history of yo-yo dieting or disordered eating, or if you carry excess body fat or have learned from blood tests that you are at risk for certain diseases, you may require a more gradual approach to becoming metabolically flexible and radically altering your body composition. However, even if you are metabolically damaged, you can still make steady progress each day without having to suffer or deprive yourself. Taking comfortable baby steps will quickly boost your confidence as well as your trust and enthusiasm for the process. Then, even if you experience the occasional slipup, such as a weekend or a vacation during which you engage in undisciplined eating, you can right the ship quickly instead of getting discouraged and sinking into self-destructive behavior patterns.

Congratulations on your interest in and enthusiasm for transforming your health. You've already taken the necessary first step toward lasting success. In the coming chapters, we will focus on an assortment of objectives that you will leverage to build the body of your dreams and enjoy a long, healthy, happy, awesome life.

Journaling Your Journey

Journaling will be a key factor in the success of your *Two Meals a Day* experience. You'll go on three distinct journal journeys.

- **Chapter-End Journal Exercises:** These will help strengthen your understanding of the concepts and your commitment to a new way of eating and way of life. Journaling will be especially important in chapter 4, which covers mindset and behavior-change concepts.

- **Gratitude Journal:** Beginning with chapter 4, you'll be asked to start a separate gratitude journal, or make distinct entries into your *Two Meals a Day* journal, as a centerpiece of living in a state of gratitude.
- **12-Day Turbocharge Journal:** Every day, you'll make a journal entry relating to each of your five daily assignments (details shortly).

The particulars of your journal are up to you. No fancy structure is necessary; just grab a blank spiral-bound notebook and write free-form observations as directed in the chapters and the 12-Day Turbocharge challenges. You may be journaling about the specifics of your kitchen and pantry purge, your efforts to improve your sleep habits and environment, or the escalation of your fasting aptitude. You can record what you eat each day to heighten awareness as you transform bad habits into good ones. You can devote special attention to areas where you struggle and provide an honest accounting of your thoughts and emotions along the way.

Journaling will help you stay accountable and provide valuable insights that you can refer to whenever you feel the need to refocus or get a motivational boost. If you have transitioned most of the communication elements in your life (e.g., calendar, to-do lists) to the digital realm, that's great. However, research from Indiana University suggests that a handwritten journal can be more effective for lifestyle transformation goals. Writing by hand requires more cognitive power, creativity, and psychic investment than typing your thoughts or reacting to a structured template such as a questionnaire. MRI imagery shows that unlike typing, writing by hand helps synchronize the analytical left brain and creative right brain, stimulating brain synapses in a manner that is similar to meditation. Writing's sequential hand movements help hone your skills for linguistic processing and working memory. Writing by hand also forces you to slow down and perhaps better appreciate the words and ideas you are creating—a different experience from hammering away on a keyboard. Neuroscientists suggest that trading in the keyboard for the pen may also improve creative expression.

Keeping a journal gives you a valuable resource to consult whenever you need a motivational boost or a course correction when you fall off track. Another way to boost the impact of your journaling is to select meaningful excerpts or summary concepts and turn them into acronyms or pithy statements that might make sense only to you. Write these on a sticky note or index card and post them in a prominent location for daily inspiration. For example, when I coached Brad while he was on the professional triathlon circuit, I would end every phone call or personal meeting with a single phrase: "Remember, patience and trust." This inspired him to write the phrase on an index card and display it at home. The comment summarized our extensive consultations relating to training strategy and season planning as well as the essential need to stay focused in the face of potential distractions or diminished confidence caused by setbacks on the racecourse.

Your journaling will align with your personal style: it's okay to be as long-winded or as succinct as you wish, and you can keep your writing completely private if you prefer. However, one thing's for sure with journaling: you gotta do it! Writing a few minutes every day is more effective than dusting off your journal once a week for a long writing session. That said, even committing to weekend entries is better than nothing. Unwinding a lifetime of subconscious programming and destroying self-limiting beliefs and behavior patterns is serious business; simply jotting down passing thoughts or puffy positive affirmations is not going to cut it.

When you can build a strong journaling habit, you can enjoy a host of long-term psychological and physical benefits, including better emotional regulation, self-awareness, and self-confidence. Journaling has also been shown to improve physical health; lower inflammation, blood pressure, and stress hormone levels; and improve insulin sensitivity, liver function, lung function, and immune cell activity. Gratitude journaling in particular has been shown to prompt spikes of the feel-good hormones dopamine, serotonin, and oxytocin. These hormones travel through neural pathways in the brain and program you to be a happier person. Keep an eye out for the exercises at the end of every chapter and get ready to fill some pages!

The 12-Day Turbocharge

You'll find this awesome twelve-day immersive experience after the seven chapters of the book. Armed with all the knowledge from your reading, you will pick the appropriate time to embark upon an intense and challenging series of daily assignments in each of five areas: food, fasting, fitness, mindset, and lifestyle. Many of the daily challenges are written exercises or actions accompanied by written exercises. While staying in turbocharge mode would be unsustainable over the long term for most of us, the idea is to expose yourself to a number of winning strategies and behaviors from which you can pick and choose and incorporate those into daily life over the long term.

CHAPTER 1

Clean Up Your Act

The first step to transforming your body into a lean, energetic, fat-burning beast is to eliminate nutrient-deficient, high-insulin-stimulating foods from your diet. You must get insulin under control, or all bets are off when it comes to building metabolic flexibility and developing your ability to fast. Our bodies are simply not designed to process the massive amount of carbohydrates in today's grain-based diet. Remember, humans evolved by consuming extremely minimal carbohydrates in the form of wild seasonal fruits, starchy tubers, and high-fiber vegetables. We evolved to burn mostly fat, exist in a state of ketosis routinely, and to live a low-stress lifestyle that doesn't require tons of glucose to sustain. Our *Homo sapiens* default genetic setting as fat burners is illustrated by the fact that you only have around a teaspoon (five grams) of glucose circulating through your entire blood volume of around five quarts (4.7 liters). This ratio is tightly regulated at all times by your liver—the control tower for the processing and distribution of nutrients into the bloodstream.

When you indulge in oatmeal breakfasts, Starbucks Frappuccinos, PowerBars, and pasta dinners, you abuse your extremely delicate hormonal mechanisms and hitch a ride on the familiar blood sugar roller coaster that makes you tired, cranky, and fat. Even if you choose healthful carbohydrates and stay away from junk, you can still develop a hyper-insulinemia problem if you eat and snack too frequently, don't move around or work out enough, or don't get adequate sleep. Remember, even when you choose slower-burning whole grains, legumes (beans, soy products, lentils), and starchy tubers (sweet potatoes, squash, and so on), it all eventually gets converted into glucose. You still need to produce a significant amount of insulin to process these carbohydrate calories over time. Add in today's liberal year-round consumption of fruit (especially the high-glycemic, low-antioxidant tropical fruits); the hidden sources of sugar in restaurant meals, condiments, sauces, and processed meals and snacks; and the insidious liquid carbohydrate calories in myriad sweetened beverages that are calorically dense but fail to satiate, and you have a huge disconnect from our genetic predisposition for health.

Metabolic syndrome is a cluster of interrelated disease conditions driven by poor diet and physical inactivity. Medical and nutrition experts agree that it is today's number one global health epidemic (yes, even more than COVID-19, because metabolic disease dramatically increases one's susceptibility to the virus and the severity of its symptoms and mortality risk) and that it's driven predominantly by excess insulin production. The Cleveland Clinic states, "The exact cause of metabolic syndrome is not known...[but] many features...are associated with 'insulin resistance.'" The five markers of metabolic syndrome are: high blood pressure, high blood glucose, excess belly fat, high triglycerides, and low HDL cholesterol. Amazingly, these are so closely tied to dietary choices that four of the five risk factors can be corrected (in most individuals) in only twenty-one days by ditching the unhealthful foods described in this chapter. The fifth, slimming your waistline, might take longer depending on your starting point. However, reducing your total insulin production will mobilize stored body fat and help you progress quickly to a healthier body mass index.

If you can lower your overall dietary insulin production, you will lower disease risk, lose excess body fat, boost immune functioning, feel better, think better, and live better. It's difficult to dispute the idea that producing the ideal minimal amount of insulin (to accomplish the job of delivering calories and nutrients to your cells) could be the single most important lifestyle practice in support of longevity. It is known in science that across all species, the individuals who produce the least amount of insulin over a lifetime live the longest. Unfortunately, under FDCS (flawed and dated conventional stupidity, remember?), prediabetic and type 2 diabetic folks are treated with prescription medication (more insulin!) and flimsy directives to eat fewer calories and exercise more. Such efforts almost always fail in the long term because they don't address the root cause: metabolic dysfunction and hormone dysregulation caused by hyperinsulinemia. Achieve metabolic flexibility, and you steer clear of this mess!

Calorie Confusion, Constraints, and Compensations

Dr. Jason Fung, a Canadian nephrologist and weight loss expert who wrote *The Obesity Code*, *The Diabetes Code*, and several books about fasting, states, "The calories in, calories out theory of obesity is one of the great failures in the history of medicine." Dr. Fung explains that a calorie-restrictive diet alone will not reduce body fat over the long term because genetically programmed survival mechanisms against starvation will start kicking in to lower your metabolic rate and drift you back toward your annoying body-composition "set point." This is the idea that whatever you do to eat fewer calories, burn more calories, or even eat more calories and burn fewer of them, your genetically influenced homeostatic drives conspire to eventually return you to a specific set point. The familial genetic attributes Mom and Dad gave you have a strong influence on your set point; Dr. Fung cites research concluding that obesity risk is 70 percent genetic.

Counterintuitive as it may seem, the calories you burn during strenuous, depleting workouts make little or no contribution to your fat-reduction goals. Countless studies reveal that exercise calories burned are offset by a corresponding increase in appetite as well as a reduction in routine caloric expenditure during the day. This shocking and counterintuitive idea is scientifically validated by what is known as the *compensation theory*. Compensations happen both consciously—rewarding yourself for that 6:00 a.m. spin class with an evening on the couch with Ben & Jerry—and subconsciously: we tend to be a bit more lazy and sluggish, eat bigger portions, and snack more frequently in the aftermath of impressive workouts.

Amazingly, humans seem to have assorted homeostatic compensatory mechanisms that effectively place a ceiling on our daily total energy expenditure (TEE). If you burn a bunch of calories at a workout, your body finds assorted ways to burn fewer calories at rest over the course of the day. This is known as the *constrained model of energy expenditure* and counters the common misconception that a devoted workout routine will speed up your metabolism at rest. These concepts have risen to prominence after a landmark 2012 study of the Hadza tribe, modern-day hunter-gatherers living in Tanzania. The study, led by American anthropologist Herman Pontzer, PhD, revealed that despite their extremely active lifestyles, which include walking between four and seven miles each day, the Hadza were found to burn around the same number of calories daily as an average urban office worker! I've actually done some caloric intake and expenditure calculations that show that

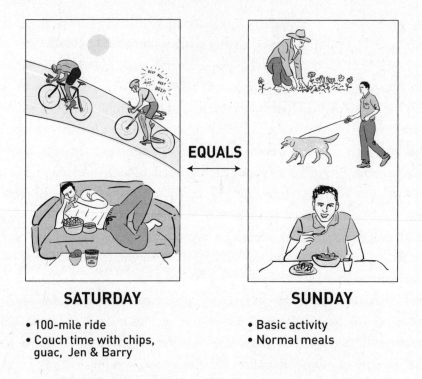

SATURDAY

- 100-mile ride
- Couch time with chips, guac, Jen & Barry

SUNDAY

- Basic activity
- Normal meals

a Saturday featuring a hundred-mile bike ride in the morning, followed by hours on the couch watching TV and slamming chips, guacamole, and recovery smoothies, is in energy balance with a Sunday of taking the dog for a walk, doing some yard work, and eating normal meal portions.

The revelation here is that the way we have fought the battle of the bulge for decades has been an ill-conceived, dismal failure. It has led to the completely flawed and psychologically harmful misconception that excess body fat is indicative of laziness and lack of discipline: eating too much and exercising too little. Dr. Fung calls this "the calorie deception." He explains that hormones influence hunger and satiety beneath your conscious awareness so that overeating, excess body fat, and diet-related disease conditions are almost entirely a result of hormone dysfunction caused by hyperinsulinemia.

I've long believed that body composition is 80 percent dependent on diet and only 20 percent on exercise and other lifestyle factors. Dr. Fung goes so far as to say that controlling insulin is *95 percent* of the solution here! Or, as my friend Eddy says, "Abs are made in the kitchen." Beyond your genetic influences, years and decades of hyperinsulinemia and the resultant hormone dysfunction will cause your set point to drift ever higher. This is where we get the widely cited statistic that American adults gain an average of a pound a year from ages twenty-five through fifty-five—by adding 1.5 pounds of fat and losing .5 pounds of muscle. This results in huge increases in disease risk and a 40 percent obesity rate for American adults today.

Even if you have lucky genetics and don't carry a lot of visible excess body fat, it's possible you are still what Dr. Phil Maffetone calls "overfat"—possessing extra fat that impairs health and fitness, especially visceral fat. Visceral fat is a distinct type of fat that accumulates around the abdominal organs as well as the heart. Visceral fat is far more destructive to health than the subcutaneous fat that typically accumulates in the hips, thighs, and rear end. This is because visceral fat releases inflammatory chemicals known as cytokines into the bloodstream, hindering fat burning, and suppressing key antiaging hormones such as testosterone and human growth hormone. The inflammatory, hormone-altering properties of visceral fat beget the accumulation of more visceral fat. In his book *The Overfat Pandemic*, Dr. Maffetone estimates that 76 percent of the world's population can be classified as overfat. As one of the world's leading experts on endurance training and a coach to many world champions in distance running and the Ironman triathlon, he also asserts that you cannot exercise your way out of an overfat condition.

So if eating less and exercising more doesn't work, what does? The research is clear: the best way to improve your body composition is to minimize your overall dietary insulin production for the rest of your life—through fasting and, as Dr. Maffetone suggests, "replacing junk food with real food." When you ditch processed foods and reduce meal frequency, you lower insulin and activate your long-dormant fat-burning genes. You will be able to maintain stable mood, appetite, and cognitive focus all day long and quickly and efficiently reduce excess body fat. Your daily caloric requirements for peak physical and cognitive functioning actually decrease. It's like upgrading to a car that gets better gas mileage. You will be able to absolutely thrive on a maximum of two meals a day and further explore the life-changing, life-extending benefits of routine fasting (i.e., going at least twelve hours without eating, between your last meal of the evening and your first meal the following day) and occasional prolonged fasting for focused fat reduction, disease prevention, and detoxification. With a sustained commitment to fasting and minimizing insulin production, you can gradually lower that stubborn metabolic set point and essentially rewind your biological clock so that you'll look and feel better than you have in years.

Disease Risks from Hyperinsulinemia

Chronic (a.k.a. systemic) inflammation is believed to be the root cause of virtually all disease and dysfunction in the body, including cancer, heart disease, and cognitive decline. Chronic inflammation indicates that the body is struggling to defend itself against a chronic stressor, such as reactive foods (e.g., gluten, peanuts, and lactose), excess exercise with insufficient recovery time, chronically elevated glucose and insulin levels, and even seasonal allergies. Because our bodies are not designed to be on the defensive 24-7, chronic inflammation eventually leads to immune suppression, digestive disturbances, hormone dysfunction, assorted minor conditions ending with "itis" (arthritis, colitis, gastritis, sinusitis), and major modern killers such as cancer, heart disease, and diseases of cognitive decline. By contrast, acute inflammation is typically desirable in the short term. Acute inflammation helps your muscles run, jump, lift, and sprint. It facilitates the containment and healing of a routine bruise, twisted ankle, or bee sting.

People with lucky genes who don't store much fat may still have metabolic dysfunction, excess visceral fat, and elevated disease risk attributable to inflammatory lifestyle practices—especially the ingestion of toxic seed oils. You may have heard of the disturbingly common occurrence of super-fit individuals dropping dead from surprise heart attacks—a result of their bodies being chronically inflamed from carb dependency and excess exercise. Over years and decades, chronic inflammation causes scarring in the heart muscle and damage to its electrical circuity. Blood tests for fasting glucose, fasting insulin, HbA1c (estimated average glucose over a long time period), triglycerides (the level of fat in the blood—elevations are driven by excess insulin), triglyceride-to-HDL ratio, and C-reactive protein (a key marker of systemic inflammation) can reveal hidden disease patterns in healthy-looking individuals who eat poorly and exercise to extremes.

Excess caloric intake and chronically high insulin levels also send genetic signals to your cells to divide at an accelerated rate. This is common during distinct growth phases of life, when accelerated cell division is desired—pregnancy, infancy, and adolescence (e.g., as a teenager tries to pack on muscle for high school sports). Otherwise, accelerated cell division, marked by the overstimulation of growth factors such as insulin-like growth factor (IGF-1) and mammalian target of rapamycin (mTOR), leads to accelerated aging. Cells throughout the body divide a finite number of times and then they die. This can be seen in the gradual deterioration of cellular functioning in muscles, organs, the immune system, and the metabolic system as the body ages. For example, the gradual weakening of the immune response—known as *immunosenescence*—is the reason elderly people are more vulnerable to infection than young people.

Glycation is another disturbing consequence of a high-carb, high-insulin-producing diet. The body's longest-lasting cells are the most vulnerable, including those of the brain, cardiovascular system, eyes, kidneys, and skin. Diabetics who can't properly regulate blood glucose commonly suffer from vision and kidney problems. It's commonplace for the elderly to have wrinkled skin, dementia, and heart disease.

Brain cells are the most sensitive to oxidation, inflammation, and glycation, and today's disturbing increase in rates of cognitive disease is being increasingly tied to nutrient-deficient, high-insulin-producing diets. The senile plaques and neurofibrallary tangles of Alzheimer's disease are believed to be driven by glycation. Neuropathologist Dr. Suzanne De La Monte, of Brown University, explains that dementia is fundamentally a metabolic disease characterized by impaired glucose metabolism in the brain, "with molecular and biochemical features that correspond with diabetes." The connection is so strong that Dr. De La Monte's team has coined the widely appropriated term "type 3 diabetes" to describe conditions of cognitive decline.

TRAINING FOR THE CORONALYMPICS

We can use COVID-19 as a model for the adverse impact of certain lifestyle practices on both infectious disease and noninfectious chronic health problems such as diabetes, heart disease, and cancer because the immune system plays a role in each of these conditions. The weakening of immune functioning driven by diet-related and lifestyle-related disease, and the impact of lifestyle on immunity, have been largely disregarded by mainstream media in favor of fear-driven coverage of the pandemic. Dr. Ronesh Sinha is going to help us expand our perspective beyond the emphasis on wearing masks and keeping six feet apart. Dr. Sinha, an internal medicine specialist and author of *The South Asian Health Solution* and the popular health blog CulturalHealthSolutions.com, operates a unique wellness program serving large employee groups at some of the world's leading technology companies in California's Silicon Valley. He sees alarming levels of metabolic dysfunction, immune suppression, and serious disease in his patients, despite the fact that they are perhaps the most affluent workers in the world (in the global tech hub, salaries are 2.5 times the US median).

It's not uncommon for Dr. Sinha to treat heart attack victims in their thirties and for seemingly trim, healthy, high-performing folks to have disastrous blood markers and medicine cabinets full of prescriptions. Despite their advanced education, many of Dr. Sinha's patients are oblivious to healthful eating guidelines and get little or no exercise. He blames their health problems on a combination of poor diet and long hours at the computer as well as on the psychological harm caused by the extreme pressures inherent in the affluent, high-tech Silicon Valley scene. He argues that even huge career rewards and incentives can have a direct adverse impact on physical health by fostering a consumerism and FOMO (fear of missing out) mindset, which elevates stress hormones and suppresses immune functioning.

Dr. Sinha's services include extended consultations with entire families, during which he urges them to clean up their diets, get moving, and get healthy. He puts an optimistic spin on the pandemic, which he nicknamed Covesity because of the strong connection between metabolic risk factors such as obesity and vulnerability to the coronavirus. He believes it can help skyrocket motivation for many couch potatoes! Dr. Sinha is getting everyone's attention by urging us to "train" for the pandemic as you would train for a sporting event. We know that an incredibly high percentage of people hospitalized with COVID-19 present with preexisting conditions such as obesity, diabetes, high blood pressure, and excess visceral fat. Dr. Sinha explains the importance of training for what he calls the Coronalympics as follows:

> The initial exposure to COVID-19, known as the viral load, is only one part of the chain of events that can lead to severe illness or death. If you come in contact with the coronavirus, the power of your immune response—specifically, the release of chemical messengers called cytokines—determines your fate. This is known as the cytokine load. If the cytokine response is too severe, your immune system will essentially attack itself, resulting in potentially fatal complications such as fluid-filled lungs and irreversible heart damage. If you can manage your cytokine load with a strong respiratory and cardiovascular system (bolstered by daily exercise) you have the potential to rebuff exposure to COVID-19 in the first place or deal with it as a minor illness versus a major life-threatening disease. The same is true not just for preventing other infections in the future but also for minimizing the risk of developing chronic illness.

Dr. Sinha suggests that you will fare much better against all manner of exposure to pathogens, ranging from the common cold to a global pandemic, if you possess three attributes: an intact immune system (which is strongly correlated with healthful eating and regular exercise), an intact respiratory immune system (again, regular exercise helps keep the sinuses and lungs clear, with strong filtration abilities), and a strong aerobic system (which builds strong accessory breathing muscles, which in turn are vital in preventing severe complications from infection). Spread the message to your friends and loved ones: you should, at the very least, increase all forms of general everyday movement and ditch the Big Three toxic modern foods, which I'll cover below.

The Big Three Toxic Modern Foods

The Big Three toxic modern foods are sugars, grains, and refined industrial seed oils. Until you rid your diet of the Big Three, you will remain stuck in carbohydrate dependency and unable to efficiently access and burn stored body fat.

The Big Three have long formed the foundation of the modern diet, to the great detriment of human health. A grain-based, high-carbohydrate diet prompts wildly excessive insulin production (in contrast to the genetically optimal ancestral diet), lifelong insidious weight gain, and an assortment of disease patterns driven by metabolic syndrome. You're probably aware of the idea that refined grains lack nutrition and spike blood sugar quickly. The metabolic response to a slice of white bread or a forkful of plain pasta is not much different from the response to a tablespoon of sugar. In white flour products, the original wheat kernel has been stripped of two of its natural components: the bran (containing fiber, vitamins, and minerals) and the germ (containing fatty acids and antioxidants). The remaining segment of the plant, the endosperm, delivers a dose of "naked" carbohydrate calories that spike blood sugar quickly.

Unfortunately, whole grains such as whole wheat bread, brown rice, rolled oats, and the like (with the bran, germ, and endosperm preserved) have been recommended as the centerpiece of a healthful diet. This is a highly problematic premise that has made the Standard American Diet (SAD) a dismal failure of phenomenal scale and severity. Indeed, whole grains, with the three segments intact, deliver incrementally more nutritional benefits and a lower initial glucose spike than refined grains, but the nutritional value of grains pales in comparison to that of truly nutrient-dense foods such as fish, eggs, liver, fermented foods such as sauerkraut and yogurt, and colorful produce. *Know this*: both whole and refined grains are a cheap source of calories that are easy to harvest, process, and transform into the highest-profit items in the grocery store, such as cookies, crackers, chips, baked goods, snacks, treats, and frozen meals. The rationale for a grain-based diet is based on decades of flawed science and manipulative marketing, driving a profit machine for food manufacturers and creating a disease paradigm. The epidemic of diet-driven metabolic syndrome is also a reliable profit center for the medical and pharmaceuticals industries.

The other huge objection to eating whole grains is that they contain natural plant toxins, a.k.a. *antinutrients* or *antigens*, which can trigger systemic inflammation, autoimmune reactions, and leaky gut syndrome. Gluten is the most prominent offender, and many sufferers have figured out how immediately destructive this agent in modern-day wheat products can be. It's becoming increasingly apparent that at some level we are all sensitive to gluten and other antinutrients found in grains, because we have not evolved to eat these unnatural modern foods and they are extremely difficult to digest. Yes, the first cultivation of grains, around ten thousand years ago—the catalyst for the advent of civilization—counts as "modern" on the evolutionary timeline.

The chronic and usually mild symptoms that we experience from consuming grains and assorted other plants that cause reactions in sensitive individuals is so widespread that we have come to believe that gas, bloating, constipation, transient abdominal pain, and occasional diarrhea are a normal part of life instead of an adverse response to the plant toxins that you have slammed down your throat every day since infancy. Millions of ancestral health enthusiasts have reported amazing healing stories after they ditched grain-based foods and emphasized evolution-tested hunter-gatherer foods. Enthusiasts of the increasingly popular carnivore diet (see page 31) are taking it a step further and restricting their intake of virtually all plant foods. The healing stories include sudden and dramatic improvements in nagging inflammatory and autoimmune conditions such as arthritis, allergies, asthma, leaky gut syndrome, assorted skin conditions, and all manner of digestive and elimination dysfunction.

It's also time to take a close look at refined, high polyunsaturated industrial seed oils, a.k.a. vegetable oils, especially because they may be a less familiar villain than sugars and grains. As Dr. Shanahan explains in *The Fatburn Fix*, refined seed oils don't spike insulin, as processed carbohydrates do, but they disrupt metabolic functioning in ways that promote insulin resistance. Seed oils are extracted from the raw materials of corn, cottonseed, safflower, soybean, sunflower, and rapeseed (from which canola oil is derived) at high temperatures with the use of harsh chemicals. This results in oxidative damage to the product, damage that is greatly exacerbated when the oil is heated for cooking or used in making assorted baked, processed, packaged, or frozen food products.

By contrast, the naturally high volume of oil in an olive, avocado, or coconut means that it can be easily extracted without the need for aggressive and harmful processes using high heat and chemical solvents. For example, you may see the designation "first cold pressed" on bottles of extra-virgin olive oil. This indicates that the olive was crushed and pressed only once, without being heated or otherwise processed. This delivers a temperature-stable oil for cooking or consuming directly—on a salad, for example. Dr. Shanahan cites research estimating that 40 percent of all the calories you consume in a restaurant meal come from the seed oils it was cooked in. Holistic health expert and best-selling author Dr. Andrew Weil declares that 20 percent of calories in the SAD come from soybean oil alone. If you visit a typical grocery store, you will see that 60 to 70 percent of all processed, packaged, and frozen foods contain one or more of these insidious health destroyers.

When you ingest refined seed oils, they are not burned for fuel the way other fats generally are because of their unnatural chemical makeup. Instead, their similarity to natural fat molecules confuses the body into integrating these agents into healthy fat cells. Unfortunately, they are very difficult to burn for energy and can greatly hamper your overall ability to burn stored body fat over time. If you have problem areas of fat accumulation that don't seem to go away even when you are losing fat in general, the cellular dysfunction caused by seed oils is likely one of the causes. Seed oils also break down into toxins that generate oxidative damage and systemic inflammation. The adverse health consequences of consuming seed oils are so immediate and extreme that Dr. Shanahan states, "They are free radicals in a bottle; literally no different than eating radiation."

When toxic oils short-circuit your fat metabolism, you become even more dependent on dietary carbohydrates for energy. Extreme biohacker and elite adventure sports athlete Ben Greenfield, author of *Boundless* and host of the Ben Greenfield Fitness podcast, observes that seed oils might be considered the gateway to insulin resistance and diabetes because of how they short-circuit fat metabolism. He notes that while refined carbohydrates get the majority of blame in this area, they are arguably less problematic because

THE BIG THREE
Toxic Modern Foods

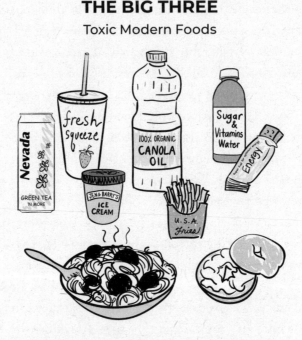

Sugars/Sweetened Beverages, Grains, Industrial Seed Oils

you can burn them off during exercise, unlike toxic and dysfunctional fat cells. Sugar and refined carbs can be highly destructive in excess but industrial seed oils are inherently destructive at any amount consumed.

I include artificial sweeteners as "sugar"—and they should be totally eliminated from the diet as well. In addition to concerns about ingesting chemical agents linked to cancer and emerging concerns about how sweeteners can harm gut bacteria, some research suggests the highly disturbing potential of sweeteners to spike insulin. In *The Obesity Code*, Dr. Fung attests that aspartame spikes insulin by 20 percent—more than plain white sugar! Consequently, sweeteners can deliver a disastrous double-whammy effect of both spiking insulin and confusing the brain's appetite center to crave real sugar. These mechanisms are part of the *cephalic response*, where the mere thinking about food, smelling food, or tasting a sweet, but non-caloric substance, stimulates the cerebral cortex to initiate certain digestive functions, such as gastrointestinal secretions and insulin release.

If you innocently down a Coke Zero or Diet Dr Pepper during an afternoon lull at the office, you are giving your brain the familiar and intensely rewarding sensation of sweetness, but without the complete satisfaction that comes with consuming actual sugar calories. Your sweet tooth will be temporarily satiated, but the insulin spike prompted by fake sugar also removes the glucose that is normally circulating in your bloodstream. This causes an energy dip and accompanying hunger spike. These dynamics compel your brain to drain the Coke Zero and subsequently desire real sugar. Long-term studies confirm that diet soda drinkers don't drink fewer calories or lose more fat than regular soda drinkers. While many other factors are in play, it's interesting to note the parallel increase in recent decades of obesity rates and diet soda consumption.

Fructose, the predominant source of carbohydrate in fruit, can also be particularly harmful to fat-reduction efforts. Fructose doesn't spike blood glucose or trigger insulin production as other forms of carbs do because it needs to be processed in the liver before it can be burned for energy. The liver is also where excess glucose is converted into triglyceride and stored as fat. This makes fructose the winner of the "carbohydrate most likely to convert into fat" award—especially if you consume lots of other carbs and don't exercise enough to deplete your glycogen stores. Apologies to the Weight Watchers folks who give fruit a zero point score, but you can overdo fruit consumption to the extent that it inhibits your fat-loss goals. (See page 34 for the best fruit options.)

Don't get me started about high-fructose corn syrup (HFCS), which delivers the worst of all possible worlds: it has the aforementioned lipogenic properties of fructose; it delivers an insulin spike (because it also contains glucose); and it lacks the protective agents in real fruit (antioxidants, fiber, and so on) that help improve digestion and moderate fructose's insulinogenic effects. HFCS has also been implicated in promoting systemic inflammation and leaky gut syndrome.

It's pretty simple to ditch toxic oils by making the right choices at restaurants and cooking with natural saturated fats (butter, ghee, coconut oil, tallow, and lard) and heart-healthful monounsaturated fats (avocado and olive oils). Because industrial seed oils are generally tasteless, it's no sacrifice to immediately and permanently eliminate them from your diet.

Sugar and grains, on the other hand, may be more difficult to eradicate. These foods have been shown to have addictive properties and stimulate your appetite, producing a desire to consume more of them. The great work of Gary Taubes (*Good Calories, Bad Calories* and *The Case Against Sugar*) and Dr. Robert Lustig (*Fat Chance* and *The Hacking of the American Mind*) contains details about the ways in which processed carbohydrate foods and beverages flood your dopamine pathways and bind with opioid receptors in the brain, delivering intense instant gratification and a drive to consume more of them. In

Dr. William Davis's bestselling book *Wheat Belly,* he presents evidence that the *gliadin* protein contained in our genetically engineered modern-day "dwarf" wheat crop stimulates the appetite receptors in the brain to the extent that you are prompted to consume an additional four hundred calories per day. On ingestion, gliadin degrades into an opioid polypeptide, crosses the blood-brain barrier, and has been linked not only to appetite stimulation but also to behavior disturbances, ADHD, allergic reactions, and impaired immune and neurological functioning.

You may struggle a bit with making these dietary changes if you habitually eat grain-based meals or if you are in the habit of soothing yourself with intensely flavorful sugary sweets and beverages or if you consume lots of processed, packaged, frozen, and fast foods laden with seed oils. The best approach is to commit to total elimination of the Big Three for a minimum of twenty-one days in order to break free from their addictive influences. Over time, sugary treats and grain foods will likely find their way back into your diet on occasion when you celebrate sensibly, but you can certainly commit to never again consuming industrial seed oils, which can be easily replaced by healthful oils.

During this initial dietary transformation, it's important to surround yourself with alternatives that are extremely nutrient-dense and vastly more nourishing at the cellular level than an ice cream or a Starbucks concoction, which delivers only a few seconds of gustatory pleasure (and minimal nourishment). Because ditching the Big Three is the first step to health, please don't worry about restricting calories, losing fat, or extended fasting just yet. As you begin your transition to metabolic flexibility and efficiency, it's important that hunger, appetite, and cravings do not derail your efforts in any way. Instead, satisfy yourself with delicious go-to meals such as an omelet for breakfast, a colorful salad for lunch, and a nice steak and vegetable dinner. If you find your energy flagging between meals or have a hankering for a snack, feel free to have some vegetables slathered in nut butter, a couple of hard-boiled eggs, a few squares of dark chocolate (with an 80 percent or higher cacao content), or even a tin of sardines. Once you become highly fat adapted and into a long-term *Two Meals a Day* routine, you'll comfortably and naturally move away from snacking, without even thinking about it.

The goal here is to achieve continued forward progress without backsliding into a carb binge or suffering from the afternoon blues or the so-called low-carb flu. That's right: contrary to Flawed Current Conventional Keto Wisdom (FCCKW—sound it out so you can memorize the acronym...), I don't believe you have to struggle or suffer in any way during your journey. Be gentle with your body and your psyche, eat plenty of nutritious food, and don't deny yourself the pleasure of enjoying meals and enjoying life. When you start skipping meals, cutting out snacks, and extending your fasting periods, your efforts should feel natural and comfortable instead of strained. This is the magic of metabolic flexibility and the reason the *Two Meals a Day* approach will work through thick and thin (including occasional setbacks and occasional indulgences and celebrations) where other dietary strategies will fail.

The idea is that after twenty-one days you will have built enough momentum to keep the sugars, grains, and seed oils out of your diet indefinitely without a second thought. Over the past decade, hundreds of thousands of ancestral-diet and health enthusiasts have experienced the amazing awakening that comes from cleaning up the way they eat. When you eat with the *Two Meals a Day* approach, you will always be satisfied because you will be giving your body the rich nutrition that it craves, and you will rarely be hungry because you are keeping insulin optimally low and thereby stabilizing appetite hormones that typically spike when you eat high-carb meals.

The Kitchen and Pantry Purge

The Big Three toxic agents are so insidious in our modern food supply, and marketed so aggressively, that they can very easily sneak into your meals and your home despite your best intentions. For example, when using the handy Starbucks mobile ordering app, the default setting for iced teas and other cold drinks in the Flavors category is "4 pumps of liquid cane sugar." You have to actually select the Flavors option, open a new window, and press the Minus button four times so that you can order a drink without added sugar. There are many fresh food preparations bathed in canola oil at natural-foods supermarkets that proudly tout their commitment to product selectivity and environmental sustainability. Read labels (see the list below for what to watch for), ask questions (track down manufacturers online if necessary), be ever-vigilant, and commit to a zero-tolerance, total-elimination policy for seed oils, chemical additives, GMOs, and generally inferior foods.

Following is a pretty extensive list of foods and beverages to eliminate, but please honor the spirit of the list when you encounter similar products that aren't specifically mentioned. When dining out, politely but assertively find out exactly what's in your meals and negotiate changes to avoid toxic ingredients. Insist that your meals be cooked in butter, lard, or olive oil instead of seed oil—or dine elsewhere.

Note that the day 1 assignment of the 12-Day Turbocharge is a determined wielding of the garbage can as you purge offenders from your refrigerator and cupboards and clear space ahead of an imminent shopping spree for nutritious ancestral foods. If you're like I am and don't want to wait another moment to clean up your act, go ahead and take immediate action with the book in one hand and the garbage can in the other. Doing some advance work before the Turbocharge will make things easier and more fluid during the intensity of the twelve-day experience.

Following, by category, is an assortment of foods to eliminate.

Industrial seed oils: Bottled cooking oils (canola, cottonseed, corn, peanut, soybean, safflower, sunflower, and anything identified as "vegetable oil" or "vegetable shortening"); condiments with those oils listed on their labels (including most mayonnaise, salad dressing, sauces, and dips, unless proudly stated otherwise on the label); buttery spreads and sprays (Smart Balance, Promise, I Can't Believe It's Not Butter); deep-fried fast food; margarine; packaged and frozen baked goods (you shouldn't be going near those anyway); leftover restaurant entrées (ask for butter next time!).

Sweets and treats: Bakery and pastry shop fare, candy and candy bars, cake, cheesecake, cookies, cupcakes, doughnuts, frozen desserts (ice cream bars, popsicles, and others), frozen yogurt, ice cream, milk chocolate, pie.

Sweeteners: All artificial sweeteners (NutraSweet, Sweet'n Low, Splenda, and others), agave products, brown sugar, cane sugar, evaporated cane juice, fructose, high-fructose corn syrup, honey, molasses, powdered sugar, raw sugar, table sugar, all syrups.

Sweetened beverages: Designer coffees (mochas, blended iced-coffee drinks); energy drinks (Red Bull, Rockstar, Monster Energy); bottled, fresh-squeezed, and refrigerated juices (acai, apple, grape, orange, pomegranate, Naked Juice, and Odwalla concoctions; Nantucket Nectars, Ocean Spray, V8); overly sweetened kombucha drinks (read labels—some are low in sugar; most are not); almond, oat, rice, soy, and other nondairy milks; powdered drink mixes (chai-flavored, coffee-flavored, hot chocolate, lemonade, iced tea); all soft drinks and diet soft drinks, including tonic water; sports performance drinks (Gatorade, Powerade, Vitaminwater); cocktails made with sweet beverages (daiquiri, eggnog, margarita);

cocktail mixes made with sugars; sweetened teas (AriZona, Honest Tea, Pure Leaf, Snapple).

Grains: Cereal, corn, pasta, rice, and wheat; bread and flour products (baguettes, crackers, croissants, Danishes, doughnuts, graham crackers, muffins, pizza, pretzels, rolls, saltines, tortillas, Triscuit, Wheat Thins); breakfast foods (Cream of Wheat, french toast, granola, grits, oatmeal, pancakes, waffles); chips (corn, potato, tortilla); cooking grains (amaranth, barley, bulgur, couscous, millet, rye); puffed snacks (Cheetos, Goldfish, Pirate's Booty, popcorn, rice cakes).

Baking ingredients: Cornmeal, cornstarch, and corn syrup; evaporated milk and condensed milk; flours made with wheat, gluten; starch; yeast.

Condiments: Review labels of condiments, sauces, spreads, and toppings. Discard those that contain sweeteners and/or industrial seed oils and choose alternative products in categories such as ketchup, mayonnaise, salad dressing, and barbecue sauce (my Primal Kitchen products are made with an avocado-oil base and are free from offensive agents); avoid all jams, jellies, and preserves (even all-fruit, no-sugar-added offerings).

Dairy products: Processed (American) cheese and cheese spreads (Velveeta); ice cream; nonfat and low-fat milks and yogurts; all other low-fat, high-carbohydrate dairy products; all nonorganic dairy products.

Discounted products: Beware of items in any category sold at a low price point or put on sale, for they are almost surely inferior in every way to a chemical-free, preservative-free, local, organic, and sustainably grown, raised, and harvested product.

Fast foods: Burgers, chicken sandwiches, fish fillets, french fries, hot dogs, onion rings, chimichangas, chalupas, churros, all deep-fried foods, and most everything offered at traditional fast-food establishments across the developed world. Note: Numerous modern fast-food chains offer much better offerings than what's available at the typical burger joint. Chipotle and other "fresh Mex" offerings are good examples.

Processed foods: High-carbohydrate energy bars, granola bars, trail mixes, processed fruit snacks, and other packaged and bulk-bin snacks made with grains and sugars; packaged, processed, frozen, and fast foods made with grains, refined oils, and/or added sugars.

Low-quality foods on the ancestral list: Conventionally raised meat and poultry from feedlot operations (choose grass-fed beef, pasture-raised fowl, and heritage breed pork instead—details in chapter 2); prepackaged meat products, such as smoked, cured, and nitrate-treated bacon; bologna, ham, hot dogs, gas-station jerky laden with preservatives, pepperoni, salami, and sausage (search for less processed options in these categories, free from nitrates and other chemicals and preservatives); nonorganic eggs, milk, and other dairy products (choose those that come from pasture-raised animals and are sustainably harvested, or at least certified organic); nonorganic produce with a high pesticide risk (those with difficult-to-wash or edible skins, such as leafy greens and berries); produce out of season or transported from distant origins (fresh local summer berries, thumbs-up; big-box-store pineapples and mangoes in wintertime, thumbs-down); nuts, seeds, and nut butters processed with oils or covered in sugary coatings; most farmed fish and imported fish (details in chapter 2).

The purpose of the aforementioned list is not to overwhelm you with what you can't eat but to show you that so many of the foods considered "normal" have been confirmed to be antithetical to health. When you eliminate these detrimental foods from your world, you create more space in your daily caloric allotment for nutrient-dense foods. While the list of preferred foods is smaller, there is an almost infinite variety of ways to enhance the flavors of these with herbs, spices, sauces, dressings, and toppings. The result is that you can make each meal or snack not only more nutritious but also more flavorful and exciting. Making this transition can deliver wonderful improvements in energy levels and chronic health conditions and prompt a natural and efficient reduction in excess body fat. Perhaps most empowering is the sensation that you are no longer dependent on food to sustain your energy and cognitive focus.

Inside your body, great things are happening when you burn clean fuels such as fat and ketones. With less oxidation, glycation, and inflammation occurring when your cells metabolize energy, you may notice better sleep, faster recovery from workouts, and increased cognitive clarity and endurance. And while a high-energy day of commuting, work, exercise, and family life can still leave you fatigued in the evening, it will be a more pleasant sensation of feeling ready to relax and wind down gracefully before bedtime. By contrast, consider how a day fueled primarily by processed carbs can leave you feeling: jittery, agitated, and craving an additional hit of sugar. Being a stress-balanced fat burner makes for a nicer evening in front of Netflix or at the card table, but more important, it helps you escape the prevailing disease patterns driven strongly by carbohydrate dependency.

Granted, ingrained habits, cultural traditions, and an actual physical dependency on carbohydrates can be difficult to overcome. Cleaning up your act is going to take commitment, focus, and resolve. Wake up every day and renew your commitment, reminding yourself why you are pursuing this dietary transformation. Through repetition and endurance, you will create powerful new habits. Instead of worrying about missing out on your old favorites, consider the kitchen and pantry purge as a clearing of space that enables you to *add* more good stuff into your daily diet!

Clean Up Your Act—Journal Exercises

1. **Lower insulin, lower body fat, lower disease risk:** List some of the main ways you believe you can minimize insulin production through dietary restrictions, modifications to your meal and snacking patterns, and improvements in your daily movement and workout habits.
2. **Kitchen and pantry purge:** Jot down your thoughts and emotions about the purge. Include a list of some of your favorite foods and beverages that are going to present the biggest challenges and areas of focus when you strive for a total elimination of the Big Three. List some replacement foods and beverages that you'll enjoy.

CHAPTER 2

Emphasize Nutrient-Dense Ancestral Foods (and Eat Your Superfoods!)

Humans evolved to digest an incredible variety of colorful, wholesome, nutrient-dense plants, animals, and even insects. The earliest *Homo sapiens* explorers left East Africa around sixty thousand years ago and proceeded to colonize the entire globe over the next forty-five thousand years. The original human migration route followed the African coastline into the present-day Middle East, then to India, Indonesia, and eventually Australia. Our ancestors enjoyed abundant marine life, rich in omega-3 fatty acids, which are lauded for their potent anti-inflammatory properties as well as their beneficial effects on cognition, immune function, cardiovascular function, and cancer prevention. Paleoanthropologists contend that gaining access to foods high in omega-3 was a prominent driver in the evolution of our outsize brains.

Wherever our ancestors settled, they made the best of what their environment offered. Those living at the northern latitudes likely consumed large amounts of oily cold-water fish and nearly zero plant carbohydrates. Equatorial peoples might have consumed plenty of carbs from wild fruits, vegetables, and starchy tubers. Those who endured long, cold, brutal battles against the elements and food scarcity surely ate nothing for long stretches. Perhaps they subsisted on assorted plant life and small game just long enough to reproduce—no doubt hoping their descendants would fare better. The takeaway from our evolutionary journey is that we're pretty damn resilient to a variety of dietary strategies and can function well even if we go long periods without having much to eat.

Today, manipulative marketing forces, media hype, and flawed science have made the topic of healthful eating more controversial and confusing than ever. For example, critics who trash the evolutionary rationale might be accused of taking insights out of context or drawing conclusions from flawed science. The saying goes, "Show me the science," but it seems as if there are studies that will validate any imaginable position these days. While we can all agree that industrial food processing and Concentrated Animal Feeding Operations (CAFO)—large livestock facilities—are bad for the body and the environment, distorted and irresponsible proclamations like "red meat causes cancer" tend to go viral without sufficient scrutiny.

An increasing amount of propaganda promoting a whole-foods, plant-based diet contends that this approach is more sustainable and more eco-friendly than an omnivorous diet—and even morally superior to it. These assumptions are aggressively countered by people with differing opinions about how and what to eat. Even among those with extremely similar big picture beliefs, the debating of the nuances can cause confusion to anyone trying to adopt a new way of eating. It's time to put a stop to this nonsense by presenting a simple plan that's inclusive to even those with radically different dietary beliefs. The *Two Meals a Day* plan works whether you're vegan, carnivore, or anything in between.

Perhaps best of all, *Two Meals a Day* puts you in the driver's seat: it lets you design your healthful, enjoyable, nutrient-dense, sustainable-for-life eating strategy. I'm continually asked to identify the best foods to eat, and many times the question seems to carry a sense of desperation. I want to put your mind at ease once and for all. Here's the deal: you never have to eat stuff you don't like; I want you to enjoy every single bite of food you put in your mouth for the rest of your life. For *Two Meals a Day* to work, there are certain indisputable rules and guidelines you must operate within, but you are free to choose the food groups, specific foods, recipes, preparation methods, and meal times (but you only get two a day!) that feel right to you. I encourage you to maintain an open mind and a willingness to experiment and continually refine and perfect your optimal eating strategy. Remember, with *Two Meals a Day*, you have the flexibility to evolve your taste preferences, adjust your diet to your fitness and health goals, and perhaps change course if you experience health disturbances that you suspect are related to certain foods.

When you establish a baseline commitment to eliminate the Big Three toxic modern foods, you'll be way out in front of the pack and well on the road to achieving your healthspan potential. From there, an assortment of disparate strategies, depending on your genetics, lifestyle factors, fitness and body-composition goals, and individual food preferences and challenges, follow. Even Dr. Peter Attia, one of the world's leading longevity physicians and an expert on extended fasting and ketogenic eating, likes to simplify his boilerplate dietary advice: "Just eat stuff your great-grandmother would have been able to eat."

Beyond eliminating the Big Three, it's essential to strive for the most wholesome, nutrient-dense options in every food category when you shop and uphold the highest standards when it comes to the restaurants and menu selections you choose. It can take a lot of work to be sure that the foods you put in your grocery bag and those that are served to you meet these high criteria. Today's food-industrial complex has bastardized many inherently healthful foods, and manipulative marketing is persuading us to eat an assortment of garbage, provided it's characterized by misleading buzzwords such as "heart-healthy," "gluten-free," "cholesterol-free," "100% real fruit," and so forth. Even the word *organic* has been ridiculously misappropriated to universally mean "healthful." We have massive marketing propaganda convincing you that heavily processed, chemical-laden meat substitutes (that even contain industrial seed oils!) are somehow better for you than real meat.

This chapter will explain how to choose wisely in each of the ancestral-inspired food categories of meat, fish, fowl, eggs, vegetables, fruits, nuts, and seeds, and healthful modern foods such as organic high-fat dairy products and high-cacao dark chocolate. I will also introduce you to some superfoods with particularly impressive nutritional benefits. Unfortunately, these superfoods are often absent from the meals of even the most health-conscious eaters. For example, our hunter-gatherer ancestors routinely consumed an entire animal in "nose-to-tail" fashion. Organs were highly prized and believed to have exceptional healing properties. Nothing went to waste—even carcasses would be boiled down for days to yield incredibly nutritious bone broth. Today, we typically consume only the muscle meats of an animal (e.g., burgers, steaks, chicken breasts and thighs) and avoid the liver and other organs, which are among the most nutrient-rich foods on the planet.

Fermented and sprouted foods were also a central element of the ancestral diet, delivering potent probiotics that are essential to the health of the gut microbiome. Today, our ability to process, pasteurize, and refrigerate food largely negates the need to sprout and ferment, and these foods have become marginalized instead of emphasized as a healthful part of a daily diet. This chapter will provide all the information and guidance you need to choose the very best foods in each category and add a superfood element to your diet that can propel you to a high level of energy, focus, health, and disease prevention.

Meat and Fowl

Animal flesh has been the centerpiece of the human diet over the course of evolutionary history and provides an array of nutritional benefits, especially the highly bioavailable complete protein that is the most important dietary requirement for health and survival. Today, meat consumption has become controversial, primarily because of highly objectionable concentrated animal feeding operations that deliver inferior products, mistreat animals, and cause environmental pollution. All the objections to eating meat, including the supposed connection between red meat and cancer, can be overcome by relying on local, sustainable, grass-fed, or certified organic meat whenever possible. You also must avoid overcooking meat (charring generates potentially carcinogenic compounds) and avoid all manner of processed meats (chemically treated hot dogs, bacon, sausage, bologna, salami, frozen meats, and almost all fast-food offerings). Granted, consuming only the cleanest meat and fowl can be expensive, but this is the food category where your selectivity matters the most.

Feedlot animals are given hormones, pesticides, and antibiotics to prevent illness and increase yield in crowded, unsanitary, polluting environments. An animal's muscle tissue and organs can be negatively affected by its malnourishment and unhealthful living conditions. If you purchase mass-market meat or fowl, you are likely getting an insulin-resistant animal (resulting from its unnatural, grain-based diet) with between ten and thirty times more pesticide exposure than you get from produce and with significantly more proinflammatory omega-6 fatty acids in its tissues. The omega-6 fats come from the accelerated fattening on fortified grains that occurs over the final months of an animal's life before slaughter. By contrast, pasture-raised and grass-fed animals have between two and six times more anti-inflammatory omega-3 and monounsaturated fats than feedlot animals, along with higher levels of other vitamins, minerals, and micronutrients, and have a much richer and more satisfying flavor.

You might be surprised to see the diminutive size of a pasture-raised chicken in your local farmer's market in comparison to the bloated offerings found at the supermarket, but the flavor intensity of a pastured chicken or bacon from a heritage breed pig will blow you away. The same is true when you taste a hamburger made of grass-fed purebred Wagyu beef and compare it to a bland fast-food burger, which actually requires meatlike flavoring chemicals just to be palatable (read Eric Schlosser's *Fast Food Nation* for details). In a single bite you will see the light and resolve to never go back to conventional meat and fowl.

The ideal choice in meat and fowl is a local animal that was 100 percent grass-fed or pasture-raised. Get familiar with your nearby farmer's markets, natural-foods grocers, and food co-ops. Talk to proprietors, because they are typically very passionate and informed about how to find the best food for you and your family. Explore specialty butchers and ethnic markets for options other than the mass-produced favorites—cow, pig, chicken, and turkey. For example, lamb, buffalo, and venison are more commonly grass-fed and sustainably harvested. There are many great internet resources, too, if your local options are limited. ThriveMarket.com, WildIdeaBuffalo.com, LoneMountainWagyu.com, ButcherBox.com, and GrasslandBeef.com can get you started on finding the best quality meat.

Food labeled with the certified USDA Organic seal is the next best choice after local, grass-fed, and pasture-raised meat or alternative meats. Chain grocers, natural-foods grocers, and even big-box stores are stocking an increasing amount of organic meat. Organic certification ensures that the animals were raised without hormones, pesticides, antibiotics, genetic engineering, irradiation, sewage sludge, or other detrimental practices and lived in humane conditions where they were able to move around freely. However, organic meat is a distant second choice to animals that were 100 percent grass-fed (cattle, buffalo, lamb) or pasture-raised (chicken, turkey, pork), because even organically raised animals likely ate a suboptimal grain-based diet and lived a primarily confined life instead of roaming in nature. Be wary of the many other descriptive phrases you might see on meat and fowl, because such claims are minimally regulated and thus of dubious value. These include "free-range," "hormone-free," "antibiotic-free," "natural diet," and the like. That said, these messages hint at an improvement over feedlot products emblazoned only with the logo of a major brand. As consumer awareness and demand increase, it's getting easier and becoming more affordable to find the very best meat and fowl, so set your standards high and do the best you can to locate grass-fed and pasture-raised meat.

Fish

Fish and other marine life have been a centerpiece of the human diet for millennia and rank among the most nutrient-dense foods on earth. Plant-based eaters can do themselves a big favor by including fish in their diets. Marine life is a fantastic source of protein;

vitamins B, D, and E; the minerals selenium, zinc, iron, magnesium, and phosphorus; and full-spectrum antioxidants. Fish are the richest dietary source of the lauded omega-3 fatty acids (especially the hard-to-find DHA and EPA types), which enhance brain and nervous system functioning, protect against cardiovascular disease, and have powerful anti-inflammatory properties.

Oily, cold-water "SMASH" fish (sardines, mackerel, anchovies, salmon [wild-caught], and herring) have the highest omega-3 values and overall health benefits. As an added convenience, canned varieties of these fish are easy to find and very affordable. The shellfish family (clams, crab, crayfish, lobster, mussels, oysters, shrimp, scallops) is also highly regarded for its unique and potent nutritional offerings. The high zinc content in oysters boosts testosterone and dopamine, giving them a well-deserved reputation as an aphrodisiac. The widely popular canned tuna is nutritious and affordable; the best varieties are white, light, and albacore. Look for label distinctions or niche brands conveying some environmental sensitivity, because the major commercial tuna providers get low scores from watchdog groups (see below).

Be sure to expand your consumption of seafood to include the nutritional superstar seaweed—namely, kombu, kelp, nori, and wakame. These seaweed varieties are the best source of dietary iodine, which is critical for healthy thyroid functioning and hard to find in other foods. Enjoy the unique flavor and phenomenal nutrient density of fish eggs (roe), such as salmon roe and caviar. They are one of the only rich dietary sources of vitamin D and are very high in omega-3s, the all-important vitamin B_{12}, and selenium. The Weston A. Price Foundation, regarded as the leading resource for the study of nutrition and health in traditional ancestral populations, confirms that our ancestors associated the consumption of fish roe with fertility; great efforts were made to find roe and feed it to women who wanted to become pregnant.

As with meat and fowl, you must strive to find the most nutritious and sustainable fish options and avoid numerous categories of low-quality fish. Avoid all packaged, processed, boxed, and frozen fish products, especially breaded and deep-fried offerings. In general, strive to avoid most types of farmed fish; fish imported from the Baltic Sea, Chile, and Asia, because of concerns about polluted waters, chemical use, and long transport times; predatory fish (king mackerel, mahi-mahi, marlin, shark, swordfish, big tuna) because of their potentially high levels of mercury and other contaminants; and fish that are endangered or caught by environmentally damaging methods (bluefin tuna, Chilean sea bass, orange roughy, red snapper). To keep informed about the frequent changes and updates in the latter category, visit MontereyBayAquarium.org, MSC.org (the Marine Stewardship Council), and EDF.org (the Environmental Defense Fund).

Most farmed fish are environmentally problematic and nutritionally inferior to wild-caught fish, but some are okay. In Nicolas Daniel's documentary, *Fillet-Oh!-Fish*, the producers say: "Through intensive farming and global pollution, the flesh of the fish we eat has turned into a deadly chemical cocktail." In particular, farmed Atlantic salmon, which comprises an estimated 90 percent of the US salmon market, should be avoided. You can be sure your restaurant is serving farmed Atlantic salmon unless it proudly specifies otherwise. Dr. Joseph Mercola, author of *Fat for Fuel* and publisher of the popular Mercola.com health information website, cites a study in which farmed Atlantic salmon were five times more toxic than any other food tested!

Farmed salmon and many other farmed fish are raised in cramped, polluted pens and exposed to high levels of dangerous chemicals (polychlorinated biphenyls [PCBs], dioxins, methylmercury, dieldrin, toxaphene, ethoxyquin). These are fat-soluble compounds that accumulate in the flesh of fatty fish such as salmon. Farmed salmon have two to five times more fat than wild fish and five times more inflammatory omega-6 fatty acids because of their junk-food diet, which typically includes refined seed oils! Like their land-based counterparts in feedlots, farmed salmon are given hormones, pesticides, and antibiotics to ward off disease in their cramped, unsanitary conditions.

There are certain categories of farmed fish with minimal toxin levels and good nutritional profiles that make them safe to consume. Stick with US sources to avoid concerns about pollution and lax chemical regulations in countries such as China, Chile, and Baltic Sea nations that export a high volume of fish. For example, farmed freshwater coho salmon is acceptable. If you see farmed "organic" salmon from British Columbia, Ireland, or Scotland, it may be a step up from mainstream farmed salmon, but there are still objections that warrant a pass on farmed salmon. If budget is a concern, try to find wild-caught salmon in a can or previously frozen, because it will be considerably less expensive than fresh wild-caught salmon.

Safe domestic farmed fish include barramundi, catfish, crayfish, rockfish, sablefish, striped bass, tilapia, trout, and most farmed shellfish. In addition, farmed shellfish are attached to a fixed object, just as they are in the wild. They don't eat artificial feed, and they have a nutritional profile similar to that of their wild counterparts. When you shop for the ever-popular shrimp (the number one seafood in the United States), be sure to choose a US-sourced product. Most shrimp is imported from unsanitary farms located in other countries.

To be sure you are getting quality products and avoiding toxic fish, stick to the SMASH hits of the fish family, keep up-to-date on sustainability from the aforementioned websites, and find a quality provider of fresh fish. With any luck you can find a specialty market in your area or a great internet resource. VitalChoice.com has a wonderful selection of high-quality seafood, for example.

Eggs

Eggs are the original superfood—the essence of life—and deliver across-the-board nutritional benefits. Egg whites contain high-quality complete protein, while the yolks are a treasure trove of antioxidants, anti-inflammatory compounds, healthful omega-3 and saturated fats, and vitamins A, E, K_2, B complex, and folate. Eggs are particularly high in choline, which boosts memory and cognition and supports cell maintenance and DNA synthesis. Eating eggs presents plant-based eaters with an opportunity to obtain nutrients that are easy to become deficient in when avoiding most animal foods. One of the most ridiculous conventional stupidities is to advise against egg consumption. Another is to eschew the yolks in favor of the whites. Meta-analyses (compilation studies of data from hundreds of individual studies) have completely refuted any connection between egg consumption and heart disease, or even egg consumption and blood cholesterol levels, and confirmed the tremendous nutritional benefits offered by eggs.

Local, farm-fresh eggs sold by hobbyists or farmer's market vendors are the premier choice in this category. The chickens enjoy an active and omnivorous outdoor lifestyle, with a diet of insects, lizards, worms, weeds, grasses, and seeds. They lay eggs with a nutrient density vastly superior to that of the eggs laid by chickens confined to industrial facilities, who consume processed feed laden with objectionable hormones, pesticides, and antibiotics. Their bright orange yolks (from the natural sources of beta-carotene in their diets) can contain up to ten times more omega-3s than egg yolks from conventionally raised hens. Anyone who has tasted a farm-fresh egg from a pasture-raised chicken can attest to the incredible flavor intensity that will make you a lifetime convert. The cost-benefit ratio—paying a few extra bucks per dozen for a superfood—is a no-brainer.

Beyond a true local farm-fresh egg, retail cartons labeled with both "pasture-raised" and "certified humane" or "animal welfare approved" are the next best choice. This indicates that the chickens were afforded significant access to pasture and the aforementioned natural food sources and that their supplemental feed was typically certified organic and of superior quality to conventional feed. Ranked next are cartons with the distinction "pasture-raised." Without the "certified humane" or "animal welfare approved" labels, their access to pasture may have been limited, and they may have consumed more feed than natural food, but they are still considered excellent. Eggs from pasture-raised hens are enjoying increasing mainstream distribution, and you should strive to avoid anything below this ranking. You can likely find the pasture-raised distinction (and the certified humane or animal welfare approved designations) on at least one brand and perhaps more at your favorite local grocer. Vital Farms distributes its pasture-raised, certified humane eggs to major national and local grocery chains and big-box stores, including Whole Foods Market, Walmart, Target, Publix, Kroger, and even Amazon Prime home delivery.

If you can't find pasture-raised eggs, certified organic eggs are the next best choice. Organic eggs are free of undesirable hormones, pesticides, and antibiotics, and the hens are probably afforded less crowded and more sanitary living conditions than conventionally raised birds. Eggs labeled with assorted unofficial designations such as "omega-3," "natural diet," "free-range," "cage-free," "vegetarian," or "hormone-free" are also likely superior to conventional eggs from a crowded indoor chicken-coop operation. However, don't be deluded by marketing terms. Omega-3 looks good on a carton, but it likely indicates that the chickens simply had some flaxseed added to their feed. Be vigilant about finding fresh eggs, because many conventional eggs can routinely be thirty days old on the store shelf. An eggshell should feel robust and take some effort to crack. It's so easy to find quality eggs that you should think "pasture-raised or bust" and never settle for a conventional egg or even a merely certified organic egg.

Another healthful and adventurous idea is to look for alternatives to chicken eggs. Duck eggs and quail eggs are typically available at natural-foods grocers, farmer's markets, and food co-ops. Try to discover emu, goose, gull, ostrich, pheasant, and turkey eggs and try them out. Alternative eggs are obviously not from feedlot operations and thus offer nutritional benefits similar to those of a pastured-chicken egg.

Vegetables

Vegetables have high levels of antioxidants, flavonoids, carotenoids, and phytonutrients that help optimize metabolic, immune, and cellular functioning. They help protect the brain and the body from the ravages of aging and oxidative stress and help nourish healthful bacteria in your gut microbiome. Vegetables grown aboveground (leafy greens, peppers, asparagus, tomatoes, and those in the cruciferous family [broccoli, cauliflower]) are high in complex carbohydrates and low in starch, with abundant fiber and water content. This means you can consume them liberally without an adverse insulin response, even if you are trying hard to reduce excess body fat or stick to keto carbohydrate limits.

Root vegetables, grown in the ground (beets, carrots, onions, parsnips, rutabagas, sweet potatoes, turnips, yams), absorb high levels of antioxidants, vitamins, and iron from the soil, making them nutritional powerhouses. In comparison to aboveground vegetables, root vegetables have a higher starch content and potentially have more carbohydrate and insulin impact. If you are trying to lose fat, they warrant moderation, but they're a great supplemental carb choice for high calorie burners. Root vegetables, along with fruits, have the fewest toxin concerns in the plant family (see below), making them a good choice for carnivore-style eaters looking to safely include plants and carbs in their meals. Exclude white varieties of potatoes from your options, because they have more starch and are highly glycemic, laden with pesticides, and less nutritious than potatoes with colored flesh.

The cruciferous family ranks particularly high on the nutrition scoreboard. Named for their cross-shaped flowers, they include arugula, broccoli, bok choy, brussels sprouts, cabbage, cauliflower, and kale. These foods have stellar anticancer, antioxidant, antimicrobial, and antiaging properties. Red-colored veggies (and fruits) are believed to help prevent prostate cancer; greens have antiaging benefits and support vision health; yellow and orange foods have antioxidant and anti-inflammatory properties. The USDA's ORAC (oxygen radical absorbance capacity) report provides antioxidant values for individual foods, but it's safe to conclude that all vegetables are teeming with micronutrients. Some of the vegetables with the highest antioxidant scores are beets, broccoli, brussels sprouts, carrots, cauliflower, eggplant, garlic, kale, onion, red bell peppers, spinach, and yellow squash.

You should be selective about your vegetables for a few reasons. To avoid pesticide risks, choose organic produce if the skin is going to be consumed or is difficult to wash. Reject the hype touting vegetable juices and powders as superfoods, because they will always be inferior to the real thing. You'll definitely get a concentrated dose of certain beneficial agents, but you'll also get a bigger sugar hit with juice and a reduction in nutritional value with a powder that's undergone even the most basic processing. Finally, if you believe you may have sensitivity to the natural toxins contained in plants, monitor your consumption of the foods in the various vegetable (and other plant food) categories to detect any adverse reactions, especially when you consume vegetables in raw form. Signs of plant reactivity include gas, bloating, and digestive pain in association with vegetable consumption as well as chronic autoimmune or inflammatory conditions that have resisted traditional medical treatment.

The best option by far is to buy local, in-season, pesticide-free vegetables grown on small farms. You can usually find these at a farmer's market or natural-foods grocer in your area. Finding locally grown, in-season produce from small farms ensures that you avoid the perils of the food-industrial complex and enjoy freshness, great flavor, and rich nutrition. Often, small farms don't go to the expense of obtaining official organic certification, but you can gain a level of comfort knowing that your product was grown in a sustainable manner free from the typical pesticides and chemicals of industrial farming.

The next best choice is to buy certified organic vegetables, which are now prevalent in national chains such as Costco, Walmart, Whole Foods Market, Target, Kroger, and others. Locally grown and certified organic produce delivers more nutritional benefits than conventionally grown products, without the increasingly disturbing health concerns associated with large-production farming, which relies on pesticides. You may be familiar with glyphosate, a toxic herbicide that is widely used for both landscaping (yards, parks, golf courses) and commercial farming. The popular weed killer Roundup is one of hundreds of products containing glyphosate. Despite growing evidence that glyphosate is a carcinogen that inflicts cellular damage at the DNA level, it remains in heavy use. Monsanto, the creator of this toxic weed treatment, has even developed genetically modified crops to withstand heavy exposure to glyphosate. This is one of those examples of conventional stupidity that I call "digging a hole to install a ladder to wash the basement windows."

Conventionally grown vegetables are also frequently raised with nutrient-deficient monocrop soil. They're picked too early, artificially ripened with ethylene gas, and shipped from distant locations to your local market. This makes them a thumbs-down in both sustainability and nutritional value. If you want vegetables whose chemical exposure risk is high—those with a large edible surface area (spinach, kale, leafy greens) or those whose skin is consumed and/or difficult to wash (bell peppers, celery, cucumbers, carrots)—be firm in your resolve to only eat local or certified organic products. Foods in these categories are also treated with some of the most powerful and toxic pesticides, so take a hard pass on these offerings. If you want vegetables (or fruits) with tough, inedible skins or rinds (avocados, squash, bananas, melons), those that are easily washable or with nonedible skins (onions, asparagus), and all nuts and seeds, the pesticide exposure risk—and the need to find organic options—is less critical.

Don't Eat Your Vegetables?

The emerging carnivore diet movement offers a surprising challenge to the widely assumed health benefits of eating vegetables and suggests that many individuals can benefit from an experimental period of total exclusion of all plant foods. This includes grains, especially, as well as legumes, vegetables, fruits, nuts, and seeds. As I mentioned in chapter 1, grains and all other plants contain natural toxins that deter predators from consuming them. These agents include lectins (gluten is a form of lectin found in wheat; other grains and legumes have high amounts of other lectins), phytates (prominent in nuts and seeds), oxalates (in leafy greens, nuts, and legumes), isothiocyanates (found in cruciferous vegetables), saponins (in beans and legumes), enzyme inhibitors (high in soybeans), phytoestrogens (in soy, corn, and flaxseeds), the tannins in fruit, and many other agents.

These toxins can be neutralized through cooking, soaking, sprouting, and fermenting—in many cases a plant is inedible or poisonous without these preparations. Nevertheless, consuming plants still delivers significant residual exposure to antinutrients, especially if consumed in raw form. The level of potential harm varies depending on the plant and the individual. For someone with celiac disease or a peanut allergy, consuming problematic foods can cause a severe immediate reaction. For others, decades-long consumption patterns can result in subclinical symptoms that are never directly associated with a specific plant but can really harm both short-term and long-term health. This was the case for me. Eating grains caused all manner of mild to moderate digestive ailments and inflammatory conditions (my "normal"), which quickly vanished when I ditched grains, in 2002.

The popularity of gluten-free, grain-free, ancestral-style eating validates that ditching all grains, or at least nasty modern dwarf wheat, can alleviate moderate digestive and inflammatory conditions and lower insulin production. Until recently, fruits, vegetables, nuts, and seeds have been touted—unchallenged—as all-powerful superfoods with nothing but high marks across the board. The increasingly popular carnivore movement, however—spearheaded by physicians and athletic role models Dr. Shawn Baker and Dr. Paul Saladino and popular blogger and decade-long adherent Amber O'Hearn—is buoyed by thousands of truly amazing stories of people who have stopped consuming plant foods and thereby healed assorted chronic illnesses or sprouted six-packs in short order. Visit Dr. Shawn Baker's MeatRx.com for hundreds of success stories in dozens of disease categories submitted by carnivore enthusiasts. Listen to Dr. Saladino's *Fundamental Health* podcast or read his book, *The Carnivore Code*, for extensive scientific support for the carnivore approach.

You may be under the assumption that chomping on a head of broccoli or downing a handful of blueberries delivers a direct dose of potent antioxidants and anti-inflammatory agents into your bloodstream. What's actually happening when you ingest high-antioxidant plant foods is that the antinutrients in the plant prompt your liver to mount an internal antioxidant defense response. We fight back against the minor poisoning, which fine-tunes the immune system and inflammatory response, delivering a net positive adaptive benefit, or *hormesis*. The same dynamic of stressing the body appropriately (hormetic stress) in order to get stronger happens when we do a set of dead lifts, sprint around the track, visit the sauna, or take a brief plunge into freezing water. By contrast, when you train too hard with insufficient recovery time, get overheated during a hot workout or competition, or get lost in a snowy forest and become hypothermic, the chronic or severe nature of the stressor obviously becomes unhealthy.

This is precisely the problem with frequently consuming plant toxins, especially in the presence of other chronic modern stressors such as junk food, sleep deficiency, excess exercise, and stressful job or relationship dynamics. For people who are not genetically adapted to efficiently digest certain plant foods, even occasional servings of bread, pasta, or raw kale smoothies is too much. For example, gluten and other lectin proteins have been shown to damage the delicate microvilli that line your small intestine. When this important barrier becomes inflamed and permeable, undigested bacteria and toxins are allowed to enter the bloodstream. This is a phenomenon known as leaky gut syndrome. When foreign agents enter the bloodstream, your body perceives this shit (sorry, but the term is apropos here) as a virus and mounts an autoimmune response. Over time, eating seemingly healthful plant foods can overwhelm the body's defenses and trigger an assortment of autoimmune and/or inflammatory reactions. Leaky gut syndrome has emerged in medical science in recent years as a likely downstream cause of all manner of chronic illnesses and diseases not just in the digestive system but also throughout the body, including allergies, arthritis, asthma, colitis, inflammatory skin conditions (acne, psoriasis), insomnia, irritable bowel syndrome, joint pain, sleep apnea, and assorted other conditions ending with "itis" (gastritis, diverticulitis).

The gas, bloating, indigestion, and transient abdominal pain that virtually all of us report occasionally or regularly can be attributed to consuming plant toxins as well as heavily processed foods. Sadly, it's so commonplace that we have collectively come to view digestive irregularities as normal and fail to make the connection between diet and our suffering. This is especially the case when we have been programmed to believe that salads and raw vegetable smoothies represent the holy grail of healthful living. Consider this quotation from an extreme healthful eating enthusiast and elite athlete friend who reports that he gets a bloated abdomen every time he consumes a smoothie packed with raw produce: "It's so healthy, it's worth it." Something's wrong with this picture!

If you have even mild recurrent digestive discomfort after meals, swings in energy, mood, or appetite during the day, or if you otherwise suspect you may be sensitive to plant toxins, you will most definitely experience a tremendous health awakening by not eating any form of nutrient-deficient, high-insulin-stimulating, leaky-gut-promoting grains. If you are interested in further exploration and optimization, consider a strict thirty-day ban on all plant foods. Many enthusiasts report vastly better digestion and elimination, an absence of gas and bloating, and even improvements in depression, anxiety, ADHD, and other mood and cognitive disturbances.

After a strict elimination period, you can experiment with reintroducing the least risky plants over time. These include fruits, starchy vegetables, cooked vegetables, and nuts, seeds, and legumes that have been soaked, sprouted, or fermented. Monitor your body carefully for any adverse gastrointestinal reactions and determine your comfort level with plant intake. I've been grain-free for nearly two decades and am pretty selective in my consumption of fruit (I eat berries in the summertime.) However, vegetable consumption has been a centerpiece of my diet with no ill effects. After all, my signature meal is the Sisson Bigass Salad (page 229), laden with my own healthful avocado oil–based dressing. Still, intrigued by the carnivore rationale in recent years, I've noticed that I've drifted away from the consumption of high volumes of vegetables and toward a meat-based, animal superfood–focused diet.

Fruit

Fruit has long been regarded as a central element of healthful eating and is a great source of broad-spectrum antioxidants and micronutrients. However, it's easy to eat too much of the wrong kinds of fruit at the wrong times, so moderation and selectivity are warranted in this category. Today's year-round availability, genetic engineering of larger, sweeter fruits grown in depleted soil, and the excessive carbohydrates in the SAD make fruit a potential trouble area. The best bets are locally grown, in-season fresh fruits with relatively high antioxidant and low glycemic values. Berries are the superstar in the fruit category and can be consumed liberally when fresh and in season. Even if you are a strict keto enthusiast, you can enjoy fresh local or certified organic blackberries, blueberries, raspberries, and strawberries in the summertime. Finding wild fruit would be the ultimate goal, but if that is not possible, seek out local farmer's market fare or certified organic products.

While I'm not too keen to split hairs about your consumption of colorful natural foods such as fruit, we have to acknowledge fruit's contribution to metabolic syndrome, a global health epidemic. Fruit can exacerbate the problem of excess body fat because it is the most lipogenic (fat-forming) of all forms of carbohydrate. Fructose is the predominant carbohydrate contained in fruit. Unlike carbohydrate sources that can be burned immediately, fructose must be first converted into glucose in the liver before those calories can be burned. The liver also happens to be the place where excess glucose is converted into triglyceride and stored in your fat cells. Unfortunately, slamming down fruit because it gets zero points from Weight Watchers can contribute directly to excess body fat and other metabolic problems. Fructose has been found to be five to ten times more likely than glucose to promote fatty liver disease and insulin resistance. Furthermore, many people have difficulty digesting fructose, especially processed fructose, such as that found in high-fructose corn syrup and processed foods—a condition known as fructose malabsorption. Symptoms include flatulence, cramps, bloating, and diarrhea, and there may be a link to depression.

Dr. David Perlmutter—a neurologist, expert in functional medicine (a.k.a. root cause–based medicine) and gut microbiome health, and author of the bestselling *Grain Brain* and related titles—recommends not eating any fruit during the winter months because doing so runs counter to our evolutionary experience. Limit your fruit consumption to seasonal and local offerings and hold off entirely if you are trying to drop excess body fat. If you have symptoms of fructose malabsorption, first eliminate all processed fructose from your diet and consider a fruit-restriction period as a test. Furthermore, understand that fruit exists on a nutritional spectrum, ranging from high antioxidant–low glycemic (the best) to low antioxidant–high glycemic (the ones to limit). Berries, lemons, limes, and stone fruits (cherries, peaches, apricots) rank among the best. Avocados are also technically fruits and rank among the true superfoods: they are obviously high antioxidant–low glycemic because of their high monounsaturated fat content. Low antioxidant–high glycemic fruits that should be moderated or avoided include tropical fruits (mangoes, papaya, pineapple), grapes, tangerines, plums, and especially dates and dried fruits because of their extremely high sugar content and caloric density (since they lack fiber and water).

If you have healthy blood profiles, an ideal body composition, and an active, physically fit lifestyle, fruit can be a dietary centerpiece and a great way to restock depleted glycogen after workouts. Remember: while the liver converts excess carbs to fat, it is also a major storage depot for glycogen. Fruit is also a sensible choice if you are concerned about plant antigens (see page 34), because fruit has much lower levels of the toxic agents that concentrate in other types of plants (grains, legumes, leafy greens, cruciferous vegetables).

Nuts, Seeds, and Their Derivative Butters

Nuts and seeds are another "life force" food category. They contain nutritious protein, fatty acids, enzymes, antioxidants, phytonutrients, and abundant vitamins and minerals. Numerous large-scale dietary studies (including the Iowa Women's Health Study, of nearly 40,000 women; the Harvard T. H. Chan School of Public Health Nurses' Health Study, of 127,000 women; and the Physicians' Health Study, of 22,000 men) suggest that regular consumption of nuts, seeds, and their derivative butters significantly reduces the risk of heart disease, diabetes, and other health problems.

These foods are extremely satiating and have been touted as an excellent snack option that will help ease the transition from carbohydrate dependency to metabolic flexibility. In the same breath, however, ancestral enthusiasts also observe that the caloric density of nuts, seeds, and their butters can compromise fat-reduction goals. Don't worry: while snacking is acceptable in the early days of your transformation, you'll leave it behind when you become fat-adapted. Furthermore, when you focus on maximizing dietary nutrient density, and the food choices and lifestyle behaviors that promote hormone optimization, your hunger and satiety signals will naturally stabilize your caloric intake and body composition.

Be sure to find options that are raw or dry-roasted, because many leading brands of packaged nuts contain refined industrial seed oils that are used during processing. Read labels carefully! Consume fresh nuts within six months or store them in the freezer to extend shelf life. If the nuts you have on hand start to smell oily or rancid, or if they develop flecks in their surface color, discard them.

The ultrapopular peanut is actually a member of the legume family and is one of the most common allergenic foods. As with all other plant foods, if you can tolerate peanuts and peanut butter without any adverse reaction, it is probably safe to enjoy them. If you have nagging autoimmune or anti-inflammatory conditions, however, peanuts are a good candidate for temporary restriction so you can assess whether they have any impact.

Nut butters are gaining in popularity. Single-serving packets are great for convenient energy on the go and are a perfect replacement for high-sugar gels. If you can find the rare but decadent delicacies macadamia nut butter and coconut butter (Brad's Macadamia Masterpiece has both, at Bradventures.com), they rank right up there with dark chocolate as a delicious, satisfying treat to replace your old sugary options.

Puree your favorite nuts in a food processor, and you have an interesting way to liven up a salad or a plate of steamed vegetables. Make nut butters a base for your Brad's NOatmeal (page 247) or spread them onto fresh vegetables. For a decadent dessert treat, spread pureed nuts on a piece of dark chocolate (one that has an 80 percent or higher cacao content) and let it melt in your mouth. Macadamia nuts are lauded for having the highest monounsaturated fat content (84 percent) of any nut or seed, while walnuts have the highest omega-3 content. Enjoy these delicious, nutritious foods, but exercise some moderation if you are trying to shed body fat.

High-Fat Dairy Products

The rule of thumb for strict Paleo adherents is to eat only foods that existed in prehistoric times, but I like to make ancestral-inspired eating as inclusive and enjoyable as possible. Certain high-fat dairy products can be enjoyed because they are nutritious and have minimal health drawbacks. However, it's very important to choose wisely. The gold standard in dairy is raw, fermented, unpasteurized, unsweetened, high-fat, low-carbohydrate, organic selections—including ghee and butter; full-fat cream, cottage cheese, and cream cheese; and raw or certified organic whole milk—from pasture-raised and grass-fed animals. You can also enjoy organic fermented dairy products, including cultured buttermilk, full-fat Greek yogurt, kefir, raw-milk cheese and aged cheese, and full-fat sour cream.

Avoid all low-fat and nonfat items, such as 2 percent and skim milk, nonfat yogurts, fruit-flavored yogurts, low-fat cottage cheese, imitation whipped cream, imitation coffee creamer, fat-free cheese, ice cream, frozen yogurt, and all other frozen dairy desserts. These products are essentially sugar bombs and can cause digestive problems and allergic reactions in many people. Avoid all nonorganic dairy products because of the manufacturers' abhorrent processing methods and the high prevalence of hormones, pesticides, and antibiotics in the animals and the end products.

Lactose is the form of carbohydrate found in dairy products, and approximately 80 percent of the global adult population has a mild to severe intolerance for it. If you have developed lactose intolerance after childhood, you may experience an assortment of digestive difficulties (gas, bloating, diarrhea, constipation, transient sharp digestive pain) after consuming high-carbohydrate milk products.

Casein is one of the two types of protein in dairy products; whey is the other. Casein is classified as either A1 or A2, and research strongly suggests that A2 casein may be much easier to digest than A1. A1 casein is believed to trigger autoimmune reactions and leaky gut syndrome in many people. Most conventional milks and dairy products in the store come from cows producing both A1 and A2 casein. You won't be able to tell the difference unless you are sourcing alternative brands specially designated as pure A2 cow's milk. A2 happens to be the form of casein in goat's milk and yogurt and sheep's milk and yogurt, which is why many lactose-intolerant folks fare much better choosing alternative milks. Dr. Steven Gundry, bestselling author of *The Plant Paradox* and *The Longevity Paradox*, believes that most lactose intolerance cases are really A1 intolerance. Most modern cattle produce A1 casein after thousands of years of selective breeding for the heartiest, highest-production animals; they just happen to be A1 producers.

Symptoms of casein sensitivity include digestive difficulties, sinus inflammation, excess mucus production, and flare-ups of autoimmune conditions such as arthritis, allergies, asthma, acne, and skin rashes. Casein is believed to stimulate opioid receptors in the brain and promote food addiction as well as contribute to mood and cognitive disturbances. By sticking to dairy options that are either fermented or have a high fat content, you can minimize or negate concerns about lactose and casein.

Most dairy products in the supermarket have been pasteurized and homogenized to protect against food-borne pathogens, improve product consistency, and extend shelf life. These high-temperature, high-pressure processes destroy many of the nutrients in dairy products as well as the enzymes and beneficial bacteria that help you digest them. Pasteurization and homogenization alter the molecular composition of milk, making the component fats, proteins, and carbohydrates difficult to digest. Studies of people suffering from lactose intolerance reveal a huge success rate in alleviating symptoms upon switching from conventional milk to raw milk. One Weston A. Price Foundation survey of seven hundred families revealed that 80 percent of lactose-intolerant participants were able to drink raw milk without difficulty; another study, from the University of Michigan, showed an 84 percent success rate. Studies of European children suggest that consuming raw milk helps protect against allergies and asthma.

Consequently, raw milk or cheese obtained directly from a local farm or trusted provider is the most nutritious choice—if you can find it. Raw milk from a grass-fed cow has across-the-board nutritional superiority to conventional pasteurized and homogenized milk, including higher levels of omega-3 fatty acids; conjugated linoleic acid (CLA) fats, which support fat metabolism; assorted fat-soluble vitamins that are hard to find in other foods; calcium; antimicrobial agents; and butyrate, to support gut health and reduce inflammation. You have likely heard dire warnings to avoid raw dairy products because of the risk of ingesting dangerous food-borne bacteria. But experts such as Chris Kresser, MS, LAc, a functional medicine educator and author of *The Paleo Cure*, have revealed these warnings to be overstated. It would indeed be ill-advised to consume raw milk from a conventionally raised cow because of their crowded, unhealthful, unsanitary feedlot environments. These concerns are why it's virtually impossible to find mass-market raw milk or other raw dairy products on store shelves. However, raw milk is invariably sourced from boutique local dairies raising grass-fed cattle in a sustainable environment that makes the risk of food-borne illness actually lower than it is in most other food categories.

If you can't find raw dairy products, be sure to choose certified organic products to avoid the many objectionable agents (hormones, pesticides, antibiotics) routinely included in their nonorganic counterparts. Being certified organic is especially important for high-fat dairy products, because toxins concentrate in the fat cells of animals. Conventional dairy products routinely contain recombinant bovine growth hormone (rBGH), dangerous chemicals such as PCBs (polychlorinated biphenyls), POPs (persistent organic pollutants) such as the evil pesticides DDE and DDT, illegal antibiotics, and other impurities.

These chemicals all increase cancer risk and cause massive health problems—so much so that you should avoid nonorganic dairy products entirely.

Fermented dairy products can qualify as superfoods because of their elevated levels of all the important nutrients and their potent anti-inflammatory and antioxidant properties. The fermentation process also offers protection against lactose and casein intolerance, even if your fermented products contain carbs and protein. The presence of lactic acid bacteria that results from the fermentation process delivers high levels of B vitamins; vitamin K_2; healthful conjugated linoleic acid; bioactive peptides, which aid in digestion; and of course the all-important probiotic bacteria strains, which nourish your gut microbiome. Fermented dairy products such as cultured buttermilk, cheese, kefir, sour cream, and yogurt have been a mainstay of ancestral diets across the globe since primal times. Kefir has been around since 10,000 BCE and is a time-honored way to help improve digestion and boost immune functioning. Enjoy the very best dairy products and be extremely disciplined in your choices—avoid all nonorganic products as well as low-fat and nonfat sugar bombs.

Dark Chocolate

Dark chocolate is a delicious and nutritious treat with numerous health benefits and a low carbohydrate content. After a short period of acclimation, it can become your go-to treat in place of the typical sweet-tooth fare that you reach for when you want a little something after dinner. Strive to consume bars that have a high cacao percentage and the "bean-to-bar" designation on the label. High cacao, bean-to-bar dark chocolate is a rich source of antioxidants (polyphenols, flavonols, catechins), numerous phytonutrients, and broad-spectrum minerals, including iron, chromium, copper, magnesium, and manganese. The ORAC antioxidant values of the cacao bean are among the highest ever measured—higher than other superfood superstars such as acai berries and blueberries. Cacao also has more flavonols than green tea. (Flavonols are bioactive compounds with assorted health and anti-inflammatory benefits, such as increasing nitric oxide levels, which improves arterial functioning.)

You may have heard about the powerful opioid peptide in chocolate called *phenylethylamine*, a.k.a. the love drug. This hormone-like substance, which also occurs naturally in your brain and body, acts as an amplifier for numerous mood-elevating neurotransmitters such as dopamine, serotonin, and norepinephrine. Sensible consumption of dark chocolate can help improve mood, focus, concentration, and motivation as well as alleviate anxiety and stress. Essentially, the potent compounds in cacao help prevent your delicate neural circuits from becoming overexcited or, alternatively, emotionally flat and burned out.

Dark chocolate is the most prominent dietary source of an agent called *theobromine*, which has cardiovascular benefits, acts as a natural stimulant and memory booster, and reduces inflammation. It also acts as an appetite suppressant. *Epicatechin* is another prominent flavonoid in dark chocolate that has been found to boost nitric oxide production. Nitric oxide helps make arteries more soft and supple, lowering blood pressure and protecting your cells against free radical damage. Other research reveals that dark chocolate can protect against heart disease by lowering oxidized LDL cholesterol (the most causative for atherosclerosis) and increasing healthful HDL cholesterol. Dark chocolate enthusiasts are amused by the legend of the late Jeanne Calment of France (1875–1997), the longest-lived human on record, who died at the age of 122. Calment reportedly consumed high volumes of olive oil and up to a kilogram (2.2 pounds) of chocolate each week!

Dark chocolate is labeled according to the percentage of ingredients, by weight, obtained from the cacao bean. A 100 percent cacao bar has no added sugar and a bitter taste. A milk chocolate or semisweet chocolate bar has sugar and milk powder added, putting it an entirely different food category from dark chocolate—i.e., a sugar bomb! Choose dark chocolate bars that contain at least 70 percent cacao and avoid many offerings labeled "dark chocolate" that can be as low as 45 percent cacao. As you acclimate your taste buds away from your go-to sweets of the past and begin to appreciate the intense, savory taste of dark chocolate, strive to progress to eating bars that are in the range of 80 to 90 percent cacao. This will ensure that you are getting the maximum nutritional value with the minimum amount of sugar. Review labels to be sure that there are more grams of fat than sugar in your bar, which should be the case with high-cacao bars.

Selectivity is warranted when choosing dark chocolate brands because many bars use large-scale processing methods and bulk ingredients of unknown origin and questionable quality control—for both the product quality and labor practices. It's common for large-scale commercial producers serving the giant candy industry to harvest substandard cacao beans, including rotten ones. Then beans are cavalierly overroasted to burn out any rotten taste and mixed with enough sugar, lactose, dextrose, corn syrup, vanilla, and artificial flavorings to create a palatable end product—with a low price and a high profit margin. Many inferior bars undergo "Dutch" (yep—a Dutch chemist named Casparus van

Houten invented the process in 1828) processing, with alkali, to reduce acidity, improve flavor, and lower processing costs. However, this substantially reduces the flavonol and polyphenol content as well. Even more disturbing is the fact that many cacao producers in African nations with minimal government regulations use child labor to harvest their crop. If you are buying a mainstream big-brand dark chocolate bar priced at around a dollar per ounce, you can assume your bar is a product of child labor. Expect to pay vastly more for an ethically sourced, high-quality dark chocolate bar—in the neighborhood of three to five dollars per ounce.

In contrast to industrialized chocolate production, the best cacao comes from small farmers methodically growing and harvesting an exquisite product through low-tech, labor-intensive fermentation and air-drying techniques. These beans are teeming with antioxidants and phytonutrients and carry subtle flavor notes of the soil, climate, and flowers and fruit of the area. This natural environmental flavoring concept—called terroir—is typically found in wine production, but it also exists in the world of elite dark chocolate bars, which can be said to offer fruity, floral, spicy, herbal, nutty, and caramel notes.

To find the best bars, look for these designations on the label: bean-to-bar, fair trade, and certified organic. Bean-to-bar means the artisanal chocolate maker sourced the beans from their origin in equatorial cacao farms and completed all the production steps in-house to get that bar into a wrapper. Consequently, you want to see "cacao beans" first in the ingredients lineup and a bare minimum of other ingredients. The best bars will typically be made of cacao beans, sugar, perhaps some cocoa butter to enhance mouthfeel, and perhaps vanilla—that's it. By contrast, the first item in a mass-produced bar might be chocolate liquor, cocoa mass, chocolate, or bittersweet chocolate, indicating that the ingredients were premixed and melted into an intermediate-stage product of obscure origin. You may also notice other objectionable ingredients in cheap bars. For example, it's common to use soy lecithin as an emulsifier: if it's in your chocolate bar, you're getting a dose of genetically modified soybeans.

The fair trade designation indicates a product made using environmental sustainability practices under equitable working conditions and without child labor. It means that farmers receive fair prices for their harvest and that the producer invests additional funds in community redevelopment. A certified organic designation assures greater oversight of the growing, harvesting, and processing procedures for the cacao beans, sugar, and any other ingredients in the bar. Bars made without synthetic pesticides, fertilizers, herbicides, and GMOs protect the farmers, the environment, and your health.

Keep in mind that many small cacao farmers, like local growers of produce, might grow their crop naturally but don't bother to apply for expensive organic certification. Read labels carefully and look for cacao beans as the lead ingredient. It is worth the effort to communicate online with favorite chocolate manufacturers to gain assurance that you are getting a clean product. Be wary of "eco-earthy" brands with touchy-feely logos and labeling—many still contain questionable ingredients despite their higher price point.

Get excited about this sensible indulgence and become a connoisseur! Search for various boutique brands of bean-to-bar dark chocolate and engage in some ceremonial taste-testing with friends and family. Focus all your senses on the experience. Break off a small square and enjoy its aroma. Instead of biting into the chocolate, allow the square to rest on your tongue and soak in the flavor until the chocolate dissolves. You'll grow to appreciate various mouthfeels, flavor profiles, and textures—and discover some favorites. Some outstanding bean-to-bar artisanal chocolate providers: Askinosie.com, CoracaoConfections .com, CreoChocolate.com, HuKitchen.com, KellerManniChocolate.com, LillieBelleFarms .com, RitualChocolate.com, and TazaChocolate.com. Visit BarAndCocoa.com for a wide selection of premium bean-to-bar products (cacao percentages range from 60 to 100 percent) from around the world.

Once you get your hands on some prized bounty, be sure to avoid the rookie mistake of refrigerating your bars. Refrigeration destabilizes the fats and sugars in the bar, causing them to rise to the surface—perhaps you've seen white streaks on bars that have been refrigerated. Store your chocolate in a cool, dry place, such as a cupboard or even a custom-built basement chocolate sanctuary. And don't forget: no biting! Just savor the flavor.

Beverages and Hydration

Forget the commercials showing sweaty athletes sucking down sugar-filled "recovery" drinks for multimillion-dollar endorsement contracts—water is the drink of champions. The main objective in this category is to avoid consuming sweetened beverages that deliver massive amounts of carbohydrates with minimal satiety. This includes coffee-shop concoctions and the huge assortment of energy drinks, sports drinks, refrigerated juice blends, and other products covered in the beverages-to-avoid section of the previous chapter. Even a fresh-squeezed vegetable or fruit medley teeming with antioxidants is going to deliver enough of a sugar hit to warrant a pass. Yes, it's natural sugar from fruit, but juicing concentrates the dose. What's more, these drinks are typically layered on top of a high-carbohydrate diet, thus making a contribution to hyperinsulinemia rather than to the vibrant health and boundless energy promised by the marketing messages.

From a foundation of adequate daily water consumption, you can also enjoy unsweetened herbal or caffeinated tea, coffee (cream is fine, but keep added sugar to a bare minimum), and homemade kombucha that has been naturally sweetened and fermented. Read labels and watch out for overly sweetened commercial kombucha offerings with excessive carbohydrate content, or cut these drinks with soda water (three parts soda to one part kombucha). Recently, the market has exploded with a range of low- or no-calorie beverages, including still and sparkling waters with fruit infusions. Stay away from products containing artificial sweeteners. It would be better to make your own cucumber-lemon water at home than go for something that often tastes ridiculously sweet because of its artificial or natural sweeteners, such as stevia. Beverages with natural, nutritious fat calories are acceptable, such as bone broth, raw milk, kefir, and unsweetened coconut and almond milk. However, these latter "drinks" might be more appropriately categorized as foods.

You may have heard various edicts about hydration, ranging from the long-standing "eight glasses a day" to "sip constantly," promulgated by fitness experts who urge you to carry a bottle around wherever you go. For the most part, simply honoring your thirst mechanism will help you hydrate effectively. Virtually everything you eat and drink has significant water content and will contribute to your hydration goals. Even coffee hydrates nearly as effectively as plain water despite its short-term diuretic effect. Bone broth, Greek yogurt, vegetables, berries, fish (comprising 65–90 percent water), and steak (around 75 percent water) all hydrate nicely. The Mayo Clinic estimates that solid foods can provide up to 20 percent of your hydration requirements.

Even if your fluid consumption varies from day to day, your kidneys and endocrine system do a marvelous job of maintaining optimal fluid and electrolyte balance in the bloodstream at all times. If you drink too much fluid, urine production increases, and more sodium is released into the bloodstream. If you're exercising on a hot day, sweating and underdrinking to the extent that your blood becomes concentrated by 2 percent, you will experience extreme thirst, compelling you to rebalance. The medical consequences of dehydration only kick in when your blood gets 5 percent concentrated, so we humans have plenty of safety-net mechanisms to ensure we are well hydrated almost all the time. After all, there were no CamelBaks or Klean Kanteens in primal times.

The picture gets a little more complex for high-performing athletes who experience increased sweat production and calorie burning. During intense or prolonged workouts, your elevated body temperature and stress hormone production can actually mute your thirst mechanism. Also, as your body perceives a high rate of fluid loss, vasopressin (an antidiuretic hormone) triggers the kidneys to dump extra fluid into the bloodstream to support your work efforts, which mutes your thirst mechanism as the kidneys are telling you, "We got this." Losing sodium and other electrolytes through sweating can create imbalances that increase dehydration risks. Your body needs to maintain a delicate and optimal water-to-sodium ratio at all times, so sodium deficiency will inhibit water absorption.

Typically, athletes who eat nutritious foods, rehydrate well after tough workouts, and respect the importance of recovery will stay well hydrated. However, a pattern of challenging workouts in hot temperatures, possibly combined with diet and fluid-intake shortcomings, can eventually cause you to start drifting into a state of chronic mild dehydration. If you commence a workout with your blood a bit concentrated, you'll probably feel fine and your body will rally to perform on demand. However, this will also increase the stress impact of the workout, extend recovery time, and set you up for real trouble at future workouts. If you attempt to rehydrate by consuming a huge volume of plain water immediately after your workout, you can overwhelm the delicate sodium-fluid balance and cause most of your chugalug to be excreted instead of absorbed by tissues throughout the body.

For optimal absorption, always include a bit of sodium with the fluid you consume. Use unprocessed pink Himalayan salt or ancient sea salt instead of iodized salt to get the benefit of dozens of additional minerals. If you work out and sweat regularly, strive to consume an additional five to ten grams (one to two teaspoons) of sodium per day. Add a pinch of salt to each cup of liquid or several good shakes from a dispenser into every liter that you drink. Adding this amount will not taste unpleasant. Then sip your fluid gradually over the next hour or two for efficient absorption. Interestingly, adding a bit of glucose or sucrose to your drink has been found to improve fluid absorption in the intestines. You can add a pinch of sugar per eight ounces of water, or try 100 percent natural coconut water (no added sweeteners), lauded for its naturally optimal sodium and electrolyte levels.

The ideal strategy here is to be mindful of hydration when you are rested instead of getting into trouble after a string of hot, strenuous workouts. If you have elevated hydration needs because of a busy job, a heavy workout schedule, or hot summer temperatures, carry around a thirty-two-ounce or forty-eight-ounce stainless steel container and sip from it throughout the day. It's widely recommended in the fitness community that you consume a large volume of water as soon as you awaken, so go for it (don't forget the salt). Resolve to never, ever drink to the point of discomfort or feeling bloated or you will risk a serious health condition called *hyponatremia*, which arises when you dilute sodium levels to the extent that you can lose consciousness or even die. Respect the difference between strategic hydration and oblivious overhydration.

Don't get too worked up about water quality and finding the absolute highest purity or buying expensive products touting magical cellular energy, alkalizing, or detoxification. If you can afford natural, mineral-rich springwater in glass bottles, you will enjoy the best taste and health benefits. If you are using municipal water, consider investing in an under-the-counter reverse osmosis system, or at least use a pitcher or refrigerator dispenser with carbon filtration.

Try to avoid consuming water out of plastic bottles except when there are no other options. Evidence is mounting about the damage caused by xenoestrogens (unnatural estrogenic compounds from industrial sources) in plastic packaging, personal care and household cleaning products, and our food supply. Ingesting these agents or absorbing them through the skin can disrupt the delicate hormone balance in both sexes with an unnatural estrogen overload.

At the very least, resolve to never allow your food or drink to touch plastic. Replace plastic plates, cups, water bottles, and food storage containers with glass or stainless-steel vessels. The most detrimental effects occur when your plastic container heats up, because this increases the release of estrogenic molecules into your food or drink. Never drink out of a plastic bottle that's been sitting in a car (even if it's cooled down), and never microwave food in plastic containers. When eating take-out meals, transfer them out of the plastic or Styrofoam and onto a proper plate to enjoy. To extend your estrogen avoidance efforts further, use eco-friendly personal care products, such as coconut oil for your face and castile soap for your body. Also make sure to avoid all foods made with soy, corn, and flax, which have one hundred times more phytoestrogens (plant-based estrogens) than other foods.

STRATEGIES TO MINIMIZE THE ADVERSE EFFECTS OF ALCOHOL

In my 2009 book, *The Primal Blueprint*, I categorized alcohol as a "sensible indulgence" for people who felt compelled to imbibe. I even sang the praises of red wine's antioxidant benefits. After much reflection, and a successful experience with abstinence a few years back to correct some sleep disturbances that I blamed on metabolizing alcohol, I now offer a more sobering take on the subject. I no longer feel the need to explicitly recommend consumption of a toxic substance that can easily interfere with your fat-reduction goals. I assert that you are better off not consuming alcohol, despite studies that suggest moderate drinkers outlive teetotalers. Nevertheless, I'm all about enjoying life and encouraging you to do the same, so if sensible alcohol consumption will likely be part of your scene, it's certainly worth addressing. I drink organic, chemical-free, sugar-free, low-alcohol red wines on a regular basis and will occasionally enjoy premium tequila and other alcoholic beverages in party settings. Let's review how to make the least detrimental alcohol choices and of course resolve to always drink moderately and responsibly.

Alcohol calories are known as the "first to burn" because they must be metabolized immediately on ingestion, thanks to their toxicity to the brain and other organs (that's why you feel the "buzz"). As your liver works hard to metabolize alcohol and detoxify your system, the burning of all other fuel sources is put on hold. Any glucose and fatty acids in the bloodstream are likely to be removed and sent to fat storage. When you finish metabolizing the alcohol calories, you will have low blood sugar and a craving for quick-energy carbohydrates. Can you say "the munchies"? Contrary to the common misconception that your body converts alcohol into sugar or fat, it is the empty-calorie, appetite-stimulating, and lipogenic properties of alcohol that make drinking a real downer for your fat-reduction goals.

The first-to-burn effects are magnified when the alcohol combines with the carbohydrates in beer, wine, and cocktails, not to mention the pizza or finger foods you might throw into the mix. Consequently, the least damaging way to consume alcohol is by drinking hard liquor, such as tequila, vodka, rum, or whiskey, on an empty stomach, independently of other calories. This strategy will also result in the most potent immediate buzz, so responsible drinking is essential. When you consume a drink in isolation (not social isolation; rather, without other calories), you are still obligated to burn off these empty calories at the expense of other fuel sources, but at least your body will get back into fat-burning mode more quickly than when you consume alcohol together with other calories.

As you strive to make choices about alcohol, it's important to consider that the hangovers we have long blamed directly on alcohol may more likely be the result of the sugar and chemical compounds consumed with it, combined with perhaps junk food, insufficient sleep, and other compounding factors. After all, there are detailed charts calculating the time required to metabolize various alcoholic beverages based on body weight. Theoretically, after you metabolize a reasonable amount of alcohol, you should be able to go about your business and awaken feeling fine after a good night's sleep. This insight—that there is more to the matter than alcohol—became clear to me after I abstained from red wine for several months and noticed some nagging digestive and sleep problems clearing up. For me, the benefits were sufficient to cause me to disavow my longtime evening-glass-of-red-wine routine. Then, at the urging of Todd White, founder of Dry Farm Wines, I tried organic, dry-farmed, chemical-free, sugar-free, low-alcohol red wines. To my delight, I experienced none of the previous symptoms that I had blamed on the wine, ignorant of the hidden sugars and chemical additives in conventionally produced wine. These days, I am careful to drink strategically: empty stomach, clean alcohol choices, no additional calories. This increases my enjoyment of the social experience and protects me from the hassle and regret of multifactorial hangovers.

Brian "Liver King" Johnson, founder of Ancestral Supplements and one of the most pure and dedicated ancestral-living humans you will find, describes an elaborate protocol for responsible drinking on his AncestralSupplements.com website. He recommends starting with an empty stomach and drinking straight Everclear: at 95 percent alcohol content (190 proof), it's known as the highest-potency alcoholic beverage on the market. Mix your shot with soda water, freshly squeezed lemon juice, and pink Himalayan salt. Take four of his desiccated grass-fed liver capsules with each drink to help the liver do its detox job. When you stop drinking, you are then to consume an assortment of supplements—more liver, liposomal glutathione, and vitamin C—and up to a dozen egg yolks! Brian reports sleeping beautifully after an evening of imbibing and popping up the next morning with zero ill effects, full of energy for a productive day. This guy is the real deal—he even makes his ice cubes from premium bottled springwater!

If you aren't inclined to take the elaborate steps recommended by the Liver King when you want to imbibe, you can at least honor a hierarchy of choices. First, thumbs-down to munchie-inducing mixed drinks, as discussed. Most of the adverse effects of drinking extend beyond the alcohol and over to the strawberry syrup in your daiquiri and the large pepperoni pizza you ordered for delivery straight to the bar. Beer is also a poor choice because of its carbohydrate and gluten content. Most commercial wines, even high-priced brands, contain moderate to incredibly high amounts of sugar, which you can't directly identify as sweetness because of the acidity and tannins in the wine. The sweetest wines contain up to 220 grams of sugar per liter—twice as much as Coca-Cola!

Also, there are often dozens of toxic, yet legally approved, chemical additives present in commercially produced wines. Some are used to disrupt the natural fermentation process that would otherwise reduce the sugar and alcohol content in the end product. This helps achieve the "bold" flavors that consumers and wine critics with a penchant for sweet flavors celebrate. If you choose to drink, your best options are sugar-free, chemical-free wine or high-quality tequila. If you want a mixed drink, blend tequila, vodka, rum, or whiskey with your choice of club soda, coconut water, ice, and herbs such as mint, basil, and ginger. Alternatively, flavor them with fresh fruits or a splash of juice. Get more suggestions in Kelly Milton's book *Paleo Happy Hour*, or find the "Paleo Drinking Cheat Sheet" at her website, PaleoGirlsKitchen.com.

Superfood: Nose-to-Tail Animal Products

The ancestral tradition of consuming the entire animal in a nose-to-tail manner has been tragically forgotten in today's DoorDash world. Instead, marketing influences lure us into choosing the speed and flavor intensity of fast-food burgers, while decades of nutritional propaganda have scared us away from eating animal fat. Today, we predominantly consume lean, high-protein muscle meats such as steak, hamburger, and chicken breast, missing out on a huge percentage of the nutritional benefits the animal has to offer. Fortunately, traditional cooking and nose-to-tail consumption are regaining popularity among ancestral health enthusiasts. You can easily find and enjoy budget-friendly animal superfoods such as organ meats (known as offal), bone-in cuts of meat, and authentic gelatinous bone broth. These foods have been a centerpiece of traditional diets across the globe for thousands of years and for eons of hunter-gatherers before that. In the modern era, traditional French cuisine is famous for its emphasis on organ meat. You can learn more in Tania Teschke's comprehensive French culture and cuisine cookbook, *The Bordeaux*

Kitchen. Or visit a Mexican *carniceria* (meat market) in your community for offerings such as lengua (tongue), sesos (brain), and tripe (stomach lining). Try making menudo (a stew made with tripe) or street tacos made with lengua or sesos.

You can start your superfood mission with liver, arguably ounce for ounce the most nutrient-dense food on the planet (salmon roe could compete here, too). As you know, the liver is the control tower that dispenses the exact amounts and types of nutrients you need into your bloodstream at all times and is the principle detoxifying organ in the body. This makes liver a treasure trove of virtually all the nutrition you need to thrive—a wise selection for a "stranded on a desert island, can only have one food" item. Like lions and other apex predators, ancient human hunters across the globe were known to consume warm liver on the spot after a kill.

Liver's nutritional profile is off the charts, with high levels of B vitamins, iron, zinc, magnesium, phosphorus, selenium, folic acid, choline, and fat-soluble vitamins (A, D, E, and K). For example, beef liver has seventeen times more B_{12} than ground beef. Liver is especially rich in retinol, the fully formed state of vitamin A, which is easily digested and assimilated, delivering comprehensive anti-inflammatory benefits. Retinol supports ocular health, increases bone density, and protects against cancer. Try coating 100 percent grass-fed beef liver in almond flour and panfrying it in butter or avocado oil. Cook only to medium rare to preserve nutrients. Hard-core ancestral folks like Brian "Liver King" Johnson and Dr. Paul Saladino enjoy their liver (and egg yolks) raw! If you have trouble with liver's strong taste, consider making a puree of liver and grass-fed hamburger and frying up some superfood burgers. Raw liver can also be more palatable (and more nutritious!) when served frozen (thawed just enough to be sliceable) and salted heavily.

Other organs such as brain, heart, kidney, oxtail (tailbone), Rocky Mountain oysters (testicle), stomach, tongue, and sweetbread (thymus or pancreas) score very well nutritionally, and can add some interesting diversity to your meal options. Find a quality butcher or natural-foods grocer in your area, or an internet resource, and dig into eating nose-to-tail. It's critical to find grass-fed organ meats, because organs contain more fat than muscles, and any toxins present tend to concentrate in fat cells. Organ meats are ridiculously affordable because they are still unpopular. While I enjoy a grass-fed rib eye or premium-quality sushi as much as anyone, pound for pound and dollar for dollar, you can't beat organ meats and canned SMASH fish for nutritional benefits. The affordability of eating this way is important, because I've weathered criticism over the years for recommending an "elitist" diet that is inaccessible to the masses. Take it as a challenge: examine your discretionary purchases and prioritize choosing the most healthful foods. If your budget is tight, you can zero in on the most affordable superfoods and still eat like a king or queen!

Bone broth and bone-in cuts of meat contain potent nutrients that are not found in other foods and can make a huge contribution to your connective-tissue health, immune functioning, and longevity. Consuming the connective tissue in these foods delivers the wondrous substance known as collagen, an emerging nutritional-supplement superstar. Collagen is a type of protein that was central to the ancestral diet but is woefully deficient in today's SAD. Collagen is critical to the integrity of your cartilage, fasciae, tendons, ligaments, bone, hair, skin, and nails. Over time, your natural internal collagen production declines (about 1.5 percent per year after age thirty), causing the wrinkled skin and brittle joints that characterize the aging process.

Collagen is believed to have a remarkable *tropic* effect in the body—the collagen you consume travels through the bloodstream and is deposited in the areas where it's needed most, such as brittle joints and tendons. Bone broth and bone-in cuts of meat are also rich in *glycosaminoglycans*, agents that help make new connective tissue and repair wounds. They act as a lubricant and shock absorber in your joints. Dr. Cate Shanahan, author of *Deep Nutrition*, explains that connective-tissue health is so important that it can be directly indicative of your rate of aging and longevity potential. Centenarians universally have excellent connective tissue. This is partly because of their genetic good fortune, but diet can also play a huge role in countering the natural decline in connective-tissue health as you age.

If you have joint issues or want smoother skin, consider taking a collagen peptide supplement in addition to consuming bone broth and bone-in meats. While research is inconclusive in this area, I became a huge collagen devotee when I experienced an incredibly rapid improvement in a decades-old Achilles tendon condition in conjunction with starting an aggressive collagen-supplement regimen. Now, not only do I get collagen from my diet, I also consume twenty to thirty grams per day in a collagen peptide supplement, as does my wife, Carrie. We're very pleased with the results and will continue this practice for the rest of our lives.

Bone broth is believed to have an assortment of healing properties. It helps neutralize white blood cell activity and open respiratory pathways to speed the healing from colds. This is why the age-old chicken soup remedy has scientific validity. While this is an emerging area of research, bone broth may have a valuable "heal and seal" effect on your gut lining, thus alleviating symptoms of leaky gut syndrome. Numerous success stories support this assertion: bone broth's salutary effects may be attributed to its high levels of glutamine, prompting intestinal cells to produce beneficial mucus that strengthens the gut lining. Bone broth is central to the highly regarded GAPS (Gut and Psychology Syndrome) healing protocol, in which participants adhere to a diet designed to combat depression, anxiety, ADHD, and autism spectrum conditions. Other potent amino acids in bone broth, such as proline and glycine, can act as inhibitory neurotransmitters, promoting good sleep and delivering an anti-inflammatory effect.

Find a quality bone broth in the store or, to minimize the impact on your budget, you can make your own. If you buy it in a store, understand the distinction between watery products sold in cartons that are often labeled "broth" but are more accurately described as chicken, beef, or vegetable *stock*. A true bone broth is typically sold in a refrigerated or frozen state. It's gelatinous at cold temperatures but heats into a hearty liquid beverage. A quality bone broth will list bones as the first ingredient and likely mention that it's been cooked a long time—essential in extracting all the connective tissue and marrow from bones. Be prepared to pay much more for a product authentically derived from joint material than you would pay for simple stock.

To make your own broth at home, save a chicken or turkey carcass or bones from steak or ribs. Or ask your butcher for inexpensive joint material—e.g., knuckles—which offer the richest source of the treasured collagen and glycosaminoglycans. For easy preparation, dump the bones in a slow cooker and cover with chicken or beef stock or water. Add a tablespoon of apple cider vinegar, which helps extract the marrow and cartilage during the long simmering time. For flavoring, throw in some chopped carrots, onions, and sweet potato, a can of tomato paste, and assorted spices, or follow your favorite recipe. Cook at low temperature for forty-eight hours, then strain the liquid into a container. For a superfood breakfast, enjoy a fresh cup of bone broth with a few pastured-hen egg yolks stirred in. When refrigerated, your broth should become gelatinous. A layer of fat may accumulate at the top, which you can scrape off and use for stovetop cooking.

Superfood: Fermented and Sprouted Products

In her bestselling book *Deep Nutrition*, Dr. Cate Shanahan identifies the four pillars of human nutrition: (1) fresh foods, such as vegetables, fruits, nuts, and seeds; (2) fermented and sprouted foods; (3) meat on the bone; and (4) organ meats. These categories might seem unusual for something as important as an all-encompassing dietary recommendation, but traditional cuisines from only one hundred years ago—not to mention the ancestral hunter-gatherer diet—were built on these cornerstones.

Unfortunately, even the most health-conscious eaters routinely fall short in the three latter categories. Fermented and sprouted foods, for example, are some of the best sources of probiotics, which nourish healthful intestinal bacteria and lay the foundation for excellent digestive, immune, hormonal, and cognitive functioning. Choose from apple cider vinegar, raw or aged cheese, kefir, kimchi, kombucha, raw milk, miso, natto, olives, pickles, sauerkraut, tempeh, and full-fat yogurt. These foods contain live cultures ready to nourish your healthful gut bacteria. Some fermented foods, including wine, beer, sourdough bread, and cacao, don't contain live-culture probiotics but still offer a variety of health benefits.

Fermentation occurs when microorganisms such as yeast and bacteria break down the original components of the food (e.g., carbohydrate) into various agents such as acids and alcohol, creating unique tastes and textures. This fermentation process generates microorganisms—probiotics—that have numerous health benefits. *Lactobacillus* and *Bifidobacterium* are two of the most common probiotics, and you often see these contained in capsule form or liquid supplements. Fermented and sprouted foods were centerpieces of the ancestral diet because these processes allow food to be preserved at room temperature for long periods of time. They also improve flavor and neutralize plant toxins. Fermentation and sprouting came in pretty handy in the days before refrigeration and helped people stay well fed during the times of year when there was no fresh food available. In fact, discovering the ability to sprout and ferment the earliest cultivated grains into bread was a driving force in the advent of civilization.

Fermented foods undergo a process called lacto-fermentation, in which they are submerged in high-concentration salt water (or brine) and sealed in an airtight container at room temperature for as long as two weeks. This anaerobic (lacking oxygen) environment allows the lactic acid bacteria to proliferate and create a fermented end product with a long shelf life. You can make your own sauerkraut, for example, by slicing up cabbage, submerging it in salt water in a mason jar, sealing the lid, and letting it sit for a couple of weeks. Vent the lid for a bit daily to prevent the jar from exploding. Once the cabbage is fermented, you can transfer it to the refrigerator. This arrests the fermentation process and extends the product life further.

The fermentation process varies depending on the food. For example, kombucha is made by preparing very strong and sweet black tea, then adding a starter culture called a

SCOBY (symbiotic culture of bacteria and yeast). It's easiest to obtain a ready-for-action SCOBY from a commercial resource or from a hobbyist who makes kombuchas. SCOBYs are plentiful because every batch of kombucha yields a "baby" SCOBY! The tea is fermented in a breathable container at room temperature for ten to fourteen days, during which time the SCOBY consumes the sugar and caffeine to produce a kombucha drink. You can then commence a second fermentation, in which you pour kombucha into sealable jars and add flavorings such as fresh lemon or lime juice, berries, ginger, jalapeño peppers, and many other creative options (explore additional choices in *The Big Book of Kombucha*, by Hannah Crum and Alex LaGory). Sealing the container at room temperature for a few days will allow some carbonation to accumulate and some of the calories from the added sugar to be consumed by the kombucha liquid, teeming with live probiotics. Then you can refrigerate your masterpiece and enjoy a delicious low-carbohydrate, high-probiotic beverage.

You can also sprout grains, legumes, and seeds at home. This neutralizes their natural toxins, improves bioavailability of the nutrients, boosts antioxidant content, and creates beneficial probiotics. First, rinse and drain raw seeds, beans, or cooking grains and soak them overnight in an open bowl or mason jar. Repeat the process a few times, then allow them to germinate in a warm, dry environment, such as a sealed mason jar. After anywhere from several days to two weeks, you will see evidence of sprouting.

The probiotics in fermented and sprouted foods are believed to promote a healthy gut microbiome. Gut health is an emerging field of medicine that many believe represents one of the greatest wellness and disease-prevention breakthroughs in decades. Dr. Timothy Noakes, the South African author of *The Real Meal Revolution*, *Lore of Running*, and *Lore of Nutrition*, who is also widely regarded as one of the world's leading experts on diet and exercise performance, offered the opinion that "insulin resistance and leaky gut are the future of medicine." The emerging field of gut microbiome research reveals a powerful gut-brain connection. Researchers are now describing the thirty-foot-long intestinal tract, filled with one hundred million cells of the enteric nervous system (ENS), as the "second brain." In the fetus, the ENS and the central nervous system develop from the same tissue, and the ENS has a sensory and neuron structure similar to that of the brain. We have all experienced the scientifically validated phenomenon of the intestinal tract being sensitive to emotions, from feeling butterflies before public speaking to suffering transient abdominal pain in conjunction with emotional pain.

Gut bacteria produce important neurotransmitters such as acetylcholine, dopamine, GABA, noradrenaline, norepinephrine, and serotonin, which play a critical role in mood stabilization, motivation, concentration, stress management, happiness, and contentment. Ninety percent of the mood-elevating neurotransmitter serotonin is made by the entero-chromaffin (EC) cells in the gut, not the brain! A dysfunctional gut microbiome—in which disease-promoting "bad" bacteria (e.g., *E.coli*, *Salmonella*, and so on), fungi, viruses, and other pathogens predominate over healthful bacteria—is being blamed as the originating cause of all manner of inflammatory, allergic, autoimmune, and mental health conditions. People with anxiety, depression, obsessive-compulsive disorder, poor emotional regulation, and mood disorders routinely have gut inflammation and bacterial imbalances. Dysfunctional gut bacteria with insufficient microbe diversity is also directly linked to obesity.

Healing your gut by eliminating foods that promote leaky gut syndrome (grains, sugars, industrial seed oils) and increasing your intake of high-probiotic foods can often result in an incredible health transformation. You may find yourself feeling more energetic than you thought possible because you had become so accustomed to a less-than-optimal baseline over the years. You may have heard of a cutting-edge medical procedure called fecal microbial transplantation (FMT). Patients with the life-threatening antibiotic-resistant illness known as *C. diff*—extremely prevalent in elderly and immunocompromised hospital patients—can receive a fecal transplant from a donor with a healthy intestinal microbiome and go from deathbed to restored health within days.

The probiotics you consume in foods and supplements take residence in your digestive tract and nourish only the good bacteria in your gut. This helps good bacteria to flourish and predominate over bad bacteria. With a healthy gut microbiome, you can absorb and assimilate the maximum amount of nutrition from your food, reduce inflammation, increase internal antioxidant production, and improve or eliminate acid reflux, acne, allergies, asthma, irritable bowel syndrome, migraines, psoriasis, systemic inflammation, and autoimmune conditions in all areas of the body. A healthy gut will produce the neurotransmitters that keep you energetic, cognitively sharp, and mood-stabilized. High microbial diversity has also been linked to being able to exercise for a long time without feeling exhausted and to improved heat tolerance during exercise.

You may have heard the term *prebiotics*, also known as resistant starch or soluble fiber. Found in certain foods, they are indigestible and pass through the small intestine to take up residence in the colon, where they act as a substrate (fuel source) for healthful bacteria. In essence, prebiotics are a fuel source for probiotics! Dietary sources of resistant starch include raw potato starch (sold prepackaged or in bulk bins at a health food store), green (unripe) bananas, and cooked and cooled russet potatoes and white rice. Interestingly, the molecular composition of the latter two items actually changes from carbohydrate (when eaten warm) into resistant starch when eaten cool or cold. Similarly, a green banana is mostly resistant starch but will eventually ripen and convert the starch into carbohydrate for a yellow end product. There are also small amounts of prebiotics in an assortment of plant-based foods, including dark chocolate. In addition to consuming a variety of the aforementioned high-probiotic foods, you can try gradually introducing prebiotics into your diet with an occasional green banana, a couple spoonfuls of cold rice or potato, or a teaspoon of raw potato starch (working up to more over time) in your smoothie or other liquids.

Superfoods and Nutrient Density

Dr. Joel Fuhrman, family physician and author of *Eat to Live* and numerous other books, coined the term *nutritarian* to describe a diet made up of foods that have a high ratio of micronutrients to calories. Dr. Fuhrman explains, "The nutrient density in your body's tissues is proportional to the nutrient density of your diet. Micronutrients fuel proper functioning of the immune system and enable the detoxification and cellular repair mechanisms that protect us from chronic diseases." Dr. Josh Axe, a functional medicine practitioner, expert in the gut microbiome, and publisher of one of the most popular natural health websites, DrAxe.com, combined Dr. Fuhrman's patented Aggregate Nutrient Density Index (ANDI) research with his own research to come up with his list of the world's top thirty most nutrient-dense foods. The list lines up very well with the information we covered in this chapter and can serve as a handy guide to ensure that you get maximum variety with your superfood intake.

Dr. Axe's Top Thirty Nutrient-Dense Foods

1. Seaweed
2. Liver (beef and chicken)
3. Kale, collards, and dandelion greens
4. Broccoli rabe
5. Exotic berries (acai, goji, camu camu)
6. Spinach, watercress, and arugula
7. Broccoli and cauliflower
8. Cabbage
9. Red bell peppers
10. Garlic
11. Parsley
12. Berries (blueberries, raspberries, blackberries—local, in-season preferred)

13. Asparagus
14. Carrots
15. Beets
16. Wild salmon and sardines
17. Bone broth
18. Grass-fed beef
19. Green beans
20. Egg yolks
21. Pumpkin
22. Lentils
23. Artichokes
24. Tomatoes
25. Wild mushrooms
26. Seeds (pumpkin, sunflower, chia, flax)
27. Raw cheese and kefir
28. Sweet potatoes
29. Black beans
30. Wild rice

Putting Food Pyramids into Perspective

The USDA Food Guide Pyramid has been the most popular visual representation of dietary strategy since the US Department of Agriculture debuted it, back in 1992. While the effects of the ubiquitous grain-based pyramid and the diet it recommended have been disastrous, it may be helpful to compare and contrast various dietary strategies using pyramid imagery.

Conventional Stupidity Pyramid

The 1992 pyramid replaced the "basic four food groups" propaganda that preceded it. This irresponsible and politically corrupt creation is tainted by flawed science (such as recently discovered unpublished data from the 1968 Minnesota Coronary Experiment and the revelation that major influencer Ancel Keys was later outed for cherry-picking data to promote his low-fat diet); elected officials with zero dietary expertise dictating dietary policy to the nation (an example is the US Senate's McGovern committee orchestrating the great shift away from butter to margarine in the early 1970s); and egregious special-interest lobbying and behind-the-scenes political maneuvering (the pyramid release was delayed at the last minute in 1991 because the secretary of agriculture, Edward Madigan, said it was "confusing to children," but skeptics noted that the cattle and dairy lobbies were applying heavy pressure at the time for better pyramid real estate).

The pyramid and its subsequent iterations would shape the dietary habits of the United States and the rest of the developed world for decades afterward. The USDA's 2005

Food Guide Pyramid
A Guide to Daily Food Choices

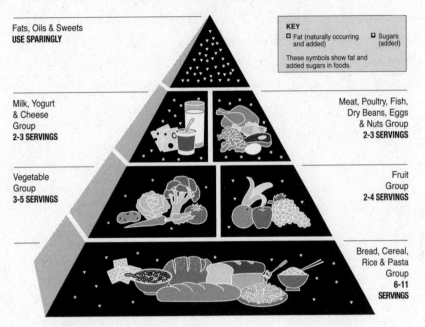

Source: U.S. Department of Agriculture/U.S. Department of Health and Human Services

revision, My Pyramid, depicts a figure ascending stairs up the side of the pyramid, so at least it's telling us to exercise off some of those refined carbs. Alas, we know this doesn't work per the flawed compensation theory of exercise!

In 2011, likely backpedaling as a result of pyramid criticisms, the USDA introduced the Choose My Plate imagery, with sections for fruits, grains, vegetables, protein, and a little dairy on the side. The presentation still promotes a high-carb, high-insulin-producing diet for an American public that now sits as the fattest and sickest population in the history of humanity (nearly three-quarters of men and 60 percent of women are classified as overweight; 40 percent of adults are obese).

Dr. Cate Shanahan minces few words when she asserts that US dietary recommendations of the past half century have been "a big giant human experiment to see how many people will die when 60 percent of their calories come from toxic junk." According to Dr. Marion Nestle, an advocate of healthful food and the author of numerous books, including *Food Politics: How the Food Industry Influences Nutrition and Health*, "The pyramid controversy focuses attention on the conflict between federal protection of the rights of food lobbyists to act in their own self-interest and federal responsibility to promote the nutritional health of the public." She also calls attention to "the inherent conflict of interest in the Department of Agriculture's dual mandates to promote U.S. agricultural products and to advise the public about healthy food choices."

Let's examine some more evolved and healthful pyramid imagery and use a Venn diagram to see the interplay between various dietary strategies that are popular today.

Primal Blueprint Food Pyramid

I first developed this pyramid back in 2007 as an antidote to the conventional stupidity pyramid. After more research and a few revisions over the years, it serves as a

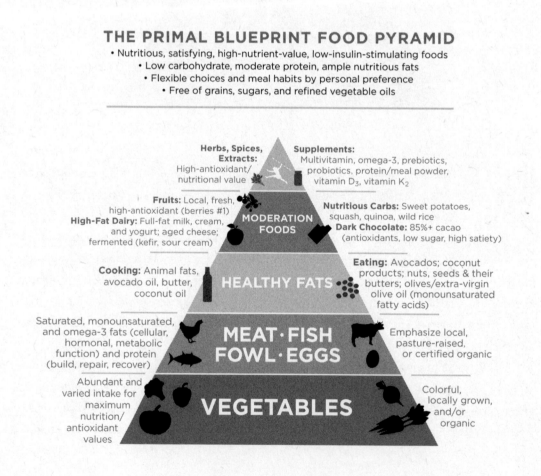

THE PRIMAL BLUEPRINT FOOD PYRAMID
- Nutritious, satisfying, high-nutrient-value, low-insulin-stimulating foods
- Low carbohydrate, moderate protein, ample nutritious fats
- Flexible choices and meal habits by personal preference
- Free of grains, sugars, and refined vegetable oils

Herbs, Spices, Extracts: High-antioxidant/ nutritional value

Supplements: Multivitamin, omega-3, prebiotics, probiotics, protein/meal powder, vitamin D$_3$, vitamin K$_2$

MODERATION FOODS

Fruits: Local, fresh, high-antioxidant (berries #1)
High-Fat Dairy: Full-fat milk, cream, and yogurt; aged cheese; fermented (kefir, sour cream)

Nutritious Carbs: Sweet potatoes, squash, quinoa, wild rice
Dark Chocolate: 85%+ cacao (antioxidants, low sugar, high satiety)

HEALTHY FATS

Cooking: Animal fats, avocado oil, butter, coconut oil

Eating: Avocados; coconut products; nuts, seeds & their butters; olives/extra-virgin olive oil (monounsaturated fatty acids)

MEAT·FISH FOWL·EGGS

Saturated, monounsaturated, and omega-3 fats (cellular, hormonal, metabolic function) and protein (build, repair, recover)

Emphasize local, pasture-raised, or certified organic

VEGETABLES

Abundant and varied intake for maximum nutrition/ antioxidant values

Colorful, locally grown, and/or organic

great visual guide to to formulating a nutritious, satisfying, ancestral-inspired diet—free from bad advice and with abundant options to honor personal preference. Visit MarksDailyApple.com or read *The Primal Blueprint* for details.

Perfect Health Food Plate

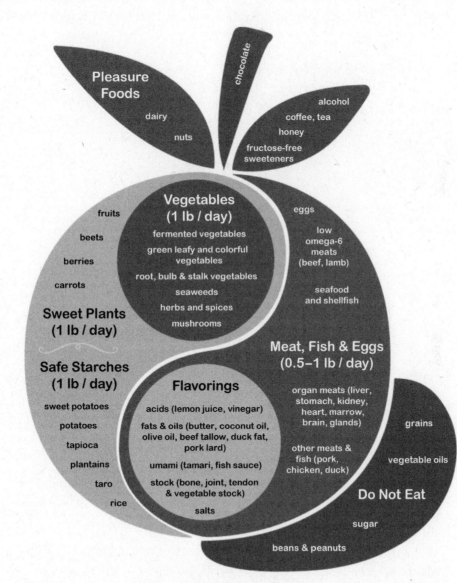

Image © 2013 PerfectHealthDiet.com

Drs. Paul Jaminet and Shou-Ching Jaminet, both trained in the sciences (astrophysics and molecular biology respectively), were drawn to the ancestral health space by Paul's successful conquering of chronic illness through dietary transformation. The coauthors of *Perfect Health Diet*, they created the Perfect Health Food Plate to help followers transition sensibly away from nutrient-deficient, inflammatory dietary patterns and reduce their risk of disease. The Jaminets' concept of "safe starches" was praised for bringing some sensibility and moderation to low-carb eating strategies. Visit PerfectHealthDiet.com for details.

Whole-Foods, Plant-Based Pyramid

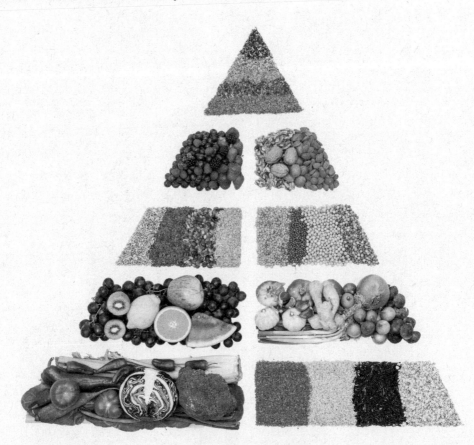

This presentation of exclusively plant-based foods depicts numerous colorful, nutritious, high-antioxidant fruits and vegetables. It also honors the many objections to consuming feedlot animal products and processed meats. Restricting nutrient-dense, sustainably raised animal foods from the diet invites criticism, but plant-based eating certainly has a strong following. People with sensitivities to gluten and other antinutrients prominent in grain foods can choose to emphasize fresh produce, nuts, and seeds. Because of the high carbohydrate content and potential difficulty obtaining sufficient protein and nutritious fats with a plant-based approach, there are risks of excess insulin production, low satiety, and consequent difficulty adhering to the diet. In addition, there is a high potential for nutrient deficiencies (especially over the long term) resulting from the exclusion of animal foods.

Carnivore Scores Chart

Carnivore is a niche dietary strategy that has exploded in popularity recently, particularly among those suffering from nagging inflammatory or autoimmune conditions possibly caused or exacerbated by the consumption of natural plant toxins. A complete restriction of plants in favor of nose-to-tail animal foods is being shown to help heal leaky gut syndrome and promote rapid healing in people who have (often unknowingly) high reactivity to plant toxins. For others, a "carnivore-ish" eating strategy is showing great effectiveness for quick and efficient fat reduction, because meals are nutrient-dense and highly satiating, while being extremely low in carbohydrate. This chart from Brad Kearns and health coach Kate Ouellette-Cretsinger ranks the most nutrient-dense categories of animal-sourced foods and makes suggestions for strategic inclusion of numerous colorful, healthful plant foods that have the least toxicity and most nutritional benefits. Visit BradKearns.com/MOFO or K84Wellness.com for details.

Food Pyramid Venn Diagram ("Pyramids in Perspective")

This presentation is inspired by a concept presented by Denise Minger in her book, *Death by Food Pyramid*. Her book explains "how shoddy science, sketchy politics, and shady special interests have ruined our health" and offers extensive historical and scientific references. Perhaps the best takeaway from this diagram is the "excluded from all" box. This is the predominant reason why *any* diet that eliminates toxic modern foods will promote fat reduction and increased energy right out of the gate.

The universal agreement that colorful, nutritious plants should be emphasized has long stood on a pedestal above the ongoing diet wars, but even this has been challenged by

CARNIVORE SCORES!

Follow this chart to eat smart; plants à la carte

MAXIMUM NUTRIENT DENSITY

GLOBAL ALL-STARS ▶ The world's most nutrient-dense foods (sorry kale, time to bail).	**Grassfed Liver** *(Bonus points: consume raw or medium rare)* Superior micronutrient profile, including off-the-charts in vitamin A and vitamin B group.	**Oysters** *(Lightly grilled, broiled, or roasted, never deep-fried)* Aphrodisiac properties are validated by the incredible zinc and B₁₂ levels.	**Salmon Roe and Caviar** Rich in iodine, choline, omega-3 fatty acids EPA and DHA.

ANIMAL ORGANS ▶ Reclaim the forgotten ancestral tradition of "like supports like."	**Liver plus Bone Broth** Heart, Kidney, Sweetbread, Rocky Mountain Oysters, Tripe Choose grassfed animals.	**Organ Supplements (Capsules)** AncestralSupplements.com: freeze-dried, 100% grassfed organs (capsules) PrimalKitchen.com: collagen peptides (powder)

WILD-CAUGHT, OILY, COLD-WATER FISH ▶ Convenient, affordable, best dietary source of omega-3s.	**"SMASH" Family** Sardines, Mackerel, Anchovies, Salmon, Herring

SHELLFISH ▶ Excellent source of monounsaturated and omega-3 fats. Choose sustainably caught/raised.	**Oysters plus Clams, Crab, Lobster, Mussels, Octopus, Scallops** Sushi bar fare!

EGGS ▶ Healthful fats, choline, B-vitamins, and life-force essence.	**Local, Certified Humane and Pasture-Raised** Vastly superior to conventional.	**Other Eggs: Goose, Duck, Quail, Ostrich** Healthier animals; no mass production.

RED MEAT ▶ Superior nutritional and fatty acid profile to poultry.	**Local or 100% Grassfed** Bone-in cuts best.	**Other Red Meat: Buffalo/Bison, Elk, Lamb, Venison** Healthier animals, no mass production.

THE STEAK LINE

Emphasize foods above line for maximum dietary nutrient density.

Chicken, Turkey, Pork Inferior nutrient density and fatty acid profile if corn/soy fed.	Local or 100% grassfed/pasture-raised poultry; heritage breed pork
Raw, Organic, High-Fat Dairy Avoid all conventional, pasteurized, and low- and non-fat products, or if allergic.	• Raw cheese (aged, hard, or brie), raw kefir, raw milk • Cream cheese, heavy cream, sour cream • Full-fat yogurt

Plant Foods Integrate strategically for recovery/glycogen reloading, to improve insulin sensitivity, optimize thyroid and adrenal function, and enjoy life!	**Avocados**	**Dark Chocolate**	**Fermented Foods**	**Fruit**
	Heart-healthy monounsaturated fats, huge potassium, high antioxidant, vitamin B6 and vitamin K.	Super high in antioxidants, flavanols, polyphenols; choose bean-to-bar, 80 percent cacao or higher.	Kefir, kimchi, kombucha, miso, natto, olives, pickles, sauerkraut, tempeh; probiotics nourish healthy gut bacteria.	Choose locally grown, in-season fruits; berries #1 for low glycemic/high antioxidant properties.
	Honey	**Nuts & Nut Butters**	**Seaweed**	**Sweet Potatoes/Squash**
	Choose raw for antioxidant, antibacterial boost. Local honey can help seasonal allergies.	Nutritious protein, fatty acids, enzymes, antioxidants, phytonutrients, vitamins and minerals (bradventures.com).	Best source of iodine, vitamin B₁₂, selenium, and omega-3.	High antioxidant, anti-inflammatory, immune-boosting, and support gut health.

Check out BradKearns.com/MOFO and K84Wellness.com for more great info and guidance.

PYRAMIDS IN PERSPECTIVE

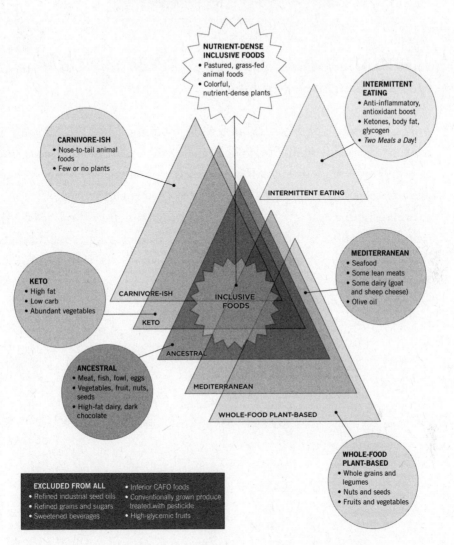

NUTRIENT-DENSE INCLUSIVE FOODS
• Pastured, grass-fed animal foods
• Colorful, nutrient-dense plants

INTERMITTENT EATING
• Anti-inflammatory, antioxidant boost
• Ketones, body fat, glycogen
• *Two Meals a Day!*

CARNIVORE-ISH
• Nose-to-tail animal foods
• Few or no plants

MEDITERRANEAN
• Seafood
• Some lean meats
• Some dairy (goat and sheep cheese)
• Olive oil

KETO
• High fat
• Low carb
• Abundant vegetables

ANCESTRAL
• Meat, fish, fowl, eggs
• Vegetables, fruit, nuts, seeds
• High-fat dairy, dark chocolate

INTERMITTENT EATING

CARNIVORE-ISH

INCLUSIVE FOODS

KETO

ANCESTRAL

MEDITERRANEAN

WHOLE-FOOD PLANT-BASED

EXCLUDED FROM ALL
• Refined industrial seed oils
• Refined grains and sugars
• Sweetened beverages
• Inferior CAFO foods
• Conventionally grown produce treated with pesticide
• High-glycemic fruits

WHOLE-FOOD PLANT-BASED
• Whole grains and legumes
• Nuts and seeds
• Fruits and vegetables

the carnivore approach, which skyrocketed in popularity in 2019. The rationale that animal foods have the most nutrient density and that plants may not be mandatory (and can even be counterproductive for sensitive folks) has forced many people—including me—to rethink the fundamentals of healthful eating. Granted, most of us may not be highly reactive to plants, but advocates recommend at least trying a carnivore experiment if you suffer from nagging inflammatory or autoimmune issues. The "carnivore-ish" triangle, which dips slightly into the whole-foods, plant-based shading, makes a concession for occasional consumption of the least offensive plants, such as fruit and starchy tubers.

Emphasize Nutrient-Dense Ancestral Foods (and Eat Your Superfoods)—Journal Exercises

1. **Ancestral foods:** List a few of your favorite foods in each of the following ancestral food categories: meat, fish, fowl, eggs, vegetables, fruits, nuts, seeds, and healthful modern foods (organic high-fat dairy products, high-cacao-percentage dark chocolate). Describe the highest-quality choices and your ideas about where to find them. For example, wild-caught Pacific salmon from Costco; 80–85 percent dark chocolate bars from LillieBelleFarms.com or Askinosie.com; sugar-free, chemical-free wines from DryFarmWines.com.
2. **Superfoods:** List some ideas for increasing your consumption of superfoods and list some sources from which you can purchase them.

CHAPTER 3

Intermittent Eating: The Fast-est Way to Health

Unlike every other diet you have encountered in your life, the *Two Meals a Day* program centers on fasting rather than on any specific foods, macronutrient ratios, or meal patterns. Fasting has profound anti-inflammatory and immune-boosting effects. It spurs the production of internal antioxidants such as *glutathione*, known as the "master antioxidant"; it optimizes the internal cellular detoxification process called *autophagy*; it enhances your all-important mitochondrial health; and it enables your brain and body to burn fat and ketones—vastly cleaner fuel sources than the glucose you burn after a high-carbohydrate meal. In these areas, fasting blows away the benefits offered by any superfood smoothie, magical jungle berry, exotic fresh-squeezed juice, or expensive detox powder or pill.

Fasting is simple, free, and easy to maintain as your baseline dietary philosophy. If you associate skipping meals with deprivation and suffering, please understand that although this may be true in a carbohydrate-dependency paradigm, it's not the case when you possess metabolic flexibility. The intermittent-eating approach is always aligned with your natural signals of hunger and satiety and should never feel like an ordeal. You will always progress at your own pace, and you can expect to make steady progress over time, to the point where something unthinkable today (such as a twenty-four-hour fast) is carried out effortlessly when you have developed sufficient metabolic flexibility.

The best way to get started with an intermittent-eating lifestyle is to simply wait until WHEN (when hunger ensues naturally) to eat your break-fast meal every day. If that doesn't work for you, you can try numerous other intermittent-eating strategies that might be a better fit for your daily work, exercise, and family routines (see chapter 5). The objective is to spend as many hours as possible in a fasted state to optimize your metabolic, immune, and cognitive functioning as well as to reconnect with your long-lost hunger and satiety signals, which have been compromised by overeating. The insight that no food or supplement will have more of a health boost than fasting should dramatically simplify your approach to healthful eating and come as a huge relief. I know it has for me.

My insatiable quest over decades to find the latest, greatest diet, superfood, or supplement and determine the best mealtimes and food combinations for performance and recovery was an arduous chore. Propaganda and flawed science compelled me to follow the conventional stupidity of a grain-based diet, which, unbeknownst to me, triggered systemic inflammation, destroyed my gut lining, and trashed my immune system. My life became extra stressful when I couldn't follow my exact plan of food choices and meal patterns, especially when traveling. I spent untold thousands of dollars on the "best" foods and supplements, trying to get an antioxidant or immune boost that can be had for free when you simply skip breakfast.

When you focus on fasting to develop metabolic flexibility, the pressure to conform to a strict meal plan or program is off. You can add a smiley face to your journal when you miss a meal instead of feeling like you have fallen behind on your nutritional requirements or set yourself up for an afternoon energy crash. If you've felt the pressure of the ketogenic approach, in which daily carb intake must be strictly limited, you can enjoy a little more flexibility at mealtimes, because aggressive fasting is a potent catalyst for ketosis. Ben Greenfield describes enjoying the best of both worlds when he engages in extended fasting, but he also enjoys celebratory evening meals with his family that feature an assortment of nutritious carbohydrates and even some carefully crafted indulgences. During his fasting periods, Ben enjoys the aforementioned autophagy and antioxidant benefits as well as the anti-inflammatory and cognitive benefits of being in ketosis. His evening meals ensure that he restocks muscle glycogen for recovery and guards against the hormonal stress of heavy training combined with heavy carb restriction. He enjoys life without stressing about dietary restrictions.

From this point forward, you can reject the inconvenient and unhealthful food-is-fuel approach to life. Instead, you can adopt the ethos that eating is one of life's greatest pleasures and choose the cleanest, tastiest, most nutritious foods you can find. You can bring mindfulness and gratitude to mealtimes instead of "hangry" emotions. You will be more in tune with your body's natural rhythms and can honor and appreciate your hunger and satiety signals without experiencing that all-too-familiar deep-seated fear of running out of energy later if you don't stuff your face during meals or carry a bunch of snacks around with you as you go through your day.

Instead of defaulting to convenient processed breakfast foods during time-crunched mornings, you can take comfort knowing that heading off to work fueled by only water, coffee, or tea is perfectly healthful. Fasting is freeing: travel can become a great opportunity for extended fasting: no more traipsing around the airport or scouring the roadside mini-mart for something decent to eat or futilely searching for foods that fit your current meal plan. Whenever you feel the slightest bit run down (scratchy throat, stuffy nose or head, elevated temperature), fasting is the best way to enhance your immune response to infection. The old wives' tale goes, "Starve a cold, feed a fever," but a more scientifically validated approach would be "Starve a cold, and all other illnesses." Leading ketogenic diet researchers are publishing studies of great promise in which they starve cancerous cells (which preferentially feed off glucose more than healthy cells do) by means of a ketogenic dietary strategy. All animals intuitively know the immunity benefits of fasting: you may have noticed your dogs and cats ignoring their food bowls when they're under the weather. While extended fasts of seventy-two hours or more have been shown to boost stem cell activity, cleanse organs of inflamed, dysfunctional cells, and regenerate white blood cells for an incredible "reset" effect, even routine short-duration fasting (e.g., a daily pattern of a sixteen-hour fast followed by an eight-hour window in which meals are consumed) will deliver amazing anti-inflammatory, antivirus, autophagy, and fat-loss benefits.

A key perk of fasting is that it boosts mitochondrial functioning, which many experts assert is one of the most prominent indicators of overall health and disease prevention. Mitochondria are the energy-producing power plants inside most of your cells. They convert oxygen and food calories into adenosine triphosphate (ATP), which powers the cells' metabolic activities. When you deplete your cells of energy, whether by fasting or by conducting a strenuous workout, it triggers a process called *mitochondrial biogenesis*—the manufacturing of new mitochondria as well as making existing mitochondria more efficient at using oxygen. You become like a solar power plant, generating a reliable source of clean-burning fuel (stored body fat and perhaps ketones, as needed) all day long. By contrast, eating too many meals and making dietary carbohydrates your primary source of energy results in inflammation, oxidative damage, and glycation. You are more like a coal plant spewing smoke and needing to constantly shovel more fuel (i.e., high-carb snacks and meals) into the fire.

METABOLIC FLEXIBILITY   VS.   CARBOHYDRATE DEPENDENCY
Solar Plant   Coal Plant

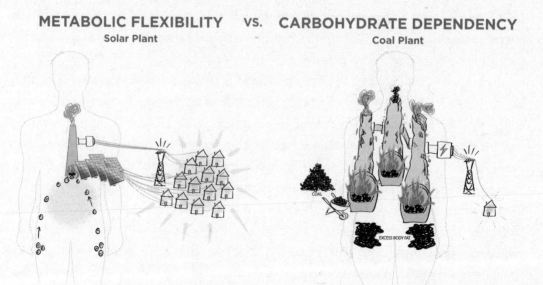

Essentially, fasting allows you to stimulate ancient pathways of cellular renewal and regeneration. Art De Vany, PhD—Paleo movement pioneer, author of *The New Evolution Diet*, and an athletic marvel in his eighties—likes to say: "We are most human when we don't eat." Of course you need to eat to provide caloric energy for a busy, active lifestyle, build and maintain lean muscle mass, and support assorted other functions in the body, but the magic happens when you follow a feast-and-famine pattern of metabolic flexibility and efficiency. We have the magnificent, genetically hardwired ability to store, manufacture, and burn various forms of energy to enjoy active, productive lifestyles—regardless of the type of calories we ingest or how frequently we ingest them. Our closed-loop functionality evolved by necessity to survive the rigors of primal life, when there was no guarantee of a "next meal."

Appreciating the elegance and efficiency of our evolutionary design includes acknowledging that humans are hardwired to overeat (particularly sugar) and store fat! There was no such thing as "three squares" ten thousand or two hundred thousand years ago. There was either food or no food, with likely tremendous fluctuation. It makes perfect sense that we evolved a brain-based mechanism that encouraged us to overeat when food was readily available and then be able to conveniently store this energy in our centers of gravity—hips, thighs, abdomen, and rear end—for future access when food was scarce. For example, our ancestors typically gorged on fresh berries and other ancient wild fruits and starchy vegetables during short summertime ripening seasons, thereby adding some extra body fat that would be used for fuel over the long, dark, cold, calorically scarce winter ahead. That's good news for our ancestors' survival, and it's good genetics to have evolved a sweet tooth. However, our ancestral pattern of seasonal consumption of wild, fibrous fruit is a far cry from consuming giant blackberries from the big-box store throughout the winter or starting your day with a green smoothie filled with more carbohydrate calories than our ancestors would eat in a day—or an entire week during wintertime. What's more, climate-controlled indoor environments and artificial lighting, which extend our days year-round, mean there is no such thing as a cold, dark, calorie-scarce winter today. In fact, from a hormonal perspective, our highly inactive, temperate, well-lit modern lifestyle locks us into the summertime carb-craving fat-storage mode twelve months of the year. Ultimately, there is little impetus for us to access and burn the abundant and clean-burning source of energy we carry around every day. Instead, we hardwire the hormonal processes that make us fat, foggy, fatigued, depressed, and ultimately diseased.

Today's obsession with the deeply flawed calories in, calories out model of metabolism ignores the genetic mechanisms that influence how the body burns and stores caloric energy. By resolving the many modern disconnects from our genetic expectations for health, it's possible to generate different hormonal signals and reclaim our *Homo sapiens* birthright to become lean, fit, strong, fat-burning beasts. We'll cover an assortment of lifestyle objectives in this book (exercise, sleep, stress management, therapeutic cold exposure, and others), but the biggest bang for your buck will come from fasting, because our modern hyperinsulinemia diet is arguably the most health-destructive genetic disconnect of them all. While the return on your fasting investment is assured, it's going to take some work and time to undo decades of ingrained food-is-fuel habits and counter the powerful influence of social conventions.

Beware of "Liquidating Your Assets"

If you attempt fasting and carb restriction while you are still carbohydrate-dependent, you are destined to struggle rather than succeed. This is a disturbingly common occurrence among people who have jumped on the ketogenic diet bandwagon or who engage in habitual crash dieting for desperation weight loss. When dietary carbohydrates have been your primary source of energy for decades, it's difficult for the body to suddenly recalibrate and start melting off body fat as promised in advertising propaganda. Instead, skipping a meal or cutting carb intake can easily cause you to feel tired, hungry, and moody. Without carbs, your bloodstream is lacking the usual steady drip of glucose, and your body isn't yet acclimated to burning stored body fat or making ketones.

If you struggle out of the gate with fasting or carb restriction, you just need to slow down the pace of your dietary transformation and allow fat-burning genetic functions to take hold in due time. If you plow ahead in crash-diet mode, the picture can start to look bleak. The energy dip caused by hypoglycemia is perceived by your primal genes as a matter of life and death, and it triggers a cascade of powerful hormonal and metabolic fight-or-flight processes, including a spike of the predominant stress hormone, cortisol. Cortisol orchestrates a key survival mechanism called *gluconeogenesis*. This is an emergency process that strips your muscles of certain amino acids, sends them to the liver to be converted into glucose, and delivers quick energy to your brain and muscles. When fight-or-flight stimulation becomes chronic, you suffer from suppressed immune functioning and system-wide inflammation, and lean muscle mass is broken down to make glucose.

Tommy Wood, MD, PhD, a pediatric research physician at the University of Washington and past president of the Physicians for Ancestral Health organization, calls chronic fight-or-flight stimulation "liquidating your assets." Overly stressful exercise patterns, toxic relationships, dysfunctional workplace dynamics, personal and family crises, and crash dieting are all examples of chronic stressors that you can cope with for a short time but that eventually lead to burnout. By contrast, an acute cortisol spike is fantastic when you toe the starting line for a race, take the stage to give an important presentation, conduct a sprint workout, or experience any other hormetic stressor—one that is optimally brief but delivers a net positive benefit.

Crash dieters typically feel great for a while. They have plenty of energy from gluconeogenesis and probably lose some body weight as well. This loss comes from a reduction in water retention and cellular inflammation and perhaps even a little fat loss, thanks to eating less food. Unfortunately, under these conditions, the fight-or-flight mechanism (designed to combat short-term, life-or-death stressors only) will eventually wear out. The result is the wholly modern condition known as burnout. The typical result of a crash diet is exhaustion, intense cravings for sugar, and an eventual return to the same body composition you had before the fight-or-flight ordeal.

The way out of this familiar trap is to unlock the vast resource of clean-burning energy that is stored body fat. Triggering the genetic mechanisms that favor fat burning (instead of carbohydrate dependency) best happens through not just diet modification, but comprehensive lifestyle change. It starts with minimizing insulin production and includes increasing all forms of general everyday movement, performing brief, high-intensity workouts, getting adequate sleep, and avoiding the aforementioned chronic stressors. Once the proper foundation is laid (ditching toxic modern foods and emphasizing nutrient-dense ancestral foods), you can establish a comfortable routine featuring increased fasting and eating two meals a day or less. On the other hand, if you are embarking on your *Two Meals a Day* journey amid a hectic, high-stress lifestyle, reducing meal frequency and cutting carbs is likely going to add more stress to an already unbalanced situation.

There are many ways to arrive at burnout besides ill-advised crash dieting. One particularly disturbing trend among extreme health and fitness enthusiasts with high motivation levels and lofty goals is pairing carb restriction with an exhausting exercise routine. A pattern of overly stressful workouts leaves you glycogen-depleted again and again, requiring massive carbohydrate consumption to refuel for the next exhausting workout. Even with a six-pack to show for your CrossFit gold star attendance or running high mileage on the road, you can still be locked into an inflammatory, carbohydrate-dependent lifestyle. If you clean up your diet but continue to engage in an extreme training program, guess where you are going to get the extra carbs you need for these workouts? That's right: liquidating your assets!

Dr. Craig Marker is a psychology professor at Mercer University in Atlanta and an elite strength coach whose recommendation of HIRT (high-intensity repeat training) instead of the more popular but more stressful HIIT (high-intensity interval training) is helping revolutionize long-standing high-intensity training strategies that are not only flawed but also dangerous. Dr. Marker explains that serious physiological damage can result from workouts that are too stressful—e.g., doing too many work efforts that last a bit too long, with rest intervals that are too short, in workouts that last too long and are repeated too frequently with insufficient recovery time between them. He adds that as you try to get through ten repeats of two-minute sprints on your Peloton screen or at the local running track, "your physiology fights to keep up by breaking down the basic components of your cells—your 'A-frames'—through chemical reactions called *disassembling* and *deamination*. This results in ammonia toxicity in the bloodstream (especially harmful to brain cells), a degradation of mitochondria, diminished ATP energy production, even at rest, and a disruption in aerobic metabolism (fat burning)."

Translation: you feel terrible for twenty-four to forty-eight hours after challenging workouts, then stabilize just enough to destroy your A-frames all over again at the next workout! Novice athletes are vastly more vulnerable to experiencing this cellular break-down than elites. In a perverse twist to the story, Dr. Marker mentions that a common side effect of extreme overtraining is weight loss—primarily from the catabolization of lean body mass. Nevertheless, fitness freaks get kudos from their peers for looking lean, but it's because they're destroying their bodies on the inside. Dr. Marker describes this dynamic as just plain "sick!"

To effectively pair cleaning up your diet with an improved training regimen, first try to make next-day muscle soreness a rare occurrence instead of something that happens routinely. Second, strive to avoid the hallowed "muscle burn" that has come to characterize an effective workout in fitness pop culture. Yuri Verkhoshansky, the late Russian sports scientist credited with inventing plyometrics, among numerous other innovations, used a sink analogy to describe how to manage lactic acid accumulation during workouts. As soon as the sink is about to overflow, you must shut off the faucet and let the water drain—back off the intensity so your body can efficiently buffer that lactic acid and not prompt the aforementioned process of cellular destruction. Dial your maximum explosive efforts back to 93 percent perceived exertion instead of 98 to 100 percent. Do sprints in the sweet spot of ten to twenty seconds, and take what Dr. Marker calls luxurious rest intervals, last-ing around five times as long as your sprint (see chapter 5).

Low-Carb Flu Who?

You may have heard of the so-called low-carb flu, which has been deemed a rite of pas-sage that must be endured when transitioning from carbohydrate dependency to efficient fat burner. Symptoms may include lethargy, headaches, brain fog, moodiness, appetite swings, and sluggish workouts that occur in conjunction with an abrupt reduction in your usual dietary carbohydrate intake. While you can expect some energy lulls and appetite spikes during the first few weeks of upregulating your fat-burning genes, your journey should absolutely not be a suffer-fest. Any symptoms of discomfort should be mild and easily alleviated by a nutrient-dense meal or nutritious snack. If you start having some rough days that affect your mood or work productivity, you should immediately revise your approach.

The most likely cause of the low-carb flu is metabolic damage from decades of high-carb, high-insulin eating, especially if you have a history of yo-yo dieting. The best strategy for avoiding the "flu" is to slow down your rate of carb restriction so your body can adjust. A grain-based, high-carbohydrate diet delivers around 250 to 500 grams of carbs per day, depending on your burn rate and your penchant for junk food. This also delivers between one thousand and two thousand calories, which can easily comprise more than half your total daily intake. By contrast, the keto template mandates that you consume 50 grams of carbs or less per day. Because the brain alone burns around 120 grams of glucose per day (nearly 500 calories!), when you aren't keto-adapted extreme carb restriction can easily trigger brain fog.

If you are trying to maintain your usual ambitious exercise program, and your muscles are used to burning carbs, you may experience the double whammy of brain fog and sluggish workouts. Instead of suffering, be sure to consume enough colorful, nutrient-dense carbs such as fresh fruit and starchy tubers to give your brain and muscles the energy they need to thrive. As your metabolic flexibility improves, it will become easier to skip meals, stabilize energy and appetite all day, perform well and recover quickly from workouts, and not have that desperate need for a snack or meal to keep the flame burning.

Another potential cause of the low-carb flu is a deficiency in sodium and other important minerals and electrolytes. This is a common problem, because ditching processed foods results in lower inflammation and less water retention throughout the body—and thus less sodium is retained in your cells. Furthermore, your dietary sodium intake drops when you eliminate processed foods that are high or extremely high in sodium. Less puffiness and less junk food are both good things: you just need to make a concerted effort to rebalance your sodium levels. Active low-carb and keto enthusiasts can benefit from consuming an additional five to ten grams (one to two teaspoons) of pure, unprocessed, noniodized mineral salt or ancient sea salt per day. Potassium and magnesium are also easily depleted when you transition to a low-carb diet, so emphasize foods or consume supplements rich in these electrolytes. This is especially important if you are an athlete who sweats frequently. Eat avocados for potassium, and use a transdermal magnesium spray at night before bed. I'll give you additional pro tips in chapter 7.

One strategy for steering clear of the low-carb flu is to make a deliberate effort to consume more nutrient-dense foods in general, because you might not be eating enough during your transition. The high satiety and deep nourishment provided by real foods, combined with lower insulin production and decreased hunger and cravings, will likely result in you needing to eat fewer calories to feel sated than you needed in the carbohydrate-dependent paradigm. Your increased metabolic efficiency may prompt a temporary compensatory reduction in your metabolic rate, which can make you feel sluggish when you try to sustain your usual exercise routine and hectic daily pace. So Dr. Tommy Wood counsels high-calorie-burning athletes transitioning out of carbohydrate dependency to eat as many nutritious calories as they can without increasing body fat. "I'll review an athlete's food journal listing two eggs and half an avocado for breakfast," Wood says. "Come on, man—eat a real breakfast! Make it six eggs and the entire avocado!" Over time, as your closed-loop system gets further refined, you will adjust to your new metabolic efficiency and be able to achieve peak cognitive and physical performance on fewer calories than you needed when you made the transition to fat-adapted athletic training.

If you are a highly motivated type, eager for quick and dramatic results, have patience and faith that this process will work for a lifetime and does not require suffering or "liquidating your assets." You don't have to worry about caloric restriction or exhaustive workouts or wonder whether your next beach-body binge program is going to work. All you need to do is respect your natural hunger and satiety signals, and you will achieve and maintain your personal ideal body composition. That said, let's also acknowledge that the hype and glitz of the fitness industry and social media put too much emphasis on aesthetics and not enough on being healthy and feeling great. When it comes to body composition, understand that results may vary according to your genetic predisposition to store fat, how much metabolic damage you have accumulated over decades of high-carb eating (and need to recover from with a sustained period of lower insulin production), and, to a lesser extent, your fitness level. Focus on making a sustained effort to feel and look your best instead of trying to measure up to airbrushed images on social media. Don't compare your rate of progress to that of others or obsess about arbitrary timelines and benchmarks.

FEMALES AND FASTING

The "liquidating assets" concept can be of particular concern to females, because the act of dropping excess body fat can run counter to the female body's most prominent natural and ancient genetic drive, which is to maintain reproductive fitness. It's a popular belief among experienced low-carb enthusiasts that, in general, males respond better to extended fasting and strict ketogenic patterns than females. A man dropping down into single-digit body fat is likely enjoying a boost in adaptive hormones such as testosterone and growth hormone (unless he's overtraining). A woman who goes deep into fasting and/or extreme exercise in pursuit of abs of steel may increase her risk of health disturbances such as amenorrhea, hypothyroidism, insomnia, declining workout performance, mood and hunger swings, and chronic fatigue. These risk factors are particularly high in women who are already lean and fit and seek marginal improvement to attain high-risk six-pack status. By contrast, women who are overfed, overweight, prediabetic, or have disease risk factors have a greater imperative to adopt the *Two Meals a Day* lifestyle. For them, there's a bigger potential upside and zero downside health risks.

The key takeaway here is you need to do this right. Everyone can benefit from fasting, especially in the age of overeating and hyperinsulinemia. To enjoy maximum benefits with minimal risk as a female, you should be in exceptional general health before beginning your *Two Meals a Day* journey—body fat under 25 percent, normal results on blood tests, and basic fitness competency. Along the way, be vigilant to avoid the pain and suffering that we typically associate with lifestyle transformation. This means paying close attention to hunger signals at all times, and eating delicious, nutrient-dense meals to the point of complete satisfaction every day. No running around feeling hungry and pushing yourself to endure your hectic daily schedule with insufficient energy.

Optimizing Your Carbohydrate Intake

If you are trying to reduce excess body fat, your strategy is straightforward: ditch the Big Three, unlock your fat-burning potential, and progress toward a *Two Meals a Day* lifestyle. After developing a high level of metabolic flexibility, you can then engage in fasting and carb restriction in order to drop excess body fat at a steady and comfortable rate until you reach what you determine to be your ideal body composition. You can enjoy plenty of colorful vegetables, but you must make fat your primary energy source through fasting (burning stored body fat) and eating meals that are high in natural, nutritious fats. It's not necessary to go looking for additional carbohydrate calories in the name of eating macronutrient-balanced meals—in fact, you don't need to look for extra carb calories at all!

You don't need to go looking for extra protein, either, which is contrary to the centerpiece of many gimmicky weight-loss diets. Because protein is the macronutrient most essential for survival, we have evolved finely tuned genetic mechanisms to ensure that we consume sufficient protein for basic health maintenance. If you underconsume protein, you'll feel terrible. You'll become emaciated and experience intense cravings for high-protein foods to correct what your genes perceive to be a matter of life and death—which it technically is if you were to continue starving yourself. On the flip side, it's difficult to overconsume protein because it is extremely satiating. You can easily go overboard on ice cream pints, but it's more difficult to do that with scrambled eggs and grass-fed steak.

If you are humming along, intermittently eating nutrient-dense foods and trying to drop some fat through carb restriction, at times you may experience afternoon energy dips or strong cravings for carbs. If the craving is legit—that is, not influenced by emotions or boredom—go ahead and indulge. Paying attention to real cravings is part of honoring your natural appetite and being metabolically flexible. I occasionally have carb cravings in the twenty-four to thirty-six hours after an intense workout, but at other times I don't. You gotta go with the flow.

When your body is calling for carbs, reach for excellent choices such as fresh seasonal berries and starchy tubers (sweet potatoes, beets, pumpkins, squash, zucchini). Quinoa and wild rice are also popular options among ancestral-inspired low-carb eaters. Quinoa is technically not a grain but a chenopod—a member of the beet and spinach family. It's gluten-free and a complete protein, with all nine essential amino acids. Wild rice, too, is technically not a grain but an aquatic grass. It has an impressive nutritional profile—no gluten or other plant toxins—and is high in protein. Other great options for supplemental carbs are the incidental carbs present in high-protein and high-fat foods, including nuts, seeds, and their derivative butters as well as high-cacao-percentage dark chocolate.

Don't worry if you depart from your fat-loss plan for a day here and there. If, for whatever reason, you indulge in some carbs, get back on track the next day and trust that your body composition will improve over time as you adhere to the big-picture principles of the *Two Meals a Day* program. Once you drop excess body fat and stabilize at your ideal body composition, you may even be able to relax your standards a bit if you feel like enjoying more of your favorite nutritious carbs or having a homemade high-carbohydrate dessert once in a while. Remember: your body has an assortment of powerful homeostatic drives that push you to a set point based on your genetics and your historic pattern of insulin production. Initially shedding excess body fat is challenging: you have to align your hunger and satiety signals, test the limits of your fasting capabilities, and at times persevere through hunger pangs for thirty to sixty minutes. If you have lofty ambitions, you can implement some advanced strategies that I'll discuss in chapter 7. Once the excess weight is off, though, it will be easier to maintain your new weight, even when you occasionally increase carb and caloric intake or reduce the amount of exercise you get.

If you are a high-calorie-burning exerciser or laborer, there are additional parameters to consider when dialing in to your ideal carb intake. While numerous high-profile endurance athletes and some strength and power athletes have made remarkable transformations and become full-on ketogenic performers, the reality for many people is that restricting carbs has the potential to interfere with workout performance and recovery. This is especially the case for people living high-stress lifestyles, who are at risk of liquidating their assets; females who are super fit; and people recovering from decades of metabolic damage, who require more time to build metabolic flexibility. Mind you, this doesn't mean that living a high-performance lifestyle compromises your path to metabolic flexibility. In fact, it means that you can achieve it even more precisely by paying close attention to the energy demands that your high-performance lifestyle dictates.

Targeting additional carbohydrate intake before and/or after ambitious workouts has been effective for many low-carbohydrate peak performers. This is especially true if you possess metabolic flexibility and don't desperately rely on carbs to keep your brain and muscles functioning all day long. Some extra carbs can give your muscles a performance boost (especially during explosive efforts) and help quickly replenish depleted glycogen after workouts. Besides, if you have just completed an intense or prolonged glycogen-depleting workout, your appetite hormones will likely send a powerful signal to your brain to eat, and often overeat, in the interest of replenishing your glycogen stores right away. As Dr. Cate Shanahan says, "When the glycogen suitcases are open, your liver and muscle storage depots take priority." When carbs have a place to go, you don't get the undesirable insulin spike that leads to energy lulls, mood and appetite disturbances, excess body fat, and disease patterns.

The idea of having empty suitcases (either because of fasting or strenuous workouts) is important to appreciate amid the frequent commentary about the destructive effects of excess carb intake and hyperinsulinemia. Carbs and insulin are only problematic when you disturb homeostasis, so if you produce an optimally minimal amount of insulin over your lifetime—just enough to deliver glucose, amino acids, fatty acids, and other nourishment to tissues and organs throughout the body and just enough to regulate enzyme activity and tightly regulate blood glucose—you are doing it right. It's important not to stress the delicate hormonal mechanisms and develop insulin resistance. The term *insulin sensitivity* describes the desirable state of cells being highly sensitive when insulin comes knocking with a delivery of nutrients for the empty suitcases.

Unfortunately, many people who are high calorie burners also sport excess body fat, despite the fact that they train for ten or even fifteen hours a week. The overwhelming reason for this is a historical pattern of producing too much insulin. As you learned from the discussion about compensation theory (see page 3), you cannot exercise your way out of a bad diet. If you are struggling to drop excess fat despite a devotion to exercise, you are going to have to cut carbs, especially nutrient-deficient grains and sugars and the performance drinks, bars, and gels that are enjoyed to egregious excess by serious exercisers. However, your first order of business is to screen for any overly stressful exercise patterns that promote carbohydrate dependency. If your mood, energy, cognitive functioning, immune functioning, and overall enjoyment of life seem to be hindered (rather than enhanced) by your workouts, you are in an overstress pattern. When this happens, you must take immediate and dramatic corrective action to reduce the degree of difficulty of your exercise regimen. If you insist on continuing with exhausting, glycogen-depleting workouts, attempts to reduce dietary carb intake are going to result in the dreaded liquidation of your assets.

If you are training sensibly, on the other hand, your next mission is to completely eliminate the sugars and grains that spike insulin and provide no nutritional benefits. Forget about dropping body fat for a moment: let's be clear that even if you are a lean, mean athletic machine, there is never any justification for consuming inflammatory, nutrient-deficient, insulin-stimulating carbohydrates. While the stress load of devoted athletic training elevates your nutritional needs in comparison to those of the sedentary dude in the next cubicle, that doesn't give you permission to eat whatever you want. Your dietary indiscretions may not show up on your waistline just yet, but bad stuff is happening inside your body when you replenish with Slurpees instead of sweet potatoes. For one thing, sugar promotes inflammation and oxidative stress. If you're trying to recover from a workout that generates its own inflammation and oxidative stress (desirable, in the case of a workout), nutrient-deficient carbs are going to hinder your recovery. You need to refill your tanks, to be sure, but the more you can stay away from junk and leverage the phenomenal anti-inflammatory and antioxidant benefits of fasting and nutrient-dense ancestral foods, the more quickly you will recover from hard training.

If you already maintain an ideal body composition, you can try the Dr. Tommy Wood strategy of eating all the nutritious carbs you desire to the point of adding a bit of body fat.

Should this occur, you can dial back your carb intake a bit, remove that unwanted pound or two or three, and get back into your groove. If you are captivated by the highly touted benefits of being in ketosis, or if you want to get down into single-digit body-fat territory as a male (a super-cut six-pack), or get below 15 percent body fat as a female (tight and toned, with visible musculature, even throughout the thighs and midsection), you can try to minimize carbs by following the commonly cited keto guidelines of fifty grams of carbohydrates per day or fewer. However, you must be sure you are training correctly—not the slightest whiff of overdoing it—and eating plenty of nutrient-dense, high-satiety meals.

FASTING FOR PEAK PERFORMANCE AND QUICKER RECOVERY? WELCOME TO THE NEXT FRONTIER OF ENDURANCE PERFORMANCE

Ultrarunner Zach Bitter is a low-carb and carnivore advocate who broke the world record for the 100-mile run with a time of eleven hours, nineteen minutes in 2019. This is a stunning pace of six minutes and forty-eight seconds per mile—running a sub-three-hour marathon back to back to back to back! Bitter reports that when he switched to a clean, low-carbohydrate eating pattern, he would awaken the morning after challenging long-distance training sessions with noticeably less joint stiffness and swelling.

Taking low-carb eating to the extreme is amateur athlete Dude Spellings of Austin, Texas. At age forty-nine, Spellings completed the epic Grand Canyon rim-to-rim-to-rim excursion—nearly fifty miles and twelve thousand feet of elevation gain—in fifteen hours. He started out fasted, remaining in a ketogenic state, and consumed only a few hundred calories of high-fat snacks during the entire journey. At the finish line, while his running partners feasted on hot pizza, Spellings decided to continue fasting overnight to help reduce inflammation and promote muscle repair. In the morning, he reported feeling fresher and less sore than he had thirteen years earlier, when he did the same crossing (and took two hours longer) as a high-carb athlete. Another historic human endurance and metabolic accomplishment was achieved in May of 2020 when Utah ultrarunner Michael McKnight completed a solo 100-mile run in the exceptional time of eighteen hours, forty minutes without consuming any calories—just water and electrolyte pills!

While these extreme performances may be hard to relate to for the average person trying to juggle health and fitness ambitions with a busy lifestyle, they offer a glimpse into the future of the way even extreme fitness goals can be pursued without compromising health. The days of pairing spin class with Jamba Juice are over. It's time to replace the "If the furnace is hot enough, anything will burn" mentality with the pursuit of metabolic efficiency—not *needing* sugar to perform, even for long-duration efforts. This movement will strike a blow to the multibillion-dollar sports nutrition industry, but its importance is underscored by the disturbing observation that even extreme fitness enthusiasts routinely carry extra body fat. This is a clear sign of a disconnect between behaviors and goals. One study revealed that 30 percent of the participants in the Cape Town Marathon (in South Africa) were above the healthful body-mass-index range. This is the same percentage as the world's population in general! In my decades hanging around triathlon race venues and fitness clubs, I have observed this phenomenon to a shocking extent. I proclaim it to be the worst-kept secret in the fitness industry. Granted, getting strong and aerobically fit is vastly superior to being sedentary, but it would be nice to enjoy a maximum payoff in aesthetics and performance (most every sport and fitness challenge rewards low body fat and a high strength-to-weight ratio) for all that hard work, wouldn't it?

Two Meals a Day Transcends the Diet Wars

For the past fifteen years I've been promoting an ancestral-style eating pattern in my books, blog articles, live events, and media appearances. I'm a huge fan of primal, Paleo, keto, and, more recently, nose-to-tail carnivorous eating. Moral and philosophical arguments aside for a moment, I don't recommend a whole-food, plant-based (a.k.a. vegetarian or vegan) diet because it excludes a huge percentage of the most nutritious foods on the planet. Since I ditched grains, sugars, and refined oils almost twenty years ago and reclaimed my health, I've been experimenting with a variety of nuanced strategies that are always ancestral-inspired.

Today, my dietary centerpieces are meat, fish, fowl, eggs, and certain vegetables. I enjoy moderate amounts of nuts, seeds (and their derivative butters), organic high-fat dairy products (cheese, cottage cheese, full-fat yogurt, raw kefir), fresh berries in season, and 80–85 percent cacao dark chocolate (which my coauthor, Brad, mails me and insists that I try). I indulge in some very well-chosen treats now and then (e.g., gelato during an Italian vacation or homemade cheesecake at a birthday party). Occasionally, I'll consume some grains as well—a carne asada street taco wrapped in a corn tortilla, a slice of warm homemade bread drowned in olive oil and balsamic vinegar, or a sushi roll with white rice. I'm too busy enjoying my life to track anything—unless I have to for a dietary analysis presentation in a book or blog post! As I've mentioned previously, my diet is a closed-loop system. Because of the excellent metabolic flexibility I've developed over the years, I can essentially generate energy independently from my calorie intake. And because I don't worry about obtaining my hour-to-hour energy requirements from food, I am able to contemplate it purely for pleasure instead of as an obligatory fuel. Granted, after a seven-day fast my tune might change a bit, but I think you get the point.

Metabolic Flexibility
Closed-Loop System

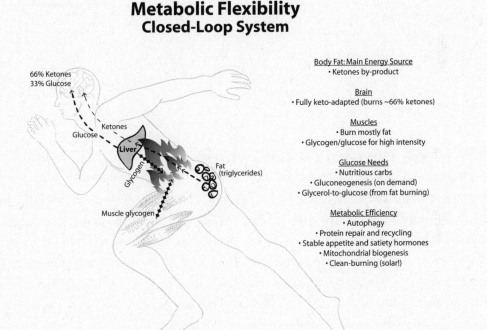

Regardless of your eating style, there are benefits to the two-meals-a-day approach. That said, if you are committed to a whole-foods, plant-based diet, I offer a few suggestions. First, consider expanding your diet to include fish and animal products (eggs, cheese) in order to improve nutrient density and ensure you are getting enough highly bioavailable protein and other important nutrients such as vitamin A, vitamin K_2, and

Carbohydrate Dependency

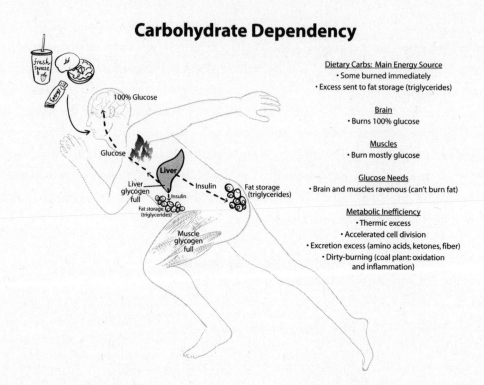

Dietary Carbs: Main Energy Source
• Some burned immediately
• Excess sent to fat storage (triglycerides)

Brain
• Burns 100% glucose

Muscles
• Burn mostly glucose

Glucose Needs
• Brain and muscles ravenous (can't burn fat)

Metabolic Inefficiency
• Thermic excess
• Accelerated cell division
• Excretion excess (amino acids, ketones, fiber)
• Dirty-burning (coal plant: oxidation and inflammation)

Labels on figure: 100% Glucose; Glucose; Liver; Liver glycogen full; Insulin; Insulin; Fat storage (triglycerides); Fat storage (triglycerides); Muscle glycogen full

choline, which are largely absent from plant foods. For example, a vegan would have to consume foods rich in beta-carotene, a plant-sourced precursor to vitamin A, and then execute a complex chain of biochemical reactions within the body to convert it to retinol, the fully formed state of vitamin A. Dr. Paul Saladino cites research suggesting that it takes twenty-one units of beta-carotene to equal the biological value of one unit of retinol. That's a lot of carrots and sweet potatoes to measure up to one serving of beef liver, the vitamin A king. Second, because as a vegetarian or vegan you consume a greater proportion of your daily calories from carbohydrates by default, you need to be sure to obtain sufficient fats from olives, coconuts, avocados, and their derivative oils. Third, you need to be sure that refined grains and sugars don't contribute to your already significant carbohydrate intake.

Beyond logistical concerns, science is now showing that genetics have a huge influence over whether you can thrive on any particular restrictive diet. Denise Minger is a recovering raw-food vegan whose namesake blog is lauded for its well-researched and often withering critique of popular diet trends. Minger describes numerous genetic attributes that can make plant-based eating a challenge, if not downright destructive to health. For example, nutrient deficiencies or common mutations in the *BCMO1* gene can compromise vitamin A conversion from plant foods, which isn't easy in the first place. An estimated 45 percent of people are "low responders" to beta-carotene. Other research identifies mutations in the *PEMT* gene that can promote choline deficiency. Genetic or lifestyle-related deficiencies in specific bacteria in your gut can inhibit your synthesis of vitamin K_2. If you have relatively few copies of the widely discussed amylase-coding gene *AMY1*, the starches you consume will more likely be stored as fat instead of metabolized.

On the other side of the debate, critics of animal-heavy diets cite research stating that certain genotypes respond unfavorably to an increase in dietary saturated fat intake. But avoiding excess animal fat is easily managed by emphasizing monounsaturated fats such as coconut products, olives, olive oil, and avocados and minimizing consumption of bacon and butter.

Beyond your particular eating style, we all need to broaden our perspective to emphasize reducing meal frequency. In *The Obesity Code* and his other books, Dr. Jason Fung strongly emphasizes that *how often you eat is just as important as the foods you choose* when it comes to fat reduction, insulin control, and disease protection. In *The Fatburn Fix*, Dr. Cate Shanahan explains that secretions of the predominant hunger hormone ghrelin are strongly tied to your circadian rhythms. If you customarily prepare a hearty breakfast every morning, you are going to be hungry when you awaken. If you like to take a 2:00 p.m. break from the office to grab a banana and an energy bar from the corner market, ghrelin will reliably spike every day at 2:00 p.m. You may have noticed this phenomenon with your pets. Every day at exactly 5:00 p.m., my goldendoodle, Shanti, heads into my office and starts to whimper theatrically—her accuracy about the time is uncanny!

If you feel some trepidation about walking away from the cultural mainstay that is snacking, realize that when you're carbohydrate-dependent, snacking is going to be part of your game because you need an energy boost when your blood glucose drops and hunger hormones spike. As soon as your focus wanes and your stomach starts growlin' from ghrelin, regardless of any stern lecture you find in a book, you are likely going to drift down to that corner market and get your favorite snack fix. As your metabolic flexibility improves, strive to confine your caloric intake to mealtimes. Eat as much as you wish in order to feel completely satisfied and happy at every meal; don't concern yourself with calorie restriction or calorie counting.

If you find yourself hankering for an afternoon snack, it's likely that your brain needs a break from tasks requiring your sustained attention. Instead of reaching for a sugary coffee concoction or high-carbohydrate "energy" bar, choose an energizing diversion such as a short walk, a yoga session, or some brief, high-intensity exercise. You'll quickly discover that your brain and body operate much better when you eat less frequently and that it is possible to thrive on a completely different eating pattern from the carbohydrate-dependency paradigm that you have been following virtually your entire life. Once you get out of your own way you can allow your magnificent evolution-honed mechanisms to assume center stage. This means getting away from an obsession with food as fuel, emphasizing intermittent eating over intermittent fasting, and improving metabolic flexibility by waiting until WHEN to enjoy your first meal.

Time-Restricted Feeding

Time-restricted feeding, a popular new concept, simply means that you consume all your calories within a specific time frame and fast during the other hours. A sixteen-eight strategy has been widely recommended in this realm, meaning sixteen hours of fasting followed by eight hours during which all meals are eaten. For example, you might finish your evening meal by 8:00 p.m., then wait until 12:00 noon the following day to break-fast. This first meal of the day opens an eating window that will close at 8:00 p.m. that evening, and then you repeat the cycle over the following days, weeks, and months—although some departures are expected because of social gatherings and special occasions. Note, though, that the strategy of eating all meals within a compressed time frame doesn't mean eating indiscriminately throughout those hours. The objective is to enjoy a maximum of two meals and no snacking inside the designated window.

A study published in 2019 in *The New England Journal of Medicine* titled "Effects of Intermittent Fasting on Health, Aging, and Disease" carried this crucial quotation from study authors Rafael de Cabo, PhD, and Mark Mattson, PhD: "Evidence is accumulating that eating in a six-hour period and fasting for 18 hours can trigger a metabolic switch from glucose-based to ketone-based energy, with increased stress resistance, increased longevity, and a decreased incidence of diseases, including cancer and obesity."

It may take some time to build sufficient metabolic flexibility to eat two meals a day in a sixteen-eight rhythm, but this is a great long-term goal. Once you feel comfortable with an eight-hour window, you can easily throw in some days that are eighteen-six, twenty-four, or even a twenty-four-hour fast as you pursue advanced body-composition, antiaging, and disease-prevention goals. I'll discuss these further in chapter 7.

One objective you can execute immediately, and honor for the rest of your life, is to limit your digestive functioning to a maximum of twelve hours per day. Your digestive system is highly attuned to your circadian rhythms. Digestive hormones and enzymes are best adapted for food intake during daylight hours, and your digestive system requires downtime just as your body in general requires sleep. The digestive circadian rhythms concept has been popularized by Dr. Satchin Panda, research professor at the Salk Institute for Biological Studies, in La Jolla, California, and author of *The Circadian Code*. Dr. Panda explains that practicing time-restricted feeding will help optimize fat metabolism, insulin sensitivity, mitochondrial functioning, immune functioning, gut microbiome diversity, inflammation control, and disease protection.

Beyond sleeping and eating rhythms, emerging research (including work from three Americans who won a 2017 Nobel Prize in Physiology or Medicine) reveals the amazing insight that every single organ and system in the body operates according to its own circadian clock. To get comprehensive, system-wide restoration every night, the idea is to synchronize the winding down of all cognitive, physical, and organ functions after dark. This means avoiding intense workouts, big meals, and anything highly stimulatory in the last few hours before bed. If you load your digestive system beyond a twelve-hour workday or eat a significant number of calories after dark, you are inviting problems. Unfortunately, Dr. Panda's research, conducted among thousands of eaters reporting to his smartphone app, myCircadianClock, reveals that the average person eats across a fifteen-hour time window each day—virtually one's entire waking hours! Furthermore, dozens of studies reveal that you are vastly more insulin-resistant after dark, meaning that evening calories are much more likely to be stored as fat.

In Dr. Panda's high-profile 2012 study involving mice, two groups ate an identical number of calories, but one group had constant access to food while the other was restricted to an eight-hour daily window. The mice with constant access became ill and obese, unlike the control group, which ate in a tighter window. Dr. Courtney Peterson, professor of nutrition science at the University of Alabama, Birmingham, repeated the theme in experiments with prediabetic men and generated similar results. Switching from a twelve-hour daily eating window to a six-hour window lowered subjects' blood pressure, insulin levels, appetite, and oxidative stress. In the evenings, they were less hungry and had increased rates of fat burning.

An important distinction to appreciate with time-restricted feeding is that your digestive clock starts when you consume any xenobiotic substance (something that requires your digestive system to metabolize), even if it has no calories. This means that black coffee, herbal tea, a vitamin pill—most anything except plain water—will initiate digestive functioning. Interesting research supports the idea that turning on your digestive clock first thing in the morning will help you become alert and energized just as exercise will. To get the best of both worlds, you can enjoy some coffee or tea when you wake up, then fast until WHEN. Dr. Michael Platt, expert in bioidentical hormone therapy and author of *Adrenalin Dominance*, recommends swallowing a spoonful of medium-chain triglyceride oil (a.k.a. MCT oil, a popular nutritional supplement available from health food stores or online) in the morning if you are fasting. This will help spur ketone production and provide energy to your brain, thereby preventing a fight-or-flight reaction in people who are vulnerable to them, including high-calorie-burning athletes (especially those in the forty-plus age group), people with thyroid or adrenal concerns, women with healthy body composition trying to lose even more fat, and people who may have a tendency to become overstressed from fasting.

16-8 Eating Pattern

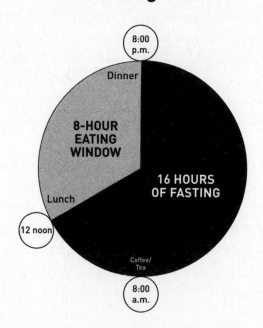

Truth be told, I add a bit of cream and a pinch of sugar to my morning coffee while "fasting" until I eat my Sisson Bigass Salad (page 229), around 1:00 p.m. Shhh—don't tell the fasting police! Activating your digestive clock upon awakening is especially helpful when you are trying to overcome jet lag and adjust to a new time zone, or if you have difficulty getting energized and feeling alert in the morning. In conjunction with initiating digestive functioning, get outside—move your body and expose your eyes to direct sunlight. These will all combine to bring you back online for a productive day.

Something that tripped me up when I was first exposed to time-restricted feeding was that I'd have days where I was sipping my coffee by 7:00 a.m. paired with late dinners and a few squares of dark chocolate while watching TV well beyond the 7:00 p.m. cutoff! Even if you dutifully eat lunch and dinner every day inside an eight-hour or even a six-hour window, you may still risk bumping up against the twelve-hour maximum limit for digestive functioning if you aren't vigilant. Granted, if you are getting the vast majority of your calories in a narrow window, this issue is not a big deal—I was able to change course (and you will be able to as well), but it is something to be mindful of so you can avoid eating too close to the cutoff time.

Intermittent Eating: The Fast-est Way to Health—Journal Exercises

1. **Metabolic Flexibility:** Describe your meal and snacking habits over the past few months and your current perceived state of metabolic flexibility. Describe your strategies for becoming more adept at fasting and time-restricted feeding over the long term. Describe lifestyle circumstances that influence your meal timing, such as workout patterns and job and family responsibilities.
2. **Fasting:** For the next week, record the duration of your daily fasts and the hours of your daily digestive functioning. Describe your exercise and activity in the morning hours and rate your level of cognitive functioning, mood, energy, and appetite prior to your first meal.

CHAPTER 4

Implement a Winning Mindset and Behavior Patterns

Over the past decade, my interactions with thousands of devoted health enthusiasts, online and in person, have revealed an elephant in the room that contributes to repeated suffering and failure: *flawed mindsets and behavior patterns* resulting from harmful subconscious childhood programming, manipulative marketing messages, unhealthful cultural influences, and ongoing failed attempts to implement and sustain healthful diet and exercise routines. In chapter 1, I urged you to ditch processed foods. Let's keep that theme alive in this chapter and clean up the self-limiting beliefs and behavior patterns that are holding you back. Time to get unstuck! This chapter will help you understand the what, why, and how of eating and living healthfully. It will help you behave in alignment with your stated goals and make empowering, conscious choices with full accountability.

Acquire Self-Knowledge

In order to truly succeed at achieving metabolic flexibility, you must attain a deep understanding of the practical aspects of healthful eating as well as the flawed subconscious programming and self-limiting beliefs and behavior patterns that are holding you back today. Having read the information about the best foods to eat for your dietary transformation, you are now, I hope, highly attuned to the best choices for your pantry and your plate. That aspect of *Two Meals a Day* is pretty straightforward. I've often joked that I can tell you everything you need to succeed in healthful eating in a single page—the additional information found in my books and on my website is intended to inspire, entertain, and deepen your knowledge of specific subjects. My elevator pitch would be: "Ditch refined sugars, grains, and seed oils; eat fewer meals and snacks; move more, sleep more, and live awesome!" However, adhering to the simple big-picture principles of healthful living can be easier said than done. It's possible to get so deep in your head that you lose connection with your heart and the power of your intuition. So before you explore the nuances of diet optimization and create a personalized meal plan, it's critical to make a simple, sustainable commitment to ditching processed foods, emphasizing wholesome, nutrient-dense ancestral foods, and honoring your natural appetite and satiety signals.

Making a commitment is the first step; the next is to marshal your resources in support of that goal. In the same way that you would clean out your pantry to make space for new, healthful foods, it's valuable to take a close look at your beliefs and attitudes—not only about food and eating habits but also about your ability to stay focused on long-term goals and resist the potential distractions and diversions of today's comfortable and indulgent modern life, all of which can send you off track.

Identifying your flawed programming, beliefs, and behaviors can be a difficult exercise to complete because most people have a tendency to harbor a negative self-image. We often succumb to FOMO via social media or unhealthy relationship dynamics; we eat for emotional comfort or snack idly. These habits and perceptions are problematic precisely because they occur subconsciously. Numerous large-scale dietary intake studies reveal that subjects have poor recall for what they eat, grossly underreport caloric intake (by an average of 30 percent!), exaggerate consumption of healthful foods, and overreport physical activity by an average of 50 percent! By conducting an honest accounting of your "issues," you can bring them into awareness and do some ambitious and sustained reprogramming. This might involve developing the ability to identify a self-critical thought and replace it with an affirmation of gratitude, or it might involve noticing a behavior such as eating too quickly and making a deliberate effort to chew each bite twenty times for the rest of the meal.

Your progress will be accelerated when you learn an assortment of techniques for taking control of your thoughts and physiology—techniques that are covered in chapter 4. For example, learning to override the initial fight-or-flight panic reaction to cold water exposure with intentional breathing techniques can help you become more resilient against all other forms of stress, distraction, emotional triggers, and self-limiting beliefs that arise during a hectic day. As you gain more control and awareness in all areas of life, you will finally be equipped to attack the causes of emotional reactivity and self-sabotage, which can be conscious (e.g., eating too much ice cream because your diet's not working anyway) and subconscious (e.g., eating for emotional comfort instead of in response to hunger).

Perhaps your top healing priority in the area of diet and failed weight-loss efforts is to acknowledge the harmful psychological effects of following conventional stupidity's calories in, calories out approach to fat reduction. You may have labeled yourself a disappointment for repeatedly flunking what you thought was a simple math problem but is in truth a hormonal problem. For the millions of people who feel discouraged, lazy, and undisciplined after failed fat-loss efforts, let's agree right now that *it's not your fault.* Gary Taubes, bestselling author of *Good Calories, Bad Calories, Why We Get Fat* and *The Case Against Sugar*, and widely regarded as one of the leading diet researchers in the world, explains it this way: "Gluttony and sloth are not causes of obesity, they are *symptoms.*"

Here's what that means: when you eat a high-carbohydrate meal, you get a quick spike of energy, then insulin floods the bloodstream to remove excess glucose. The resulting abrupt drop in glucose causes your body to become starved for energy—a sugar crash. Granted, you have abundant energy locked away in your fat stores, but it's inaccessible because of the elevated insulin. Without ample energy circulating in your bloodstream, you are too tired to exercise. Instead, appetite hormones spike as your body becomes desperate for energy, and you repeat this glucose-insulin roller coaster all day long.

Hyperinsulinemia also hinders the signaling ability of the key satiety and fat-storage hormone called leptin. Leptin tells you when you are full and whether you burn fat or store it. It is regarded as the preeminent hormone in controlling the deepest human genetic drive for both males and females: to be fit for reproduction. With leptin signaling disrupted, you are more likely to overeat and store the excess calories as fat. Repeat after me: *excess body fat is a result of hormone dysfunction caused by hyperinsulinemia—not lack of willpower or discipline.* When you lower insulin by ditching processed carbs and eating less frequently (assisted by complementary lifestyle behaviors), your body will respond by naturally optimizing appetite and satiety hormones so that you don't overeat or get fat.

Knowing that it's mostly about insulin, and much less about balancing the equation by restricting calories or burning extra calories, still puts the responsibility on you, but it's in the proper context. It gives you a complete understanding of the choices that support health and ideal body composition and those that hinder it. You can filter out the incessant onslaught of flawed science and marketing hype that tries to push you back toward the erroneous concept of calories in, calories out in order to market regimented diet and fitness programming—programming that will ultimately lead to failure, making you feel lazy and undisciplined and leading you to repeat the cycle with new flawed programming. Instead, you can excel any time you want by fasting instead of eating and/or eating a sequence of low-insulin-producing meals. You can take comfort knowing that regaining your health doesn't require pain, suffering, and sacrifice but rather making choices aligned with your human genetic predisposition for health. Relax, eat (real foods) to your heart's content, and explore your potential for an amazing new body!

Cultivate Compassion and Gratitude

Armed with the understanding that it's not your fault, you can decide that it's time to wholeheartedly forgive yourself for past mistakes and failures, whether in the realm of diet and weight loss, fitness goals, or other personal growth ambitions. Wherever you are today is a perfectly acceptable starting point for your growth and transformation. Self-compassion entails eradicating the slightest traces of guilt and self-pity from your consciousness. You'll learn about turnaround statements shortly, and journal entries of compassion and forgiveness are also effective. If you can't seem to get away from nagging guilt, it may be sobering to understand that guilt gives you an excuse to remain stuck and/ or perpetuate your guilt-producing behaviors in the future. Your guilt serves as a protection mechanism for your ego, preventing you from facing the reality that you are sabotaging your own behavior goals. Imagine if you were on a strict diet and departed from it during a weak moment to inhale a fresh-baked cookie. In the aftermath, you might experience feelings of guilt, shame, and remorse. These emotions actually protect your fragile ego: you don't have to feel like a lazy, undisciplined slob—too weak to turn down a cookie while on a diet. The feeling of guilt "proves" that you're a caring, disciplined, successful person who has made an incredibly uncharacteristic mistake worthy of extreme remorse in light of your high standards.

Can you detect the dysfunctional dynamic in play here? Harboring a negative, self-defeating mindset, you may be more likely to plunge off the deep end and devour an entire pint of Ben & Jerry's on the heels of the cookie. The conjuring of guilt, shame, and remorse for consorting with Ben & Jerry proves that you're not lazy or lacking willpower. Rather, you're just someone who has once again made a grave transgression against your shining reputation and honorable intentions. The cycle repeats every time there's a smell of a new cookie—shame and guilt instead of compassion and gratitude.

The same guilt dynamic might apply to areas where you procrastinate. For example, perhaps Grandma loves to receive handwritten letters from you at the nursing home. You know she checks her mail slot every day in anticipation of hearing from you, but you've been too busy to write recently and feel guilty accordingly. Because you're consumed with guilt over your procrastination, it's clear you are not a selfish and uncaring grandchild. Your guilt protects your fragile ego and effectively allows you to continue to leave Grandma hanging. Granted, guilt can often be leveraged into motivation, but the examples here reveal how easy it is to slip into a rut and stay there through compensatory mental gymnastics.

This is not to suggest that you should suppress your emotional reaction or give yourself a free pass every time you screw up. Dan Millman, megabestselling author of *Way of the Peaceful Warrior* and numerous sequels in the franchise, suggests that we treat emotions just as we treat the weather. When you experience a pouring rain of emotions, deal with whatever form they take—pouring rain cannot be ignored or rationalized away. However, you know that the rain will pass and you will carry on with your life. Acknowledge your "negative" emotions honestly, have compassion for your mistakes, and welcome all life experiences as opportunities for personal growth. When you struggle and feel stuck in pessimism, cultivating gratitude is your path to success. However bad you feel, it could be worse! By honing the skill to conjure gratitude on demand (instead of guilt on demand), you open the door to a healthier disposition and avoid feeling like a victim when life doesn't go as planned. As my wife, Carrie, likes to say (and has written on the kitchen message board), your thoughts—not what's happened to you—are the source of all your pain. If this sounds trite, respected research suggests that merely forming a grateful thought initiates genetic signaling that influences cellular functioning throughout your body, lowers stress hormones, and promotes relaxation.

Thoughts of gratitude are wonderful, but keeping a written journal can have an even greater impact on reorienting your brain toward happiness and contentment. Anything goes when it comes to your daily gratitude entries. One day you might wax poetic about how happy you are to be alive and breathing oxygen with two lungs; the next day you might be grateful for your new X3 Bar home exercise apparatus. Even if you can only muster ten seconds for a one-liner, make a gratitude journal entry every single day.

When you make gratitude a daily practice, you boost your potential for happiness;

gain greater control over emotions such as anger, jealousy, frustration, and regret; reduce aggression; improve empathy; and even sleep more soundly. Dr. Robert Emmons, professor of psychology at the University of California at Davis, author of *Gratitude Works!: A 21-Day Program for Creating Emotional Prosperity*, and widely regarded as the world's leading scientific expert on gratitude, offers an assortment of suggestions to cultivate a rewarding gratitude practice. First, as I mentioned in the introduction, use a handwritten journal for maximum effectiveness. Second, whatever's happening now, try to remember a time when things were worse and be thankful you got through it and that things are better today. Third, surround yourself with visual reminders, such as a sticky note with a short inspirational phrase on it or an hourglass on your desk to remind you that retirement is a year away. Fourth, fake it till you make it. If you're having a rough day, get out there and smile, say thank you, and perform a random act of kindness. These behaviors will trigger gratitude hormones and brighten your day. Finally, keep life fresh and exciting so you can cultivate gratitude for new adventures and circumstances.

Control Your Thoughts and Physiology

Dr. Bruce Lipton, author of *The Biology of Belief*, is recognized for his breakthrough research in stem cell biology, revealing the influence of psychology and spirituality on everyday cellular functioning. It's clear how environmental inputs such as food, exercise, and medication affect cell functioning, but the field of quantum biology proves that we can also influence cellular functioning with our thoughts. Think about how you feel when you get a phone call with great news: instantly happy and energetic. When bad news comes, on the other hand, you can quickly become depressed and exhausted. Lipton describes what's happening inside your body in reaction to experiences: perception switches located on your cell membranes interpret your positive or negative thoughts and trigger the production of either mood-elevating hormones such as serotonin or, alternatively, stress hormones such as cortisol.

Peak-performance guru Tony Robbins promotes a practice called priming, which involves breathing, visualization, gratitude, and relaxation exercises to reprogram the subconscious mind toward "love, passion, and success." Meditative practices of this nature have been strongly validated by science and are shown to be highly effective. Consider the amazing exploits of Dutch extreme athlete Wim Hof, a.k.a. the Iceman. Hof conducts special breathing exercises of "controlled hyperventilation" to override programmed human physiology and enable superhuman feats of cold tolerance and endurance. He has set more than two dozen Guinness World Records, including spending an hour and fifty-three minutes submerged to the neck in ice and climbing to 23,600 feet on Mount Everest wearing only shorts and shoes.

Perhaps most remarkable is Hof's ability to quickly train novices to perform similar feats using his method of intentional breathing. In 2016, he led a group of twenty-six ordinary climbers to the summit of Mount Kilimanjaro (19,340 feet, or 5,895 meters) in only forty-eight hours. This is a fraction of the typical summit excursion time, made possible by the Hof breathing exercises, which enabled the group to bypass the usual mandatory periods of acclimation to rising altitudes. Nearly half the group climbed wearing only shorts, withstanding temperatures of minus four degrees Fahrenheit (minus twenty degrees Celsius). Hof's successes demonstrate the ability of the conscious mind to override our genetically programmed fight-or-flight panic reaction when we encounter a stressor such as cold water or air or high altitude.

The idea that conscious behaviors such as priming and intentional breathing can influence your biology is a profound realization to embrace when you apply it to all areas of your life. When you can meditate, breathe, or merely think your way into a default state of love and gratitude, you become a master over your emotions and promote health and longevity. You can actually program your cells in the direction of renewal and regeneration. By contrast, if you make no effort to control your thoughts, breathing, or emotional reactivity, your cells will drift repeatedly into fight-or-flight mode as you battle to just get through another day.

Dr. Lipton validates this concept by explaining that our cells have three categories of perceptions: a growth response, a neutral response, and a protection response. He identifies love as the most powerful trigger of a growth response, promoting health and longevity, and fear as the most powerful trigger of a protection response—the essence of fight-or-flight survival mode. Interestingly, the HPA (hypothalamic-pituitary-adrenal) axis carries out both growth and protection responses in the body. Cells cannot multitask; they are either in growth mode, protection mode, or "listening to elevator music" mode— Dr. Lipton's characterization of a neutral stimulus. When a threatening environmental stimulus hits the hypothalamus (the brain's control tower for assorted hormonal and metabolic functions), it signals the pituitary gland (the master gland coordinating activity in trillions of cells) to mount a protective fight-or-flight response. The pituitary signals the adrenal glands to flood the bloodstream with stress hormones. You are now in battle mode at the direct expense of immune protection and longevity.

A protection response can happen during a traffic jam, an argument with a loved one, or upon receiving critical feedback from your boss at work. As you recount such an event to supporters and confidants, you'll likely gain validation that you were justified in mounting a protection response. However, the core message of the work of Dr. Lipton and others, including bestselling mind-body author Deepak Chopra, MD, is that you have the power to send your perception switches a different message. A traffic jam can be a great opportunity to practice some relaxation breathing and catch up with distant loved ones during a hands-free phone call. An argument with your partner? Author David Deida gives men some choice advice in his book *The Way of the Superior Man*. A heated emotional exchange is a great opportunity to "lean into [a woman's] radiant feminine energy," including the emotional intensity she brings to an argument, and shower her with love and humor. Paraphrasing Deida's message, we can conclude that only a lesser man would respond with a protection response!

Dr. Lipton contends that by the time we reach age thirty-five, 95 percent of our thoughts and actions originate from the habitual programming of the subconscious mind that occurred from infancy through age seven. This is a combination of memorized behaviors, emotional reactions, beliefs, and perceptions. As children, we were open and receptive—virtual sponges—absorbing the environmental influences that shape our lifelong beliefs and behavior patterns. Unfortunately, for many people, some or perhaps most of childhood programming was not positive or supportive. When a teacher criticizes a student or a peer teases a playmate, these experiences become embedded in the subconscious and can manifest themselves as negative self-talk and self-sabotage over the ensuing decades. Brain research reveals that our subconscious thoughts are extremely repetitive (98 percent of today's thoughts are identical to yesterday's) and largely negative (80 percent).

This means that transformation in any area of life, from breaking bad habits to forming an empowering new self-image, requires disconnecting from the subconscious and engaging in a state of conscious awareness. For example, if you eat too quickly, you can attempt to reprogram this habit by deliberately counting twenty chews every time you take a bite of food. Dr. Lipton describes the two primary ways to reprogram the subconscious as *habituation* (repetition of desired behaviors until they become habit) and *hypnosis* (accessing the sponge mindset you had as a child with an experienced therapist in order to revise the programming). The 12-Day Turbocharge (see page 172) will feature assignments to help you identify flawed beliefs and behaviors and cultivate the ability to take control of your thoughts and physiology.

Formulating a Plan of Action

The essence of this chapter is to identify specific self-limiting thoughts and beliefs as well as flawed behavior patterns against which you will take corrective action. You can begin work on this immediately if you choose, and you will be given specific assignments in this area during the 12-Day Turbocharge. You likely have an assortment of issues that will come to mind quickly. For reference and inspiration, following are some of the most common areas of struggle for people seeking health and dietary transformation.

- **Total eradication of the Big Three:** Acknowledge that marketing forces and cultural traditions are conspiring against you when it comes to cleaning up your act. While part of the allure of sweets, treats, and comfort foods comes from their intense flavor, you are also getting hit with a barrage of advertising as well as cultural influences that connect indulgent foods to celebration and fond memories. The best way to combat these forces is to commit to total elimination so that you don't have to waste any decision-making energy or willpower on resisting the temptation of your old favorites. When a bag of peanuts is dangled in front of someone with a severe peanut allergy on an airplane flight, the allergic person politely refuses the peanuts. There is no pondering, temptation, or FOMO, because the certainty of suffering vastly outweighs the pleasure of having a snack. Adopting a mindset of "these foods are off limits for me" out of the gate is the easiest way to succeed.
- **Self-image:** We are bombarded with advertising and social media commentary designed to elicit fear, insecurity, and desperation in order to command our attention and stimulate product sales. It's critical to escape the airbrushed world of models, fitness icons, and hucksters and redirect your attention to feelings of compassion and gratitude for wherever you are today. While there have been some controversies and misinterpretations associated with the body positivity movement, let's agree that you can exist in a state of gratitude and still pursue goals and dreams of looking and feeling better by improving your overall health.

- **Eating environment:** The two branches of the autonomic nervous system are the sympathetic, nicknamed fight or flight, and the parasympathetic, nicknamed rest and digest. It's essential that you create a calm, quiet, relaxing, celebratory environment every time you eat a bite of food. Next, resolve to eat at a comfortable pace, chewing each bite a minimum of twenty times to allow your salivary enzymes to play their important role in digestion. When you eat in a highly stimulating environment, such as while driving, working at your desk, or even watching television, you compromise healthy digestive functioning and risk regressing into bad habits such as overeating and idle snacking. When you improve metabolic flexibility and get into a *Two Meals a Day* groove, you will naturally gain an increased appreciation for eating as one of the great pleasures of life. Feeling a bit hungry at mealtime will help you execute this goal of optimizing your environment and eating pace.
- **Mindfulness:** In addition to eating in a relaxed, celebratory environment and avoiding the insulinogenic effects of snacking, make an effort to give your full attention and awareness to every bite of food that you eat. It's nice to relax in front of the television with a meal or treat, but please make a concerted effort, at least over the short term, to transform eating into a meditative exercise. Enjoy meals as a social connection, but eliminate all other potential distractions so you can concentrate on your intense enjoyment of the food.

You may have read an assortment of proclamations about how long it takes to form a new habit—twenty-one days, thirty days, and six weeks are all referenced frequently. The truth is that despite more than a century of extensive study of human behavior, there is no simple answer. Your personality type, stress level, attitude, and the degree of difficulty of the objective at hand make it impossible to pinpoint a theoretical finish line where you can relax and switch over to autopilot. For example, if you are attempting to create a habit of doing something that you dislike just because it's good for you, you are very likely to fail over the long term. The same is true for attempting to implement a habit of doing something you honestly don't think is important. We may come into conflict with a partner when we engage in behaviors such as squeezing the toothpaste in the middle of the tube, leaving dirty dishes in the sink, and not shutting off the lights in a room we've just left because these actions, which may be unimportant to you but are potentially important to your partner, are ingrained so deeply into your subconscious that you're not aware of doing them, despite how much they may annoy your partner and others.

Consequently, the attributes of successful habit formation include the following.

- **Importance:** The more meaning and value you place on developing a certain habit, the better your chance of success. If you are not great about cleaning up after yourself in the kitchen, but it's important to your partner, it's time to change your ways and make it important. Bestselling author and marriage expert Dr. John Gottman describes three levels of relationship progression: first getting your own needs met, then meeting your partner's needs, and finally having *your partner's needs become your own*. Go all out here and make your partner's kitchen cleanliness wishes your own!

- **Consciousness:** By definition, habit formation entails consciously and repeatedly behaving in a certain way until it becomes programmed into habit. This means that every time you engage in an activity, you must pay attention and think about what you're doing. It might help your progress to create triggers that take you out of that 95 percent autopilot mode and into mindfulness—perhaps a sticky note with a reminder about the toothpaste tube or singing a silly song about clean dishes when you're tidying up the kitchen.

- **Repetition and endurance:** If you tidy up the kitchen sink one night and proclaim yourself a changed human, you are probably going to disappoint yourself and others over time. As athletes in technique-dependent sports know better than most, reprogramming your subconscious to correct technique flaws and improve performance can be very frustrating. One day you feel like you're in the zone and in total command, and the next time out you have regressed. It's important to understand that forming a habit requires an ongoing commitment to importance, consciousness, and repetition and endurance. The powerful pull of the subconscious is always lurking, ready to sabotage your progress. Make a renewed commitment each day, and don't take any improvements in behavior for granted. If you experience any backsliding, apply your wonderful weapons of compassion and gratitude and get back on track the next time.

There is a Zen saying: "The way you do one thing is the way you do everything." The more you can move the needle away from that 95 percent subconscious-behavior mode into mindfulness, the greater your potential for long-term health, happiness, and contentment. Your efforts to transform your diet can become a catalyst for transformation in every other area of life. As we learned from Wim Hof, simply gaining mastery over breathing can enable a novice enthusiast to perform superhuman feats in a short time.

Believe!

Belief is about envisioning an awesome new future in which both your body and your mind are transformed. You can feel empowered knowing that success is completely under your control: it's a matter of making choices that align with optimal gene expression and avoiding choices that harm your health. Buoyed by the compassion and gratitude you are currently cultivating, and the honest identification of the flawed subconscious programming that is holding you back, you can put an end to the denial, excuses, and blame that have hindered your past progress. With heightened awareness, you can catch the self-destructive thoughts, statements, and behaviors that crop up reflexively throughout the day and reframe them into empowering new beliefs—affirmations and winning behaviors that you will eventually embrace as habit.

Dave Rossi, leadership and performance coach and author of *The Imperative Habit*, suggests that when you experience the inevitable fears and anxieties that crop up in the process of life transformation, you must actively redirect your focus to your *values and vision*. For example, if you feel frustrated by a lack of progress with fat reduction, you calmly acknowledge your frustration without judgment. Then turn your attention to how much better you feel each day after making healthful food choices (values) and trust that results will happen over the long term (vision).

Get inspired by connecting with real people leading busy lives filled with challenges, limitations, and distractions who are nevertheless achieving remarkable transformation. Reach out to people in your social circle or community whom you admire for their commitment to healthful living and elicit their support and guidance. Consider hiring a coach or trainer to get some personalized attention. Enlist a buddy to become your accountability partner, even if you can't eat or exercise together regularly. Take a look at the Success Stories section of MarksDailyApple.com to see the thousands of stunning before-and-after photos and impassioned stories from people who have reclaimed their health and transformed their bodies. When I first met Tara Grant, author of *The Hidden Plague*, she weighed 268 pounds and was suffering from the serious skin disease called hidradenitis suppurativa (HS). Besides the hidden plague of HS, she had assorted other inflammatory and autoimmune conditions requiring prescription medication, which hindered her ability to simply get through the day as a busy mom. Her book details an amazing journey of healing, mainly through dietary transformation and a hopeful attitude. Tara dropped a total of 125 pounds and has kept it off for a decade and counting. Her HS affliction, one that traditional medical authorities classify as "incurable" and usually treat with potent antibiotics, anti-inflammatory drugs, and surgery, is in long-term remission.

Nailing this objective of believing in yourself and harnessing your boundless potential requires a delicate balance between having compassion and gratitude for where you are today and tapping into the sustained focus, discipline, and motivation necessary to do better. Many people get tripped up by engaging in wishful thinking while still harboring negativity and self-limiting beliefs. True believers emanate compassion and gratitude and never linger in the disgust, resentment, and shame that can sabotage progress.

It takes work to break free from self-limiting beliefs, not only because of their embedded programming but also because we have been socialized to believe that negative energy can be a useful motivational tool. Sports coaches are lauded for their win-at-all-costs intensity; helicopter parents use conditional praise and veiled criticism to extract inauthentic results; high-energy trainers badger their clients to push ever harder; social media preys on our insecurities and cultivates FOMO. Feeling shame and guilt can get you off the couch and into the gym, and it can keep you away from the refrigerator for a succession of evenings, but it's a flimsy motivator in comparison to empowering beliefs. Often, after temporary success is obtained, a rebound effect of rebellion and regression occurs. When you love yourself as you are and love the process of self-improvement, you heighten your odds of succeeding with long-term lifestyle transformation.

My hope is that this material is getting you focused, inspired, and motivated, but honestly it is a huge challenge, and the stakes are high. Your flawed programming, beliefs, and behavior patterns have become part of your identity to the point where it can be difficult to appreciate the extent to which your thoughts control your behavior. As Jack Canfield, megabestselling author of the Chicken Soup for the Soul series, suggests, "If you want to find happiness in life...put a muzzle on that inner critic and transform it into an encouraging, loving, and positive inner coach." The inner critic can be incredibly destructive; Canfield cites research concluding that we talk to ourselves around fifty thousand times per day and that 80 percent of that self-talk is negative.

It's a common notion in spiritual psychology that the affluence and love we achieve in life equates to our level of self-worth. In his book *The Big Leap*, psychologist Gay

Hendricks advances the compelling argument that we bump up against an "upper limit" in life—"an inner thermostat setting that determines how much love, success, and creativity we allow ourselves to enjoy.... Unfortunately, [that] thermostat setting usually gets programmed in early childhood.... Once programmed, our Upper Limit thermostat setting holds us back from enjoying all the love, financial abundance, and creativity that's rightfully ours."

To transform any limiting belief into a positive one, Jack Canfield recommends identifying the belief you would like to change, determining how that belief limits you, and deciding how you would rather be, act, or feel. Then create a "turnaround statement" that affirms or gives you permission to be, act, and feel in a new way. Implant the statement into your subconscious mind by repeating the statement for two to three minutes several times per day for a minimum of thirty days. If this stuff sounds silly and you don't think it will work, you're right! It's not going to work for you with that attitude. If you believe deeply that this can work, that you deserve to transform, and that you will make a full commitment to the process, you are going to prove yourself right. Go for it!

Implement a Winning Mindset and Behavior Patterns— Journal Exercises

1. **Gratitude journal:** Get your gratitude journal started with a bang by spending ten to twenty minutes describing a handful of life circumstances you are grateful for right now. Commit to making an entry every day for the duration of your *Two Meals a Day* experience, including the culminating 12-Day Turbocharge.

2. **Self-knowledge:** Describe some ways that reading *Two Meals a Day* has helped you become enlightened or compelled to challenge fixed beliefs about healthful eating and healthful food choices. Describe some ways in which your new knowledge will affect your eating habits over the long term.

3. **Compassion and gratitude:** List a few past mistakes or failures that have been eating at you for a while. Resolve to let them go and give yourself a fresh start and a blank-slate mindset.

4. **New thoughts and actions:** List any self-limiting thoughts, beliefs, or behavior patterns that have negatively affected your health in the past. Describe how you are going to bring them into your awareness and take corrective action on the

spot (e.g., chewing more slowly at meals) as well as how you will sustain these new thoughts and actions by means of repetition and endurance.

5. **Believe!** Create some specific turnaround statements for the challenges you are tackling. Write them (or meaningful abbreviations of them) on index cards or sticky notes and display them in a prominent place for daily reflection.

CHAPTER 5

Follow a Fat-Burning Lifestyle

Complementary lifestyle practices are essential to honing your fasting and fat-burning skills. This chapter will address your evening sleep habits as well as ways in which you can get sufficient rest, recovery, and general downtime after exercise stress, draining workdays, and the insidious current health challenge of hyperconnectivity. You will also learn how to tackle the critical fat-burning objective of increasing all forms of general everyday movement and integrate brief, intense workouts into your routine to help turbo-charge fat burning around the clock.

Sleep Like a Champ

A good night's sleep allows your brain and body to repair and rejuvenate itself from a stressful modern life. It is the centerpiece of a healthful lifestyle—the one health practice from which all others emanate. If you aren't sleeping adequately, it's not even worth attempting dietary transformation or fine-tuning the particulars of your exercise program. The biggest modern challenge to healthful sleep is that we flood our evenings with artificial light and digital stimulation for many hours after the sun sets. This violently disrupts our all-important circadian rhythms and the extremely delicate hormonal functions that for millions of years have been calibrated to the rising and setting of the sun. Mobile devices and digital stimulation in general have compromised human sleep more severely than anything else in the history of humanity. The previous generation might have occasionally stayed up past bedtime watching a late show on television, but our ability to enjoy on-demand programming 24-7 and operate mobile devices constantly tempts us to sacrifice sleep for further stimulation.

We pay lip service to the importance of sleep, but we allow the insidious "autoplay next episode" feature to turn us into binge-watchers. We keep our phones at our bedsides so we can react to social media alerts and text message dings during that precious wind-down time when melatonin is supposed to be flooding our bloodstreams, lowering blood pressure and body temperature and generally making us feel sleepy. Research cited by Dr. Jason Fung in *The Obesity Code* reveals that Americans slept for an average of nine hours per night in 1910, eight to nine hours per night by 1960, and seven hours per night by 1995. Today, 30 percent of adults sleep for fewer than six hours per night. This has disastrous implications for general health and disease risk and is specifically destructive to the ability to drop excess body fat and build metabolic flexibility. Dr. Fung explains that a single night of insufficient sleep can spike cortisol by 100 percent, putting you on the path to carbohydrate cravings, overeating, and suppressed immune functioning the next day. Numerous longitudinal studies of large population groups validate the idea that sleep deprivation is directly associated with insulin resistance, obesity, and elevated disease risk.

Optimizing sleep requires minimizing artificial light and digital stimulation after dark, creating an ideal sleeping environment, and developing habits that keep you aligned with your circadian rhythms. Practicing the following will help you get sleepy on cue in the evening, cycle optimally through all the stages of sleep overnight, and awaken near sunrise feeling refreshed and energized for a happy, productive day.

Create an Ideal Sleep Environment

1. **Make your bedroom a sanctuary.** Along with getting in closer alignment with your circadian rhythms, it's essential to create an optimal sleeping environment—a bedroom sanctuary that serves as a shrine to rest and relaxation. Keep your bedroom simple, tidy, clutter-free, and reserved for sleeping only (okay, intimacy, too). Try searching Google or Pinterest for "minimalist bedroom" imagery to get inspired. The goal is to achieve a psychological transition between the liveliness of your home and the resting place of your bedroom. Absolutely no television, computer, work desk, or clutter allowed. Studies suggest

that just looking at a pile of clutter or an unfinished home improvement project can provoke a stress-hormone response at the subconscious level.

2. **Achieve total darkness.** Ensure that your room is completely dark when you turn out the lights. Even minor light disturbances can disrupt sleep, not just through your eyes but also through light receptors located on skin cells throughout the body. A study referenced in the book *Lights Out: Sleep, Sugar, and Survival*, by T. S. Wiley with Bent Formby, PhD, revealed that flashing a single beam of light on the back of the knee was sufficient to disrupt melatonin production. Extreme biohacker Dr. Jack Kruse cites extensive research indicating that restorative hormones such as testosterone and human growth hormone surge between midnight and 3:00 a.m. but require total darkness for maximum effectiveness.

    Get the best blackout curtains or room-darkening blinds you can find, and make sure they fit perfectly. Cover plug-in devices that emit tiny charging indicator lights with electrical tape or get them out of the bedroom. If you must get up in a dark room, put a small red LED flashlight at your bedside instead of flipping on overhead lights or using a bright phone screen to light your way.

3. **Stay cool.** Low ambient temperature and lower-than-daytime body temperature are triggers for optimal sleep. As we approach bedtime, circadian influences cause a gradual decline in body temperature and heat production and an increase in heat dissipation. As you progress through a night of sleep, thermosensitive cells in the hypothalamus also help coordinate the efficient cycling through all stages of sleep. Consequently, it's important not to undermine these delicate processes by cranking up the thermostat before bed or snuggling under too many layers of bedding, which can increase body temperature.

    Maintain a bedroom temperature of between sixty and sixty-eight degrees Fahrenheit (sixteen and twenty degrees Celsius) year-round. The ideal setup is to balance a cool core temperature (via breathing cool air and lying on a cool mattress) with comfortably warm skin (via just the right amount of nightclothes and blankets). Your brain needs a temperature drop of between two and three degrees Fahrenheit in order to go to sleep. Consider investing in the best mattress you can afford (it's only for one-third of your life!) that has breathable materials to dissipate excess heat. If you want further temperature optimization or have trouble with overheating, night sweats, or insomnia, consider investing in a chiliPAD (ChiliTechnology.com). This is a water-cooled mattress cover that can be programmed to attain specific temperatures at specific hours. Lying on a precooled mattress helps you lower your core temperature in order to facilitate sleep and prevents the common occurrence of getting too warm under the covers at night, thereby disrupting sleep. *Full disclosure*: I slept so well on a prototype chiliPAD that I became an investor in the company!

In general, try to err on the cool side with your clothing and room temperatures in the final hours before getting into bed and covering up. Surprisingly, if you take a warm bath before bed, the vasodilation of your skin surface will cause heat to dissipate the moment you exit the warm tub. The net effect will be to lower your core temperature. As you approach morning, your body temperature will naturally rise in preparation for awakening.

4. **Make it quiet.** Your sleep sanctuary must be quiet to ensure that the brain goes off-line and encounters no interference during your night of restoration. If you live in a rural area where there is complete silence overnight, that's great. People who live in urban areas may benefit from devices that use noise-canceling technology or produce white noise. The idea is that your brain quickly becomes accustomed to a consistent, soothing tone that will drown out any acute, unpredictable noises that might occur during the night—a snoring partner, a whimpering dog, urban traffic, or industrial sounds. The best choice might be a combination HEPA air filter and ionizer that energizes and purifies indoor air and blows like a fan. A tabletop fan, humidifier or dehumidifier (depending on how you want to optimize your room with respect to your climate), or dedicated white-noise machine also works well. When traveling, I like the convenience of a smartphone app that emits nature sounds such as ocean waves or rainfall.

Evening Behaviors and Preparing for Bed

1. **Celebrate the sunset.** I realize that evenings are a time to enjoy social gatherings, celebratory meals, and digital entertainment, so I don't want to cramp your style too much. However, I want you to do something every single day for the rest of your life: *celebrate the sunset*! This wondrous daily occurrence is quite a sight when you're out hiking or fishing, but it also has profound implications for

important biological processes. For billions of years, the rising and setting of the sun has calibrated the cellular functions of every living organism on earth. Our hormone secretions, cognitive processes, cellular-repair functions, and immune responses are tied to a circadian rhythm.

When the sun sets, your mind and body begin a natural and graceful transition into mellow evening mode and eventually sleep. Do the best you can to not interfere with this biological drive: finish workouts, meals, and screen entertainment as early in the evening as possible. Never view emotionally intense programming, engage in arguments, or discuss stressful personal financial or household matters in the evening hours. Make sunset a revered occasion, and table anything that can be considered highly stimulating until the next day.

2. **Minimize blue light exposure.** The most urgent health priority after dark is to greatly minimize your exposure to the artificial "blue light" that is emitted by screens and indoor lighting. Blue light is the highest-energy wavelength of visible light; the sky and the ocean look blue because high-energy, short-wavelength blue light scatters more easily than other visible light when it hits air or water in the atmosphere. Humans benefit from extensive exposure to the blue light in sunshine during the daytime, but blasting our eyeballs with bright indoor lights and screen emissions all day long and into the night has been shown to increase the risk of macular degeneration.

Our circadian rhythms are counting on zero blue light after dark, so indoor lighting and digital screens have a highly destructive effect on various hormonal functions. They have a particularly negative effect on dim light melatonin onset (DLMO), which is an important circadian process that helps you wind down cognitive and metabolic activity; lower heart rate, blood pressure, and body temperature; and eventually get you feeling sluggish and drowsy so you can cycle through various sleep stages, from REM to deep sleep. Research suggests that routine evening screen use can suppress melatonin levels by 50 percent. Melatonin is the hormone that induces sleepiness, but it also delivers potent antioxidant, anti-inflammatory, cell-repair, and genetic-regulation benefits. Hours of bright light and digital stimulation after dark override many other extremely delicate and health-critical circadian functions relating to rest and restoration. Instead of the genetically programmed wind-down that happens naturally after dark, continuous light exposure causes spikes in cortisol and ghrelin, generates an increase in insulin resistance, and hampers leptin signaling. In essence, blue light exposure at night can lead to sugar cravings and fat storage.

Fortunately, you can implement an assortment of strategies to minimize evening light exposure. Light sources that emit orange, yellow, or red hues do not disrupt melatonin production the same way blue light does. It makes sense that we have genetically adapted to firelight! Replace some of your regular lightbulbs with orange bulbs (sold as "bug" bulbs at home supply stores), or try the newly popular vintage tungsten bulbs, which have an orange filament visible inside the glass. The orange glow of Himalayan salt lamps evokes nature and tranquility. Salt lamps are also believed to attract airborne pathogens, trap them, and release energetically charged air molecules known as negative ions into stagnant indoor air. You can also wear the rose-, orange-, or yellow-lens glasses that are rated with UV protection during the evening hours, especially if you are watching television or using your phone or computer. A light lens color allows you to see well indoors, and the UV protection blocks most or all of the harmful blue light. Visit RAOptics.com to shop for stylish pairs or get inexpensive UVEX lenses online. Make sure your eyewear has a UV protection rating. If you insist on using screens after dark, download the free program f.lux (JustGetFlux.com) or purchase the inexpensive and more sophisticated IrisTech (IrisTech.co) software. Always enable the Night Shift feature on iOS devices or Night Mode on Android. These technologies help soften the intensity of the light emitting from your screen so that it's better synchronized to the nature of the light in your environment.

If you are working on a machine running f.lux software at precisely sunset, you'll notice an elegant shifting of the screen's "color temperature," a description of a light source's warmth (orange/yellow hues) or coolness (blue hues). Color temperature is measured on a scale of Kelvin ("K") degrees. For reference, candlelight is 1900K, sunny blue sky is 10000K, while a typical LCD computer monitor runs at 6500K. Hence, at sunset, f.lux kicks in to make your computer light emission warmer, or lower on the Kelvin scale.

When it's time to go to sleep, use a high-quality sleep mask if you struggle to fall asleep, have a partner staying up late, or sleep during the daytime because of your work schedule.

3. **Put away your mobile device.** Because mobile devices are easy to use and held close to your eyes, using them around bedtime is particularly harmful. A

Harvard study revealed that habitual nighttime screen use (in comparison to nighttime reading of printed material) contributes to making you feel groggy the following morning. You will also take longer to feel fully energized. Kids are especially sensitive to evening light exposure from electronic devices. Preschool children who were exposed to bright light for one hour before bed experienced a near-total suppression of melatonin that lasted for an hour after the exposure.

If you wake during the night and reach for your phone to check the time, that temporary blast of light can suppress melatonin and spike stress hormones, keeping you awake. Checking the time can also produce anxiety about how soon your alarm will be going off. And if you get drawn into a text message or news alert in the middle of the night, your brain will quickly exit rest mode and the turbines will start spinning. This is harmful because the brain needs sustained downtime to detoxify. During a continuous period of sleep, the rate of neuron firing decreases and the volume of extracellular space between neurons increases by a whopping 60 percent. This allows the glymphatic system to flush out neurotoxic waste products that accumulate while the brain is firing hard during the day. If possible, charge your phone outside the bedroom so you won't be tempted or disturbed by it.

4. **Conduct bedtime rituals.** Do your best to create a mellow evening experience, but at the very least dedicate the final hour before bed to calming behaviors and rituals. In her bestselling book *The Sleep Revolution*, entrepreneur Arianna Huffington explains that bedtime rituals trigger the brain and body to calm down and prepare for sleep. Her favorite is to "gently escort all your devices completely out of your bedroom" when it's time to wind down. If you have trouble falling or staying asleep, implement a deliberate sequence of relaxing behaviors that appeal to you. Perhaps a brief foam-rolling session, a quick trip around the block with the dog, or a candlelight bath. Then change into your pajamas, read for a bit in bed using a strap-on headlamp or book light, and turn off the lights at the same time every evening. Mark Manson, *New York Times* bestselling author of *The Subtle Art of Not Giving a F*uck* and *Everything Is F*ucked: A Book About Hope*, describes rituals as "visual and experiential representations of what we deem important." By implementing your custom-designed bedtime ritual and doing it every night without a second thought, you create a positive feedback loop with your actions. You prove to yourself that you value and prioritize your rest.

Be aware that minimizing artificial light and digital stimulation after dark is going to cramp your style more in the winter than in the summer. This aligns with our evolutionary experience: our ancestors slept more, exercised less, and ate less (especially carbs, as previously mentioned) in the winter. Give yourself a proper winter instead of lighting up your life for hours and hours after dark. In the summertime, you can do just fine with more activity and less sleep. In *Lights Out*, authors Wiley and Formby suggest that eight hours of sleep is a good goal in the summer but that we humans may need up to nine and a half hours per night in the winter!

And finally, when you arise from a good night's sleep...

5. **Celebrate the sunrise.** Optimizing evening sleep actually begins first thing in the morning with going outside and exposing your eyeballs to direct sunlight. When natural sunlight hits your retina, it travels down the optic nerve to the suprachiasmatic nucleus (SCN), in the hypothalamus. The SCN is considered the "master clock" of your circadian rhythm. It responds to light exposure by kick-starting and synchronizing an assortment of desirable cognitive, hormonal, and endocrine functions. For example, the SCN triggers a spike of energizing hormones such as serotonin, cortisol, and adenosine in the morning, making you feel alert and energized for a productive day. Darkness in the evening prompts the conversion of serotonin into melatonin, the hormone that makes you feel sleepy and influences dozens of other repair and restoration functions overnight. The SCN morning mechanisms are most potent right around sunrise, so getting to bed at the appropriate time, awakening as close as possible to dawn, and getting outside immediately will help you leverage your genetic potential for high-energy days.

Rest, Recovery, and Downtime

Getting out of bed after a good sleep and going full throttle until you collapse into bed again is behavior that is not aligned with health. It's essential to include actual downtime throughout the day—napping, resting, relaxing, daydreaming, contemplating nature, and generally unplugging from hyperconnectivity. Our brains are not capable of processing the massive amount of stimulation we face all day long without a breather.

While it might be easy to neglect downtime in order to accomplish more, more, more during each jam-packed day, it's important to realize that the hectic pace of modern life is a massive disconnect from our ancestral experience as hunter-gatherers. Humans are definitely adapted for brief bursts of peak physical and cognitive performance, and our ancestors had incredible amounts of rest, relaxation, and leisure time to balance the effects of the often harsh life-or-death challenges of primal life. Studies of the !Kung bush people, modern-day hunter-gatherers living in southern Africa's Kalahari Desert, have found that they spend three hours a day tending to basic needs and habitat chores and five hours a day hunting and gathering food. On the other side of the coin, they spend a whopping six hours per day in leisure activity (play, family connection, group socializing) and ten hours sleeping or napping. Even the patterns of our parents' and grandparents' generations were incredibly different from our patterns today. Hard work and intense concentration were part of the picture, but there was much more time for leisure, relaxation, and rejuvenation.

Today, we have effectively crowded out every opportunity for stillness, contemplation, and cognitive refreshment with the use of mobile and other electronic devices. Hyperconnectivity is alluring and addictive because the stimulation that arrives from text messages and social media posts delivers what psychologists call "intermittent variable rewards." The quintessential example of an intermittent variable reward is the highly addictive slot machine. Obtaining instant gratification from mobile technology delivers a burst of the feel-good neurotransmitter dopamine in the brain. In Dr. Robert Lustig's book *The Hacking of the American Mind*, he explains that repeatedly flooding the brain with dopamine suppresses the brain's receptors for serotonin, the neurotransmitter responsible for long-term happiness and contentment. The great philosophers throughout history have recognized that a life well lived entails persevering through difficult challenges and setbacks in order to solve problems and make a contribution to something greater than ourselves. Unfortunately, overdosing on dopamine makes us incapable of focusing attention on tasks that are less exciting but potentially vastly more meaningful and ultimately more rewarding.

Beyond hyperconnectivity, Dr. Lustig mentions many other dopamine triggers, including sugar, caffeine, illegal drugs, prescription antidepressants, excessive exercise, and the disturbing combination of video games and internet pornography—as well as the insidious marketing forces that entice us to indulge in them. Dr. John Gray, the number one bestselling relationship author of all time and the creator of the *Men Are from Mars, Women Are from Venus* franchise, contends that the latter two have particularly dire consequences for society. They hijack and satisfy the young male's most prominent biological drives to the extent that his motivation to pursue real-life career goals and relationships is diminished. The following suggestions will help you obtain the rest, recovery, and downtime necessary to combat the nonstop stimulation of modern life.

1. **Discipline your use of technology.** Mobile connectivity is one of the greatest technological breakthroughs of our lifetime, but with amazing progress comes a serious downside. Hyperconnectivity is compromising our live, interpersonal relationships and leading to record rates of loneliness, isolation, anxiety, and depression. Our dopamine fixation inhibits not only the happiness and contentment generated by serotonin-boosting pursuits but also the sense of love and connection delivered by the social bonding hormone oxytocin. Because the comparatively humdrum social interactions that stimulate oxytocin are no match for the dopamine hits delivered by our Twitter feeds, we withdraw into social isolation without realizing it.

   Your health and well-being depend on your developing the extreme discipline necessary to power down technology at the appropriate times. Like Mister Rogers changing out of work clothes and donning his signature sweater upon arriving home, you can perhaps implement some distinct transitions and boundaries so that personal, social, and family times are free from digital interference. The French government is on board with this thinking, having instituted the El Khomri law in 2017. Known as the "right to disconnect," the measure promotes work-life balance in concert with France's government-mandated thirty-five-hour workweek and five weeks of annual vacation.

   Powering down during family time and other live, interpersonal social interactions after a busy workday is an obvious choice, but it's also important to exercise restraint when powering up in the morning. A study conducted by the prominent global market research firm International Data Corporation revealed that 79 percent of Americans check their smartphones within fifteen minutes of awakening, and 46 percent check them before getting out of bed. When you engage with a device as soon as you wake up, you lock your brain into reactive, short-attention-span, dopamine-craving mode. In doing so, you compromise your capacity to engage in more desirable executive functions in the morning, such as strategically planning your day. Psychiatrist Nikole Benders-Hadi believes that when you immediately reach for the phone, "the information overload that hits before you're fully awake...interferes with your ability to prioritize tasks...[and] you are more likely to increase stress and feel overwhelmed."

Consider establishing a deliberate, custom-designed morning routine of enjoyable activities that quickly boost energy and mood, including light yoga stretches, flexibility and mobility exercises, a meditation session, writing in your gratitude journal, or leashing up the dog for a quick stroll. Create a specific and repeatable routine that you can follow habitually without needing to muster motivation, willpower, or creative energy. Do it every single day without fail so there is zero potential for distraction—everything else can wait. When you make a habit of a proactive morning routine instead of a reactive reach for intermittent variable rewards, you will become more focused and resilient against all other forms of potential distraction that await you during your busy day.

2. **Appreciate nature.** Getting outdoors into fresh air, sunlight, and open space has an immediate and profound calming effect on your mind and body. Researchers in Japan have produced extensive evidence showing that even a short immersion in a natural environment prompts a reduction in stress hormones, heart rate, and blood pressure and facilitates the transition from sympathetic to parasympathetic functioning. One study revealed that a three-day visit to the forest, including daily walks, resulted in a 50 percent rise in natural killer (NK) cell activity in the immune system, and the beneficial effects lasted for a full month afterward! The Japanese have a national public health program called Shinrin-yoku, translated as "forest bathing." At hundreds of designated therapy bases across the country, participants can enjoy an expert-guided nature walk, enroll in health classes, and even receive medical checkups. England, Norway, the Netherlands, Scotland, and the United States all have ambitious nature-immersion programs integrated into traditional medical care. Dr. Daphne Miller of the University of California at San Francisco coined the term *park prescription*, explaining that "nature has the possibility to be a health care intervention, a prescription, almost like a pill. In many of the studies, there is a dose response relationship. The more you get, the better the outcome.... So don't be surprised if, at your next visit to the doctor, you are handed a trail map and itinerary along with your lab slip."

University of Michigan psychologists Rachel and (the late) Stephen Kaplan promoted their "attention restoration theory" as a way of recovering from "directed attention fatigue" caused by being bombarded with intense and constantly varied stimulation from a computer screen; the average email-centric office worker switches browser windows thirty-seven times per hour! By contrast, taking in the sight of a magnificent forest, mountain landscape, or large body of water allows your senses to engage in a passive manner, triggering a significant drop in cortisol, blood pressure, and heart rate. Retired neuroscience professor Michael Merzenich said, "The smooth surface of the ocean rarely surprises, which is also soothing. When it's landmark-free, it's naturally calming to us, much like closing your eyes is calming."

In contrast to watching the sun set over the ocean, the unnatural and unrelenting stimulus of urban life and digital technology forces us into a hypervigilant, hypersensitive, high-stress mode of mega information processing. This stimulus lights up the primitive, reactive part of the brain known as the amygdala and promotes sympathetic nervous system dominance. When it's time for peak performance, this is great. We don't want our basketball referees, computer programmers, and ER staff to be in stargazing mode! However, humans are not designed for unrelenting fight-or-flight stimulation. Directed attention fatigue makes us impulsive, distractible, and irritable. The potential for novel stimulation and distractibility offered by mobile devices makes this a serious health concern unlike any that has been seen before.

Neuron functioning is replenished not only through evening sleep and napping but also when you engage with nature in a cognitive mode that is different from directed attention, something the Kaplans call fascination. The higher the fascination value, the greater the benefit. That's why visiting Niagara Falls, the Grand Canyon, or Yosemite's Half Dome is often described as breathtaking. Less intense nature experiences can still deliver fantastic benefits. If all that's convenient is a city park, playground, or backyard, try to appreciate the experience to the fullest. Leave your phone behind and become fascinated by the flowers in the garden, the hummingbird at the feeder, and other nuances that are easy to miss when you rush through life. Devote some time every day to immersing yourself in your natural environment in order to express your full humanity—and especially to decompress from the incredibly unnatural and highly stimulating environments that have become the new normal. Amazingly, research shows that you can even obtain restorative benefits from a simulation of nature, such as a screen saver, a poster, or a mini fountain at your desk.

3. **Nap when you need to.** Your body experiences a natural dip in circadian functioning and an increase in homeostatic sleep drive around six to eight hours after awakening. For some people, the dip is mild or even unnoticeable. For those who are more sensitive, or who experience disturbances to evening sleep or have an insulin response triggered by a midday meal, the afternoon blues are enough to significantly lower energy, mood, and productivity. Dr. David Dinges, a sleep expert at University of Pennsylvania medical school, whose laboratory studies how sleep affects neurobehavioral, cognitive, immune, inflammatory, endocrine, metabolic, and genetic functioning, estimates that between 15 and 20 percent of the population is highly sensitive, calling them "closet nappers." Dr. Sara Mednick, a Harvard-trained psychologist studying sleep at the University of California at Riverside and the author of *Take a Nap! Change Your Life*, estimates that up to 50 percent of the population is genetically predisposed to napping. According to Dr. Mednick, when we go looking for alternative ways to keep alert, such as caffeinated drinks, we—"the Walking Tired"—suffer huge productivity losses.

What's more, many anthropologists and historians observe that humans have long been habituated to, and may have some genetic aptitude for, biphasic sleeping habits; sleeping for one (long) phase in the evening and a second (shorter) sleep phase in the afternoon. This dynamic was believed to be the norm in prehistoric times, where evening sleep was likely routinely interrupted to tend to a fire, care for infants, or keep watch for danger. Biphasic sleep was also the norm up until the Industrial Revolution. A. Roger Ekirch, author of *At Day's Close: Night in Times Past,* explains that the working class of the Middle Ages would fall asleep soon after dark, then naturally awaken in the middle of the night and enjoy what was essentially their only leisure time. Erkich's detailed historical analysis of hundreds of diaries, court documents, medical books, and literature from centuries ago revealed that night was a time for sex, prayer, writing, interpreting dreams, visiting neighbors, or even petty crimes. Modern research on subjects deprived of light for weeks at a time reveals that humans seem to naturally drift toward a similar sleep pattern to the one described by Erkich.

This evidence suggests that today's norm of a single sustained monophasic evening sleep period is a product of the industrial age more than genetics. Extended workdays that preclude napping, combined with artificially lit evenings that keep us awake long past sunset, conspire to make us tired enough to crash until morning. While it's not likely society will transform to make polyphasic sleep the norm once again, you can do your best to optimize health in modern life by committing to dark, mellow evenings and taking an afternoon nap whenever you experience even a slight decline in mood, energy, or focus during the afternoon. Extensive research, especially among peak performers such as NASA astronauts and elite athletes, confirms that naps deliver comprehensive improvements in alertness, productivity, concentration, memory, mood, metabolic functioning, and physical performance.

Have you ever felt "fried" during or after a hectic day of hyperconnectivity and multitasking? This aptly named feeling occurs when the sodium-potassium pumps that enable your brain neurons to fire their electrical impulses become depleted through excessive use. Maintaining an optimal ion balance is critical to efficient energy processing in all cells. In the brain, sodium-potassium pump operations account for 70 percent of total energy output. A twenty-minute nap is not too much to ask for anyone and constitutes sufficient time to help replenish and reboot those fried electrical circuits. Your reward when you return to work is a tremendous and immediate boost in alertness. That said, even a ten-minute nap has been found to deliver increases in energy and cognitive performance lasting for two and a half hours after the nap. Another study revealed that simply anticipating a nap can lower blood pressure! If you are feeling really trashed (perhaps from jet lag), battling a minor illness, or struggling in the aftermath of an extreme physical effort, a nap of ninety minutes will enable you to complete a full sleep cycle, as you do repeatedly overnight.

Whenever you feel the need to nap, try to find a quiet area away from your workplace and initiate some ritual behavior triggers that tell your brain and body it's nap time. Start by donning a quality eye mask to block out light, then launch a smartphone app with sounds of ocean waves or a rainfall. If you can't fall asleep on cue, take comfort knowing that merely disengaging from peak cognitive functioning for a respite delivers substantial restorative benefits. Over time, you can expect to become more adept at nodding off and enjoying maximum cellular, hormonal, and physiological benefits. If you don't have a convenient napping location where you work, at the very least arrange for some do-not-disturb time and make sure you are able to rest your head on your desk, aircraft tray table, or other stationary object (support from your hands and arms is fine).

Unfortunately, there seems to be a lot of pushback about napping: many people claim they don't need naps or insist they can't fall asleep even when they try. I propose that we might be too tired to realize when we really need a nap—or at least a break from the computer screen. Sleep deprivation hinders assorted executive functions, such as self-awareness, impulse control, and the ability to resist distractions. A twenty-minute nap that could have set you up for a productive afternoon instead becomes twenty minutes wasted on clickbait and Instagram scrolling, followed by hours of slightly or severely diminished cognitive sharpness as you limp to the finish line of the workday.

What if you proactively added a nap to your daily schedule, perhaps in place of your routine stop at the coffee shop for a latte? Research suggests that making napping a habit can turn you into a happier person. In their bestselling parenting book, *NurtureShock*, authors Po Bronson and Ashley Merryman explain that insufficient sleep inhibits our ability to store and recall pleasant memories: "Negative stimuli get processed by the amygdala; positive or neutral memories get processed by the hippocampus. Sleep deprivation hits the hippocampus harder than the amygdala. The result is that sleep-deprived people fail to recall pleasant memories yet recall gloomy memories just fine." The idea is that your evening sleep won't always be ideal, so napping is a great opportunity to shore up any transient deficiencies in optimum sleep. This makes you a more focused, disciplined, energetic, and hippocampusly happy person.

Increase General Everyday Movement

Our ancestors were in near constant movement all day long in order to thrive in a survival-of-the-fittest hunter-gatherer existence. When we move our bodies in various ways, we support the complex and synchronous interactions between organs and systems throughout the body that enable peak cognitive and physical performance. When we anchor our modern human butts on a chair for hours on end in the name of productivity, the vitality of the human organism gets severely compromised. This includes quick and significant declines in cognitive, metabolic, and musculoskeletal functioning.

Being still also sabotages your fat-reduction goals. As little as twenty minutes of sitting has been shown to cause a significant decrease in glucose tolerance and an increase in insulin resistance. Sitting for longer periods triggers a series of unfortunate metabolic events. Spending a full day at your desk results in a 50 percent reduction in the enzyme activity that converts triglycerides (the stored form of fat) into free fatty acids to burn for energy. As you learned from the discussion of the compensation theory, losing excess body fat is not a matter of eating less and working out more but rather of hormone optimization. It's not about the calories that you burn during workouts, it's about maintaining an active lifestyle to send the right signals to your genes. It takes climbing twenty flights of stairs to burn off the calories in one slice of bread, but when you build lifelong habits of movement instead of stillness—taking the stairs instead of the elevator—you send signals to your genes to burn fat instead of sugar.

If you declare your workday to be too jam-packed to allow regular movement breaks, note that prolonged stillness causes drastically diminished cognitive performance and increases distractibility and fatigue. Studies confirm that spending a few hours at your desk during a busy morning results in a reduction in blood flow and oxygen delivery to the brain as well as a disruption in neurotransmitter signaling that invites mood swings and depression. Even more disturbing is the fact that a stillness-oriented lifestyle can result in long-term damage to the brain's temporal lobes, which are responsible for memory. Research has confirmed a direct link between inactivity and diminished brain functioning as well as elevated risk of dementia. A 2017 study conducted at UCLA revealed that senior citizens who fall short of a modest minimum activity level—four thousand steps per day—had thinner hippocampi, slower processing speeds, inferior working memory for quick decisions, and inferior memory consolidation compared to their active counterparts.

You can counteract brain drain extremely well by taking frequent movement breaks for walking and other activities. This has been found to be vastly more effective than cranking away for hours, then taking an extended break. Even a single moderate-intensity walk has been shown to boost production of the lauded *brain-derived neurotrophic factor* (BDNF). Nicknamed "Miracle-Gro for the brain" by Harvard psychiatry professor Dr. John Ratey, BDNF helps you build new neurons and improve the firing of existing neurons, increase blood circulation and oxygen delivery throughout the body, reduce depression and anxiety, and improve neuroplasticity. This describes the brain's ability to form new connections and pathways throughout life, making you more adaptable to everyday stress and inevitable change.

Prolonged sitting also causes an assortment of musculoskeletal and cardiovascular problems. Hip flexors and hamstrings shorten and tighten. Gluteal muscles are deactivated, making your balance and gait unstable during exercise. The lack of engagement of the abdominal core muscles (which are constantly activated when standing, walking, and performing all manner of physical work) promotes an assortment of postural imbalances and puts excessive strain on the spine and back muscles.

Biomechanist Katy Bowman, author of *Move Your DNA*, *Don't Just Sit There*, and numerous other books about healthful movement, explains: "Cells are always responding to mechanical input via a process called *mechanotransduction*. When individual cells are unmoved or undermoved, they adapt to repetitive positioning by changing their cellular makeup and literally becoming sticky and stiff. Even those who are superfit can have certain muscles and joints with reduced range of motion and an actual hardening of arterial walls in certain areas; for example, sitting in a chair all day with bent knees." It's indeed possible to possess cardiovascular fitness (an aptitude for grueling endurance workouts) but have poor cardiovascular health, evidenced by an inability to efficiently deliver oxygen to all your organs and tissues.

Bowman promotes a "Nutritious Movement" concept that compels us to broaden our perspective beyond the pursuit of narrow fitness goals through traditional workouts on the track or in the gym. While there are many benefits to becoming fit or superfit, our *Homo sapiens* genes crave a life of constant movement and variation. Because most of us are obligated to sit with keyboard and screen to get work done, the objective is to minimize the negative effects of commuting, office work, and our propensity to indulge in screen entertainment during leisure time. You can do this by finding assorted ways to increase the frequency and variety of your daily movement patterns. Fitness freaks should pay special attention. Often people who follow a devoted fitness regimen and have lofty athletic goals are guilty of taking free license to be lazy outside of workouts instead of achieving a modest quota of general everyday movement.

Just F---ing Walk

Just f---ing walk (JFW) is my way of expressing what should form the centerpiece of your daily movement objective. Walking is the quintessential human form of locomotion, and it has been disastrously neglected in modern life. Our primal ancestors walked for miles every single day as an integral part of survival. Dr. Loren Cordain cites research revealing that modern-day hunter-gatherers walk between 3.7 and nine miles each day in search of food, water, and wood. Mothers carry their children for the first four years, logging some three thousand miles. You may have heard the popular recommendation to take ten thousand steps (around five miles) per day? Americans average only half that, amounting to a paltry 2.5 miles per day. This is below what's needed to avoid the label "sedentary." Americans are lagging behind countries such as Australia and Switzerland, whose citizens walk nearly twice as far as we do each day. We are certainly far more inactive than our parents' and grandparents' generations: after all, traditional Amish farmers walk nearly four times more than their high-tech counterparts today.

While the physical health risks of sedentary living are well publicized, there are also intangible costs when we marginalize walking in modern life. Granted, it's tough to imagine following in the footsteps of Henry David Thoreau, who famously stated, "I cannot preserve my health and spirits, unless I spend four hours a day at least—and it is commonly more than that—sauntering through the woods and over the hills and fields, absolutely free from all worldly engagement." However, we can all reflect on the pointed observation from author Rebecca Solnit in her book *Wanderlust*: "Walking as a cultural activity, as a pleasure, as travel, as a way of getting around, is fading, and with it goes an ancient and profound relationship between body, world, and imagination."

Walking is a topic near and dear to my heart, because I experienced a profound revelation after my move from Malibu to Miami Beach. As you may have heard, nobody walks in LA. This is particularly true in Malibu, where the busy Pacific Coast Highway—wholly unfit for pedestrians—is the obligatory route to and from anywhere. My high-density high-rise living in Miami Beach offers the opposite experience. Carrie and I walk everywhere, to the tune of at least five miles each day, not counting our designated workouts. I rarely drive unless I'm headed out of town or catching a ride home via Uber after walking to the supermarket. I feel more connected to my community than I ever did during my car-centric decades in Malibu. I notice that I can process emotions and complex work challenges better when I'm on the move. It also seems like I have a higher baseline of cardiovascular fitness, better posture, more flexibility, and better core stability from which to launch all my other workouts, all thanks to my daily walking habit.

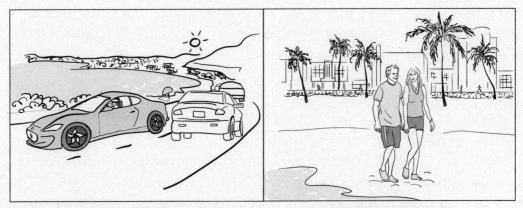

Pacific Coast Highway (PCH), Malibu, CA
Pedestrians? Can't Happen!

South Beach, Miami, FL
Walking Wonderland!

Workday Breaks

Your brain is capable of focusing intently on a peak cognitive task for approximately twenty minutes before your cognitive processing power begins to decline. Consequently, make an effort to briefly get away from your screen and move your body a bit every twenty minutes. You will get a boost of energy even if you stand up briefly to balance on one leg or do a few of Katy Bowman's "wall angels" (like snow angels, but those sweeping arm movements are made against and along a wall), which help counteract all that hunching over the keyboard. To combat eye strain, try the optometrist-recommended 20-20-20 strategy: take a screen break every twenty minutes to gaze at an object twenty feet away for twenty seconds. Do this while you complete a set of twenty deep squats—the Sisson 20-20-20-20!

Every hour, take a more structured five-minute break from sitting and your screen, ideally getting outside for a quick stroll or making a brief but intense physical effort at something (for example, climbing a few flights of stairs or doing twenty deep squats). I like to get outdoors and take a few passes on my slackline (a wide, loose, low tightrope) to help "balance" my time in the office. Whenever possible, I take phone calls outdoors while walking around the neighborhood or doing gentle stretches or strengthening exercises at home. Please also strive for a formal midday break of thirty minutes or more to completely disengage from technology and your workplace environment and get some much-needed mind and body restoration. This might entail a nap, a workout, or a stroll through the park to watch the birds. If you spend lots of evening leisure time in front of a screen, take breaks between episodes to bust out a five-minute foam-rolling session, micro workout, or yoga sequence (great ways to trigger parasympathetic functioning). Or take the dog for a lap around the block.

Workplace Variation

The increasingly popular stand-up desk experience is a great way to engage the muscle groups that go soft while sitting as well as increase your metabolic rate by 10 percent. However, Katy Bowman warns that merely switching from sitting to standing is not the solution, because you are still maintaining fixed positions for too long. This also applies to ergonomic chairs and custom-fitted workstations. According to Bowman, "They keep you more comfortable, so you remain sedentary for much longer before noticing the adverse effects!" Instead, strive to achieve maximum variation in the position and movement of your body throughout the workday. Bowman recommends arranging to spend work time sitting on the floor, kneeling, sitting on an exercise ball, and standing up in addition to sitting on a chair. Get a pull-up bar or at least regularly reach up and touch or hang a bit on the doorway whenever you walk through. If you're too short to reach a door frame, bend at the waist and reach forward to grab and pull on your desk, counter, or other stable object. "A dynamic work environment helps your body assume many different geometries throughout the day, which loads your cells differently and keeps your whole body, and the trillions of cellular bodies that comprise it, moving more and moving better," explains Bowman.

A high-tech hydraulic unit like the VariDesk is a great way to frequently alternate between sitting and standing. You can also use an ordinary footstool or stack of boxes to quickly elevate your keyboard and monitor. I use Focal Upright's Locus workstation, where I can stand and work at a slightly angled desk (that looks like a drafting table) but also have the option to lean back into a small pogo stick–style seat and place my feet on an elevated slanted board. While standing, you can bring in a stool or chair to elevate either leg, varying the load and engaging different muscles. You can mix things up in any chair as well by alternating between sitting on the front edge with a straight spine and sliding all the way to the back to straighten your spine against the backrest.

Taking into account any constraints at your workplace, see if you can arrange to sit on the floor or use a BOSU ball—a semicircular inflatable plastic ball with a flat bottom. Put your laptop or keyboard and monitor on a coffee table, bench, or stool and type away! If you can't do this at work, at least get a "low desk" for home. Using the wonderful terrestrial resistance provided by "ground reaction force" (your body weight in contact with the floor), you can alternately compress and stretch muscles and connective tissue all over your body. Consider how lowering yourself into a squatting position restricts blood flow along the tibialis anterior (front of the leg) until you feel the burn and exit the stretch, thereby achieving a "rebound" effect that has been shown to speed tissue healing and improve tissue integrity.

I'm so enamored of this subject that I coauthored a couple of scientific papers with performance and rehabilitation conditioning scientist Matt Wallden about the health benefits of assuming archetypal human resting positions. Search YouTube for "Mark Sisson archetypal rest postures" to learn how to long-sit, high-kneel, low-kneel, side-sit, and sit cross-legged to achieve a passive stretching and strengthening effect while working at a low desk. Use these ideas as a baseline, but realize that anything goes in pursuit of variation. When you can partner creative workstation efforts with frequent movement breaks throughout the day, you will quickly notice an improvement in focus as well as in metabolic and musculoskeletal functioning. You'll also notice that you're less distractible and don't feel fried at the end of the day. When I started using a stand-up desk, around 2010, I experienced an immediate improvement in the chronic hip flexor stiffness that had plagued me for decades despite devoted stretching. If you spend many hours each day in front of a screen, strive to achieve the most dynamic, least destructive experience you possibly can.

Yoga, Pilates, Tai Chi

If you can get into the groove of regular instructor-led classes in formal disciplines such as yoga, Pilates, or tai chi, that's fantastic. If you're too busy to make it to hourlong classes, try picking and choosing some of your favorite moves and piecing together mini routines you can do at home. YouTube is a good resource to help you learn the basics of do-it-yourself movement sessions. Search YouTube for "yoga sun salutation" to learn a series of graceful full-body movements that even a novice can master quickly. Yoga's flowing movement sequences, along with its intentional inhalations on stretching and exhalations on compressing, deliver a meditative mind-body benefit. Depending on your approach, you can achieve a purely relaxed parasympathetic session or a fantastic cardiovascular and musculoskeletal workout. Enthusiasts of hot yoga enjoy additional detoxification, immune strengthening, and mood-elevating benefits generated by the body's adaptive response to the stress of exercising in the heat.

Tai chi is practiced by millions of people every day across the world and has scientifically validated health benefits. Dr. Peter Wayne, author of *The Harvard Medical School Guide to Tai Chi*, calls tai chi "meditation on wheels." He explains, "You're getting all the cognitive pieces you might get from meditation—mental clarity and focus and positive thoughts and lower stress—but you're also getting physical exercise." Dr. Michael Irwin, psychiatry professor and director of the Mindful Awareness Research Center at UCLA, has published numerous studies about the health benefits of tai chi. A group of breast cancer survivors with insomnia who practiced tai chi experienced improvement in their levels of depression, fatigue, and inflammation—important in reducing their risk of cancer recurrence. Dr. Irwin explains that tai chi helps moderate sympathetic nervous system activity, delivering the incidental benefit of improved cardiovascular functioning at a level similar to walking or jogging. For the elderly, tai chi helps improve the important longevity factors of balance and mobility. It's sobering to realize that the US Centers for Disease Control lists falling as the number one cause of injury and death in Americans over age sixty-five. Tai chi has also been shown to alleviate symptoms of arthritis and improve heart and kidney functioning. Search YouTube for "tai chi for beginners" and find some great ways to get started.

Foam Rolling

Foam rolling—using a cylindrical foam or rubber tube to massage your muscles—counts toward your movement objectives and is a great way to wind down after workouts or a stressful day. Technically called self-myofascial release, rolling the large muscle groups of the body increases oxygen delivery and blood circulation and enhances the functioning of the lymphatic system. Even a brief session of five to ten minutes with a specially designed foam or rubber tube or rubber ball boosts circulation throughout the rolled muscle groups for up to thirty minutes afterward. Activating lymphatic functioning provides an important boost to the immune system, because the lymphatic system helps speed the removal of toxins and waste products from muscles and tissues throughout your body. The added benefit of foam rolling is that it quickly stimulates parasympathetic activity for a beautiful relaxation experience. This happens because the discomfort associated with applying pressure through tight spots causes painkilling endorphins to flood the bloodstream. You get instant relief from aching muscles and a calming sensation in your central nervous system.

For an effective session, roll along the large muscle groups of the upper and lower body, starting from the pelvis and rolling either up or down, away from your center. When you find a particularly tight spot, known as a trigger point, isolate it with extra pressure for an extended period of time. Working through a trigger point can help relieve referred pain—that is, pain felt in a part of the body resulting from an injury or imbalance in a different area. For example, rolling along the side quadriceps (vastus lateralis) can address painful IT band syndrome, in which pain occurs near the knee joint. Skip rolling on joints and connective tissue and focus on the big muscles. You can even roll through your abdomen, giving your organs an effective massage and a boost in circulation and oxygen. While it may be hard to imagine, you should be able to roll with deep pressure along entire muscle groups all over the body without experiencing pain. I know—try telling that to the calf muscles! With devoted practice, you will make tremendous progress in your ability to withstand deep pressure and should notice an improvement in mobility and a reduction in injuries when you engage in activity.

Active Leisure (Dancing, Gardening, Sex, Home Improvement Projects, Golf, Other Low-Energy-Expenditure Sports, and Sex)

You may have seen those charts showing that gardening for an hour burns three hundred calories, while a medium Jamba Juice and a PowerBar deliver around six hundred calories—and feel the urge to head right over to a sweaty, grueling boot-camp class that burns seven hundred calories. But as you've learned, when you're trying to improve your health, the emphasis must be placed on hormone optimization instead of calorie tallies. In this context, a variety of movements make an excellent contribution to the ultimate goal of hormone optimization. And there are many additional benefits to moving around outdoors, in open space, including breathing fresh air and getting some much-needed sunlight. JFW and anything you can do beyond that will help improve your balance and spatial awareness—which are important for all manner of fitness activities, for everyday home chores, and as protection against the high-morbidity risk of falling.

Even if you're engaging in active leisure indoors, you are still enjoying many benefits and achieving a critical counterpoint to days of hyperconnectivity. Little things like straightening up the garage or throwing the ball for the dog in the yard help improve balance, spatial awareness, mobility, and flexibility. I find that routine household chores can have a meditative effect in which the brain can relax into repetitive mind-body behaviors without the intensity that's demanded when you engage in peak cognitive tasks. When you realize that a life of near constant movement is essential to your humanity as well as a necessary component of metabolic flexibility, peak physical and cognitive performance, happiness, and longevity, it makes it easy to get moving.

Comfortably Paced Cardiovascular Workouts

By being sedentary and living life primarily indoors, we have eliminated many natural opportunities to get cardiovascular exercise, so it's important to engage in two to five hours per week of structured cardiovascular workouts in the activity of your choice: walking, jogging (if you are really fit), bicycling, swimming, participating in water sports such as stand-up paddling (my personal favorite!), and using cardio machines in the gym. The

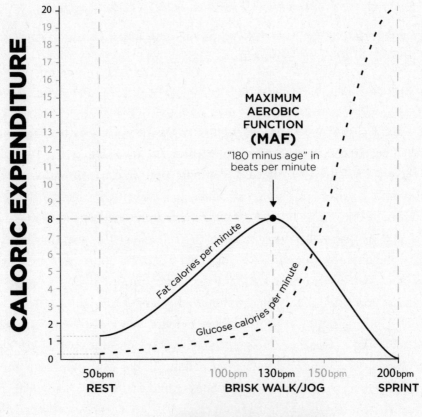

most important element of these sessions is that you exercise in the aerobic heart rate zone. This entails a *very* comfortably paced workout that emphasizes fat burning, supports general health and immune functioning, and leaves you feeling refreshed and energized at the end instead of fatigued. Dr. Phil Maffetone, author of *The Big Book of Endurance Training and Racing*, is regarded as a pioneer in fat-adapted endurance training and has coached many world champion endurance athletes. His "180 minus age" formula identifies the heart rate (180 minus age in beats per minute) corresponding with your maximum aerobic function (MAF). For example, a fifty-year-old would calculate 180 minus 50, or 130, for her MAF heart rate in beats per minute. This is the heart rate where you are burning the maximum amount of fat calories per minute, with a minimal amount of anaerobic stimulation or glucose burning.

In this example, the maximum number of fat calories are burned at a heart rate of 130 beats per minute. Increasing the heart rate and picking up the pace would obviously result in more calories being burned per minute, but a rapidly increasing percentage of them would come from glucose rather than fat. At your MAF heart rate, the effort is surprisingly easy, so that most exercisers of all ability levels routinely exceed MAF by ten, twenty, or even thirty beats at a typical workout. This is particularly true if you participate in instructor-led group classes at the gym or join social running and cycling groups on the road. At these higher heart rates, you experience the familiar perceived exertion levels, and the workout can be described as medium to difficult. These sessions invigorate you and give you a sense of satisfaction with a job well done, but they also generate a bit more stress hormones and cellular waste products and require a longer recovery time. Working at this elevated heart rate also compromises your metabolic flexibility goals because it promotes glucose burning—both during the workout and around the clock. It's not about burning more calories by going faster; rather, it's about burning mostly fat while you work out so you can improve your fat metabolism at rest.

Please understand that individual workouts that exceed MAF heart rate are no trouble to complete, and going a little or a lot harder than MAF once in a while can prompt a desirable fitness adaptation. The problem comes when exceeding MAF becomes the norm, because this almost always leads to breakdown, burnout, illness, and injury. By slowing down and conducting workouts at or anywhere below your MAF heart rate (remember, all manner of everyday movement delivers valuable cardiovascular and fat-burning benefits), you increase energy and alertness all day long, boost immune functioning, optimize hormonal functioning (particularly the reproductive hormones testosterone and estrogen, which are so sensitive to overstress patterns), and promote neurotransmitter balance for better mood stability, concentration, and a baseline happy disposition. By contrast, you may know from personal experience that overly ambitious workouts give you an endorphin buzz for a couple of hours afterward but often prompt afternoon blues, sugar cravings, evening exhaustion, and the previously mentioned cellular destruction and ammonia toxicity in the ensuing days.

Disciplining yourself to conduct almost all your cardio workouts at MAF heart rates works for everyone, from novices to hard-core athletes with ambitious athletic goals. A novice who associates exercise with suffering will be pleased to discover that properly paced workouts can be enjoyable and energizing. Competitive types should note that the training patterns and performances of elite athletes in every endurance sport for the past sixty years have proved that slowing down helps you go faster on the racecourse. This is because aerobic training allows you to continually improve your aerobic capacity without the interruptions of high-stress workouts that cause cell destruction, suppressed immune functioning, hormone imbalances, and extended recovery times.

The MAF Test to Measure Aerobic Improvement, Protect Against Overtraining, and Keep You Focused and Motivated

For motivated types who have difficultly slowing down, obtaining tangible proof of your fitness progress can help keep you on track. The best way to quantify aerobic improvement is to regularly perform a maximum aerobic functioning (MAF) test. (Note: You'll conduct this test on day 2 of the 12-Day Turbocharge.) While the test is not strenuous, improving your speed at a comfortable aerobic pace obviously improves your competitive potential in any activity requiring a modicum of endurance—i.e., virtually every athletic endeavor! If you deliver a slower time in an MAF test, this is a strong indication that you are suffering from overstress or overtraining patterns and require more rest and recovery.

The MAF test entails timing yourself over a fixed course at a fixed heart rate and repeating the exact same protocol every six weeks or so to track improvement or regression. Choose the activity of your highest competency and preference, whether it's jogging, cycling up a hill, or exercising on cardio machines that measure output in speed or distance. You can use a stationary bike, a rowing machine, an elliptical machine, or—my personal favorite—a VersaClimber. For the most accurate results, choose a distance or course that takes at least ten minutes to complete. This might involve jogging four to six laps around a running track, cycling from the base of a hill to a specific landmark, or using a cardio machine to achieve a specific measured performance. Ten minutes is sufficient for a novice, while experienced athletes can choose a longer duration. Try to maintain a heart rate as close as possible to "180 minus age" in beats per minute for the entirety of the test. Your heart rate is bound to bounce above and below that number a bit; do the best you can to regulate your pace throughout. Hint: this means you will likely have to slow down a bit toward the end to ensure that your heart rate (not your pace) is consistent.

Regularly performing the MAF test will keep you honest and committed to the big-picture objective of steadily building your aerobic capacity without the interruptions caused by high-stress workouts that require extended recovery time. Building aerobic capacity requires extreme patience and restraint: you must resist the temptation to push the pace in pursuit of a shortcut to fitness breakthroughs. Having quantifiable proof that you are getting faster and more aerobically efficient will help you see the light at the end of the tunnel.

You'll need to use a wireless heart-rate monitor with a chest transmitter to ensure the most accurate readings over time. This technology is superior to the pulse meters on the Apple Watch and other devices as well as to the pulse trackers built into treadmills and other cardio machines. Polar is the leading brand of wireless heart-rate monitors, and basic models like the Polar FT1 can be found online for $50 to $75. Get your unit as soon as possible and become familiar with it so you'll be ready during the Turbocharge. Feel free to perform an MAF test at your earliest convenience, because this will give you another comparative data point in addition to the Turbocharge tests.

Don't be dissuaded by the misdirected competitive energy that many recreational performers exhibit during training, pushing themselves to the point of breakdown. Consider the example of Eliud Kipchoge, from Kenya, a world and Olympic champion marathoner who broke the unfathomable two-hour-marathon barrier in 2019. Kipchoge published his training log on the internet for all to scrutinize, and the insights were astounding. Veteran observers were shocked to discover that Kipchoge runs well within his capacity at virtually every workout. Much of his training is done at around 80 percent of maximum effort (very similar to the MAF calculation) with extremely minimal variation from week to week. Even when pushing the absolute limits of human endurance, Kipchoge avoids the common crash-and-burn patterns of exhaustion, overtraining, illness, and injury typically experienced by other endurance runners.

One young friend of mine, an accomplished American collegiate runner with a sub-four-minute mile to his credit but still well below international elite caliber, was astonished to discover that his big workouts were tougher than those of the greatest endurance runner of all time! The next time you are doing a jog-walk and feeling frustrated that you are hardly getting a workout, yet your heart-monitor alarm is beeping at your aerobic max, consider that in relative terms, you are pushing your body harder than an elite athlete does. Remember, pushing hard more than occasionally is not only unnecessary but also highly counterproductive to your fat-burning goals and hormonal health. Slow down, burn fat, have fun, live awesome!

Conduct Brief, Intense Workouts

We have a genetic imperative to challenge our bodies on a regular basis with intense bursts of muscular strength and all-out sprinting. These types of efforts—brief in duration and explosive in nature, elicit a comprehensive adaptive response in organs and systems throughout the body. You become physically stronger, more resilient to all forms of stress, accelerate fat metabolism around the clock, build or preserve lean muscle mass, increase bone density, optimize hormonal and neurotransmitter functioning, grow more brain neurons, stimulate mitochondrial biogenesis, enhance the functional capacity of your organs to operate above their baseline (a.k.a. your *organ reserve*, a key longevity attribute), strengthen your cardiovascular system, enhance immune functioning, and essentially escape from the accelerated demise into feeble old age that is the norm today.

Unfortunately, the comforts, conveniences, and luxuries of modern life have us neglecting this key component of health, vitality, disease prevention, and longevity more than ever. Because modern humans no longer face the major environmental selection pressures that drove human evolution—starvation and predator danger—evolution has officially ceased, and modern humans have literally gone soft. While none of us is interested in battling a mighty woolly beast for tonight's dinner, we must find ways to approximate the challenges that made our ancestors lean, strong, fast, and resilient in order to avoid the atrophy that we erroneously associate with chronological aging today. While chronological aging will always have some influence on declining peak performance over the years, honoring the natural law of "use it or lose it" can help you greatly neutralize the impact of your birthday candles and ensure that you remain strong and powerful throughout life.

While many fitness enthusiasts do well with cardiovascular exercise (provided they slow down into the MAF heart rate zone!), it's less common to perform the brief, explosive efforts that deliver perhaps the most time-efficient return on your health-boosting investment. The good news is that you can transform your physique and your physiology by doing just a couple of deliberate strength workouts a week, lasting between ten and thirty minutes; a brief sprint session each week (with just one to two minutes of maximum effort in total); and a weekly sprinkling of micro workouts, which are rapidly becoming the most exciting emerging trend in fitness.

It's time to do away with any doubts you may have about going hard and acknowledge that explosive efforts are essential for everyone, not just bros in muscle shirts. Research shows that senior citizens have the ability to make faster incremental gains in strength and power than any other age group and can attain strength standards and sex hormone levels in blood tests that are similar to those of unfit people who are decades younger. Numerous studies of large population groups reveal a direct correlation between longevity and attributes such as grip strength, squat competency, and push-up competency. Arguably, the older we get, the more we stand to gain from intense exercise, because it staves off the most prominent ravages of aging—*sarcopenia* (muscle loss) and declines in balance and motor control, which lead to falling.

Integrating intense exercise into your lifestyle can be simple and, most important, sustainable. First, intense workouts can be scaled to your current level of fitness. Strength training can use your own body weight as well as low-tech stretch bands and tubes. Sprinting can be done with no-impact or low-impact exercises, although maximum benefits come from weight-bearing sprints. Choose an entry point that seems comfortable to you and try new things as you build confidence over time.

Most important, your workouts must be structured correctly. You'll get the most benefit from workouts that are less than thirty minutes in duration and feature brief, explosive efforts with sufficient rest between them. This is how you trigger a desirable temporary fight-or-flight hormone surge for comprehensive adaptive and antiaging benefits. This contrasts with the popular HIIT (high-intensity interval training) format characteristic of most group exercise classes, endurance running clubs, instructor-guided video programming (such as stationary cycling and other home-based workouts), and team sport practices. HIIT workouts typically involve an excessive number of work efforts that last a bit too long with insufficient rest between them. As you learned from the discussion of liquidating your assets (see page 70), the cumulative fatigue from the intervals and the extended duration of the workout can often result in cellular destruction, chronic glycogen depletion (and major sugar cravings), and exhaustion. Following are some suggestions for effective strength and sprint workouts.

Strength Training Options

There are many strength training methods that can produce excellent results, provided you adhere to some big-picture recommendations. The best movements are sweeping, full-body functional movements that recruit numerous large muscle groups—those that correspond to real-life physical activity. Examples include squats, dead lifts, leg presses, box jumps, push-ups, pull-ups, overhead presses, rope climbs, kettlebell swings, sweeping movements with cables, straps, or stretch cords, and much more. By contrast, working isolated muscle groups within a confined range of motion using a dumbbell or a machine is certainly better than sitting at home, but you'll enjoy more sport-specific fitness, antiaging, and injury-prevention benefits when you perform compound movements. Whatever type of exercise you choose, always strive to execute the explosive movements with excellent form. If you notice your technique or explosiveness compromised by cumulative fatigue, it's time to end the set and eventually end the workout.

Choose workouts that you enjoy and that are convenient and sustainable. Home fitness systems and machine circuits at the gym provide a measure of safety and ease of use for novices. Lifting free weights on a barbell requires precise technique and carries a relatively high risk of injury, causing many people to avoid it. However, people who get serious about lifting are enthralled by the wide-ranging physical and psychological benefits of living a strong, confident, resilient life. Start with some basic two-handed kettlebell swings, and you may quickly become interested in doing more heavy lifting. If you want to try the popular CrossFit scene or other branded fitness programs such as Orangetheory Fitness or F45 Training, perhaps you'll form a community bond in addition to getting in top shape.

Be advised, however, that a typical instructor-guided group workout lasts a bit too long for my liking and invites injury, burnout, and attrition. I know it's uncomfortable to imagine bailing out of a high-energy group class at the two-thirds mark, but I urge you to take full responsibility for your workout decisions and have the courage to follow your intuition. If you notice your form breaking, muscle groups tightening, concentration wavering, or a spike in your rate of perceived exertion in the latter stages of a group workout, cut it short and realize that you have very likely hit the sweet spot for workout effectiveness. When I was an elite marathoner and triathlete, my peers and I tried to honor the mantra "It's better to be 10 percent undertrained than 2 percent overtrained."

Resistance bands, tubes, and cords offer an easy, convenient, and affordable way to conduct a great strength training session at home or when traveling. You can perform all manner of resistance exercises with less risk of muscle soreness and injury than you incur when lifting heavy weights. Everything will fit into a small basket (or backpack when traveling), and each item costs less than a month's gym membership. The StretchCordz product is made with rubber tubing of various thicknesses, featuring an attachment strap in the middle and handles on both ends. Mini bands (Perform Better is a leading brand) strap around your ankles and offer an excellent way to activate your long-lost gluteal muscles and get your world rocked in less than a minute. The X3 Bar uses thick resistance bands to facilitate an assortment of full-body exercises that simulate lifting a heavy bar: squats, dead lifts, bench presses, overhead presses, and more, but with less risk of injury and muscle soreness. In all these examples, you can get products of various thicknesses (i.e., degrees of resistance) to align with your experience level.

I'm a huge fan of both gym machines and free weights, and my neighborhood gym has been a favorite social hub for me for decades. I work really hard a couple of days a week in thirty-minute sessions featuring compound movements such as heavy squats and dead lifts combined with multiple sets of pull-ups. I visit the gym on other days to socialize, pedal the stationary bike, and do exercises for flexibility, mobility, and injury prevention that aren't particularly strenuous. Even when my schedule is crazy with travel or other activities that disrupt my routine, I find it ridiculously easy to maintain my strength, power output, and ideal body composition, including single-digit body fat and sufficient lean muscle mass, even in my sixties. I'm certain this is because I organize my training schedule correctly, regulate my competitive intensity, and never exhaust myself in the heat of the moment—stuff I often did as a younger athlete.

Primal Essential Movements

The easiest entry point to weight training is to start lifting your own body weight in what I call the primal essential movements (PEM): push-ups, pull-ups, squats, and planks.

These are the quintessential human movements that we have been doing some variation of for a couple of million years. Collectively, they work every major muscle group using full-body functional motions that have direct application to the activities of everyday life. Don't worry—if you can't do a pull-up or a deep squat right now, my system has easier progression exercises. The method can be scaled down for a true beginner, or degrees of difficulty can be added for fitness experts. You can do chair-assisted pull-ups, pole-assisted squats, or knee push-ups, gradually increasing competency as you progress to being able to complete a proper pull-up or deep squat. Search YouTube for "Mark Sisson primal essential movements" to get a demonstration of how to do each baseline movement and progression exercises correctly.

Micro Workouts

I contend that micro workouts are one of the most exciting fitness breakthroughs of the century. I know the century is kinda young, but micro workouts are a fantastic antidote to the hazards of sedentary daily routines. These exercises are brief bouts of explosive effort that you integrate gracefully into your routine at home or at the office. They are easy to incorporate into daily life, don't require an expert level of fitness, and provide relief from the disturbing trend in mainstream fitness toward prolonged workouts that are depleting and exhausting.

The rules are flexible—a micro workout can be anything that gets you up and moving. For example, twenty deep squats at your desk, a set of pull-ups on the pull-up bar hanging in your closet, a trip down the hall and back with mini bands around your ankles, or some kettlebell swings in your yard whenever you take out the garbage. You can also do micro workouts oriented toward flexibility, mobility, and balance. For example, you can do a sequence of dynamic stretches, karate kicks, leg swings, and lunges. Hold on to your desk or a lamppost in the parking lot at first and try to progress to the point where you can execute difficult one-legged maneuvers in open space. If you are having a hectic workday, jump up from your desk, scramble down a few flights of stairs, do a set of dips on a courtyard bench, and hustle back upstairs to your office. You will gain an immediate boost in cognitive function from increased blood flow and oxygen delivery to the brain. You'll also spike neurotransmitters that elevate mood, improve focus, and turbocharge fat burning for hours afterward. Little efforts indeed make a huge cumulative difference over time. Dr. Michael Roizen, coauthor (with television personality Dr. Mehmet Oz) of *You: The*

Owner's Manual and leader of the Cleveland Clinic Wellness Institute, reports that simply jumping up and down twenty times every morning and every evening has been shown to help preserve bone density in the spine and the lower extremities.

Instead of feeling time pressure and a sense that you "need" to squeeze three trips to the gym per week into your packed schedule, just commit to taking breaks from prolonged periods of stillness and performing a few micro workouts every day. Integrate some carefully considered incentives, rewards, and benchmarks that keep you accountable. Create visual cues, such as a kettlebell placed en route to the garbage bin, a pull-up bar in a doorway, or StretchCordz and ankle bands left in plain sight instead of in a drawer. Put some incentives in place, such as breaking for lunch (or should I say break-fast?) only when you have completed a stair sprint or some exercises with the bands and cords. Put a sticky note in your office as a reminder that you can't leave for the day until you complete fifty deep squats. On the other side of the coin, I also like to use micro workouts as a reward for reaching milestones with my peak cognitive tasks. Finish writing that presentation, then head outside for a few kettlebell swings! If you're going to binge-watch your favorite Netflix series, implement a rule that you must perform a micro workout between each episode.

The suggestion to use visual cues and prop placement may seem simplistic, but these things can have an extremely beneficial psychological impact. Lindsay Taylor, PhD, my Primal Blueprint colleague and coauthor of *The Keto Reset Diet Cookbook* and *The Keto Reset Instant Pot Cookbook*, a social psychologist by training, explains.

All our behaviors are triggered by something, whether we're conscious of it or not. We can improve our goal-setting and decision-making capabilities by optimizing our environment and making behavior triggers obvious. Keeping your fitness gear out in the open plants a suggestion in your brain that exercise is important, convenient, and accessible right now. It still takes discipline to get started, but once you start, you'll most likely finish. Even a small obstacle, such as having to unpack or set up fitness gear, can make you less likely to do it. Similarly, leaving a plate of cookies on the table makes you more likely to grab one!

Micro workouts deliver numerous distinct and awesome benefits: first, when you add up the energy expenditure over a long time period, you obtain an incredible cumulative training benefit. Do a single set of twelve pull-ups four days a week, and you have hoisted your body weight over a bar 2,500 times in a year! Second, your efforts raise the baseline from which you can launch your ambitious full-scale workouts or athletic competitions without compromising your readiness for these sessions. If you include flexibility and mobility movements in your micro workouts, you get the added benefit of reducing injury risk when you conduct a challenging session. Search YouTube for "Brad Kearns morning routine" to see a sequence of leg flexibility and mobility and core strengthening moves he designed to support his sprint and high-jump workouts.

Third, micro workouts can get you fit or even superfit without prompting the stress-hormone production and cellular depletion that occur when you conduct prolonged and exhausting workouts at the gym. Fourth, your micro workouts help you achieve the health objectives of increasing general everyday movement and taking frequent breaks from peak cognitive tasks. Sets of deep squats or pull-ups are a great complement to a midday stroll around the office courtyard or a walk with the dog around the block. Develop the habit of busting out for a minute here, a minute there, and for six minutes now and then during your busy day. Even if you claim to be too busy, you must acknowledge that the improvements in cognitive function prompted by micro workouts make the time investment worthwhile.

If you are already fit and have a good strength-training routine going, you should have no problem grabbing a heavy kettlebell for some swings or doing a set of dead lifts without a formal warm-up. If you are at a basic competency level with strength training and/or spend a lot of time sitting during the day, take a minute or two to walk around and do a few warm-up moves, such as working with skinnier Stretch Cordz or doing some half squats before you go deep into a full squat. The fitness "truism" that you need an elaborate and prolonged warm-up before a workout makes sense only in the context of our highly sedentary daily lives. As Dr. Art De Vany likes to say, "The lion doesn't have to stretch before chasing his prey, and neither should you."

In recent years, I've noticed a phenomenal improvement in my lifelong morning creaking and cracking, general everyday stiffness, and the need for an extended warm-up before my Ultimate Frisbee matches. This is a pleasant surprise for someone in my age group, because it seems that I've halted a steady decline in my flexibility and mobility, which was happening over decades. I attribute my improvement to several things: switching to a Focal Upright desk during the workday; spending more time in my archetypal resting positions while reading, watching TV, or taking phone calls; integrating micro workouts into my workday with great devotion (including dynamic stretching and balancing moves on my beloved slackline); taking thirty grams of collagen peptide supplements for several years running; and eradicating all refined seed oils from my diet for two decades running. I can't say I'm bouncing around the house like a gymnast or gracefully holding difficult yoga poses—my running odometer has too many miles on it to allow that. However, I feel more nimble, energetic, springy, and athletic thanks to these practices, which are independent from my longtime devotion to athletic training.

It's time to reframe your notion of what it means to live a healthful, fit lifestyle. It's less about hitting arbitrary mileage goals or maintaining a stellar attendance record at the gym than it is about movement frequency and variation all day long. Following are Katy Bowman's insights on the matter.

Adapting your body to move more is actually pretty easy. Adapting your life to accommodate more movement is more challenging, because we live in an overwhelmingly sedentary culture. But just as you can build muscles for squatting or walking or hanging, you can build your "making time for movement" muscle. The rewards are so immediate and plentiful that the effort will feel worth it. The more you can invite your friends and family along with you, the easier all-day movement will be. We were built to move frequently, move in many different ways, and move with others.

We have movement frequency, movement variation, and "movement accuracy," a term I first heard from former US Olympic 1,500-meter runner Michael Stember when he was teaching recreational enthusiasts how to run with proper technique. When doing anything from walking down the street to performing magnificent athletic feats, be mindful of exhibiting good posture and maintaining a balanced center of gravity. Cultivate a straight and elongated spine when standing, sitting, lying down, and engaging in all manner of athletic movement. Engage your core at all times to provide a stable base for your extremities—a bit while standing and more intently while lifting weights or performing an athletic move. If you have nagging back pain, muscle weakness or imbalance, or poor flexibility, learn more about movement accuracy from books such as Esther Gokhale's *8 Steps to a Pain-Free Back* and Dr. Kelly Starrett's *Becoming a Supple Leopard* as well as Katy Bowman's *Move Your DNA* and *Dynamic Aging*.

Sprinting

Sprinting is the ultimate primal workout, honoring our ancestors' need to summon occasional all-out bursts of energy that for them often had life-or-death consequences. Sprinting can take place during high-impact running on flat ground, lower-impact hill or stair running, and low- or no-impact activities such as stationary bike, cardio machine, rowing, or swimming. Even a brief workout of short-duration sprints delivers profound hormonal, neuroendocrine, metabolic, and antiaging benefits. Becoming proficient in sprinting improves your performance and reduces your rate of perceived exertion at all other speeds below sprinting. Sprinting will also help you shed excess body fat more effectively than any other workout, because the genetic signaling prompted by nearly all-out explosive effort lasts for many hours after the workout. Although you aren't burning a ton of calories during a short session, it's the hormone optimization that sets you up for body-composition breakthroughs. I'll discuss sprinting as an advanced strategy for fat reduction in chapter 7.

It's critical to conduct sprint workouts correctly in order to avoid the burnout risks associated with overly stressful HIIT sessions. The high degree of difficulty associated with sprinting necessitates that you feel 100 percent rested, motivated, and pumped up to deliver a peak effort every time you start a workout. One sprint session a week is plenty for most everyone. If you have any indication of subpar immunity (sore throat, stuffy head), muscle soreness or stiffness (even minor), diminished motivation, or slight fatigue at rest, delay your planned sprint workout until you are chomping at the bit to open the throttle.

A deliberate preparatory sequence is also a valuable way to gauge your readiness to perform your main set of near-maximum-effort sprints. A warm-up period consisting of slow jogging, dynamic stretching, preparatory technique drills, and wind sprints is necessary to reduce injury risk and deliver a peak performance. Dynamic stretching means that the resistance during the stretch comes from extending your range of motion. Examples include lunge walks, arm circles, and high-knee jogging. Preparatory technique drills focus on a certain element of correct sprinting form to improve your technique. Examples include a hopping drill to exaggerate knee drive, a high-heel, high-toe drill to exaggerate the correct dorsiflexion of the foot on the recovery phase of the stride, and many more. Search YouTube for "Brad Kearns running technique drills, beginner" and "Brad Kearns running technique drills, advanced" to get some great ideas.

Wind sprints are brief accelerations toward maximum speed followed by a gradual deceleration into jogging, or the equivalent on a bicycle or cardio machine. Focus on executing good technique and engaging all the relevant muscle groups smoothly. You should feel alert, snappy, and explosive during warm-up to ensure a safe and effective sprint workout. If your coordination is off or your legs feel heavy, save the hard stuff for another day. Believe me—simply completing some technique drills and wind sprints makes for an outstanding high-intensity workout.

Your primary set will consist of four to ten sprints of between ten and twenty seconds each. Go with fewer reps of shorter duration for high-impact running or if you are a novice sprinter. Do more reps of longer duration for low-impact sprints or if your competitive goals are related to endurance events. After each sprint, it's important to take what Dr. Craig Marker describes as "luxurious" rest intervals. Your respiration should return to near normal, and you should feel completely refreshed and focused, ready to deliver another *effort of consistent quality*, and continue in this rhythm for the duration of the workout. This will typically entail between sixty and ninety seconds of rest between each sprint, around a five-to-one ratio of work to rest.

Sprinting for between ten and twenty seconds seems to be the sweet spot for excellent fitness adaptation without the cellular destruction that occurs at an exponential rate when you try to sprint for longer than twenty seconds. What's more, any effort longer than twenty seconds is not a true sprint, because humans are incapable of sustaining maximum output for longer than around seven seconds. Indeed, when you see Usain Bolt pull ahead of the pack in the final stages of the Olympic 100-meter final, what's actually happening is that he is decelerating less than his competitors! Whether you are a novice or a high-level athlete, these parameters constitute a wonderful template for a true sprint workout that develops explosive power without the cumulative fatigue and cellular destruction of prolonged, exhausting workouts. As you improve your fitness, you will simply go faster instead of trying to sprint for longer distances, complete more reps, or take shorter rest intervals.

Delivering an "effort of consistent quality" means meeting a uniform performance standard (e.g., taking fifteen seconds to complete an eighty-meter sprint) at a uniform rate of perceived exertion (e.g., you declare it to be a 93 out of 100 percent) with each sprint. If your sixth sprint of eighty meters takes seventeen or eighteen seconds to complete, or if you have to notch it up to a subjective 97 percent perceived exertion level to finish in fifteen or sixteen seconds, it's time to end the workout. You should also end it immediately if you experience any new muscle stiffness or pain, a fatigue-induced breakdown in your technique, any sort of dizziness, nausea, or difficulty catching your breath during the recovery period, or central nervous system fatigue, in which your focus or motivation to continue declines. For many fitness enthusiasts brought up with a "no pain, no gain" mentality, it will require some discipline and ego restraint to execute sprint sessions correctly. Take inspiration from elite-level sprinters who routinely curtail workouts or even withdraw from big races at the last minute if they notice so much as a twinge in their hamstrings.

The final element of an excellent sprint workout is a proper cooldown, in which you jog or otherwise deliver a minimum effort for between seven and ten minutes until you stop sweating and help your heart rate, respiration, and metabolic functions calm down gradually. By the end of your cooldown, you should be able to breathe and speak normally, feel satisfied and a bit euphoric from an optimal level of workout stress, and feel pleasantly fatigued but not trashed. You should be able to walk away from the track with a little bounce in your step and an eagerness to return soon.

Sprinting on flat ground delivers the most benefits, including strengthening connective tissue, increasing bone density, and prompting maximum genetic signaling for fat reduction. Because it involves high-impact trauma, it also has the highest risk of injury. If you are a novice, are overweight, or have injury-risk concerns, you can build momentum with low-impact or no-impact sprints (performed on cardio machines or stationary bikes or executed while rowing or swimming, for example). Following those types of workouts, you can progress to sprinting uphill or up flights of stairs. After several excellent sessions with no pain or injury flare-ups, you can introduce some wind sprints on flat ground, perhaps in conjunction with stair or uphill sprint workouts. After some adaptation to wind sprints, you can ease into the world of high-impact sprinting and continue to progress to a full-length workout.

Emphasize Recovery

Fitness enthusiasts deserve accolades for countering the couch potato cultural norm, but the subsection of highly motivated, goal-oriented folks in the endurance, group exercise, and CrossFit communities also share a personality tendency to overdo it. Overly stressful exercise patterns have been shown to suppress immune function, suppress important adaptive hormones such as testosterone and human growth hormone, and increase your risk of cardiac disease attributable to repeated scarring and inflammation of the heart muscle during strenuous workouts and not taking sufficient rest between such efforts. Whether your fitness pursuits actually accelerate the aging process instead of delivering the intended benefits comes down to how well you pace yourself during workouts and manage the delicate balance between stress and rest. The central theme of my book *Primal Endurance* is that by honing your aerobic development without the stress and extended recovery time of more difficult sessions, you can actually go faster on the racecourse.

The "no pain, no gain" workout mentality is slowly but surely fading from prominence, but some remnants may still reside deep in your psyche, if not your social media feed. Know this: your training program does not have to be exhausting in order to be effective, and you don't have to destroy yourself in big workouts in order to achieve fitness breakthroughs or toughen up for competition. In my time as an elite athlete and in my decades of coaching elite professionals, I have noticed time and again that the athletes who are the most intuitive, willing to adjust plans on the fly, and able to properly regulate competitive intensity in training are the ones who bring home the gold. They are able to dig deep in important competitions precisely because they have not abused their reserves of energy and willpower repeatedly in training.

I suggest thinking about your workouts as falling into three categories: break even, breakthrough, and recovery. A break-even workout is one that maintains your fitness at a comfortable pace and with moderate effort. A breakthrough workout is one that's difficult and challenging enough to stimulate a fitness improvement. These are done only occasionally, and you must feel 100 percent rested and energized for maximum effort. Recovery workouts are of shorter duration and require less effort than a break-even workout so that they are truly restorative.

Surprising as it may seem, easy to supereasy recovery sessions make a significant contribution to your fitness because they make you more resilient for difficult workouts. They also reduce injury risk by strengthening joints and connective tissue, help hardwire correct technique into your central nervous system, and improve your mood, enjoyment of exercise, and overall sense of well-being. We often glamorize the most difficult workouts, but it's simply not possible to run twenty miles, cycle one hundred miles, or deliver a new personal best for a CrossFit benchmark workout without putting in the preparatory effort of easier training sessions.

Joel Jamieson, leading strength and conditioning coach and trainer of MMA world champion fighters (8WeeksOut.com), is lauded for placing recovery at the center of an effective training program. He promotes a specially designed "rebound workout" that can help you recover more effectively than total rest! This is a radical insight that Jamieson has validated with heart rate variability (HRV) tests. Elements of a rebound workout include dynamic stretching, mobility and flexibility drills, foam rolling, and deep-breathing exercises that boost blood circulation and oxygen delivery without stressing the body. You can also include a handful of very brief explosive efforts (no-impact) followed by long rest intervals—for example, sprinting for ten seconds (at below maximum effort) on a stationary bike, followed by easy pedaling for a minute during which you make a concerted effort to lower your heart rate as quickly as possible. The sprint will cause a brief fight-or-flight reaction, while the recovery period generates a compensatory "rebound" response that stimulates parasympathetic function. Hone this skill of lowering your heart rate during these sets in the gym and you can use it when faced with other forms of stress (a traffic jam, a workplace conflict, and others that arise during a hectic day).

Low-intensity movement is the best way to recover from hard training, so keep JFW a priority. Spend a little extra time doing flexibility and mobility drills in conjunction with your formal workouts and in micro workouts. Promote recovery by never extending yourself too far in the first place. Don't conduct high-intensity sessions if you are sore, stiff, feeling sluggish at rest, or have signs of compromised immunity. Stay under control during your most intense efforts, focusing on preserving explosiveness and executing precise form at all times. Monitor fatigue as your workouts progress, and pull the plug if you notice muscle tightness, form breaking, or negative emotions arising. Exercise extreme restraint and discipline during aerobic workouts to stay at or below your "180 minus age" MAF heart rate for the duration of nearly every workout. Even brief forays into glucose-burning zones make it difficult to return to fat burning when you slow down and thus ruin the intended metabolic benefits of the workout. Try your hand at some rebound-style workouts and see if you can finish the session feeling better than when you started.

Follow a Fat-Burning Lifestyle—Journal Exercises

1. **Sleep environment:** Describe your current sleep environment and the ways you can improve it to create a true sleep sanctuary. Mention specific ideas for reducing light (e.g., salt lamp, orange bulbs, room-darkening blinds), eliminating clutter, and optimizing room and body temperature.
2. **Evening routine:** Describe your current evening routine and the ways you can minimize artificial light and digital stimulation after dark. Note specific ideas for

replacing screen engagement with calm, mellow activities (socializing, dog walking, reading, foam rolling, and others).

3. **Rest, recovery, and downtime:** Describe your current relationship with technology, including areas of weakness that increase stress, reduce productivity, and hamper recovery. List some specific ideas for being more disciplined and structured in order to reduce distractibility and hyperconnectivity—for example, batching email interaction to better focus on peak-performance tasks, establishing strict off hours for technology, and building in routines for exercise and nature immersion to ensure that you succeed.

4. **General everyday movement:** Describe your current movement habits and develop specific ideas for increasing all forms of general everyday movement. Start with ideas for more walking, then include other movement endeavors that are both appealing and doable—for example, participating in formal movement practices (yoga, Pilates), taking frequent breaks from prolonged periods of stillness, and designing some micro workouts to conduct over the course of the workday and during leisurely evenings.

5. **Comfortably paced cardiovascular workouts:** Describe your current cardiovascular exercise routine and ideas for improving your commitment to comfortably paced cardio. Note whether you adhere to the "180 minus age" heart rate guideline and how you might improve your adherence to it if necessary.

6. **Brief, intense workouts:** Describe your current high-intensity training patterns and devise ideas for improving your commitment to properly conducted sprint and strength workouts. Describe any necessary modifications to your current workouts and/or the type and frequency of workouts to add to your routine. Address the concept of micro workouts with thoughts about ways to integrate them into your lifestyle.

7. **Recovery:** Write down any areas of particular concern—those where your stress-rest balance is lacking. List specific ideas for integrating more rest, recovery, and downtime into your lifestyle.

CHAPTER 6

Put Two Meals a Day into Play

For the most part, you can maintain your existing dietary beliefs and enjoy your favorite meals (assuming you eliminate toxic foods and emphasize healthful foods, of course!) while you pursue your overarching goal of reducing the total number of meals you consume—this week, this month, and for the rest of your life. The timing of your two meals (maximum) each day can be adjusted to align with your daily schedule and personal preference. For example, you could routinely fast in the morning, eat a nutritious lunch meal, and enjoy a delicious evening meal with family. People with a hectic daily work schedule might prefer a hearty breakfast and an earlyish dinner on most workdays. When you have established a good rhythm of eating a maximum of two meals a day without snacking, you can throw in some days of extended fasting. This could consist of a single centerpiece meal along with a light snack or high-fat beverage in the morning. Following are some suggested *Two Meals a Day* patterns that you might like to test over time as you dial in a long-term strategy that works best for you and your lifestyle.

Gradual Progression

If you have metabolic damage from a history of yo-yo dieting, difficulty dropping excess body fat, or disease risk factors revealed by blood tests, or if you are currently eating more than two meals a day and/or snacking frequently and routinely eating outside a twelve-hour daily window, it may be best to follow a gradual progression to reach a baseline of two daily meals with no snacking in between. Instead of getting overwhelmed with too many objectives at once, try tackling them in the following order.

1. **Mind your twelve-hour digestive window.** Getting this right will make it easier to eventually eradicate snacking. When it's time to relax and enjoy a show or socialize after dinner, brush your teeth first so you won't be tempted to munch on something.

2. **Ditch the Big Three**. As you learned in chapter 2, this doesn't necessarily have to coincide with an extreme reduction in your carbohydrate intake, and it certainly doesn't mean caloric restriction. Enjoy a sufficient amount of colorful, nutritious carbs in order to reduce or eliminate the risks of experiencing the symptoms of low-carb flu.

3. **Address snacking.** At first, do whatever it takes to keep the Big Three out of your life and avoid backsliding into carb binges. If your energy dips between meals, go ahead and snack, but make sure you emphasize nutritious high-fat foods (e.g., macadamia nuts, nut butters, dark chocolate, hard-boiled eggs, leftover steak). Over time, strive to cut back and eventually eliminate snacking. Realize that the desire to snack is often driven by forces other than hunger, such as boredom or the need for a cognitive break. Replace snacks with micro workouts! Of course, a snack can take the place of one of your meals when you get further down the road of metabolic flexibility.

4. **Honor your natural hunger and satiety signals.** Eat all your meals in a calm, quiet setting. Eliminate distractions such as televisions, computer screens, and even reading. Chew each bite extensively and savor the entire experience. Notice the point at which you are satisfied (it is often long before you're "full") and leave the rest of the food on your plate.

5. **Test *WHEN*.** Delaying your first meal of the day until you're truly hungry takes the pressure off because you know you can eat anytime. By contrast, pushing to achieve a 16-8 eating window before you're ready can lead to obsessing about the clock and developing an unhealthy relationship with food. All your progressions should feel natural, comfortable, and easy to sustain. If you are able to easily delay your first meal until around midday, getting into a *Two Meals a Day* groove will be much easier.

Break-Fast *WHEN*—When Hunger Ensues Naturally

The most simple, sustainable, and quantifiable strategy for boosting metabolic flexibility is to delay your first meal of the day until you experience true sensations of hunger. While this might not be optimal for certain people who have limited time or access to food at midday and need to fuel up at home before heading out, it seems to be the most popular and convenient long-term strategy. After not eating for eight hours overnight, you awaken in a prime fat-burning state. You are slightly glycogen depleted, which typically prompts the production of ketones in the liver. This happens to a mild extent if you aren't keto-adapted or to a significant extent if you are aligned with ketogenic dietary guidelines. With fat burning heightened in the morning, you are ready for hours of productivity without the potential interference of having to prepare and digest a meal. Mornings are a great time to build more metabolic flexibility by leveraging the overnight fasting period. You certainly don't have a huge need for immediate calories until you spend a few hours burning stored energy and working up an appetite.

If you wake up and inhale a great American high-carbohydrate "most important" morning meal (juice, toast, oatmeal, cereal, and other carb-rich foods), you immediately override all the momentum toward fat burning resulting from your overnight fast and switch into carb dependency mode. By midmorning, after you burn through breakfast calories and produce the requisite amount of insulin to deal with the carbohydrate load, you might get hungry for a snack or notice your mind wandering to thoughts of lunch. You have boarded the glucose-insulin roller coaster and will remain on it for the rest of the day—and potentially for the rest of your life, unless you escape these SAD dietary patterns. If you eat a nutrient-dense breakfast with ample fat and protein, free from refined carbohydrates, you won't get the insulin crash but you'll still stop burning body fat and making ketones in favor of burning off the meal. That said, enjoying a nutritious morning meal is not necessarily a bad thing, and it may be an effective strategy for you to consider based on your daily schedule.

If you do a decent job with the five steps in the "gradual progression" section (page 144), you should be able to last at least a couple of hours after waking before you feel a need to eat. With continued effort, virtually anyone can progress to the point where the break-fast meal is eaten around noon. Obviously, this sets you up for smashing success with the *Two Meals a Day* strategy. If you want to activate your digestive circadian rhythms in the morning to help get all your cylinders firing, enjoy some coffee or tea or other low-calorie beverage. I contend that the cream and sugar in my morning coffee is inconsequential to my compressed-eating-window goal because I burn the minimal sixty or so calories they add to my coffee in a short time.

When you implement the WHEN strategy, resolve to stay active in the morning, but save your high-intensity workouts for a later hour, when your metabolic flexibility is exceptional. Walking or doing a low-level cardio session is not strenuous enough to spike appetite and will further optimize your fat-burning state. If you've eaten a morning meal for decades, you may experience a circadian-influenced ghrelin spike in the morning. See if you can ignore it, knowing it will subside in less than twenty minutes. Instead, try to energize yourself with a walk, a micro workout, or an engrossing cognitive task. As midday nears, you'll realize at a certain point that you really would love some food to sustain you. Relish the experience of eating in order to actually quell hunger, not because it's a certain time of day or you simply need a break from work.

If you are trying to drop excess body fat, make occasional efforts to extend yourself past that hunger point for another thirty to sixty minutes before you enjoy a meal. Be cautious with this advanced strategy; it can easily backfire by causing you to overeat during your narrow time window. Resolve to get really comfortable with a 16-8 baseline, then go beyond that once in a while in pursuit of body-composition improvements. Remember to focus on lowering insulin through fasting and eliminating refined carbs. Don't try to combine extended fasting with eating fewer calories, because this will potentially lower your metabolic rate and make you feel sluggish.

Morning-Evening Pattern

A morning-evening strategy is appropriate for people with physically demanding jobs, people who have difficulty making time for meals or gaining access to healthful food at midday, athletes seeking to optimize meal and workout timing, and people working in a fast-paced, high-stress office environment that's difficult to unplug from. If you aren't able to take at least thirty minutes to mentally and physically disengage from your workplace and put yourself in a quiet, relaxing environment, even a nutritious meal may not be advised. Remember: the sympathetic nervous system's fight-or-flight mechanism directly contradicts the parasympathetic system function nicknamed "rest and digest." When you adopt the morning-evening pattern, you can set your digestive circadian rhythms and fuel yourself for a high-energy day before leaving home, then focus on your core daily responsibilities without interruption. When you get home and transition into relaxation mode after a busy day of physical and/or mental demands, you can enjoy a celebratory dinner and stay in alignment with the *Two Meals a Day* template.

While the morning-evening pattern may run counter to my previous point about fat burning being disturbed by eating first thing in the morning, if you fully commit to the morning-evening pattern you will be okay. By powering through productive daytime hours (including perhaps an ambitious workout) without a midday meal, you are turbocharging fat burning and depleting glycogen to make high-octane ketones for brain superfuel—the same benefits that accrue when you fast in the morning until WHEN. Although completing a sixteen-hour overnight fast is definitely a feat of metabolic flexibility, it's arguably just as impressive to complete a ten-hour fast during waking hours of much higher calorie burning.

In further support of a morning-evening pattern, you are more insulin sensitive in the morning than at any other time of day. This means that your cells are more receptive to the signaling of insulin, so a little goes a long way to get the job done. If you eat two identical meals, one in the morning and one at nighttime, you will likely experience more fluctuation in blood glucose, produce more insulin, and be more likely to store ingested calories as fat instead of burn them with the food you eat in the evening. In contrast, whatever you eat in the morning is going to be burned off quickly as you get busy!

Athletes have found success with the Morning-Evening pattern to deliver pre-workout calories in the morning and promote recovery with the evening meal. My longtime work colleague Brian McAndrew, who makes me sound and look good on podcasts and YouTube videos, is a strict devotee of keto and carnivore-style eating (he coauthored *Keto Cooking for Cool Dudes* and *Carnivore Cooking for Cool Dudes* with Brad). Brian is also a serious powerlifter who spends up to two hours in the gym working hard several days a week. Brian's workout typically comes around midday, after he has had sufficient time to digest a morning meal. His high protein breakfasts (see his books for some incredibly creative ideas perfect for athletes) deliver a steady drip of amino acids that negate the need for using protein supplements before or after workouts. Come early evening, he will enjoy another substantial meal, ensuring full replenishment from his big workouts and giving him enough time to digest without interfering with bedtime.

Dr. Art De Vany also favors a Morning-Evening meal pattern sandwiching a midday workout. He likes to have fasted before exercise to send a "renewal signal" to his cells, then fast for at least four hours after an intense workout to maximize the benefits of autophagy and mitochondrial biogenesis. Dr. De Vany explains that a long interval between meals promotes *proteostasis* (protein homeostasis)—the stabilization of the critical operations of protein making and (desirable) protein degradation in cells throughout the body. By contrast, eating too much too often can cause dysregulated protein production and degradation, which is the essence of accelerated aging, cognitive decline, and increased cancer risk. (Hence one of my brilliant subtitle suggestions that didn't make the final cut: "Quit Eating So Much Goddamn Food!") Depleting cellular energy through fasting or strenuous workouts is like having a quality control inspector visit the assembly line to ensure that everything is going efficiently and stays in proper working order.

Let's break this down a little further: when you starve your cells of energy by fasting or conducting an intense or prolonged workout, or especially when you combine the two (something I do nearly every day), you achieve a tremendous repair-and-renewal effect that constitutes antiaging at its finest. In addition, Dr. De Vany sees this pattern of fasting, exercise, and controlled nutrition as a cure for depression: "Starve and exercise!" He explains that starvation, through the aforementioned cellular detoxification process called autophagy (see page 65), eats up some of the dysfunctional synapses in your brain. "For every damaged molecule," he says, "there's a damaged thought. A depressed brain or a brain that has post-traumatic stress—those are injured neurons inside the brain, and you just need to get rid of the dysfunctional molecules that are causing those neurons to malfunction.... First heal the brain. You heal it with neurotrophic factors. Be outside. New thoughts, new patterns of behavior.... Being outside is enormously effective. There's stimuli you can't even relate to, but you perceive them. Your unconscious brain is what's going to heal you first."

Intuitive Strategy

In the intuitive approach, your eating decisions are driven mainly by your hunger and satiety signals as well as by your mood, environment, and daily variation in sleep, work, exercise, and socializing habits. An intuitive strategy frees you from the often hidden stresses and hassles of adhering to a meal schedule and allows you to just go with the flow every day. As you might imagine, this is most effective when your outstanding metabolic flexibility allows you to thrive whether or not you eat regular meals. At the highest level of sophistication, meals are eaten only when you're hungry and able to consume the most nutritious and desirable food possible in a relaxed meal setting.

When you follow an intuitive strategy, you'll find yourself skipping or delaying meals without realizing it. You'll break free from the cultural attachment to certain foods at breakfast, lunch, and dinner. You might enjoy some steak in the morning and eggs in the evening. Maybe you'll feel like having a few squares of dark chocolate at 10:45 a.m. instead of a sit-down breakfast or lunch. Then you'll enjoy a hearty early dinner. Maybe you'll occasionally skip dinner and go to sleep early because you're tired rather than microwaving something unimpressive and then munching down a bowl of popcorn and watching Netflix because these have become your nightly habits. If you are eating intuitively, when you decide to indulge, you'll be able to do so wholeheartedly, with deep appreciation for every aspect of the experience. Contrast this with the guilty-pleasure mindset we've been socialized to adopt whenever we indulge. As you learned in chapter 4, shame and guilt can compromise much of your enjoyment and help you get stuck in a pattern of rebellious behavior.

Essentially, the intuitive strategy allows you to break free from any and all attachments relating to food. Ascending to the point where you can adopt this strategy acknowledges that controlling caloric intake does not mean you are in control of your life (a concept that anorexics fail to embrace, to their extreme detriment); eschewing animal foods does not equal moral superiority; and your six-pack is not who you are, it's just something you wear well! When the smoke clears, you are left with pure awareness of your true caloric energy needs and pure appreciation for the foods and meal circumstances that you enjoy.

Granted, it's certainly less objectionable to be emotionally attached to a 16-8 meal pattern than it is to be addicted to carbs. Ditto for being wedded to an identity as a planet-conscious vegetarian or a six-pack wearer instead of a glutton. However, as your friendly neighborhood Zen Buddhist will remind you, attachment inevitably leads to suffering. In a world driven by instant gratification, hyperconnectivity, and consumerism, we are all programmed to cultivate unhealthy attachments to all kinds of crap, and food is one of the most destructive items on the list. If you can take some baby steps to break free from emotional attachments to eating, your metabolic flexibility may very well serve as a catalyst for more flexibility and more peace of mind in many other areas of life.

Along these lines, the intuitive strategy might be the most effective way to drop excess body fat and keep it off forever—even better than a hard-core 16-8 pattern or precise carb restriction along keto guidelines. Over the years, I've counseled numerous highly disciplined people frustrated by fat-loss stalls. They typically claim to be doing everything right. On further examination, unhealthy emotional attachments will be uncovered (to the clock, to favorite foods that are "approved" as healthful, or even to excessive and counterproductive calorie burning), or we'll expose lingering self-limiting beliefs and behavior patterns that are playing out behind the scenes. One common example is harboring a subconscious belief that you're undeserving of a sexy physique, or that LGN (looking good naked) is a silly and superficial goal compared to high-minded ideals such as avoiding vanity at all costs. By the way, I've found LGN to be one of the most effective motivators of them all!

Being completely free from any rigidity or quantification reduces the risk of the incredibly common backsliding and rebellious behavior that occur in reaction to restrictive and regimented programs. Even if you're highly fat-adapted and possess excellent discipline, focus, self-awareness, and knowledge of healthful eating, it's easy to fall into attachment patterns that hinder your progress—for example, eating habitually at noon because it marks the end of your 16-8 fasting window or overindulging in "approved" high-fat snacks to cope with feelings of deprivation after abstaining from your previous favorite snacks and treats. When you can transcend these and other pitfalls of regimentation, excessive self-quantification, and general attachment to food, meals, and results on the bathroom scale, dropping excess body fat and keeping it off happens in the background without your having to think about it.

Unfortunately, the freedom of the intuitive strategy has a perilous flip side, because you are liberated from some of the guidelines and restrictions that have kept you accountable. When you are not obsessed with your 16-8 goals, you may find yourself not eating until 2:00 p.m. one day, but the possibility exists that you won't be compelled to wait until 12:00 noon to eat on other days. It may be helpful to understand that the intuitive strategy is not a loosey-goosey strategy! In this context, the cavalier use of the old advice *everything in moderation* really bugs me. Today, given the epidemic rates of diet-related disease (not to mention the coronavirus pandemic, which preferentially attacks people suffering from obesity, diabetes, high blood pressure, and weakened cardiovascular and immune systems), I believe an extreme commitment to healthful eating is warranted. As Oscar Wilde said, "Everything in moderation, *including* moderation."

While I want you to enjoy your life, and enjoy that omelet Cousin Babby prepared for you at 10:00 a.m. during her visit, even if you are on a 16-8 plan, an occasional departure from your winning template is different from using hall passes left and right to avoid best practices. If you feel like you need the safety net of adhering to a 16-8 window, or the fifty-carbohydrate-grams-per-day ketogenic diet limit, or the rule that ice cream is not allowed into the house, I understand. Strict parameters are warranted when you're trying to ditch carb dependency, reduce excess body fat, or achieve specific athletic goals.

I implement a variety of guidelines, incentives, and rewards to keep me honest with my eating choices, help me resist the distraction of YouTube videos (I favor stuff like electric hydrofoiling, stand-up paddling, or Laird Hamilton and Kai Lenny big-wave surfing), and curb the inclination to slack off on the final sets of my workout. However, I also know how to relax, unwind, unplug, and embrace the times when my intuition guides me in a direction other than strictly pursuing peak efficiency every day in every way. As I said at the outset of the book, I've been there and done that with my extreme marathon training regimen, which destroyed my body instead of leading me to Olympic glory.

I believe the secret to optimizing your caloric intake and meal patterns is your incredibly sensitive and finely tuned genetic signals of hunger and satiety. You really can't go wrong when you relax, put the food scales and calculators away, detach from emotional, cultural, and environmental triggers for eating (and overeating!), and allow your long-lost hunger and satiety signals to return to center stage. You get to appreciate food as nourishment for a healthy, fit, energetic life instead of another example of modern-day excess. A beautiful balance point is achieved when you are "hungry enough" for nearly every meal you sit down to and eat "just enough" to feel satisfied instead of full (you don't want to be full of food as well as regret for overdoing it and spoiling the experience).

You can strive for the same balance point in your sex life, workout patterns, Netflix viewing, and even your standard of living. Sociologists and statisticians have long asserted that once you attain a certain reasonable income level—one that meets your basic needs and allows you to enjoy some comforts and leisure opportunities—more money simply does not buy more happiness. Reflecting on the fact that my own standard of living and career complexity have steadily escalated over the years, I realize that my thoughts and emotions about the stresses—and successes—of entrepreneurial life have stayed exactly the same. It's just the number of zeros on the figures involved that have changed.

Commit to the hard work of developing metabolic flexibility, because this is the necessary prerequisite for breaking free from regimented meals and carbohydrate dependency and the flawed psychology that goes hand in hand with them. It's impossible to free yourself from obsession with and attachment to food when you are literally dependent on regular meals for energy. When you have built some momentum, see how it feels to relax a bit and go with the flow!

Put Two Meals a Day into Play—Journal Exercise

Strategy and Progression: Describe your present eating style, including your typical window for digestive function and calorie consumption. Plot out a realistic progression from the present to an eventual pattern of two meals a day (maximum) and no snacking. Describe your preferred strategy, whether break-fast WHEN, morning-evening, or intuitive. Include details about your daily work and exercise schedule and how you believe your strategy will work effectively.

CHAPTER 7

Advanced Strategies for Fat Reduction

As you may have discovered, calorie restriction paired with ambitious caloric expenditure does not work for fat reduction, as we have been led to believe. The compensation theory sabotages the best-laid plans of even people with maximum discipline and willpower. As I mentioned in the introduction, the metabolic set point theory is legitimate, and it takes a concerted effort to alter your genetic predispositions. If you have made a valiant effort to achieve the objectives covered in the previous chapters and have either hit a plateau or aspire to even better results, you can try some advanced strategies. In this chapter, I'll cover a progression of fasted workouts, extended fasting periods, sprinting, and the exciting cutting-edge strategy of cold exposure to trigger fat reduction. During your 12-Day Turbocharge, you'll dabble in some of the techniques covered here; this chapter is designed to provide further detail and guidance for implementation of these strategies over the long term.

These techniques are not easy, but they work. It's important to adopt an empowering mindset in which you fully buy into what you're doing, embrace the challenge, appreciate the process regardless of the outcome, and respect the fact that big success requires big commitment. For example, I believe that working through hunger now and then delivers profound psychological benefits. Coming from my background as an extreme calorie-burning and calorie-consuming athlete who was literally dependent upon carbohydrates to perform, I feel like pushing the limits of my hunger now and then proves to me that I am no longer at the mercy of food to survive and thrive. I'm no longer beholden to the dogma of conventional stupidity that brainwashed me to worship a false god—that is, the calories in, calories out model of energy expenditure. Embracing hunger once in a while also gives me a renewed appreciation for the beauty of mealtimes and eating delicious food. Anytime we take something for granted—whether it's a relationship, an airline flight being on time, a reliable internet connection, or a meal—our appreciation of it can easily be diminished. With our constant access to all manner of ready-made meals and snacks, it's easy to become disconnected from the satisfaction of working hard to procure food for a nourishing meal. When you can experience sensations of true hunger occasionally, and then let these hormonal processes play out for a bit before extinguishing them, you become a more mindful, grateful, and intuitive eater.

Following are some ways to signal your genes to shed excess body fat relatively quickly. Once you reach your body-composition goal, you should be able to maintain your new physique indefinitely without much trouble. Even if you back off from these advanced strategies, reduce your exercise volume, and/or get a little loose with your diet, your homeostatic drives and compensatory processes will help keep your body-fat percentage within a tight range. These are the same compensatory mechanisms that make it tough to shed fat in the first place! That said, if your future involves a sustained increase in dietary insulin production, you will gradually accumulate body fat in response. To keep your body composition in check, focus on lowering your theoretical insulin AUC (area under the curve) value. This means producing an optimally minimal amount of insulin, just enough to get the job done; best achieved by fasting routinely and avoiding refined carbohydrates and industrial oils. Don't stress about being superconsistent with your workout caloric expenditure, or cutting back on the amount of nutrient-dense food you enjoy. Enjoy your life, including celebratory dining and taking relaxing breaks from extreme devotion to workouts. If you harbor fears about getting soft, imagine your hand on a dial that you simply have to turn down a few notches to lower insulin production and accelerate fat burning.

Fasted Workouts

When you exercise in a fasted state, then wait between one and four hours before eating, you are forcing your body to accelerate fat burning to meet your energy needs. As you learned earlier, starving your cells of energy through the combination of fasting and burning calories through exercise prompts mitochondrial biogenesis—the making of new energy-producing mitochondria in your cells. As presented in the solar-plant-versus-coal-plant illustration in chapter 3 (see page 68), fat requires mitochondria to be burned for energy, but glucose can be burned directly in the cell without mitochondria. The better your mitochondria work, the better you burn the clean fuels of fat and ketones around the clock.

Fasted workouts constitute an advanced strategy, because if you haven't built the metabolic machinery to burn fat—the solar power plant—you risk triggering fight-or-flight gluconeogenesis to meet your high-glucose energy requirements during and in the hours after the workout. A carb-dependent athlete attempting a fasted workout or a fasting period after a workout is merely increasing the stress impact of the workout and extending recovery time. Until that athlete's diet (and high-stress, sugar-burning lifestyle habits) are transformed, he or she will not gain the benefits of fasted workouts. Assuming you can comfortably operate in a 16-8 compressed eating window with a somewhat active morning of working and perhaps some light exercise, you can take the next step and conduct a morning workout after an overnight fast, then continue fasting afterward for a period of time, usually at least one hour and eventually up to four—a bit of a challenge but not too daunting. Then, just as you can when you're progressing toward a 16-8 pattern, you can enjoy a satisfying meal when you experience true sensations of hunger.

The fasted workouts strategy has four variables: the duration of your fast before the workout, the duration of your fast after the workout, the degree of difficulty of the workout, and the total duration of the fast. Experiment and determine what's best for you. Following is a suggested progression that gets you started and continues all the way to the highest degree of difficulty and maximum fat-reduction benefits.

1. **Overnight Fast, Moderate Workout:** You should be able to comfortably complete a recovery or break-even workout in a twelve-hour overnight fasted state (see page 159). Your energy expenditure was minimal overnight, so you still have sufficient liver and muscle glycogen to perform an aerobic session of up to sixty minutes or a brief, intense session lasting twenty minutes or less. If you are hungry for breakfast immediately afterward, go ahead and enjoy your meal.

2. **Overnight Fast, Moderate Workout—Post-Workout WHEN Fast:** Conduct an aerobic session of no more than sixty minutes or a high-intensity glycolytic (glucose-burning) workout of no more than twenty minutes. This could be a sprint session or some intense strength training in the gym. See how long you can comfortably last after a moderate workout until you get hungry. Even fasting

for an hour of power before sitting down to a meal constitutes a great stimulus for metabolic flexibility.

3. **Overnight Fast, Difficult Workout:** This workout is of sufficient duration and/or intensity to significantly deplete glycogen. This might entail a high-intensity session of up to forty minutes or an aerobic session of up to two hours. Again, if you have to eat immediately following your workout, go ahead. An omelet or other low-carb meal would be ideal, but if you are craving carbs, eat to feel fully satisfied and energized for some productive hours ahead. Strive to eventually minimize the carb content of this post-workout meal in order to progress to the next level.

4. **Overnight Fast, Difficult Workout—Post-Workout WHEN Fast:** Welcome to the amazing new dimension of the fat-adapted athlete! The overnight fast and difficult workout are sure to significantly deplete glycogen. This means the post-exercise fasting period is being fueled by accelerated fat burning and ketone production. See if you can last at least an hour before enjoying a satisfying meal. You'll maximize the benefits of the post-exercise spike of adaptive hormones such as testosterone and human growth hormone, something that can be muted by insulin if you eat right away.

5. **Overnight Fast, Difficult Workout—Post-Workout Extended Fast:** This is pretty advanced, so only take it on when you're ready! This level offers amazing potential for fat reduction. I've known many athletes who are able to shed several pounds of fat in a single week by stacking ambitious workouts on top of extended fasting. While I've frequently emphasized feeling comfortable and proceeding at a careful pace to avoid liquidating your assets, you can get more aggressive at this level.

When that inevitable sensation of hunger eventually arrives, one, two, or four hours after your big workout, see if you can persevere through the hunger spike for a while longer. Find something to keep you busy, such as an engaging work project, a phone call, or an outdoor stroll. I find that taking a brief break from my office to ascend some stairs or conduct a micro workout can propel me into a different metabolic state right away. I feel a burst of alertness that lasts for around half an hour afterward, likely because of a boost in fat burning and ketone production. And while riding out a ghrelin spike is no joke, I can attest that it reliably subsides after fifteen minutes, especially if you engage in some form of movement as soon as you get hungry.

Making Incremental Gains When You're Already Fit

When you implement advanced strategies to achieve a bridesmaid-body break-through in time for the wedding, you should be aware that you may not be able to sustain your very most impressive physique indefinitely. Tour de France athletes trying to shed the last few pounds of fat in the final run-up before the three-week event will pedal for up to six hours and then starve themselves for a few hours afterward. This is the only way to trigger further fat reduction when they are already in the single-digit range. However, these elite performers know that they can only sustain extremely low body-fat levels for the duration of the three-week tour, after which they naturally recal-ibrate to normal caloric intake and a slightly higher body-fat percentage.

However, even when you temporarily push the boundaries of your metabolic flex-ibility and then recalibrate to baseline, you will help optimize your body composition for years and decades to come. Consider the hypothetical example of a fit male stuck at 14 percent body fat despite devoted training and responsible eating. Implementing the basics of the *Two Meals a Day* program (cutting out the Big Three offensive foods, eating fewer meals, and fasting more) should enable him to quickly reach and maintain 12 percent body fat. Going from 14 percent to 12 is pretty straightforward, but making incremental gains from there requires temporarily going outside the comfort zone with a burst of fasted workouts, a few twenty-four-hour fasts, or an aggressive cold therapy regimen (see page 165). With diligent implementation of these advanced strategies, he might be able to achieve 9 percent body fat temporarily. After dipping down into unsustainable territory for a bit, he will predictably drift up to a higher percentage over time. However, the adaptive response to his efforts can help shave his long-term set point down from 12 percent to 11 percent.

This possibility is supported by studies on fasting, insulin sensitivity, and nutri-tional ketosis. When you lower insulin production (even temporarily), you improve insu-lin sensitivity. The positive feedback loop of needing less insulin to get the job done allows you to build on your metabolic flexibility; it's the opposite of the escalating dis-ease processes driven by insulin resistance. When you fast and restrict carbohydrates enough to trigger ketone production, you enjoy an assortment of downstream genetic signaling benefits that can help improve body composition. Ketones have profound protein-sparing effects, switching on genes that help build and preserve muscle tis-sue. Ketones deliver anti-inflammatory effects that are more potent than prescrip-tion drugs, enhance fat burning, and help prevent the accumulation of inflammatory visceral fat. Ketones trigger mitochondrial biogenesis, making you better at burning fat and less reliant upon dietary carbohydrates as an energy source. These benefits also allow you to train harder and recover faster, so you can burn more fat and build more muscle. Success with metabolic flexibility begets more success, including the ability to get a tiny bit leaner and fitter over time instead of the more common steady decline in fitness and accumulation of fat as we age.

Extended Fasting

You should only consider extended fasting when you have exceptional all-around health and immune function. If you started your *Two Meals a Day* journey unfit, obese, with a history of metabolic damage from yo-yo dieting, or with thyroid, adrenal, autoimmune, or inflammatory health conditions, focus on the gradual progression presented in chapter 6: establish a twelve-hour digestive window, ditch the Big Three toxic modern foods, tighten up your snacking habits, honor your natural hunger and satiety signals, then venture gently and gracefully into the world of WHEN. Strive to get into a 16-8 routine and enjoy your new life of metabolic flexibility. You can certainly expect to achieve a gradual and sustained reduction in excess body fat over time, but aggressive efforts to shed fat are not advised if you have a history of metabolic damage. You can certainly explore occasional longer fasting periods, and they will likely happen from time to time naturally. However, there is no urgency to push yourself beyond a 16-8 pattern for at least a year after you first transition away from carbohydrate dependency.

If you already fast on an extended basis from time to time, are a serious fitness enthusiast, and/or have low body fat, you should easily be able to introduce 20-4 days or even occasional days of twenty-four-hour fasts. Interestingly, if you already have excellent metabolic flexibility and body composition, you stand to benefit less from extended fasting than someone who aspires to these characteristics. This is especially the case for fit females, who can easily overstress themselves if they layer extended fasting on top of a heavy training schedule. Remember that the six-pack female celebrated on magazine covers and viral social media posts is swimming upstream against the single most powerful female human genetic drive, which is to maintain reproductive fitness and fertility. Female fertility is predicated on consuming ample nutritious calories and maintaining a reasonable level of body fat, well above the typical magazine-cover specs. Trying to shed more body fat can easily become a fight-or-flight exercise with negative repercussions.

That said, if you feel as though you're not quite "there" yet and aspire to break through frustrating weight-loss plateaus or shed some of the highly undesirable and health-destructive belly fat (a.k.a. visceral fat) that seems to creep up as the decades pass, extended fasting can lead to major breakthroughs. If you are experienced and comfortable with a 16-8 pattern, try a twenty-hour fast (e.g., an 8:00 p.m. dinner followed by fasting until 4:00 p.m. the following day). Pick a day of minimal overall stress and conduct only a moderate morning workout. Remember the rules of fasting: you never want to force it or struggle through declining energy, brain fog, or prolonged hunger sensations. See how long you can last while feeling great, performing great, and not really thinking much about food. As you learned from our previous discussion of the circadian-influenced appetite hormone ghrelin, you may experience sensations of hunger around 12:00 noon if you're accustomed to eating around that time. Trust that the discomfort of the rumbling stomach will subside in minutes, especially if you redirect your attention and energy to a quick stroll or micro workout.

You may have heard directives to break a lengthy fast with easy-to-digest foods such as smoothies and soups. I wouldn't worry too much about that after a twenty-hour fast. Choose an appealing celebratory meal—you deserve it! However, please resist the temptation to overeat after an extended fast. Sit down in a quiet, low-stress eating environment, chew at a deliberate pace, and enjoy the experience with full attention and awareness.

Twenty-Four Hours and Beyond

When you have successfully completed a couple of twenty-hour fasts, you can aspire for the esteemed twenty-four-hour fast. Challenge your mind and body to not eat for an entire day and see how you feel. Try fasting from an early dinner to another early dinner. Several of my friends and thought leaders in the ancestral health scene do this on a regular basis, and some of them fast for much longer. The founder of Dry Farm Wines, Todd White, fasts for twenty-three hours every day! Each evening, he enjoys a celebratory dinner (usually with work colleagues, and with plenty of wine flowing in the name of product R&D) and doesn't eat again until the following evening. Todd reports that the logistics of his day are much easier: instead of spending time prepping and eating meals, he has convenient blocks of time available for meditation, focused work, and high-intensity workouts.

The OMAD (one meal a day) strategy is becoming increasingly popular among metabolically flexible folks seeking to maximize the benefits of fasting, accelerate fat metabolism, and burn high-octane ketones in the brain. It's common practice throughout Europe to consume coffee in the morning and then a celebratory meal after work. Dr. Cate Shanahan, an OMAD devotee herself, likes to pair a high-fat morning coffee (with added cream and/or MCT oil) with what she calls an early evening supermeal.

Dr. Peter Attia conducts a quarterly five-day fast while carefully tracking numerous blood, metabolic, and athletic performance metrics. Brian "Liver King" Johnson and his wife, Barbara, also conduct a five-day, water-only fast every quarter. Get this: the Johnsons' fasting period starts not with a Last Supper–style feast but with a grueling, glycogen-depleting workout that Brian describes as a "failed hunt." The idea is to simulate conditions that our ancestors likely endured regularly. Brian and Barbara report that after a few days of refeeding and returning to full-scale athletic training following the five-day fast, they experience a reliable boost in fitness benchmarks and daily energy levels. Dr. John Jaquish, inventor of the X3 Bar strength-training device and author of *Weight Training Is a Waste of Time*, follows a continual forty-eight-hour fasting protocol, eating a large, all-meat meal every two days. At 240 pounds and single-digit body fat, John's nutritional requirements are substantial, but his closed-loop functionality allows him to thrive and perform and recover from awesome workouts while deeply fasted.

The research of Dr. Valter Longo, director of the Longevity Institute at the University of Southern California and author of *The Longevity Diet*, reveals that organs temporarily shrink during an extended fast. This is a consequence of the shedding of damaged, inflamed cellular material resulting from the stress of everyday life. Research also confirms that the important internal detox processes of *autophagy* (cell repair) and *apoptosis* (desirable programmed death of damaged, dysfunctional, and precancerous cells) are markedly accelerated during extended fasts, during which the hormetic stressor of starving your organs of their usual supply of caloric energy prompts stem cells to spring into action and initiate comprehensive renewal and repair processes.

Dr. Longo's research touts an assortment of extra benefits from prolonged fasts. Even a twenty-four-hour fast will not fully deplete muscle and liver glycogen, so fasting for two days and beyond will prompt additional spikes in fat burning and ketone production. In particular, glycogen-depleting fasts will spur the burning of stubborn visceral fat. Other observed benefits include lower inflammatory markers (such as C-reactive protein, a.k.a. hs-CRP); lower blood pressure; lower glucose, insulin, and triglyceride levels; a reduction in the growth factor IGF-1 (which delivers antiaging and disease-prevention benefits); and a boost in production of the precious BDNF—brain derived neurotrophic factor, a.k.a. Miracle-Gro for the brain.

KEEPING FASTING IN PERSPECTIVE

Some extreme health enthusiasts and biohackers suggest that seventy-two is the magic number—the minimum fasting hours necessary to trigger profound autophagy and anti-inflammatory benefits, but I'd like to back off from any "more is better" proclamations. Instead of trying to break records, focus on the long haul. Try to establish a 16-8 rhythm and/or a fractal, intuitive pattern featuring long fasting periods, delicious meals, and no snacking. Imagine checking in with yourself seven months from now—or seven years from now—and feeling comfortable with your routine.

If you attempt an extended fast, be sure that your energy and cognition remain steady for the duration. Save the really difficult workouts for another time; limit yourself to comfortably paced aerobic exercise and micro workouts. When your fasts extend beyond twenty-four hours, you start to produce higher levels of energizing hormones such as cortisol, adrenaline, and norepinephrine to keep your resting metabolic rate high in the absence of taking in calories. These are the same hormones that spike when you exercise, and the combined stressors can easily trigger a burnout condition after the fast, which could take the form of overeating and/or experiencing fatigue in the days thereafter. Finally, if you have a history of or tendency toward disordered eating, psychologists advise against attempting extended fasts because of their potential negative psychological consequences.

Sprinting

At my interactions with live audiences, I invariably get questions about how to deal with frustrating weight-loss plateaus. My favorite response is, "Nothing cuts you up like sprinting." If you have done the hard work of transforming your diet and building metabolic flexibility, sprinting can help shed those final few pounds of stubborn fat. In comparison to burning calories with hours and hours of cardio every week, you can potentially obtain a tenfold return on your investment with sprinting. Here's the opening sentence of a study published in the *Journal of Obesity* titled "High-Intensity Intermittent Exercise and Fat Loss": "The effect of regular aerobic exercise on body fat is negligible; however, other forms of exercise may have a greater impact on body composition." Prolonged workouts can deliver many physical and psychological benefits, but they won't melt the fat away. Sprinting will, provided you conduct the workouts correctly and have built metabolic flexibility (see page 138 for more information about the way sprinting turbocharges fat burning).

The magic of sprinting comes from adaptive responses to the training stimulus as well as from the so-called afterburn effect. Afterburn refers to the fact that your metabolic rate is elevated for as long as seventy-two hours after even a short-duration sprint workout because of a phenomenon known as *excess post-exercise oxygen consumption* (EPOC). As your body works to return to homeostasis, extra oxygen is used for the purposes of hormone balancing, glycogen renewal, cell repair, muscle protein synthesis, ATP replenishment, and increased fatty acid oxidation. The adaptive response to sprinting describes powerful genetic signaling and hormonal cascades that help change your body so you can perform better the next time out. This includes improving oxygen delivery to muscles, recruiting more explosive muscle fibers, and shedding unnecessary body fat.

While adaptive responses are triggered by prolonged cardiovascular workouts and even piano lessons, these activities don't lead to fat reduction as much as sprinting does. You can get away with carrying excess body fat while engaging in lower-impact or lower-intensity activities, but the penalty is much more severe when you're sprinting. You are training to accelerate quickly at the start, pump the arms aggressively, strike the ground with maximum propulsive force in every stride (Usain Bolt's force production is more than one thousand pounds per stride—five times his body weight!), and command the stabilizer muscles to maintain a balanced center of gravity throughout the effort. Even the slightest bit of wasted energy, such as a wayward arm swing or transporting a payload of jiggly abdominal fat that makes zero contribution to forward propulsion, will have a huge adverse effect on your ability to generate top speed. The same dynamic holds true for any fitness endeavor or athletic event that entails jumping off the ground. Look at the chiseled physique of an Olympic diver or the skeletal frame of an elite high jumper. But don't worry if your physique is not quite Olympic caliber when you start. Do the best you can, knowing that continued improvement will be the reward for your commitment to something that's likely out of your comfort zone.

The profound genetic signaling for fat loss prompted by sprinting is why you never see a fat sprinter or jumper! By contrast, at the starting line of even the most challenging endurance events, such as a marathon, trail ultramarathon, or Ironman triathlon, you will notice that the majority of the participants carry a little or a lot of excess body fat. This is likely because of carbohydrate-dependent eating patterns and the compensatory responses of reduced everyday activity and increased caloric intake prompted by prolonged, depleting workouts. What's more, the disturbingly common chronic cardio patterns followed by serious endurance athletes and group exercise devotees can actually send genetic signals to overeat in an attempt to survive the stress on the body caused by exhausting workouts that deplete muscle glycogen. The end result of extreme endurance training is little or no genetic signaling to shed fat. Many extreme exercisers have been shocked when they shed excess body fat by training *less* and making only modest dietary adjustments.

Follow the instructions in chapter 5 for properly conducting a sprint workout, with the emphasis on consistent, high-quality efforts and plenty of rest between them. You want a complete absence of the cumulative fatigue and cellular depletion that comes with a stressful HIIT workout, because this kicks you into compensation mode (less activity, more appetite) in the hours afterward. Because the caloric energy demands of a sprint workout are minimal, you can sprint in a fasted state. In fact, being fasted when you sprint is likely the best idea, because you will eliminate the risk of stomach distress caused by eating too soon before a workout. In addition, because of the extreme metabolic demands of a sprint workout, it's best to wait at least an hour afterward, and maybe longer, before eating again. It's likely that your appetite will be muted because of elevated body temperature and stress hormone levels after a sprint session. Following the suggestions to fast before and a bit after your session automatically creates a nice level-5 experience (see page 157)—a fasted morning plus a difficult workout plus a post-exercise fasting period.

The adaptive benefits of sprint workouts are maximized when you engage in weight-bearing sprints. If, because of an insufficient fitness level or injury risk concerns, you must start with low-impact or no-impact sprinting on a bike or cardio machine, strive to make continued progress toward running sprints on flat ground. While sprinting once a week is recommended, you can add a second sprint session during aggressive short-term fat-reduction efforts. If you do running sprints, start by adding a low-impact or no-impact session on a bike or cardio machine. If you think you can handle a second high-impact sprint session, try doing only the running technique drills and wind sprints described in chapter 5 (see page 138). These are plenty strenuous enough to stimulate the adaptive hormonal response but will minimize the risk of injury and burnout that can crop up when you sprint too frequently.

Remember, it's all about the genetic signaling, and a little goes a long way. As you gain competence, don't be tempted to throw in longer sprints, more reps, or shorter rest periods. Just enjoy getting faster as you perform your template workout. Stick to the plan and watch the fat reliably melt away over time. If your sprint sessions are resulting in more than minor muscle soreness or next-day fatigue, tone down your efforts so that you can feel "okay" the next day. A message of caution for those who are brave and driven enough to venture out to the track and sprint: overly stressful workouts (e.g., too many and/or too lengthy sprints, and/or insufficient rest periods between efforts) trigger excess stress hormone production and a compensation response. Well-executed explosive workouts stimulate a desirable spike in adaptive hormones (followed by a quick return to homeostasis) and efficient fat reduction. Brief, explosive micro workouts can also be a great catalyst for fat reduction. While sprint running requires extensive warm-up and preparatory drills, doing anything explosive for ten seconds counts as a form of sprinting in this context, including a set of deep squats, pulling StretchCordz or mini bands, and swinging a kettlebell. Adhere to the protocol described in chapter 5 (see page 134).

Cold Exposure

Anecdotal evidence and cutting-edge science are revealing the incredible potential of therapeutic cold exposure, a.k.a. cold thermogenesis, to stimulate fat reduction independently, and as a complement to, diet and exercise efforts. Exposure to cold water is particularly therapeutic because its greater molecular density (versus air) drains body heat twenty-five times faster than exposure to cold air. Taking a cold shower—or, better yet, plunging into a tub of near-freezing water for a few minutes every morning—triggers an intense hormonal response. You experience an immediate and sharp increase in alertness and motivation as well as accelerated fat metabolism for hours afterward. Exposure to cold prompts your body to burn fat calories in an attempt to stay warm. Ray Cronise, a former NASA research scientist and prominent biohacker, lost twenty-seven pounds in six weeks with cold-activation techniques consisting of hot-cold contrast showers, "shiver walks" (outdoor walks underdressed), and sleeping in chilly conditions. Cronise describes the technique as "thermal loading" to increase metabolic rate.

Note: If you have preexisting health conditions such as thyroid or adrenal dysfunction, or if you have any symptoms of minor illness, hold off on cold exposure until you regain your basic level of health.

Therapeutic exposure to cold helps counterbalance yet another genetic disconnect from our ancestral past—our virtually 24-7 existence in comfortable, temperature-stable environments. As mentioned in T. S. Wiley's *Lights Out: Sleep, Sugar, and Survival,* we are locked year-round into a hormonal "summer mode" of sugar eating and fat storage in preparation for a cold, calorically scarce winter. Alas, that winter experience never comes—from a genetic-signaling perspective. We must acknowledge that modern humans have literally gone soft because of our obsession with comfort, convenience, luxury, and instant gratification.

Granted, no one wants to rewind the evolutionary timeline and experience the harsh natural selection pressures our ancestors faced. However, when we recoil at the mere mention of a cold shower or a quick plunge into a chilly river at the end of a hike, it's clear we have lost some of the edge that makes us human. Our lack of interest in the daily challenges that have made us—in the words of Brian "Liver King" Johnson—"the baddest mammalian predators to ever walk the earth" has resulted in accelerated aging and increased risk of disease.

Like fasting, cold exposure provides a window into our ancestral past, for primal humans were routinely subjected to cold temperatures. Experts believe that cold exposure was a significant driver of an assortment of evolutionary adaptations, including optimizing endocrine and immune functioning and honing the ultimate survival attribute of efficient fat burning. Our adaptation to cold temperatures is most likely why we possess a special type of fat known as brown adipose tissue (BAT). Unlike regular "white" fat, which we store on our bodies and burn for energy, BAT exists primarily to keep us warm. Research shows that hormetic exposure to cold activates brown fat, triggering an increase in the burning of regular body fat.

Besides brown fat activation, a cold plunge delivers a fantastic burst of energy, alertness, and euphoria. You are tapping into ancient adaptive processes and response mechanisms that are hardwired into our genes. One prominent Finnish study revealed that immersion into forty-degree-Fahrenheit water (4.4 degrees Celsius) for even as few as twenty seconds spikes the prominent mood, focusing, and motivation hormone norepinephrine by 200 to 300 percent for up to one hour! Cold exposure also delivers profound anti-inflammatory, immune-boosting effects, including an increase in the production of the internal superantioxidant glutathione. Cold exposure also prompts the release of the vaunted cold-shock proteins, which facilitate an assortment of repair processes in brain synapses and muscle tissue.

The vasoconstriction and vasodilation that result from cold exposure serve to strengthen your cardiovascular system. This counters the common quip that jumping in an ice bath or a frozen lake will give you a heart attack! Getting cold and rewarming also triggers a pumping reaction throughout the lymphatic system, providing a potent detoxification effect and a boost in white blood cell and killer T cell immune functioning. The common misconception that getting cold will cause you to catch a cold is disproved by a study of winter swimming devotees revealing that they experienced 40 percent fewer respiratory tract infections than a control population. Cold exposure followed by sun exposure also helps boost vitamin D production, something of particular benefit in minimizing the risk of contracting any viral infection—yes, including global pandemic infections. Cold therapy enthusiasts also enjoy numerous psychological benefits. When you can develop the discipline to turn that handle to cold for the last two minutes of your shower—or jump into an icy body of water, an ice bath, or a chest freezer filled with water that's in the thirties, forties, or fifties for a few or several minutes—you develop focus and resilience that carry over into all other peak-performance endeavors in life.

If you're still on the fence instead of stripped down and immersed in your closest chilly river, let's emphasize the importance of keeping your cold exposure short enough to trigger an adaptive benefit without its seeming like an unpleasant ordeal. Remember, twenty seconds of immersion into forty-degree-Fahrenheit (4.4-degree-Celsius) water delivers a huge hormone boost, so you can assume that one to two minutes at fifty-five degrees Fahrenheit will do the same. The optimally brief fight-or-flight stimulation makes you naturally more alert and energized after you get out of the water and start working to return to homeostasis. If you were to remain in the cold tub until you became truly uncomfortable and started to shiver, you might overstress the delicate fight-or-flight mechanisms in the same manner as you would by undergoing an exhausting workout or a stressful personal or work situation. A good benchmark to follow is to leave the water before you start shivering. Research suggests that muscles start to burn more energy and produce extra heat *before* you start shivering, so no need to try to set records.

The best strategy for taking a cold plunge is to cultivate a focused, positive, resilient mindset; become intent on executing the mission without wimping out. Whether you are in the shower, a cold tub, or a frigid body of water, using intentional breathing will help you withstand the initial shock response that typically occurs when you enter. You have probably had the experience of jumping into cold water, screaming reflexively, exiting immediately, and making a beeline for the nearest towel, tub, or hot shower. You can easily mitigate that panic reaction by taking deep, diaphragmatic breaths for the duration of your time in the water. Begin an aggressive inhalation by first inflating the abdomen, followed by the chest cavity. This will enable the diaphragm muscle and the oxygen-rich lower lobes of the lungs to fully engage for the most efficient breathing.

Commit to a reasonable goal of staying under the showerhead for two minutes or completing twenty breath cycles before leaving a cold tub or body of water. If you feel as if you are about to shiver, get out immediately and try to do a bit better next time. At my health club, I have access to a therapeutic cold plunge maintained at forty-eight degrees Fahrenheit (nine degrees Celsius). I enjoy hot-to-cold contrast therapy, in which I start with ten minutes in the sauna, then sit up to my neck (important because brown fat is concentrated in the upper back) in the cold pool for five to seven minutes, then finish with a few minutes of rewarming in the hot spa. It's been fun to notice my tolerance naturally increase over time. At first, I could last comfortably in the cold pool for around two minutes; now seven is no problem.

Getting Started with Therapeutic Cold Exposure

1. **Contrast showers:** Get your feet wet with this health practice by switching between cold and hot water for thirty seconds at a time during your daily shower(s). You'll likely find it a bit uncomfortable at first, but after a few days you'll get used to it and deeply appreciate the refreshing energy boost you obtain from some basic cold exposure.

2. **Cold finish/cold showers:** After a handful of contrast showers, try to end every shower with two minutes of full-blast cold. After a handful of those, you can progress to taking a cold-only shower for a few minutes.

3. **Ice baths or plunges:** Once you become a cold shower expert, consider upping your game to a bathtub or outdoor livestock tank filled with ice water, or finding an appropriate lake, river, or ocean for a cold plunge. In general, anything under sixty degrees Fahrenheit (fifteen degrees Celsius) is suitable for cold therapy.

4. **Chest freezer:** Perhaps you will one day consider the ultimate affordable 24/7 home therapy experience—a chest freezer filled with water chilled to your

desired temperature! Search YouTube for "chest freezer cold water therapy Brad Kearns" to learn how to get a chest freezer setup going.

5. **Cryotherapy:** The increasingly popular practice of visiting a cryotherapy center for a short session inside an extremely cold air chamber is also an option. Some purists claim that water offers more health benefits, and the high cost of memberships or single visits can be a deterrent.

Note: Greetings from Miami! This progression guide assumes that you are doing your cold exposure and then heading into a day amidst pleasant indoor or outdoor temperatures. If this is the case, rewarming naturally over time (including doing some light exercise or adding a clothing layer if necessary) will help maximize the fat burning benefits. If you are showering and then heading into the elements to install snow chains or work in an unheated warehouse, you may want to make cold exposure a seasonal practice or pair your sessions with rewarming via a hot shower or a sauna (as with the popular practice of contrast therapy).

Let your personal preference and your natural tolerance dictate the details of your regimen. Over time, you may notice a natural inclination to use colder temperatures and/or remain in the water for more time. Advanced enthusiasts will spend five to seven minutes in water in the thirties, ten minutes in water in the forties, and up to twenty minutes in water in the fifty-to-sixty-degree range. However, if you overdo it to the point of shivering and/or feeling punky for a while afterward, you will trigger protective mechanisms that actually reduce your energy, mood, and cognitive functioning in the hours following your cold exposure in reaction to what was perceived as a life-or-death threat.

Losing Excess Body Fat

In the excitement of adding cold exposure to the list of cutting-edge biohacking practices, we've forgotten to figure compensation theory insights into the equation. Cold exposure certainly activates brown fat and increases the burning of (white) body fat, but it's also clear from science and anecdotal evidence that cold exposure can stimulate appetite. Brad and I have conducted experiments to validate this insight. At anywhere from twenty minutes to one hour after a devoted cold session, a hunger-inducing ghrelin spike reliably occurs. This is independent from circadian-influenced ghrelin spikes and seems to occur distinctly in tandem with cold exposure sessions. Research reveals that cold exposure causes a drop in blood glucose (because muscles are burning extra glucose—and fat—to rewarm), a likely reason for an ensuing appetite spike. Perhaps you can recall a time when you followed a hard day of skiing or chopping wood in the wintertime with a massive meal or string of meals? As your body burns calories to rewarm, appetite mechanisms command you to consume more calories to fuel the suddenly raging fire.

If you are serious about dropping excess body fat once and for all, my suggestion is to try to fast for a few hours after your cold exposure session, overriding any ghrelin spike that comes your way. After that unpleasant spike passes and your stomach quiets down, realizing that no food is coming anytime soon, your body will kick into accelerated fat burning and ketone production. This may give you a nice burst of mental clarity, or at least stabilize your mood, energy levels, and cognitive functioning for a few hours. Ben Greenfield, one of the pioneers in popularizing cold exposure in recent years, reports interesting data from the continuous blood glucose monitor he wore for two weeks while engaging in cold exposure. He claims the single most potent stabilizer of his blood glucose levels every day was his four-minute morning cold plunge!

For fat reduction, it's best to try to rewarm naturally instead of jumping right into a hot shower or undergoing the hot-to-cold contrast therapy I described. In mixing hot and cold, I'm going more for relaxation than fat reduction. Some extreme cold enthusiasts deliberately underdress after their sessions in an attempt to leverage the benefits for a longer time period. They also conduct independent efforts to run the thermostat in their homes a little cold in the spirit of Ray Cronise's shiver walks. If you decide to dabble in therapeutic mild cold stress, be sure to keep your hands and head warm if you underdress or expose yourself to low temperatures for an extended period of time. This will reassure your brain that you are in no thermic danger and keep calorie burning elevated. Performing a handful of cold exposure sessions, as well as extended fasting sessions each week, can rank up there close to sprinting as a fat reduction secret weapon, so go for it!

Advanced Strategies for Fat Reduction—Journal Exercises

1. **Fasted workouts:** Describe your current experience and competence level with fasted workouts. Using the ideas in this chapter as suggestions, list a progression of increasingly difficult fasted workouts to strive for in the months ahead.

2. **Extended fasting:** Describe your current experience and competence level with extended fasting. List a progression of extended fasting efforts to strive for in the months ahead.

3. **Sprinting:** Describe your current experience and competence level with sprinting. List ways to incorporate sprinting into your current fitness regimen, including specifics of a starting-point workout and a sensible progression to a more challenging session in the months ahead.

4. **Cold exposure:** Describe your current experience and competence level with cold exposure. List a progression of cold exposure efforts to strive for in the months ahead.

The 12-Day Turbocharge

I hope your journey through this book so far has been as interactive and multidimensional as possible. This was the intention with the journal assignments at the end of each chapter and the encouragement to immediately do things such as ditch junk foods, optimize your sleep environment, monitor your exercise heart rate, and so on. Now it's time to plunge into the *Two Meals a Day* lifestyle in an intense and dramatic manner. It's time for the 12-Day Turbocharge! This stand-alone program draws upon all the knowledge and practical suggestions you have been exposed to in this book to create an experience designed to get you inspired and focused on long-term lifestyle transformation.

Every day for twelve days, you'll tackle an assignment in each of five areas: food, fasting, fitness, mindset, and lifestyle. Plan on devoting one to two hours per day to completing your action and journaling assignments. I recommend starting day 1 on a Monday so that weekend-appropriate challenges will fall on days 6 and 7. If you lag behind or face logistical challenges preventing you from completing an assignment, take note and make a commitment to do so as soon as possible. If it's appropriate and possible to double up and finish the missed challenge the following day or the day after, that's the best choice for continuity. If you can't squeeze the challenge in during the twelve-day block, be sure to complete it as soon as possible after that.

You'll want everything in your life to be just right when you commence the Turbocharge. Pick a start time when you feel focused, energized, and motivated to tackle a brief but challenging immersive experience. Make sure that your overall life stress levels are low and you aren't dealing with any unusual burdens or obligations. If you have travel plans, are hosting out-of-town family or friends, or have nagging injuries that hinder your workouts, wait until things normalize before commencing the Turbocharge. Everything should feel comfortable as you proceed with your typical day-to-day routine at home.

Following is a list of what you'll need to ensure an enjoyable and successful Turbocharge. Please do the necessary research, organizing, scheduling, and purchasing beforehand.

Food and Fasting

- Serviceable kitchen with basic cookware and appliances
- Budget allocation for nutritious foods and celebratory meal preparations
- Natural-foods grocer and/or internet resource for high-quality foods
- Healthful cooking oils such as extra-virgin olive oil, avocado oil, and coconut oil as well as saturated fats such as butter, ghee, and lard

Fitness

- Wireless heart-rate monitor with chest strap transmitter and watch (the Polar FT1 model is affordable and accurate)
- Local venue for sprint workouts and MAF tests, such as a running track or a flat, smooth path or trail
- Local venue or internet resource for a formal movement class (yoga, Pilates, tai chi)
- Ideas and logistics for a grand play adventure in nature on day 7
- Equipment for a workplace variation project on day 8 (stand-up desk, low desk, micro-workout gear)

Mindset

- Spiral notebooks or other blank books for your *Two Meals a Day* and gratitude journals
- Vision board supplies: magazines, poster board, glue, art supplies, and/or digital imagery for a creating a "mind movie"

Lifestyle

- Blue-light-minimizing eyewear and/or light sources (orange or yellow UV-blocking lenses, orange lightbulbs, salt lamp)

■ Cold exposure venue (ice bath or natural body of water under sixty degrees Fahrenheit—river, lake, ocean)

Day 1

Food: Kitchen and Pantry Purge

I hope you took immediate action to partially or completely rid your home of detrimental processed foods when you read about the kitchen and pantry purge in chapter 1. But whatever state your fridge and pantry are in right now, it's time to finish the job! Discard all forms of refined industrial seed oils, grains, and sugars (see pages 16 and 17). If any of these agents are still leaking into the picture, it's time to commit to zero tolerance for the Big Three for the duration of the 12-Day Turbocharge.

The major problem area to focus on is dining out, because your restaurant's salmon and broccoli plate or your take-out carne asada and guacamole is likely to have been prepared with industrial seed oils. Read labels when you purchase exotic herbal teas, kombuchas, or any offerings on the Starbucks menu, because added sugar is commonplace. Notice how much better you feel getting off the blood-sugar roller coaster during the Turbocharge, and with any luck you will sustain long-term elimination of these foods or at least use them sparingly.

Fasting: Twelve-Hour Digestive Circadian Rhythm

Limit all manner of digestive functioning to a maximum of twelve hours today. This is a challenge you will carry forward for the entire Turbocharge and beyond. Pay particular attention to the fact that your digestive clock starts with the processing of any xenobiotic substance, even if it has no calories (e.g., coffee, tea, vitamins, etc.). From this baseline, the fasting category will involve consuming calories in a compressed window of time, trying a couple of extended fasts, and integrating workouts into your fasting period.

Fitness: Aerobic Workout at MAF Heart Rate

Calculate your "180 minus age" maximum aerobic function (MAF) heart rate in beats per minute. For example, a forty-two-year-old exerciser would have an MAF heart rate of 138 beats per minute (180 minus 42 equals 138). It's extremely important to obtain an accurate measurement of your heart rate for all your cardiovascular workouts to ensure that you experience their intended metabolic benefits—promoting fat burning instead of sugar burning. As I said in chapter 5 (page 129), the most accurate heart-rate measuring requires the use of a wireless heart-rate monitor with a chest transmitter and watch.

I hope that you picked one up and will strap it on every time you conduct a cardio workout forevermore. Yes, it's that important. It's simply too difficult to rely on perceived exertion or manual spot checks of your pulse rate, because it's easy to drift above MAF without a noticeable increase in perceived exertion. Even athletes with decades of experience require a constant reminder, in the form of a beeper alarm, to avoid exceeding their aerobic maximums. If you choose not to buy a wireless unit, you can perform the workout using gym equipment that's equipped with a pulse meter or by using a suitably equipped wristwatch. A truly MAF workout should feel comfortable at all times; you should be able to recite the alphabet or converse with an exercise partner without running short of breath.

Mindset: 12-Day Turbocharge Journal and Gratitude Journal

Start new sections in your *Two Meals a Day* journal to cover the assignments in the 12-Day Turbocharge—or start a brand-new journal if you wish to keep them separate. Similarly, start a separate gratitude journal or clearly designate the journal pages you use for gratitude entries.

Turbocharge journal: List some flaws, frailties, bad habits, past mistakes, and failures that you can forgive yourself for right now. These could be diet failures, flaking out on exercise ambitions, or aspects of your daily routine that have drifted into the "need to improve" category.

Gratitude journal: Make a list of several lifestyle circumstances you are grateful for as well as several health attributes you are grateful for. If you aren't quite where you want to be with your present level of health, energy, and body composition, acknowledge the remarkable ability of the human body to respond to environmental signals and transform.

Lifestyle: Take a "Before" Photo

Snap a "before" photo in front of a full-length mirror wearing minimal clothing. Approach the experience without negativity and resolve to use the photo to keep you grateful, motivated, and accountable as you strive for body and life transformation goals.

Create a sleep sanctuary. Get rid of paperwork, piles of clutter, and any TV or computer screens in your bedroom. Tidy up your closet, bathroom, and nightstand areas as you strive for a minimalist effect. When in doubt, or if you haven't used something in a while, toss it! Strive to achieve complete nighttime darkness in the room. Use temporary window coverings while you look for permanent solutions such as new blackout curtains. Remove or tape over all minor light emissions and get rid of night-lights. Get a red or amber flashlight (far less disruptive to melatonin than the blue-light emissions of a regular flashlight) and place it at your bedside to use if you need to get up in the dark. Assess the noise level in your room and get a combination HEPA air filter–ionizer, a humidifier or dehumidifier (depending on your environment), or fan to emit white noise as desired. Find the most distant location you can tolerate to plug in your mobile device—ideally, in the hallway. If that isn't possible, charge your phone out of reach of your bedside. This will minimize EMF (electromagnetic field) exposure and help you resist the temptation to check your phone at bedtime or first thing in the morning.

Journal

- Food: Comment on your once-and-for-all kitchen and pantry purge, including an itemized list of stuff you tossed. If you took care of business in chapter 1, write about how your diet change has affected energy, mood, and cognitive performance to date.
- Fasting: Note your digestive function start time and end time.
- Fitness: Note your MAF heart rate calculations and workout notes.
- Mindset: Write your Turbocharge and gratitude journal entries.
- Lifestyle: Comment about your "before" photo and sleep sanctuary efforts.

Day 2

Food: Restock Healthful Foods

If you purged your kitchen and pantry and restocked them back when you read chapters 1 and 2, this action item won't be as daunting as doing it in real time during the Turbocharge. If you indeed have built some momentum with plenty of nutritious options in the home and an absence of processed junk, go buy some extra special items today. But if today is ground zero for a restock, it's time to go on a shopping spree for delicious, high-quality, nutrient-dense ancestral foods. Locate the best natural-foods market in your community and talk with the staff to get recommendations for and insights into the most healthful options in each food category. Determine whether there is a co-op or farmer's market in your area where you can buy fresh foods every week. Try some internet resources for specialty items and ways to shore up deficiencies in your local stores, referring to the many suggestions presented by category in chapter 2 and recapped in the day 5 material (page 183).

Fasting: 14-10 Eating Pattern

Strive to complete a fourteen-hour overnight fasting period before consuming your first calories of the day. Expect to feel alert, energetic, and focused without food during the morning hours. This is representative of adequate metabolic flexibility—you are burning body fat and perhaps making some ketones as reliable sources of energy before your first meal. If you find yourself struggling with low energy, mood swings, brain fog, or sugar cravings during the fasting period, go ahead and eat your first meal and record the duration of your fast. If necessary, downscale the rest of the fasting assignments so you don't exceed your capabilities and trigger your body's fight-or-flight response.

Fitness: Aerobic and Strength Assessments

Conduct a maximum aerobic function test by covering a predetermined distance or along a route that takes around ten minutes to complete. Maintain a heart rate as close as possible to your MAF calculation of "180 minus age" in beats per minute. Repeat the test every four to six weeks over the exact same course and distance.

Your strength assessment will consist of a single set of each of the primal essential movements: push-ups, pull-ups, squats, and planks (see page 133). Do as many reps as you can until failure with each exercise. Rest at least five minutes between exercises to ensure a fresh, high-quality effort. Record the results in your journal and repeat the test every four to six weeks. Expect to improve your results over time as you adhere to an effective strength-training routine. If you have distinct athletic goals or performance markers that you currently keep track of, feel free to choose alternative assessments, such as a timed 400-meter sprint or a set of bench presses or dead lifts. As it is in the MAF test, the key is to repeat the exact same strength assessments in order to accurately track improvement or regression.

Mindset: Identify Self-Limiting Beliefs and Behavior Patterns

Complete this journal exercise with total honesty and objectivity. Make one list of self-limiting thoughts and beliefs and another list of self-limiting behaviors. For example, harboring a negative body image goes in the former category, while eating too fast goes in the latter category. In addition to the overt issues you are currently dealing with daily, spend some time in reflection in order to assess whether there is anything lurking in your subconscious that can be added to the list. Write a brief explanation of the specifics of each item. For example, you may note a connection between eating too fast and growing up in a large family where you had to compete for food at the table.

Lifestyle: Dark, Quiet, Mellow Evening

Dedicate the final two hours before bedtime to winding down—no screens, no excitement, and minimal light (use UV-blocking orange or yellow lenses and/or orange or yellow light sources). Choose mellow activities such as quiet socializing, a neighborhood stroll, foam rolling, drawing or practicing other art forms, taking a warm bath, giving or receiving a massage, or reading in bed. Tomorrow you will pick and choose a few of your favorite activities to create a soothing bedtime ritual that you will repeat each evening.

Journal

- Food: Comment on restocking your kitchen and make an itemized list of foods you purchased and the sources you used.
- Fasting: Note the start time and end time of your eating window, and include a subjective evaluation of your 14-10 experience.
- Fitness: Record the results of your MAF test and strength assessments.
- Mindset: Complete the self-limiting beliefs and behaviors journal assignments.
- Lifestyle: Make notes about your mellow evening, particularly what you enjoyed most, so that you might integrate that into tomorrow's evening routine.

Day 3

Food: Healthful Recipe Research

Spend thirty to sixty minutes reviewing the recipes in this book, and/or other cookbooks that interest you, and list half a dozen of the most appealing—those that have the potential to become go-to meals for you and your family. Identify one meal that you'll prepare for a celebratory dinner for family and friends on day 6, and invite your guests today. Compile a list of ingredients from your recipe choices and purchase them on your next shopping trip.

Fasting: 14-10 Eating Pattern

Complete another day of 14-10 fasting and eating, because the challenges will escalate quickly during the Turbocharge.

Fitness: Introductory Sprint Workout

Perform the following in sequence for a safe and effective sprint session:

- aerobic warm-up,
- dynamic stretching (search for "Brad Kearns pre-workout dynamic stretching routine" on YouTube),
- preparatory technique drills (search for "Brad Kearns running technique drills" on YouTube), and
- six brief accelerations—wind sprints—lasting around five seconds each.

For the main set of sprints, perform explosive efforts that are well within your capabilities, and leave the workout feeling pleasantly fatigued and satisfied instead of depleted and exhausted. With the success of this effort, you will conduct a full-length sprint workout on day 8. If you struggle a bit today, just repeat this workout on day 8. Escalate the degree of difficulty of your sprint workout only when you feel well prepared and 100 percent rested and motivated for a peak-performance effort.

Mindset: Destroy and Reframe Self-Limiting Beliefs and Behaviors

Address each self-limiting belief and behavior on yesterday's list and implement the Jack Canfield strategy of describing how it limits you and deciding how you would rather be, act, or feel (see page 101). Then create a turnaround statement that affirms your desire to transform. Be precise with your language so you can "buy into" new beliefs and behaviors that seem realistic and doable. Here's an example: if you harbor a negative body image, this may repeatedly discourage you from adhering to dietary restrictions or a regular exercise routine. When you encounter the slightest bit of resistance that requires discipline and resolve to overcome, your negative body image will sabotage your best intentions, and you'll regress back to your undesirable baseline. Knowing that a negative body image won't just vanish with a breezy affirmation, perhaps you can form a new belief: you can make steady progress with sustained effort. Even if you dislike or hate what you see in the mirror right now, you can still completely buy into this new belief, which affirms that steady progress is possible. This will free to you to take necessary action and stay the course, even through adversity.

Lifestyle: Create a Soothing Bedtime Ritual

Today you can string together a few of your favorite evening pastimes that don't involve screens and create a template for a soothing bedtime ritual that you will repeat each evening. Perhaps some things really clicked for you during last night's exercise, and you can draw upon a lifetime of experience with activities that make you feel calm and relaxed. Perform the same sequence every evening until it becomes automatic. When it's time to commence the ritual, going through the motions without having to use brainpower to remember what's next will serve to deeply relax your mind and body in preparation for sleep. You will likely be amazed at the benefits of making a deliberate transition out of the dynamic and highly stimulatory nature of hectic modern life into a ritualistic pattern that delivers some of the same mind-body-connection benefits as a session of yoga, tai chi, or meditation.

Your ritual might best start with a phone alarm reminding you that it's time to begin. From there, perhaps you'll choose to take the dog out for a ten-minute stroll around the block, return home and brew some herbal tea, spend five minutes foam rolling, then make entries in your gratitude journal while you enjoy the tea. After that, head to the bedroom for lights-out.

Options abound for putting together a sequence that's relaxing and pleasurable. In the wintertime, my go-to evening ritual is a lengthy soak in the hot tub with my wife, Carrie, followed by a five-minute plunge into a cold pool, followed by a few minutes of rewarming in the spa. After a quick shower, I hop on a temperature-cooled mattress (ChiliTechnology.com), spend fifteen to thirty minutes reading (using a small headlamp in a dark room), and then it's lights-out. In the summer, Carrie and I will grab our dog, Shanti, for a final romp around the neighborhood (which takes between five and twenty minutes—depending upon the number of interesting neighborhood smells apparently). Back home, I'll take a five-minute cold shower, then enjoy some final reading. The cold shower and year-round cooled mattress help facilitate a lowering of body temperature—one of the key triggers for melatonin release and sleepiness.

Whatever sequence you put together, make sure the duration is short enough to easily manage every night. Feel free to add or subtract certain elements over time, but make sure you always have a repeatable template in place.

Journal

- Food: List the recipes you found and make a list of ingredients to shop for.
- Fasting: Note the start time and end time of your caloric consumption and subjectively evaluate the 14-10 window.
- Fitness: Record details of your sprint workout—reps, duration, recovery intervals—and make a subjective evaluation of its effectiveness.
- Mindset: Complete your self-limiting beliefs and behaviors journal assignments.
- Lifestyle: Write a detailed description of your soothing bedtime ritual and comment upon the experience.

Day 4

Food: Freshly Prepared Food—Not Packaged, Processed, or Frozen

Prepare all your meals from scratch and consume only fresh foods today. Obviously, some packaged foods—such as eggs in a carton, meat in a wrapper, and other fresh, minimally processed items—are fine, as is the incidental use of healthful sauces, dressings, and toppings (read labels to avoid products that contain sweeteners and industrial seed oils).

Fasting: 14-10 with No Snacking

Time to up the ante gracefully in terms of your metabolic flexibility. Maintain a fourteen-hour fasting window, as you did on the previous two days, but inside your ten-hour eating window, don't consume any calories between meals. With any luck you were dissuaded from snacking as soon as you read the introduction to this book, but today it's time to clean up any loose ends in this area and make a concerted effort to catch yourself, even if you reach for something insignificant, such as a handful of nuts.

Fitness: Micro Workouts

Today you will delve deep into the wonderful world of micro workouts (see page 134) by performing a minimum of five distinct sessions lasting between one and five minutes each. Do a micro workout upon awakening to get the energy flowing, then use them as strategic breaks from prolonged periods of stillness during the workday. String together a few brief, explosive exercises or perform a sequence of flexibility and mobility movements. As I hope you will discover today, a minimal time investment can have a huge impact on your energy, cognitive focus, overall mood, and sense of well-being.

Record the specifics of each micro workout in your journal. See if you can formulate a handful of go-to sequences that you can repeat without having to exert any cognitive or creative effort. For example, jumping up from your desk to perform twenty deep squats, make twenty wall angels, and climb five flights of stairs can become your set routine for the workplace.

Mindset: Turnaround Statements—Subconscious Programming

Review the turnaround statements you generated yesterday and implement Jack Canfield's recommendation to repeat each statement for two to three minutes several times per day for a minimum of thirty days. Today, conduct a minimum of five sessions, and strive to do the same each day for the next thirty days. Bookmark the journal page(s) where you wrote your turnaround statements for easy reference.

Lifestyle: Create a Winning Morning Routine

Experiment with a few different ideas, then lock into a deliberate sequence of activities that you can form into a daily morning habit over the next few weeks. Ideally, the routine will involve exposure to direct sunlight and movement to get blood and oxygen flowing throughout the body. Perhaps you'll favor taking a quick stroll outdoors, completing a series of simple yoga moves on the lawn, then sitting on the patio for a few minutes with a cup of tea and your gratitude journal. Athletes might design a customized flexibility and mobility routine, including some light strengthening exercises, and end with a couple of minutes of cold exposure (see page 165). Keep your phone on the sidelines and discover a few morning behaviors that make you feel good. Adding elements that require counting (e.g., ten sun salutations, holding a back arch for a count of twenty, writing three gratitude journal entries, taking a cold shower for two minutes) improves the mindfulness aspect of the morning ritual. Over the next few weeks, dial in a defined routine that you can execute on autopilot every day.

It's critical to make absolutely sure your routine is short and simple enough to be sustainable over the long run. Tone down your eagerness to plunge into the "ideal" morning routine and err on the conservative side when you create your first template. You must apply the commitment and discipline necessary to repeat the sequence each day until it becomes programmed into habit. Once a strong habit is in place, you may choose to increase the duration or degree of difficulty of the template as desired, making it much more likely to succeed. If you blast out of the gate with an hour of power during the 12-Day Turbocharge, real life has a way of messing with your grand ambitions.

Listen to "The Lasting Benefits of a Morning Routine"—the December 10, 2019, episode of Brad's *Get Over Yourself* podcast—as he details his four-year journey of creating and sustaining an increasingly elaborate daily routine that involves flexibility, mobility, core strengthening, and injury prevention. He describes starting out with a modest sequence of moves designed to prevent injury during sprinting and jumping. When filming it for YouTube (search for "Brad Kearns morning routine"), he was surprised to learn that what he thought was a five-minute session to get the blood flowing actually lasted twelve minutes! After two years of consistent daily execution, Brad was compelled to add a couple of new movements specific to his fitness goals, then a couple more in the following months, and a couple more further down the road. Today, his daily routine lasts thirty-five minutes, and optional add-on items frequently make it last forty-five minutes. What started as a simple alternative to reaching for the phone upon awakening has evolved into quite a strenuous and effective workout. Completing the sequence each day has dramatically elevated the platform from which Brad launches his formal sessions of sprinting and high jumping.

Journal

- Food: Describe the fresh meals you prepared and make a subjective evaluation of the experience.
- Fasting: Note the start time and end time of your caloric consumption and subjectively evaluate the 14-10-and-no-snacking experience.
- Fitness: Write a detailed description of each micro workout. Create some more fun workouts to add to your template in the future.
- Mindset: Comment on the turnaround statement exercise.
- Lifestyle: Write a detailed description of every element of your morning routine. Create a repeatable routine for the future.

Day 5

Food: A Deep Dive into Superfoods and Premium Foods

Spend some time exploring local grocery options and the internet for foods such as grass-fed organ meats, wild-caught seafood, first-cold-pressed olive and avocado oils, artisan bean-to-bar chocolate, and other premium-quality products (see chapter 2). Prepare some recipes using ingredients that are a step up from the usual supermarket offerings. See if you can develop a deep interest in a certain product category and learn how it's grown, harvested, and marketed, just as a wine connoisseur would study a particular varietal.

For meat, try ButcherBox.com, LoneMountainWagyu.com, GrasslandBeef.com, ThriveMarket.com, WildIdeaBuffalo.com, and ForceOfNature.com.

For artisan chocolate, try Askinosie.com, CoracaoConfections.com, CreoChocolate .com, HuKitchen.com, KellerManniChocolate.com, LillieBelleFarms.com, RitualChoco late.com, and TazaChocolate.com.

For seafood, try VitalChoice.com.

Visit Amazon.com's grocery section to find some excellent cold-pressed oils and other premium products.

Fasting: 16-8 Eating Pattern

The 16-8 eating pattern typically entails finishing eating by 8:00 p.m. and consuming your first calories at 12:00 noon the next day. If you prefer to pursue a morning-evening meal pattern, as described in chapter 6, keep this challenge as a 14-10 pattern with no snacking or midday meal in between.

Fitness: Breakthrough Aerobic Workout

Extend the duration of your typical cardiovascular session to achieve a fitness breakthrough. When you feel fully rested and energized for a challenging session, try to go one and a half times your normal duration—or beyond! Be sure to maintain your heart rate at "180 minus age" in beats per minute (or below) at all times to stimulate maximum fat burning and minimal glucose burning.

Mindset: Step-by-Step Action Plans

After reviewing your mindset assignments of the previous three days, list up to three beliefs or behavior patterns that you intend to change. Create a detailed step-by-step plan of action for each one. Describe how you are going to increase the importance and prioritization of the goal as well as the repetition and endurance necessary to succeed. If you plan to shop for more healthful foods, for example, list the local stores or internet resources that you intend to patronize. If you are going for physique transformation, try to get as specific as possible about your goal. Instead of a general statement such as "I want to look good in a bikini by summer," state your desired new waist or dress size or a fitness benchmark you want to attain.

Lifestyle: Advanced Strategies—Cold Exposure Session 1

It's time to take the cold plunge! Get comfortable in your warm shower, then begin some deep, diaphragmatic breaths, put your hand on the nozzle, and crank the handle all the way to cold and leave it there for two minutes. It's very important to breathe your way through this challenge so you override the predictable panic reaction that happens when the cold water hits. Set a goal of two minutes, but if you begin to shiver or feel truly uncomfortable, know that you can stop and try to go longer next time. If it's wintertime and you're heading out into cold weather, it's okay to finish up with hot water. But if you aren't facing harsh conditions, strive to rewarm naturally over the ensuing thirty minutes by dressing warmly or doing some light exercise.

If you have sufficient confidence to take on a more ambitious challenge, find a cold ocean, river, or lake nearby and enjoy a dip. You can also purchase twenty to forty pounds of ice and fill your bathtub for a brief immersion. Breathe deeply throughout the experience and get out before you start shivering.

Journal

- Food: List the details of your food sources and purchases.
- Fasting: Note the start time and end time of your caloric consumption and subjectively evaluate the 16-8 experience.
- Fitness: Record the details of your breakthrough aerobic workout, including heart rate and perceived rate of exertion. Strive to perform a breakthrough session once a month, and gradually extend the duration of your workout over time.
- Mindset: Create step-by-step action plans, as directed on page 184.
- Lifestyle: Note the duration and other details of the cold plunge and write a subjective evaluation of the experience.

Day 6

Food: Celebratory Meal

Shop for fresh ingredients and prepare a celebratory meal from scratch. If you want to ask guests or children to contribute a side dish or healthful dessert, go ahead. See if you can steer a bit of the dinner conversation toward your 12-Day Turbocharge adventure! Note that day 11 features another celebratory meal. You don't have to make a big fuss each time, but see if you can have one grand gathering and perhaps a smaller gathering on the days that are most convenient for you.

Fasting: 16-8, No Snacking

Spend another day in the 16-8 pattern, paying special attention to avoiding calories between meals.

Fitness: Formal Movement Class

Do your best to find an instructor-guided yoga, Pilates, tai chi, or barre session with other students in a convenient location. If it's not possible to join a class, search YouTube for a good video and follow along at home. There is an assortment of excellent options on You-Tube, so try searching for "hatha yoga for beginners," "restorative yoga for beginners," "tai chi for beginners," "Pilates at home for beginners," or "barre at home for beginners." Give the session your full attention and energy, with no distractions. Focus on the restorative benefits of these practices and be sure to stay within your current fitness capabilities.

Set a long-term goal of attending a formal class on a regular basis—at least twice a month or, ideally, at least once per week. Also, pick and choose your favorite elements of guided classes and create your own mini session that you can use as part of your morning routine or as a micro workout. Search YouTube for "sun salutation for beginners"—that's a great mini session of flowing yoga poses that integrates breathing and stretching for excellent mind-body benefits.

Mindset: Subconscious Programming—Note Card, Vision Board, Mind Movie

For each of yesterday's step-by-step action plans, create a brief statement and/or acronym that is meaningful and inspirational to you. Write these comments on a sticky note or index card and place it in a location where you will see it often during the day. Take things a step further by creating a vision board, a.k.a. a dream board, relating to your future goals. This popular practice entails gathering photographs, magazine clippings, drawings, and affirmations in a collage and displaying it in an ideal spot for frequent viewing.

If a digital experience interests you, you can use a simple slide show or more advanced video production software (iMovie, Final Cut Pro, Photoshop Elements) to create a "mind movie," as recommended by Dr. Joe Dispenza—neuroscientist, peak-performance expert, and bestselling author of *Becoming Supernatural.* Compile imagery representative of your "perfect life"—perhaps photographs of homes, cars, vacations, social gatherings, or fitness accomplishments such as climbing a mountain—into a three-minute presentation that you'll watch repeatedly. Viewing your index card, vision board, and/or mind movie on a regular basis will deliver inspirational reminders of your goals, commitments, values, and vision. This will help increase motivation, improve accountability, and counter the self-limiting subconscious programming that keeps you from feeling deserving of realizing your dreams.

Lifestyle: Nap Like a Champ

Take advantage of your Saturday and enjoy a world-class nap. Create an environment as dark and quiet as possible; you may need to use a white noise machine in the afternoon. Lie down for at least thirty minutes—up to an hour or longer if desired. Try not to use an alarm unless absolutely necessary. Take the pressure off and allow your body to awaken naturally. Even if you can't fall asleep, just relax with a blindfold or eyeshade over your eyes and do some intentional breathing to calm your mind and enjoy some valuable downtime.

Journal

- Food: Jot down details about the preparation and enjoyment of your celebratory meal.
- Fasting: Note the start time and end time of your caloric consumption and subjectively evaluate the 16-8 experience.
- Fitness: Comment about your formal movement class.
- Mindset: Make detailed notes about the visuals you want to include on your note card, vision board, or mind movie as a catalyst for starting and completing the project.
- Lifestyle: Write down your thoughts about your nap.

Day 7

Food: Hara Hachi Bun Me

Hara hachi bun me is the 2,500-year-old Confucian practice of eating meals only to the point of feeling 80 percent full. The practice remains a cultural mainstay in the longevity hotbed of Okinawa and in religious and spiritual traditions such as Zen and Ayurveda. The Blue Zones longevity movement identifies this practice of eating to satisfaction—but not fullness—as one of the Power 9 attributes common to long-lived populations across the globe. Once you attain satisfactory metabolic flexibility, you can use the practice of hara hachi bun me to drop excess body fat. While I would consider my metabolic flexibility to be outstanding, I'll certainly acknowledge that there is room for improvement when it comes to my eating environment, pace, and tendency to eat a bit beyond satisfaction out of reflex.

Today, make a concerted effort to eat your meals in a calm, quiet setting. Chew each bite twenty times or more to activate the salivary enzymes and facilitate proper digestion. Pay close attention to the point at which you achieve satisfaction and start implementing a habit of pushing the plate away when you're 80 percent full instead of routinely finishing everything on it.

Fasting: 16-8 with Fasted Morning Aerobic Workout

Conduct a break-even workout of moderate duration and difficulty. Take care to keep your heart rate at or below "180 minus age" in beats per minute for the duration of the session.

Fitness: Play Adventure in Nature

Knock off several health objectives at once with an outing in which you can enjoy sunlight, fresh air, cardiovascular exercise, and the beauty of nature. Try to include some brief, high-intensity, explosive bursts of strength or speed. Two of my favorite recreational endeavors are stand-up paddling (SUP) and Ultimate Frisbee. My weekly Ultimate match is a seven-on-seven battle royale with a very high level of physical exertion and competitive intensity. It's an absolute blast to take the field with accomplished athletes half my age and try to hang in there. My SUP outings are a more peaceful and solitary interaction with the ocean. It's the single best calming experience I've ever discovered, and it also delivers a very good cardiovascular workout, upper-body and core strengthening session, and total-body proprioception and balance challenge.

It's great to get out with family and friends for the occasional grand adventure, in which you learn a new activity such as SUP or rock climbing. However, your play outings don't have to be complex, competitive, or expensive. A lengthy hike with a picnic midway can be as rejuvenating as a day at a luxury spa. The main objective is to escape the pressures and predictability of your daily routine, take a distinct break from hyperconnectivity, and get your body moving in a beautiful natural setting.

Mindset: Winning Logistics and Visual Cues

You can work hard to reframe self-limiting beliefs and devise a lovely step-by-step process to reach your goals, but if your daily environment is not fully functional and supportive, it can greatly inhibit your chances of success. Today, spend some time rearranging your home and workplace in a way that will support and encourage you to adhere to your health and fitness goals. Make sure your food-preparation and dining areas are clean, tidy, well organized, and fully stocked with the books, tools, appliances, and ingredients you need to prepare delicious meals. Create inviting micro workout spaces at home and at work, with gear placed in plain sight to entice you to partake at any time. Post a list of exercises in your micro workout area and a shopping list of healthful foods on the fridge. Place an index card or a sticky note on your computer with a few trigger phrases that will help you stay focused on high-priority work, avoid distractions, and take frequent breaks. Create a note on your mobile device describing your favorite workout parameters and benchmarks for easy reference when you get to the gym or Pilates class. Stay focused, motivated, and accountable by operating in an environment designed for success!

Lifestyle: Screen and News Fast

Today, do the best you can to put your devices away and enjoy a Sunday filled with outdoor activity, in-person socializing, reading, hobbies, or solo reflective time. Today's play adventure will automatically facilitate your success. Look at your phone and computer only when absolutely necessary. In addition, take a daylong break from consuming broadcast and internet news. A large percentage of news and clickbait is designed to elicit fear and anxiety through sensationalist, high-shock-value programming. Instead of monitoring the pulse of the crazy world, take a breather and relish the simple pleasures of being present and attentive to your immediate environment.

Journal

- ▪ Food: Comment about your hara hachi bun me experience.
- ▪ Fasting: Note the start time and end time of your caloric consumption and subjectively evaluate the 16-8 experience and your aerobic workout.
- ▪ Fitness: Comment on your grand play adventure in nature.
- ▪ Mindset: Record details of your efforts to optimize environmental logistics and create visual cues.
- ▪ Lifestyle: Write down thoughts about your screen and news fast.

Day 8

Food: Heightened Awareness

Put several challenges into play today as you escalate the degree of difficulty of your Turbocharge: do not snack; practice hara hachi bun me eating; consume only freshly prepared foods; and spend time looking and/or shopping for interesting new recipes.

Fasting: 16-8 with Fasted Sprint Workout

You are ready for the 16-8 with fasted sprint workout challenge—provided you conduct the sprint workout properly! Make sure the session is not exhausting and depleting by adhering to the parameters detailed in chapter 5 (see page 138) and in today's fitness challenge (see below). In the hours after the workout, try to move frequently. This will help speed recovery, boost fat burning, and make you less likely to succumb to carbohydrate cravings.

Fitness: Conduct a Full Sprint Workout

Hopefully you can conduct a running workout but choose no-impact or low-impact activities if necessary. Go through an aerobic warm-up, including dynamic stretching, preparatory drills, six wind sprints lasting five to seven seconds each, and then perform a main set of between four and ten sprints at 95 percent effort (see page 71 for guidelines). Focus on being explosive, preserving excellent form, and staying within your capabilities. Sprint for ten to twenty seconds (closer to ten if you're running, closer to twenty for no-impact or low-impact sprints), then enjoy luxurious rest intervals that are at least five times longer than your sprint.

As soon as you finish the session or as soon as you get home, lie down with your feet elevated and breathe deeply for ten minutes. Dr. Jannine Krause, functional medicine physician and host of *The Health Fix* podcast, cites research concluding that this mini nap session shortly after a high-intensity workout will help you achieve a rebound parasympathetic response to the sympathetic stimulation of the workout. This will help you return to homeostasis more quickly and speed your rate of recovery from these stressful but highly beneficial workouts.

Mindset: Turnaround Behaviors and Habit Formation

Today you will bring your turnaround statements to life by choosing three actions designed to deactivate flawed subconscious programming and establish empowering new habits. Start by reciting a turnaround statement of your choice, as described in the day 4 mindset assignment (see page 182). Immediately afterward, take an action that supports the turnaround statement. Repeat this process three times over the course of the day. If you are working on not becoming distracted by and reactive to technology first thing in the morning, for example, perhaps you have formulated a turnaround statement saying that you always prioritize fitness over tech addiction. Recite the statement, then commence the morning routine you designed on day 4. If you're trying to break the habit of idle snacking in the afternoon, say, recite your turnaround statement, then immediately conduct a micro workout as a replacement for a snack.

Lifestyle: Nature Immersion

Get out of your work environment at lunchtime and try to find the most immersive nature experience in your vicinity. If you are in a highly urban setting, such as a downtown high-rise, do the best you can to simulate nature. The fern grotto and indoor fountain in your building lobby were designed for just this reason—as proxies for the benefits of the outdoors. Take inspiration from Japan's forest-bathing practices and imagine yourself decreasing stress hormones, lowering blood pressure, and stabilizing your mood—a parasympathetic reset that will bring the necessary balance to your hectic workday. As you learned in chapter 5, the best results occur when you can become truly fascinated, so give nature the undivided attention of all your senses and leave your digital device behind.

Journal

- ■ Food: Comment about your combination challenge (no snacks, eat only until 80 percent full, limit yourself to fresh foods, research grocery and internet options).

- Fasting: Note the start time and end time of your caloric consumption and subjectively evaluate the 16-8 protocol with the fasted sprint workout.
- Fitness: Write down details of your sprint workout—reps, duration, recovery interval, and a subjective evaluation of the experience.
- Mindset: Note your thoughts about today's turnaround statements paired with behaviors.
- Lifestyle: Write down your thoughts about your nature immersion.

Day 9

Food: Intense Scrutiny

Now that your pantry is cleaned out—whether you did it on day 1 or after reading chapter 1—and now that you've had some time to live with the new foods in your home, it's time to closely examine your kitchen for any lingering problem foods. It's likely that you have items in the pantry or fridge that contain processed sugars, grains, or objectionable oils. Review the labels and see if you can find anything else to toss. Write some notes in your journal about your dining-out habits over the past nine days and consider whether any entrees or prepared foods might have contained ingredients that you vowed to eliminate. This exercise is designed to help you to refine your game so that in the future, your seed oil consumption will be near zero and sugars and grains will be only occasional indulgences.

Fasting: 18-6 Eating Pattern

Did you read that carefully? An eighteen-hour fast followed by a six-hour eating window! This should be no problem for you at this point, but we'll pair this escalated effort with moderate exercise to be sure you can handle it.

Fitness: Recovery Workout

Start with some intentional breathing and dynamic stretching (search YouTube for "Brad Kearns dynamic stretching routine to start your day"). If you have a foam roller, spend five minutes doing a full-body roll over the big muscle groups. When you find a "trigger point" of tightness, apply direct pressure to that spot for ten seconds, then resume rolling along the full length of the muscle group. Be sure to breathe deeply through the discomfort when you hit a trigger point.

Next, try a short sequence of brief bursts of intensity paired with lengthy recovery intervals. For example, get on a stationary bike, elliptical machine, rowing machine, or anything else that's no-impact—or jump in the swimming pool—and sprint at 85 percent effort for five seconds. Spend the next sixty seconds breathing deeply and focusing on lowering your heart rate. Try to get into a trancelike state in which you command your respiration and heart rate to lower quickly. Repeat this sprint-and-recover sequence up to six times. This strategy will hone your ability to stimulate parasympathetic activity so you can relax on cue whenever you experience any form of fight-or-flight stimulation—an argument, a hectic situation at work, a traffic jam, and so forth. Finish your workout with some nonstrenuous flexibility and mobility drills and dynamic stretching.

Mindset: Mind-Control Exercise

Choose one of the practices described in chapter 4 or chapter 7 for today's project. The objective of this exercise is to experience how the mind can influence cellular function. Try an intentional breathing exercise (search YouTube for "guided Wim Hof breathing"); take a cold shower or cold plunge (search YouTube for "Brad Kearns chest freezer cold water therapy"); or go through a priming exercise (search YouTube for "Tony Robbins guided morning routine"). Alternatively, challenge yourself to face a stressful everyday situation with a resolve to control your attitude and emotions. If your rush-hour commute stresses you out, hop into the slow lane, relax your ETA expectations, and enjoy an audiobook or podcast. In this manner, you transform an experience that you (and most all of us!) deem to be inherently stressful and turn it into a pleasure cruise. If you have a strained relationship with a friend, family member, or work colleague, initiate a telephone or in-person conversation in which you commit to staying positive, polite, respectful, and validating. Set an intention for healing and progressing instead of falling back into familiar dysfunctional patterns. If necessary, "fake it till you make it," advice legitimized by bestselling relationship author Dr. John Gray.

Lifestyle: Disciplined Use of Technology

Execute some heroic acts of discipline and restraint with your screen use today. Complete your morning movement routine and enjoy some personal or social time without taking so much as a glance at any digital device. If you typically listen to music or podcasts while exercising, spend today's workout listening instead to your breath and increasing your awareness of technique and muscle movement. When the workday is done, implement a hard stop by powering down or theatrically shutting the laptop lid. Make sure you're finished with all screens at least ninety minutes before bedtime and devote the final segment of your evening to socializing and your soothing bedtime ritual.

Journal

- Food: Comment about your second kitchen purge and your recent dining-out habits.
- Fasting: Note the start time and end time of your caloric consumption and subjectively evaluate the 18-6 window.
- Fitness: Describe every element of the recovery workout in detail and make a subjective evaluation of the experience.
- Mindset: Evaluate the mind-control challenge(s) you took on today and what you learned from the experience.
- Lifestyle: Write about your disciplined use of technology.

Day 10

Food: New Recipe, Celebratory Meal

Try an interesting new recipe from the offerings in this book or another book of your choice. Host another gathering or serve the dish to the usual diners at home. During your preparation, see if you can slow things down and appreciate the meditative aspects of mundane vegetable chopping or pot stirring. Notice how being hands-on and engaged from start to finish creates a vastly richer dining experience than ordering takeout.

Fasting: Day Off!

You deserve a day off from the escalating fasting challenges. Keep to your maximum digestive-function of window of twelve hours, though. Get ready for a twenty-four-hour effort on day 12!

Fitness: Workplace Variation

Follow the recommended 20-20-20 strategy for your eyes (take a screen break every twenty minutes to gaze at an object twenty feet away for twenty seconds) and do some brief counterbalancing exercises such as making wall angels. Take a five-minute break every hour, getting up from your desk for a quick visit outdoors and/or a brief micro workout. Take an extensive midday break to get into fresh air and open space and recharge your cognitive batteries.

Extend today's assignment by creating a few alternative arrangements for your traditional work desk, both at the office and at home. Devise a makeshift stand-up desk or create a low desk by placing your laptop on a coffee table, then sitting on a stool, a BOSU ball, or the floor. Experiment for the next several days as you consider your preferences for a dynamic work environment. Remember, variation is the key. A hydraulic worktable that easily shifts from stand-up to sit-down is fantastic, and a BOSU ball makes the low-desk experience inviting and fun.

Mindset: Mindful Meals

Enjoy both your meals today with full attention, awareness, and gratitude—including, of course, the meal you prepare from scratch—for a start-to-finish gratitude experience. During the meal, engage all your senses with a deep appreciation for the nourishment and the effort you made to create something special. See if you can encourage your dining companions to depart from the typical rushed and distracted mealtime dynamics and enjoy a sophisticated culinary celebration.

Lifestyle: Creating Prioritized To-Do Lists

Spend five to ten minutes first thing in the morning and five to ten minutes as soon as you begin work to create prioritized to-do lists for both your personal life and your work. Get everything that's rolling around in your head down on paper, then carefully rank the tasks in order of priority. You may want to split the prioritized to-do items into short-term (within a week) and long-term tasks. As you go about your day, refer to the lists frequently and methodically proceed through each task in order. Notice how easy it is to get pulled into doing stuff that's not on the lists or spend excess time and effort on low-priority tasks. Take some notes along the way to identify both struggles and successes.

You can enter your initial to-do lists in your handwritten journal today, but consider transferring them over to digital to-do lists for long-term reference. This way, you can easily add, delete, and rearrange the order of priority. Consider using an application that automatically synchronizes data across devices, such as Apple's Notes app or the popular Evernote app, which offers free and premium versions for all platforms. If you are a dyed-in-the-wool devotee of a low-tech FranklinCovey planner, Moleskine book, or other paper product, that's fine, too. Just make a point to spend some extra time today in planning mode.

Journal

- Food: Comment about the new recipe you tried and the celebratory meal you enjoyed.
- Fasting: Write about what it felt like to take a day off.
- Fitness: Note your thoughts about your movement breaks and workplace variation efforts.
- Mindset: Record details about your mindful dining experiences.
- Lifestyle: Create to-do lists as directed and subjectively evaluate the experience.

Day 11

Food: Foods to Avoid—Review

Spend some time today reviewing the kitchen and pantry purge section of chapter 1, which lists the specific items and brands to avoid in various food categories. Frequent review will help you commit the best foods for success to memory so your decision making at the supermarket and online can feel automatic and effortless.

Fasting: Twelve-Hour Digestive Circadian Rhythm

Another easy day as you gear up for a twenty-four-hour fast tomorrow. But remember to keep your digestive-function window at twelve hours.

Fitness: Extended Walking Day

Get out and explore your community on foot as you never have before. Throw some incentives into the mix, such as walking at least a mile (and maybe much more if you can handle it) to a nice restaurant or, okay, even a gourmet dessert joint. Get your entire family involved and resolve to integrate more pedestrian experiences into family life.

Mindset: Gratitude Exercise

Celebrate the accomplishment of reaching this point in the challenging 12-Day Turbocharge! Spend 5 to 10 minutes journaling thoughts of gratitude about your 12-Day

Turbocharge experience. Ideally, conduct this exercise in a calm, quiet, relaxing natural setting. Replay some of the highlights of the challenges you have conquered so far, and be sure to maintain a smile throughout!

Lifestyle: Advanced Strategies—Cold Exposure Session 2

Time to up the ante a bit from your first foray into the cold by spending longer in the shower or going for a full immersion in an ice tub or perhaps a natural body of water that's well under sixty degrees Fahrenheit (fifteen degrees Celsius). Remember to execute deep, diaphragmatic breaths throughout your exposure to override a potential shock reaction to the cold.

Appreciate the indirect benefits of cold exposure: improved focus, discipline, and stress tolerance in all areas of life. Tony Robbins, a daily practitioner of cold exposure (he has custom pools built at all seven of his luxury residences around the world), describes it as "my mind telling my body what to do; to not hesitate but to act."

Journal

- Food: Comment about your review of foods to avoid—compliance, concerns, specific foods.
- Fasting: Write about what it felt like to take a day off.
- Fitness: Write about your extended walk.
- Mindset: Make gratitude entries in your journal as suggested above.
- Lifestyle: Note the specifics of your cold exposure—venue, duration, temperature, and a subjective evaluation of the experience.

Day 12

Food: Ancestral Foods and Superfoods—Review

Spend some time today reviewing the information in chapter 2 about choosing the very best foods in each of the major categories: meat, fowl, fish, eggs, vegetables, fruits, nuts and seeds, organic high-fat dairy products, dark chocolate, beverages, alcohol, and superfoods—i.e., nose-to-tail animal products and fermented and sprouted foods. Comment in your journal about your compliance, preferences, and favorite sources for various products.

Fasting: Twenty-Four-Hour Fast

Consider fasting between an early dinner and an early dinner the next day, and make sure you have a low-stress day ahead of you. Gentle movement, such as JFW, will make the experience easier by boosting fat burning, while fight-or-flight stimulation of any kind will promote carbohydrate cravings. Remember: any effort to improve metabolic flexibility represents progress, so if you reach twenty hours and start to feel uncomfortable, it's okay to enjoy a small snack such as a high-fat beverage (kefir, raw milk, a protein smoothie) or a couple of squares of dark chocolate, then see if you can carry on for a bit more. You'll know when you really need to eat a proper meal. That said, if a ghrelin spike occurs, see if you can endure fifteen to twenty minutes of discomfort in pursuit of a fasting breakthrough.

As you gain experience with extended fasts, you will also gain confidence that you can execute them anytime. I've done a fair number of deliberate twenty-four-hour fasts for therapeutic purposes, but I've also had countless occasions when I've gone from twenty-one to twenty-four hours between meals without realizing it, whether because I'm traveling, staying busy, or having a low-appetite or low-energy-expenditure day in the office or at home.

Fitness: Recovery Workout and Evening Stroll After Dinner

Implement some of the techniques you tried on your day 9 recovery workout in an abbreviated session or another full-length session if you desire. This, too, will boost fat burning and help you sustain energy during your twenty-four-hour fast. After your break-fast or early dinner, take a leisurely stroll through the neighborhood. Remember, a fifteen-minute walk at a slow pace is enough to reduce the insulin response to the meal by half!

Mindset and Lifestyle: Detailed Journaling

Spend thirty to sixty minutes writing about all aspects of your experience during the 12-Day Turbocharge. Divide your comments into five areas, each relating to one of the daily assignments: food, fasting, fitness, mindset, and lifestyle. Dedicate the first couple of pages to data compilation, so you can easily access the information in the future: your MAF (maximum aerobic functioning) numbers and PEM (primal essential movements) assessments, your morning routine and evening ritual, and anything else you'll want to refer to.

Journal

- Food: Comment on your review of ancestral foods and superfoods—compliance, concerns, specific items.
- Fasting: Evaluate your twenty-four-hour fast—the degree of difficulty, its effects on energy and cognition, and your overall thoughts about the experience.
- Fitness: Write about your recovery workout and after-dinner stroll.
- Mindset and lifestyle: Carry out your journal assignments as suggested.

The Future

Congratulations on completing the Turbocharge! You may be ready for a break, but I hope you feel energized and inspired by the previous twelve days. Although it's not realistic to exist in Turbocharge mode indefinitely, the experience is intended to help you dial in a winning daily routine that feels comfortable and sustainable. Along those lines, let's recap the important objectives in each category—goals that will sustain you over the long haul. If you are able to more or less adhere to the following recommendations for the rest of your life, you dramatically improve your odds of living a long, healthy, happy life and avoiding the epidemic of diet-and-lifestyle-related disease that has become the norm today.

Food and Fasting

Ditch the Big Three: Establish zero tolerance for industrial seed oils. If a bottled, packaged, or frozen product contains them, don't buy it. If you're dining out, make the necessary inquiries so you can steer clear of them. When in doubt, assume something's made with toxic oils. If sweetened beverages, sugary treats, and refined grains work their way into your diet, make sure they are never anything more than occasional indulgences.

Establish a twelve-hour digestive circadian rhythm: There is really no reason to depart from this for more than one day, ever. Even if you are in full-fledged vacation mode with evenings of revelry, you can pair these occasions nicely with extended fasting the next day.

Don't snack: Eat delicious, satisfying, nutrient-dense meals so you don't have the inclination to snack. Consider snacking to be an occasional indulgence or a way to replace one of your two meals.

Eat intermittently: Get into a good rhythm in which fasting is the norm, you eat when you're hungry, you finish when you're satisfied (not full), and food is always a celebration. This might be a 16-8 pattern, a morning-evening pattern, or a more fractal and intuitive pattern. As you improve metabolic flexibility, two daily meals are likely to become a maximum rather than an average.

Fitness

JFW: Make walking a centerpiece of your human experience. Orchestrate strategies and situations that obligate you to walk more, such as always parking at the outer edges of parking lots, taking stairs instead of elevators, and honoring a solemn vow as a dog owner to always give your animal the exercise it deserves, no matter what. Set up a blaring alarm inside your head that goes off after one hour of stillness. The only way to turn it off is to get up and JFW!

Implement a morning movement routine: Create a methodical sequence of movements that is energizing, easily repeatable, and indefinitely sustainable. If you can only spare five minutes, commit to making it happen every single day. Begin immediately upon awakening; include exposure to direct sunlight. Repeat the exact same moves every day, although it's okay to revise the sequence over time.

Conduct aerobic workouts: Respect the distinction between an optimal aerobic, fat-burning workout and one that's slightly too stressful and causes a spike in glucose burning. Always monitor your heart rate to stay at or below "180 minus age," except on rare occasions such as during a competition or a breakthrough workout. Strive to accumulate between two and five hours of structured aerobic exercise each week. In addition to your JFW efforts, this will help you maintain your status as a healthy, active human.

Conduct high-intensity workouts: Conduct brief, intense strength and sprint workouts that boost antiaging hormones and dramatically improve fitness and body composition but are not exhausting or depleting. Emphasize explosiveness, excellent technique, and staying in control instead of the dated and destructive "no pain, no gain" approach. Two strength sessions lasting between ten and thirty minutes each per week, and one sprint session with only a couple of minutes of explosive effort in a total workout time of twenty minutes, is plenty.

Conduct micro workouts: Elevate your fitness baseline and help meet your daily movement requirements with brief bouts of explosive effort that deliver an awesome cumulative fitness benefit without the risk of breakdown and burnout that happens as a result of doing too many overly stressful full-length workouts with insufficient recovery between them. Micro workouts are also a great way to refresh your cognitive batteries and boost fat burning during the workday.

Workplace variation: Avoid prolonged periods of stillness by taking regular breaks for walks, doing flexibility and mobility exercises, and making time for micro workouts. Create alternative workstation options such as a stand-up desk and a low desk, and strive to vary your positioning as much as possible over the course of the workday.

Recovery: Make recovery a central element of your exercise program. Avoid exhausting workout patterns and perform high-intensity sessions only when you're well rested and energized. Then conduct specially designed recovery workouts that trigger parasympathetic function.

Mindset

Destroy and reframe self-limiting beliefs and behaviors: Recite your turnaround statements for two to three minutes at least once a day—ideally, twice a day—for at least the next thirty days. Each day, combine this verbal exercise with an activity from one of your step-by-step action plans.

Program your subconscious: In tandem with the aforementioned verbal and physical exercises, program your subconscious by creating a dream board, mind movie, or a visual cue, such as an index card displaying meaningful acronyms. Honor the power of these tools by keeping them in sight and revising them as needed. Consider branching out into other strategies such as playing subliminal audio recordings designed for specific life goals, engaging in guided meditation, and even hiring a life coach, spiritual guide, or other peak-performance expert.

Maintain your journal: Commit to some form of handwritten journaling in pursuit of peak performance and living in gratitude. Establish a schedule and guidelines that feel natural and easy to maintain, but keep your commitment no matter what. Again, if you only have five minutes to spare, open up your journal and write something every day to turn this behavior into a rewarding habit.

Sharpen your awareness: Pay careful attention to negative self-talk and self-limiting or self-sabotaging behavior patterns so that you catch self-sabotage every time, call it out, and replace it with a turnaround statement or empowering behavior. Notice the destructive effects of commiserating, complaining, and validating negative attitudes among your family, friends, and coworkers and resolve to never add fuel to the fire or attempt the typically losing proposition of policing others' mindsets! Instead, offer thoughtful statements that are either neutral or empowering and redirect the focus of the conversation away from negativity.

Lifestyle

Engage in sufficient rest, recovery, and downtime: Optimize your sleep environment, minimize artificial light and digital stimulation after dark, and enjoy quiet, dark, mellow evenings with a soothing bedtime ritual. Nap when necessary and spend time in nature to lower stress.

Discipline your use of technology: Honor distinct off hours from hyperconnectivity to enjoy in-person social interactions and solo reflective time. Spend a little time every day maintaining prioritized to-do lists before you dive into reactive stimulus.

Try cold exposure: Conduct brief, therapeutic cold exposure sessions to enjoy a hormone boost, improve focus and discipline, become more resilient to all forms of life stress, and boost fat burning.

Good luck with your continued quest for health, happiness, and longevity! Your interest and enthusiasm is greatly appreciated. For support and inspiration along the way, visit TwoMealsADayBook.com, MarksDailyApple.com, or BradKearns.com.

Frequently Asked Questions

Fasting

How do I know I'm ready for fasting? I don't want to trigger the fight-or-flight response and liquidate my assets!

You must be in good general metabolic health before you consider an ambitious fasting protocol. This means you are free from inflammatory, autoimmune, thyroid, adrenal, and leaky gut conditions; have stable mood and energy levels during the day; and can delay a meal for a couple of hours without too much trouble. If you suspect you have any of the aforementioned issues, first strive to ditch the Big Three toxic modern foods and spend some time detoxing and nourishing your depleted cells with healthful foods. Follow the gradual progression presented in chapter 6 and trust that the process will deliver results over the long run. Remember that progress comes in many forms and follows many time frames. Even if your fasting efforts don't go as planned, setbacks and recalibrations can deliver a net positive benefit. When you feel ready for the challenge, take the pressure off with a WHEN approach that doesn't enforce rigid timelines.

I enjoy snacking. I feel like it gives me an energy boost and a break from my stressful workday. Can I continue?

There is tremendous value in rituals that support a balance between stress and rest and provide a break from prolonged periods of stillness and sustained cognitive efforts. The comforts associated with a snack break have made it a cultural mainstay since the Industrial Revolution. But be aware that snacking can really mess up your fat-reduction goals, because a snack of any kind will halt the burning of body fat and prompt an insulin release.

Consider replacing between-meal caloric consumption with something that delivers similar benefits, such as a micro workout, a sequence of flexibility and mobility exercises, a stroll around the block in the sunshine, or even a short nap. A movement break of any kind will improve blood circulation and oxygen delivery to the brain and body and upregulate fat metabolism. You'll get a natural boost in energy and cognition without the downsides of snacking. That said, if you are metabolically flexible and satisfied with your current body composition, an occasional nutrient-dense snack such as a handful of macadamia nuts, a few squares of dark chocolate, or a hard-boiled egg is of minimal concern. Besides, with metabolic flexibility, you will likely not have a hankering to snack in the first place!

Fat Reduction

I'm a competitive athlete who follows an ambitious training regimen that exceeds ten hours per week. However, I still carry some excess body fat. Can the **Two Meals a Day** *approach help me?*

It's extremely common among devoted fitness enthusiasts in the endurance sports, CrossFit, and group-exercise communities to carry excess body fat despite their high- or even mega-calorie-burning regimens. This can feel extremely frustrating when you devote extensive time and energy to fitness but don't see the results in your physique. Many blame bad luck with genetics when it's more accurately attributed to overly stressful training patterns and lifestyle circumstances causing chronic elevation of stress hormones. A sympathetic-dominant fight-or-flight existence dysregulates your appetite and satiety hormones, prompts compensatory mechanisms that stall fat loss, and locks you into carbohydrate dependency—even as you burn a ton of calories and regularly deplete glycogen. Know this theorem: extreme exercise drives laziness, sugar cravings, fat storage, and elevated disease risk.

If you suffer from daily fluctuations in energy, mood, appetite, and cognitive functioning, have difficulty skipping even a single meal, habitually snack throughout the day, or require extra calories to get through a workout of sixty to ninety minutes, these are signs that you are metabolically inflexible despite your high fitness level. Not only is this keeping your spare inner tube afloat, it's also hampering your performance and health in many ways. For one, the need to consume calories before, during, and after exercise can traumatize your digestive tract. Some 30 percent of participants in the Hawaii Ironman World Championships report moderate to severe digestive distress during the competition. Second, you are burning more dirty fuel and generating more inflammation and free radicals than you would if you were burning mostly body fat instead of ingested sugar. This diet-induced oxidation and inflammation increases the stress impact of the workout and delays recovery. Keep in mind the example of fat-adapted endurance machine Dude Spellings *fasting* to facilitate recovery after his Grand Canyon double crossing (see page 79).

Finally, your carbohydrate-dependent diet and exercise patterns are increasing your risk of diet-related disease, including type 2 diabetes! Countless high-performing athletes have received the shocking news that they are prediabetic and hyperinsulinemic despite their devotion to training. Dr. Timothy Noakes is a notable example: his prediabetes diagnosis despite decades of ultramarathon running compelled him to rethink the foundation of his life's work—studying endurance exercise physiology within the restrictions and distortions created by the carbohydrate-dependency paradigm. Sorry for the metaphor, but your high-calorie-burning and high-calorie-eating lifestyle essentially has you stuck on a treadmill of futility—manifested graphically in the presence of excess body fat on many a sweaty, hardworking fitness enthusiast.

Turning things around as an athlete is easy because your physical fitness can help accelerate your metabolic fitness when you change your diet. Following is a suggested plan to get the body you deserve from all your hard work.

1. **Ditch grains, sugars, and refined industrial seed oils from your diet.** Give yourself a fighting chance at becoming metabolically flexible by getting the junk out of your diet. This includes sugary bars, gels, and beverages. If you "need" these to finish your workouts, you are doing the wrong workouts!
2. **Eliminate even the slightest whiff of overtraining.** Maintain MAF heart rates during aerobic sessions, eliminate depleting, exhausting HIIT sessions in favor of HIRT sessions (see page 71), shorten the duration and reduce the frequency of high-intensity workouts, and integrate more micro workouts into your regimen.

3. **Increase general everyday movement.** Prolonged sitting causes sugar cravings and fat storage. Movement promotes fat burning.
4. **Prioritize sleep.** Sleep deficiencies elevate stress hormones and compromise fat burning. Adequate sleep helps stabilize appetite and satiety hormones and promotes fat burning.
5. **Manage stress.** Hectic, fight-or-flight days promote carbohydrate dependency. Rest, recovery, relaxation, and a healthful balance between stress and rest promote fat burning.

Once you get these five objectives handled, you can consider strategic reductions of carbohydrate intake along with a WHEN strategy. Compared to starving yourself and pushing harder in workouts, this is going to feel ridiculously easy. It's also going to bring results when you stick with it!

How can you say that increasing calorie burning and decreasing caloric intake won't lead to fat reduction? Calories in, calories out must be literally accurate, right?

Dr. Jason Fung's *The Obesity Code* cites extensive research to validate the incredibly counterintuitive concept that you won't lose fat by simply eating less and exercising more. One way to think about this is to consider how unfathomable it is to match caloric intake with caloric expenditure every single day over the long term. If calories in, calories out were literally true, with no compensating variables, your body weight should fluctuate ten or twenty pounds in either direction every year! But as I said in chapter 1, we have an array of compensatory mechanisms and homeostatic drives that conspire to keep us hovering around our body-composition set point. Your set point is greatly influenced by genetics combined with lifestyle behaviors, either favorable or destructive. The vast majority of us can reflect on our appearance as teenagers to get a hint of our genetic influences toward storing fat or staying lean (unless we already screwed things up before adolescence). The steady accumulation of additional body fat over the decades beyond our youthful prime represents mainly the effects of an inflammatory, high-insulin-producing diet and, to a lesser extent, contributory lifestyle behaviors.

While it's sobering to consider the ineffectiveness of calorie restriction combined with calorie burning for fat reduction, research also reveals that study subjects who eat more and exercise less don't *add* excess body fat at the expected rate.

For example, if there are 3,500 calories in a pound of fat and you were to experiment with eating 350 excess calories per day, you should predictably gain a pound of fat every ten days. Instead, the same compensatory mechanisms that prevent you from losing fat also prevent you from gaining it. For example, excess caloric intake prompts an increase in heart rate, respiration, body temperature, and metabolic rate in general. You may find yourself more active and fidgety throughout the day after overeating.

A phenomenon known as the thermic effect of food, a.k.a. diet-induced thermogenesis, accounts for between 5 and 10 percent of calories you ingest. Using our example, if you burn 2,000 calories per day and add the extra 350 for a total of 2,350 calories, as many as 235 of those calories are burned during the process of digesting, absorbing, and storing the calories you consumed! Protein has an especially significant thermic effect: an estimated 25 percent of protein calories are allocated to their digestion. Metabolic flexibility also significantly increases the thermic effect of food. Researchers have observed two to three times the rate of diet-induced thermogenesis in lean people than in obese people.

This is not to say that long-term overeating is advisable—there are many adverse health consequences of overeating independent of its effects on body fat and metabolic rate. After all, insulin resistance essentially occurs when the body becomes worn out by overeating and incessant insulin production, thus allowing the disease patterns of metabolic syndrome to develop. The takeaway here is to realize that fat reduction is about hormone optimization (mainly, lowering insulin) rather than the calories in, calories out equation. Instead of calories in versus calories out, it would be more accurate to call it calories stored versus calories burned.

If it's not about calories in, calories out, what is the secret to shedding excess body fat?

Engage in lifestyle behaviors that signal your genes to burn fat instead of store it by lowering dietary insulin production through routine fasting and the elimination of refined carbohydrates and industrial seed oils. When you lower insulin, you become able to access and burn stored body fat and bring it to the forefront as your preferred energy source—not ingested calories. Instead of responding to the urgent need to keep awake, focused, and energized all day via clockwork meals and frequent snacks, transition your dietary goals to the following.

- Enjoy life, with meals as a centerpiece of celebration and social connection.
- Obtain the protein you need for everyday metabolic functioning and repairing and maintaining organs and tissues.
- Obtain essential fatty acids in support of cardiovascular, reproductive, immune-system, nervous-system, hormonal, and general metabolic health.
- Obtain nutrient-dense dietary carbohydrates as desired, ranging from zero to an ancestrally inspired maximum of around 150 grams (six hundred calories) per day. This is pursuant to the first goal of enjoying life and to optimize athletic performance and recovery.

The loss of excess body fat results from honoring your authentic hunger signals with nutrient-dense foods, eating meals to the point of satiety, and allowing the magic of metabolic flexibility to create a natural, moderate caloric deficit so that you achieve a reliable reduction in excess body fat over time. This is not going to be a linear reduction because of the many compensatory variables I've discussed at length. Rather, metabolic flexibility allows you to progress to a healthy metabolic and hormonal state in which you can gracefully burn a variety of fuel sources as needed. When you commit to the *Two Meals a Day* program and bank long hours in a fasted state every day, this is naturally going to bring stored body fat to center stage.

If you are "doing everything right" for months on end and are still frustrated about your excess body fat, you can put advanced strategies into play as detailed in chapter 7 (and covered in the next question!).

Okay, I've done everything right and still can't drop the final seven pounds. I have eliminated processed carbohydrates, only eat two meals a day, and get an excellent blend of cardio and high-intensity workouts each week. What can I do in order to make further progress?

The advanced strategies covered in chapter 7 really work, but only if you are highly fat-adapted. Otherwise, any concerted effort to drop fat will prompt a stress response and/or compensatory mechanisms will kick in. First, follow the general rule of thumb that your fat-loss efforts should not entail pain, suffering, or sacrifice. Rather, they require increased attention to detail, mindfulness during meals, and the application of breakthrough strategies as needed. Second, when you are hitting the most important objectives nicely, adding a few of the peripherals (sleep, parasympathetic activities) can often be the catalyst for a breakthrough. These are often overlooked because of our flawed notion that it's all about calories. Adopt a holistic, patient, confident belief that sending the right signals to your genes all day long will reliably change your body composition. If you have great indicators of fat adaptation from doing everything right, consider the following ideas to achieve a breakthrough.

- Pair morning cold exposure with fasting until 12:00 noon.
- Fast until WHEN, then wait another fifteen to sixty minutes before eating.
- Conduct a high-impact sprint workout once a week consisting of explosive, short-duration efforts with extensive rest in between.
- Conduct a low-impact sprint workout once a week: bicycle, cardio machine, water sport, or uphill sprints.
- Include micro workouts in your regimen. Remember, it's not about the calories: it's about genetic signaling. Can a few sessions a day lasting between one and five minutes each really make a big difference? Absolutely!
- Practice hara hachi bun me at all meals. Create a calm, quiet, distraction-free environment and chew each bite twenty times to facilitate this goal.
- Sleep more. Hormone optimization requires complete restoration overnight. Minimize artificial light and digital stimulation in the final two hours before bedtime so you will get sleepy on cue.
- Engage in parasympathetic activities. These calibrate you toward fat burning and away from sugar cravings and cortisol-driven appetite spikes. Add more leisurely walks, foam rolling, massage, intentional breathing, and restorative exercise—such as yoga and rebound workouts—to your daily routine.
- Experiment with increased carb intake. Leanne Vogel, author of the *The Keto Diet* and *Keto for Women*, recommends a strategic increase in carbohydrate intake designed to fine-tune insulin sensitivity, help rebalance hormones, and spur additional fat reduction after a plateau. She explains that this is particularly beneficial for females and that there are thousands of success stories that validate this as a viable technique. Start by consuming half your body weight in carb grams at your evening meal one day a week.

I'm still not completely buying the idea that it's almost all about insulin. Over the years, I've noticed that my body weight aligns very closely with my weekly training hours.

Indeed, many athletic types have challenged my assertion that body composition is 80 percent diet and 20 percent exercise, sleep, and lifestyle. There are several nuances here worth discussing. First, we must acknowledge that you can gain or lose a significant amount of body weight in a short time through variations in diet, exercise, and natural hormonal cycles. For example, if you conduct a strenuous, hourlong, glycogen-depleting workout at a high sweat rate, it's possible to lose up to ten pounds! You can lose up to two liters of fluid per hour in sweat. Each liter weighs a kilogram (dig the metric system!), so you'd weigh 4.4 pounds less on the scale.

If you are fully glycogen-loaded and deplete yourself during the workout, this can reduce your weight by another five pounds. This is because every gram of stored glycogen binds with three to four grams of water, and we can store around five hundred grams of glycogen in the liver and muscles. You can gain most of this weight back in the ensuing hours of rehydration and eating hearty meals. On the flip side, if you go on a weeklong cruise and stuff your face without exercising, you can exceed your routine baseline weight by seven to ten pounds because of increased glycogen storage and fluid retention in cells throughout the body—plus adding a pound or two of fat.

Consequently, it's far more valuable to deemphasize body weight in favor of tracking body-fat percentage. While technology is improving, making body fat easier to track without expensive testing, it's more convenient and likely more motivating to use subjective tools such as a tight-fitting pair of pants or a daily (or weekly) LGN checkup in front of a mirror. If you have veins and a specific amount of muscle definition visible through the abdomen when you are at your best, you can snap a photo and establish some visual benchmarks. While we have heard plenty of admonitions against worshipping the bathroom scale, or even owning a scale, Dr. Ronesh Sinha makes an excellent counterpoint. He says that checking the scale daily helps him track his rate of glycogen replenishment: when he hits the high end of his typical five-pound body-weight range, he knows it's time for more exercise and less indulgence. If he weighs in at the low range, he can help reduce overtraining risk by backing off from depleting workouts and restocking with nutrient-dense carbohydrates.

If you are enamored of the low scale numbers that appear when you are in heavy training, reflect on the commentary about liquidating your assets, because this is likely a prominent contributor to your number. If you want to look defined instead of emaciated, and feel vibrant and energetic at rest instead of sluggish and skinny from too much training, adjust your exercise energy expenditure to a manageable level and make a point of consuming ample amounts of nutritious foods of all kinds. Surprising as it may seem, reducing training volume and increasing your intake of nutritious calories can often promote a reduction in excess body fat, because your body becomes a less stressed, less inflamed, better fat-burning machine at rest. This is particularly the case when you're trying to burn off inflammatory belly fat, which accumulates as a result of overly stressful lifestyle behaviors of all kinds.

So does working out make any kind of contribution to my body-composition goals?

Yes indeed! Your workout regimen can benefit your body composition by increasing fat metabolism at rest, stabilizing your energy, mood, and appetite during the day, and inspiring you to choose healthful foods and consume fewer total calories because you feel healthy, vibrant, and energetic. By contrast, insufficient daily movement or a drastic reduction in your workout routine can easily cause you to gain excess body fat because inactivity can promote insulin resistance, carbohydrate cravings, and less discipline with food choices and portion sizes. Also, if you are able to neutralize these factors, you should easily be able to maintain an ideal body composition independent of fluctuations in the amount you exercise. For example, my body-fat percentage is around the same as it was when I was an elite marathon runner and Ironman triathlete decades ago. Today, I eat far fewer calories, burn far fewer calories, and produce far less insulin than I did as an endurance machine, and I am vastly healthier in many respects.

What is the best way to lose excess body fat without causing compensation-theory rebounds?

To avoid triggering fight-or-flight or compensation-theory mechanisms that will arrest fat loss, consider one of the following two strategies to get the job done.

First, you can achieve a mild average caloric deficit each day that's not stressful or difficult to adhere to and that you barely notice. Top trainers in weight-dependent combat sports recommend a maximum daily deficit of three hundred calories. This under-the-radar strategy guards against triggering compensatory reductions in calorie burning, especially if you throw in days when you eat in caloric balance. Granted, it's difficult if not impossible to accurately achieve a mild caloric deficit, but if you are just mindful to back off a bit in the spirit of hara hachi bun me, this strategy can be very effective.

Another option is a short-term, hard-core approach in which you aggressively restrict caloric intake, override appetite spikes, and get the fat off quickly. This strategy is obviously unsustainable both from a willpower perspective and from a compensation-theory perspective, because counterbalancing forces eventually kick in. However, the short-duration approach can be appealing to certain personality types who don't have the patience or the precision to try for a sustained three-hundred-calorie daily deficit. Increased frequency of cold water therapy and sprint workouts can be very helpful during these aggressive fat-reduction efforts.

The total energy expenditure (TEE) theory doesn't make sense. I'm way more active than my neighbor and must burn way more daily calories!

Superfit folks experience an assortment of metabolic efficiencies that make their daily caloric expenditure only marginally higher than that of sedentary folks. After his revelatory study of the Hadza in Tanzania, Dr. Herman Pontzer conducted a study among hundreds of modern citizens revealing that moderately active folks burn only around two hundred more calories per day than inactive folks. Increasing exercise beyond moderate levels did not increase calorie burning, disproving the common belief that a devoted exercise regimen creates a "metabolic advantage." What's more, if your caloric expenditure is unusually high for a day or a week, all manner of powerful compensatory mechanisms kick in to keep you calibrated at a metabolic set point. This is represented in the illustration on page 4, showing the parity between Saturday (a one-hundred-mile bike ride paired with laziness and extra food) and Sunday (increased general movement and a sensible caloric intake). If you are still shaking your head, consider that an hour of vigorous exercise burns around 650 calories. If you average out that caloric expenditure over the other twenty-three hours of the day, your burn rate increases by only twenty-seven calories per hour. This doesn't put you much ahead of your inactive neighbor, who will reliably close that gap by burning more calories than you do while grocery shopping or climbing a flight of stairs.

Macronutrients

You say don't worry about counting calories, tracking macronutrient ratios, or measuring ketones, but I feel like quantification has helped me succeed in the past.

Tracking can be especially valuable in the early stages of transforming your diet or exercise program, because it will help increase your knowledge base in support of adhering to your stated goals and eventually transitioning to an intuitive approach. Over the long term, though, following a rigid program can demand too much brainpower and willpower. It can feel like an increasing logistical hassle and entail too much suffering and sacrifice. These bring a high risk of burnout and backsliding into old habits.

I want to empower you to take responsibility for your health and implement an intuitive approach to eating, exercise, and living an awesome life. The power of knowledge, self-awareness, and tangible results from your healthful lifestyle habits will keep you on track without having to sweat the small stuff or painstakingly record every bite of food you eat or mile you run. That said, certain personalities seem to respond better to quantification, because it can provide valuable accountability and a sense of security. If you insist that you do better when tracking data, by all means go ahead. Just try to maintain a healthy perspective so that your tracking is, for the most part, a recording of past behaviors that were informed by intuition and common sense. This is better than being a slave to rigid standards that you track. This approach can often provoke obsessions, insecurities, and other negative energy that leads you to make poor decisions.

I'm confused about the role of carbohydrate intake in fat loss and peak performance. The keto philosophy is to strictly limit carbs, but other experts suggest that carbs are important, especially for females.

Indeed, the diet wars have become increasingly annoying and confusing to the average person, who can't spend all day reviewing the research. The starting point for this conversation is the assertion that there is never any justification for consuming nutrient-deficient refined carbohydrates. Even if you are a high-performing athlete with low body fat, refined carbs promote oxidation and inflammation, which will suppress immune functioning and delay recovery.

Optimizing carb intake depends on numerous personal variables, including your genetics, fitness goals, and stress levels. Perhaps the most significant variable is your body composition and whether you aspire to reduce excess body fat. If you are trying to drop fat, the most reliable path is to lower insulin production through fasting and restriction of carbs and industrial oils. This may include temporarily limiting your intake of fruit, sweet potatoes, and starchy tubers as well as nuts, seeds, dark chocolate, and high-fat dairy products. Once you have attained your ideal body composition, you can try to reintroduce nutritious carbs and see how you tolerate them. You may notice some beneficial effects, such as improved mood and faster recovery from workouts. If you notice any adverse effects, such as fatigue after meals or an increase in body fat, you can dial things back in search of your ideal pattern. Perhaps the best recommendation is to stay in close touch with your natural appetite signals and notice when you crave carbs as well as when your carb intake has had adverse effects. The brain is very good at directing you to consume the precise nutrients you need at all times, unless you abuse your delicate appetite and satiety mechanisms by overeating.

I'm a hard-training athlete, and I'm worried that fasting and cutting carbs will affect my performance.

The world of fat-adapted athletic training is proving that amazing achievements are possible without stuffing carbs down your face before, during, and after workouts. Dr. Jeff Volek's highly regarded FASTER study (fat adapted substrate use in trained elite runners) revealed that highly trained endurance runners can burn vastly more fat calories per minute than was previously believed to be humanly possible and that glycogen replenishment can occur after depleting workouts even when little or no carbohydrates are eaten! Replenishment happens through the internal processes such as gluconeogenesis (converting ingested protein into glucose for immediate energy, mainly for the brain) and separating the glycerol molecules from triglycerides and sending them to the liver to be converted into glycogen.

Becoming a fat-adapted athlete requires devoted dietary transformation as well as a sensible training program with sufficient aerobic (fat-burning) cardio workouts and brief, high-intensity sessions that aren't overly stressful and depleting. If you have a high-carb, high-insulin-producing diet, extreme exercise habits, and/or an overly stressful lifestyle, you have a high probability of crashing and burning if you abruptly ditch carbs and try to maintain your high-stress ways. The best approach is to tackle dietary transformation first, perhaps in conjunction with a temporary reduction in both training hours and intensity. A correct approach to diet modification and training should unlock incredible performance benefits, including reduction in body fat, better control of inflammation, and faster recovery time. As you proceed on the path to becoming a fully fat-adapted athlete, consider the commentary from Dr. Tommy Wood in chapter 2 about eating enough nutritious foods to fuel your performance and recovery needs. In particular, pay attention to your natural appetite signals and honor any authentic cravings for carbohydrates that might occur in the aftermath of strenuous workouts.

Is keto an all-or-nothing proposition in which there exists a no-man's-land for carbohydrate intake?

If you are fully committed to ketogenic eating, you can enter into an alternative metabolic paradigm wherein your muscles burn fatty acids at a high rate and preserve glycogen efficiently, and your brain burns mostly ketones and minimal glucose. If your approach is flawed, you can indeed exist in a no-man's-land where your carbohydrate intake is insufficient to supply your energy needs but your fat- and ketone-burning skills are not sufficient to pick up the slack.

This phenomenon is of particular concern to athletes with high calorie-burning requirements. Dr. Stephen Phinney and Dr. Jeff Volek, authors of *The Art and Science of Low Carbohydrate Performance*, have published research revealing that an undesirable "tug-of-war" effect can happen in the early stages of becoming fat- and keto-adapted. This occurs when the muscles don't have enough of their usual supply of glucose (but don't yet burn fatty acids efficiently), so your workout performance suffers. Meanwhile, your brain doesn't have enough glucose, but it's not getting any ketones, either. The double whammy of the afternoon blues and lousy workouts is no fun. To stay out of no-man's-land, consider toning down your workout energy expenditure for the first three weeks of your transition away from high-carbohydrate eating patterns. Focusing on low-intensity aerobic activity and keeping any high-intensity stuff really brief (e.g., micro workouts) will ensure that your brain gets the glucose it needs. Meanwhile, for your diet, engage in fasting and carb restriction with enough discipline to trigger ketone production.

Is low carb just for endurance athletes, or can strength and power athletes benefit, too?

Athletes in the strength and power realm have not embraced low carb or keto as enthusiastically as endurance athletes, likely because of the significant glycolytic demands of high-intensity workouts and the perceived need for more dietary carbohydrates. However, research and anecdotal evidence reveals that a fat-adapted approach can be effective for high-intensity exercise as well. KetoGains .com kingpin Luis Villasenor has been in strict ketosis for nearly two decades while performing at a high level in bodybuilding and power lifting and maintaining an extremely lean, muscular physique. He has helped many strength and power athletes succeed without having to resort to the flawed and dated strategy of stuffing down maximum carbs and protein all day long. Early keto diet promoter Danny Vega (host of the Fat Fueled Family podcast with his wife Maura) has been performing magnificent feats of strength, sporting an eye-popping physique, and guiding enthusiasts of all levels to drop excess body fat safely with a keto approach.

Succeeding as a low-carb strength and power athlete entails first getting good at burning fat at rest. This will reduce your glucose needs during the walk from the parking lot to the gym, during your fifteen minutes of warm-up exercises, and even in the middle of explosive efforts. With a fat-burning, carbohydrate-sparing baseline, you will have plenty of glucose available for even the toughest workouts. Second, workouts must be brief, featuring explosive efforts with plenty of rest between them. Avoiding the prolonged, exhausting, depleting sessions that are so common in weight rooms and group exercise classes will also reduce your desperate need to refuel with carbs during and immediately after workouts. Third, taking sufficient recovery time between tough high-intensity sessions will ensure that you refuel with glycogen (even on a low- or very-low-carb diet) before you attempt another grueling session. Fourth, make your dietary transition as comfortable as possible by toning down your workout routine for at least the first three weeks of restricting dietary carbohydrates. Finally, be mindful of boosting sodium and electrolyte intake so you don't become depleted by the combination of a new diet along with sweating during tough workouts.

I've heard various recommendations about protein consumption. What does the Two Meals a Day *program suggest?*

In brief, don't worry too much about protein, because your natural appetite and homeostatic mechanisms do a great job naturally optimizing your protein consumption. Most experts recommend consuming an average of 0.7 grams of protein per pound of lean body mass (1.54 grams per kilo) per day. This is easy to achieve automatically with just about any diet, with the exception of an extremely restrictive plan such as a vegan or a deliberately low-protein diet. Because protein is the most urgent dietary requirement for survival, we have powerful mechanisms that cause us to crave high-protein foods if we get into a pattern of underconsumption. Dietary protein deficiency will cause you to catabolize lean muscle mass and throw off an assortment of critical repair and renewal functions. This promotes extreme fatigue, makes you look emaciated and unhealthy, and drives strong cravings for high-protein foods.

While it's unsustainable to exist in a state of chronic protein deficiency, you can still get into trouble by trending on the low side of your basic requirements. This may cause transient muscle catabolization that's hard to notice (or, worse, you might grow fond of your low scale number and skinny appearance), a slight decline in peak performance capabilities, and slower recovery from workouts. You might have days or weeks when you feel terrible, then okay for a bit, then terrible again. If you insist on following a restrictive diet (including ignoring cravings for protein-rich foods that aren't on your "list"), you can experience a long, slow candle burn over months or years to the extent that a deficient state becomes your new normal.

Many experts recommend that hard-training athletes consume an average of around one gram of protein per pound of total body weight (2.2 grams per kilo). A higher intake is also commonly recommended for the elderly, because they don't synthesize protein as efficiently and because they want to guard against the huge mortality risk factor of sarcopenia (loss of muscle mass). On average, carnivore diet proponents, like Dr. Shawn Baker and William Shewfelt routinely consume significantly more than one gram of protein per pound of body weight daily, asserting that 1.2 grams per pound is safe and effective. Mainstream authorities have long argued that increased protein intake can be stressful for the liver and kidneys charged with excreting the excess and that it can cause an overstimulation of growth factors in the bloodstream, such as mTOR and IGF-1. This chronic overstimulation can lead to accelerated, unregulated cell division and increased cancer risk. Again, these warnings may be most relevant in extreme cases, such as those of bodybuilders who consume triple their body weight in grams of protein per day.

There has been a recent trend (which I support) of backing off from the dire warnings about excess protein with the acknowledgment that if you are healthy and active, you probably don't have to worry much about consuming excess protein. For one, protein's extremely high satiety factor will naturally regulate your intake of high-protein foods. Also, if your carbohydrate intake is low, extra protein can be used to help restock glycogen via gluconeogenesis. I've discussed gluconeogenesis as a negative thing—when you strip down lean muscle mass to make sugar for your ravenous brain—but gluconeogenesis that uses ingested protein is a highly efficient way to restock glycogen. Gluconeogenesis is believed to be a demand-driven process, meaning that you make only the exact amount of glucose you need to perform at your best and recover efficiently.

Note that daily protein targets are expressed as an average, because your body has assorted protein-sparing and protein-shedding mechanisms to help balance temporary dietary fluctuations. For example, the lauded fasting benefit of auto-phagy involves repairing and recycling amino acids. If you aren't getting any protein at mealtime, your body makes do very nicely working with what's available. If you consume more protein than your body needs now and then, you will reduce hunger, trigger a temporary increase in metabolic rate as you repair and/or build lean muscle mass (per the aforementioned thermic effect of protein—burning as much as 25 percent of its own calories), and perhaps engage gluconeogenesis if necessary—all helping to promote long-term homeostasis.

I love bread, seem to suffer no ill effects from it, and am willing to allocate a portion of my daily carbohydrate budget to some premium-quality bread. Is this okay?

If you choose to indulge in favorite foods that are off the ancestral template, be sure to carefully select the highest-quality and least detrimental foods in that category. Enjoy the experience to the fullest and treat it as a rare and celebratory event. There is a huge difference between that and mindlessly allowing nutrient-deficient foods to remain in your diet just because of your ingrained habits and/or because they provide a few moments of gustatory pleasure—this will often result in hours of not feeling great after indulging.

Rapid-Fire Round

I'm a fit female who wants to drop a few more pounds. How can I tell if I'm doing it safely?

Carefully monitor yourself for fatigue and/or sugar cravings at the end of workouts and at rest. Notice if you have reduced motivation to exercise, fluctuations in mood, energy levels, and cognitive function during the day, and sleep disturbances at night. These are all signs that the combination of carbohydrate restriction, calorie restriction, and ambitious workouts are becoming too stressful and therefore counterproductive.

How can I tell if I'm overfat?

Dr. Phil Maffetone recommends that your waist measurement be half your height in inches or less. Anything outside this range he deems overfat. He also asserts that 91 percent of the global population falls into this category. Dr. Ronesh Sinha looks for the male waist-to-hip ratio of .95 or below. For females, Dr. Sinha wants a waist of less than thirty-five inches, with a waist-to-hip ratio of .85 or below. For example, waist measurement in inches should be slightly or significantly less than hip measurement in inches—e.g., a thirty-two-inch waist to thirty-six-inch hips is a .88 ratio.

How can I tell if my high-intensity workouts are too stressful?

Watch for these symptoms and take immediate corrective action if you experience them:

- routine muscle soreness after workouts;
- fatigue and negative attitude immediately after workouts;

- mood swings, sugar cravings, and afternoon blues anywhere from twelve to forty-eight hours after workouts;
- frequent muscle burn during workouts;
- compromised form during resistance efforts or sprints in the latter stages of workouts;
- feelings of apprehension before workouts.

Never perform a breakthrough session unless you are 100 percent rested and motivated beforehand. Take luxurious rest intervals that allow you to feel completely refreshed and energized to perform the next work effort at the same quality standard. Typically, this entails a rest interval five times longer than the sprint effort (e.g., sprint twelve seconds, rest for a minute). End the workout before (or right when) your form breaks or your energy or performance standard drops off noticeably.

How can I tell if I'm sodium-depleted?

Watch for these symptoms and take immediate corrective action if you notice them:

- dizziness upon standing;
- excessive thirst;
- muscle spasms or cramps;
- restlessness, irritability, and fatigue during the day;
- afternoon blues or sugar cravings.

If you are making an abrupt transition from carb dependency to ancestral-style eating, add between five and ten grams (depending on your activity level) of high-quality mineral salt or ancient sea salt to your beverages each day. If you suspect you are sodium-deficient, add more until the thought or sight of salt seems distasteful or until you feel fully hydrated and are voiding clear urine frequently throughout the day.

I experienced years of metabolic damage from carb dependency and yo-yo dieting. How long will it take me to become a fat-burning beast?

After three weeks of total elimination of the Big Three toxic modern foods, you should experience massive improvements in your ability to regulate energy, mood, and appetite during the day. If your metabolic damage is severe, it may take between six and twelve months to fully optimize fat-burning genetic mechanisms and be completely free of carbohydrate dependency. It is only then that you should attempt strategic reduction of excess body fat via extended fasting and further carbohydrate restriction.

I thought insulin was important for building and maintaining muscle mass, recovering from workouts, balancing hormones, and other health functions.

Indeed, insulin is an important anabolic/anticatabolic hormone responsible for delivering glucose and amino acids to cells throughout the body. The concern and caution about insulin result from the fact that hyperinsulinemia (harmful chronic overproduction of insulin) is so prevalent. The big-picture health goal is to produce an optimally minimal amount of insulin—enough to get the job done without disturbing homeostasis.

How do I know whether my insulin production is okay or excessive?

If you carry excess body fat (per the Dr. Maffetone and Dr. Sinha calculations; see page 219)—especially visceral fat, around the midsection—it's likely that you have been chronically overproducing insulin. If you obtain a fasting insulin blood test, strive to get under 8.0 urgently. A count of under 3.0 is excellent. Because insulin offers many health, performance, and recovery benefits, it may be best to adopt a feast-or-famine eating strategy, wherein you eat nutritious meals, produce sufficient insulin to promote homeostasis, and concurrently strive to bank long hours in a fasted state between your nutrient-dense meals.

How can fruit be worse than other carbs when it has so many nutritional benefits?

Although fruit is highly lipogenic (that is, it has a high propensity to be converted into fat), the negative effects of fruit consumption happen largely when too many other forms of carbohydrates are consumed in concert with fruit. If your glycogen tanks are full, fruit is easily converted to fat. If your carb intake is sensible, fruit consumption has many advantages over other carbs. Consuming whole fresh fruit gives you fiber, water, and micronutrients that contribute to satiety in a way that processed carbohydrates do not. Furthermore, concerns about the autoimmune and inflammatory effects of plant antigens in grains, legumes, nuts, seeds, and vegetables are greatly minimized with fruit.

How can I tell if I'm liquidating my assets?

Be on the lookout for these symptoms and take immediate corrective action if you notice them:

- sugar cravings immediately after high-intensity workouts;
- delayed fatigue twenty-four to seventy-two hours after high-intensity workouts;
- overeating at your break-fast meal after an aggressive fasting effort;
- hectic weekdays paired with weekends of exhaustion and burnout;
- periods of excess energy during hectic days—feeling fidgety, hurried, distractible, and not very hungry;
- an excess of fight-or-flight stimulation (hectic workday, high-intensity workouts, high-shock-value entertainment) as well as insufficient parasympathetic stimulation (foam rolling, yoga, meditation, walking, nature immersion).

Most of us in modern life are at constant risk of becoming overstressed and liquidating our assets, leading to eventual burnout. It's critical to make devoted efforts to conduct morning and evening rituals, schedule downtime from technology, take regular movement breaks, and draw a series of deep, diaphragmatic breaths whenever you become overstimulated and frazzled.

Two Meals a Day Recipes

Brad's "NOatmeal"

4 servings

Made with healthful fats and protein and just enough natural sweetness, this oatmeal is easy to make and incredibly rich and satisfying. Vary the amount of nut butter according to your preferred consistency. Double or triple the recipe to have a ready-made supply for busy mornings.

Prep time: 5 minutes
Cooking time: 7 minutes

1 cup unsweetened coconut or almond milk

4 large egg yolks

2 teaspoons pure vanilla extract

2 teaspoons cinnamon

½ cup pureed nuts of your choice

3 tablespoons nut butter, such as Brad's Macadamia Masterpiece (available at Bradventures.com), or more or less to taste

In a large saucepan, combine milk, egg yolks, vanilla, and cinnamon and mix well. Simmer on low heat for about five minutes, stirring occasionally. When the mixture is warm and well blended, add nuts and nut butter and stir a couple more minutes until the desired consistency is reached. Keep in mind that the mixture will thicken significantly after being removed from the heat, so err on the watery side when you pull the pan off the stove.

Macronutrient Information

Total calories: 331
Fat: 23 grams / 207 calories

Carbs: 20 grams / 80 calories
Protein: 11 grams / 44 calories

Breakfast Hash and Broiled Eggs

2 servings

Hashes are often prepared with shredded potatoes, but why not experiment and use brussels sprouts? If you can't find brussels sprouts, a big bag of preshredded cabbage is a nice low-carb alternative.

Prep time: 10 minutes
Cooking time: 15–18 minutes

1 pound bulk pork sausage

2 tablespoons butter

4 ounces fresh mushrooms, diced

1 small shallot, minced

2 cups quartered brussels sprouts

4 garlic cloves, minced

Salt and pepper to taste

4 large pastured eggs

2 ounces crumbled goat cheese

Preheat the broiler to its highest setting.

In a large ovenproof skillet, cook the sausage over medium heat, breaking it up into bite-size pieces, until cooked through. Using a slotted spoon, remove the meat from the pan and set aside.

To the fat remaining in the skillet, add butter and mushrooms and cook on medium-high heat until golden brown. Add the shallot, brussels sprouts, and garlic. Sauté until the brussels sprouts are tender and the shallot is translucent, about 5 minutes. Season with salt and pepper. Transfer the cooked sausage back into the skillet and toss to combine. Taste and adjust seasoning.

Make four wells in the sausage mixture. Crack an egg into each well, season with salt and pepper, and place the pan on the middle rack of the oven. Broil for 3–5 minutes, depending on how runny you like the yolks. Top with crumbled cheese and serve immediately.

Macronutrient Information

Total calories: 2,408
Fat: 180 grams / 1,620 calories

Carbs: 63 grams / 252 calories
Protein: 134 grams / 536 calories

Hearty Farmer's Market Breakfast Casserole

4 servings

Filled with vegetables, herbs, and lots of protein, this dish will keep you full and grounded all morning. You'll love it so much that you'll be tempted to eat it for dinner!

Prep time: 12 minutes
Cooking time: 30 minutes

1 pound bulk pork sausage

1 red or green bell pepper, seeded and diced

1 medium zucchini, diced

1 medium onion, diced

4 garlic cloves, minced

8 large pastured eggs

1 cup shredded Cheddar cheese, divided

¼ cup chopped fresh basil

¼ cup minced fresh parsley

2 teaspoons salt

½ teaspoon pepper

½ cup heavy cream or unsweetened coconut cream

2 scallions, thinly sliced

Preheat oven to 375°F.

In a large pan over medium heat, brown the sausage, breaking it up into bite-size pieces. Increase the heat to medium-high and add the bell pepper, zucchini, onion, and garlic and sauté for 5 minutes.

Meanwhile, in a large bowl, whisk together the eggs, ½ cup cheese, basil, parsley, salt, pepper, and cream. Transfer the cooked sausage mixture to a 9-inch pie pan. Pour the egg mixture over the top and sprinkle with scallions and remaining cheese. Bake for 25 minutes, or until golden brown and just set.

Macronutrient Information

Total calories: 765
Fat: 61 grams / 549 calories

Carbs: 13 grams / 52 calories
Protein: 41 grams / 164 calories

Chaffle Avocado Toast

2 servings

Who says you have to fill your waffle iron with nutrient-deficient grains and sweeteners? Haul that thing back out of the dark cupboard corner and try the increasingly popular "chaffle"—a cheese waffle! This deliciously crispy concoction is topped with healthful fats, vegetables, and protein.

Prep time: 10 minutes
Cooking time: 15 minutes

2 large pastured eggs

1 cup shredded cheese, such as Cheddar or a mixture of half Parmesan and half mozzarella

½ teaspoon pepper

1 scallion, thinly sliced

4 slices uncured bacon

1 avocado

¼ teaspoon salt

¼ teaspoon garlic powder

4-inch section cucumber, peeled and thinly sliced

2 lemon wedges

Pinch of red pepper flakes

In a medium bowl, combine the eggs with the shredded cheese, pepper, and scallion. Pour the batter into a waffle maker and cook according to the manufacturer's directions—in two batches if necessary (see note below)—until golden brown. Transfer to a wire rack.

Meanwhile, in a large skillet over medium heat, cook the bacon, chop it, then set aside. In a small bowl, mash the avocado flesh with salt and garlic powder.

To assemble, layer cucumber slices on top of the chaffles, followed by the avocado mixture, chopped bacon, a squeeze of fresh lemon juice, and a pinch of red pepper flakes.

Make a double or triple batch of chaffles, then store them in the freezer. When you're ready to eat, simply pop them in the toaster.

Macronutrient Information

Total calories: 520
Fat: 40 grams / 360 calories

Carbs: 14 grams / 56 calories
Protein: 26 grams / 104 calories

Creamy Chicken Tortilla Soup

4 servings

You won't miss tortilla chips when you experience this incredibly intense and diverse blend of flavors and toppings.

Prep time: 15 minutes
Cooking time: 25 minutes

- 2 tablespoons lard or beef tallow
- 1 medium onion, diced
- 8 boneless, skinless chicken thighs, cut into 1-inch cubes
- 2 tablespoons tomato paste
- 4 ounces canned diced green chilies
- 2 tablespoons cumin
- 1 tablespoon coriander
- 1 tablespoon dried oregano
- 1 tablespoon chili powder
- 1 teaspoon smoked paprika
- 2 teaspoons salt
- 1 teaspoon pepper
- 8 garlic cloves, minced
- 2 medium zucchini, quartered lengthwise and sliced
- 2 carrots, halved and sliced lengthwise
- 1 small head green, white, or red cabbage, chopped
- 4 cups chicken bone broth
- 1 cup chopped fresh cilantro leaves
- ½ cup thinly sliced scallions
- 1 cup full-fat sour cream
- Sliced fresh jalapeño peppers, sliced black olives, shredded cheese, diced onion, and sliced avocado for topping

In a large soup pot over medium-high heat, melt the lard. Add the onion and sauté until translucent, about 3 minutes. Add the diced chicken thighs, tomato paste, green chilies, cumin, coriander, oregano, chili powder, smoked paprika, salt, and pepper. Stir to combine and sauté until the chicken is almost cooked through, about 10 minutes.

Add the garlic, zucchini, carrots, cabbage, and bone broth. Bring to a boil, then reduce to a simmer. Simmer for 10 minutes, or until the vegetables are crisp-tender.

Stir in the cilantro, scallions, and sour cream. Taste and adjust seasoning. Serve with the toppings on the side.

Macronutrient Information

Total calories: 623
Fat: 31 grams / 279 calories

Carbs: 34 grams / 136 calories
Protein: 52 grams / 208 calories

Tuscan Sausage Soup

4 servings

The combination of fatty Italian sausage, sun-dried tomatoes, and dry Parmesan cheese in this hearty one-pot recipe is going to blow you away. Let this one bubble for a while in your kitchen, so the delicious aroma drifts through your home as you cultivate gratitude for the opportunity to eat such delicious food.

Prep time: 10 minutes
Cooking time: 25 minutes

2 pounds spicy bulk Italian sausage

2 tablespoons extra-virgin olive oil

1 large onion, diced

6 garlic cloves, minced

2 medium zucchini, diced

½ cup sun-dried tomatoes packed in olive oil, drained and minced

¼ cup chopped fresh basil

½ cup chopped fresh parsley

1 teaspoon dried oregano

1 teaspoon salt

½ teaspoon pepper

6 cups chicken bone broth

4 cups fresh spinach leaves

¼ cup grated Parmesan cheese

In a large soup pot over medium heat, cook the sausage, breaking it into bite-size pieces. Just before it's cooked through, transfer to a bowl using a slotted spoon, reserving the fat in the pot.

Increase the heat to medium-high, add the olive oil and onion, and cook until translucent, about 3 minutes. Add the garlic, zucchini, sun-dried tomatoes, basil, parsley, dried oregano, salt, and pepper. Toss to coat and cook for an additional 5 minutes.

Transfer the sausage back into the pot and cover with the broth. Bring to a boil, then reduce heat to a simmer. Add the spinach and stir just to wilt. Remove from the heat, add the grated Parmesan, and serve hot.

Macronutrient Information

Total calories: 613
Fat: 45 grams / 405 calories

Carbs: 18 grams / 72 calories
Protein: 34 grams / 136 calories

Sisson Bigass Salad

2 servings

This is just one of many variations of my centerpiece midday or evening meal. Experiment with steak, chicken, turkey, and other meats in place of the tuna, and an assortment of colorful vegetables and/or dressings.

Prep time: 10 minutes

3–4 cups shredded lettuce or mixed greens

1–2 cups sliced fresh vegetables, such as fresh mushrooms, bell peppers, carrots, beets, and tomatoes

¼ cup shredded Cheddar cheese (optional)

1 5-ounce can sustainably harvested tuna packed in water, drained

¼ cup nuts, such as walnuts, pecans, or almonds

2 tablespoons sunflower or pumpkin seeds

2 tablespoons avocado oil–based salad dressing, such as Primal Kitchen Balsamic Vinaigrette and Marinade or Primal Kitchen Green Goddess

In a large shallow bowl, or a resealable storage container, layer the lettuce, vegetables, and cheese (if desired), in that order. Flake the tuna over the top. The salad can be stored or transported at this point.

When you're ready to eat, sprinkle the nuts and seeds over the top and drizzle with the dressing.

Macronutrient Information

Total calories: 879
Fat: 63 grams / 567 calories

Carbs: 24 grams / 96 calories
Protein: 54 grams / 216 calories

Caribbean Taco Salad

2 servings

If you've never tried combining chili powder and cinnamon, this salad is going to make you an instant convert—ground turkey will never taste better! Put on some reggae music and drift off on your own island fantasy.

Prep time: 10 minutes
Cooking time: 10 minutes

2 tablespoons butter

1 20-ounce package ground turkey

1 teaspoon salt

½ teaspoon pepper

1 tablespoon cumin

1 teaspoon dried oregano

1 teaspoon chili powder

½ teaspoon paprika

½ teaspoon onion powder

¼ teaspoon cayenne pepper

¼ teaspoon cinnamon

4 garlic cloves, minced

½ teaspoon grated fresh ginger

1 green or red bell pepper, seeded and diced

Zest of 1 lime

Juice of 2 limes

¼ cup extra-virgin olive oil

2 cups thinly sliced green cabbage

2 cups baby spinach leaves

¼ cup thinly sliced scallions

½ cup chopped fresh cilantro leaves

In a large skillet over medium-high heat, melt the butter. Add the turkey, salt, pepper, cumin, oregano, chili powder, paprika, onion powder, cayenne, and cinnamon. Cook, breaking up into small bits, until the meat is cooked through.

Add the garlic, ginger, and bell pepper and cook until fragrant, about 1 minute. Add the lime zest and juice, and olive oil. Toss to combine.

In a medium bowl, combine the cabbage and spinach. Top with the meat mixture, scallions, and cilantro.

Macronutrient Information

Total calories: 1,193
Fat: 89 grams / 801 calories

Carbs: 22 grams / 88 calories
Protein: 76 grams / 304 calories

Curried Chicken Salad

2 servings

Bibb lettuce is the best nest for this tasty meal, but crunchy cabbage will work, as will a bed of mixed greens. The chopped nuts help jazz up the texture and increase satiety.

Prep time: 5 minutes
Cooking time: 15 minutes

8 boneless, skinless chicken thighs, cut into 1-inch cubes

Salt and pepper to taste

1 green bell pepper, seeded and diced

2 stalks celery, diced

2 scallions, thinly sliced

½ cup chopped nuts, such as macadamia or pecans

2 large romaine or Bibb lettuce leaves

For the dressing

1 cup avocado oil–based mayonnaise, such as Primal Kitchen Mayo

Zest of 1 lemon

Juice of ½ lemon

1 tablespoon curry powder

½ teaspoon garlic powder

½ teaspoon salt

½ teaspoon pepper

Preheat the oven to 425°F. Line a baking sheet with parchment paper.

Arrange the chicken pieces on the prepared pan and season with salt and pepper. Bake for 15 minutes, until the internal temperature reaches 160°F. Remove from oven and allow to cool for 5 minutes.

While the chicken bakes, make the dressing: whisk together the mayonnaise, lemon zest and juice, curry powder, garlic powder, salt, and pepper in a medium bowl.

Add the bell pepper, celery, scallions, and chopped nuts. Add the cooled chicken, toss to coat, and adjust seasoning.

Place a lettuce leaf on each of two serving plates, top with salad, and serve.

Macronutrient Information

Total calories: 1,118
Fat: 85 grams / 765 calories

Carbs: 14 grams / 56 calories
Protein: 82 grams / 328 calories

Tuna Salad with Cucumber "Chips"

2 servings

Keep canned tuna in your pantry to use as a quick and versatile meal base. Look for label designations such as "line caught" or "pole caught" to avoid problems associated with industrialized tuna operations. Combined with mayonnaise and avocado, this salad is amazing served with your favorite low-carb crudités, such as the cucumber suggested here or radish, jicama, and bell pepper.

Prep time: 5 minutes

12 ounces sustainably harvested canned tuna packed in water, drained

4 stalks celery, diced small

2 scallions, thinly sliced

Zest and juice of 1 small lemon

½ avocado, mashed

½ cup avocado oil–based mayonnaise, such as Primal Kitchen Mayo

1 teaspoon everything bagel seasoning

½ teaspoon pepper

1 English cucumber, sliced on the diagonal

Combine the tuna, celery, scallions, lemon zest and juice, avocado, mayonnaise, bagel seasoning, and pepper in a medium bowl. Serve sliced cucumber on the side.

Macronutrient Information

Total calories: 735
Fat: 59 grams / 531 calories

Carbs: 9 grams / 36 calories
Protein: 42 grams / 168 calories

Taco Salad

2 servings

Who needs a tortilla when you can enjoy the varied and intense flavors and textures in this ultrasophisticated spin on a popular staple? Again, nothing you'll find in a restaurant will ever compare to this, so make a huge batch of it and enjoy it all week.

Prep time: 15 minutes
Cooking time: 10 minutes

1½ pounds ground beef

4 garlic cloves, minced

1 tablespoon cumin

1 teaspoon coriander

1 teaspoon chili powder

2 teaspoons salt

½ teaspoon pepper

4 cups chopped leafy greens, such as romaine, spinach, or kale

2 cups shredded green cabbage

2 ounces fresh white button mushrooms, thinly sliced

½ cup fresh cherry tomatoes, halved

1 avocado, diced

2 stalks celery, thinly sliced

1 cup shredded Cheddar cheese

½ cup full-fat sour cream

½ cup prepared salsa

1 cup chopped fresh cilantro leaves

1 bunch scallions, thinly sliced

Juice of 2 limes

In a large skillet over medium heat, combine the ground beef, garlic, cumin, coriander, chili powder, salt, and pepper. Sauté, mixing thoroughly, until the meat is cooked through. Remove from the heat and set aside.

In a large bowl, layer the greens, cabbage, mushrooms, tomatoes, avocado, celery, and cheese.

To make the dressing, whisk together the sour cream, salsa, cilantro, scallions, and lime juice in a small bowl. Spoon the beef mixture over the greens and vegetables and generously drizzle with dressing.

Macronutrient Information

Total calories: 1,453
Fat: 97 grams / 873 calories

Carbs: 37 grams / 148 calories
Protein: 108 grams / 432 calories

Green Chili Chicken Chili

4 servings

This one-pot chicken-and-vegetable dish hits the spot, bursting with flavors from spicy pork sausage, comforting bone broth, and a big dose of dried and fresh herbs and spices.

Prep time: 8 minutes
Cooking time: 30 minutes

2 tablespoons extra-virgin olive oil or lard

1 large yellow onion, chopped

6 garlic cloves, minced

1 pound boneless, skinless chicken thighs, cut into 1-inch cubes

1 pound ground chicken

1 pound spicy bulk sausage

2 medium zucchini, diced

2 cans (14 ounces each) diced green chilies

2 tablespoons cumin

1 tablespoon dried oregano

1 teaspoon coriander

¼ teaspoon cayenne pepper

4 cups chicken bone broth

1 cup chopped fresh cilantro leaves

½ cup thinly sliced scallions

Sliced fresh or pickled jalapeño peppers, full-fat sour cream, shredded cheese, diced black olives, and sliced avocado for topping

Heat the oil in a large stock pot over medium heat. Add the onion and garlic and cook 3 minutes. Add the chicken thighs, ground chicken, and sausage. Cook about 8 minutes, stirring to break up, until almost fully cooked.

Add the zucchini, green chilies, cumin, oregano, coriander, cayenne pepper, and bone broth. Bring to a boil, reduce heat, and simmer, uncovered, for 10 minutes. Remove from the heat, adjust seasoning, and add the cilantro and scallions. Serve hot with toppings on the side.

Macronutrient Information

Total calories: 993
Fat: 61 grams / 549 calories

Carbs: 23 grams / 92 calories
Protein: 88 grams / 352 calories

Caribbean Seafood Stew

2 servings

Not only is this dish poppin' with exotic flavors, it's also super quick to prepare, thanks to fast-cooking red snapper.

Prep time: 10 minutes
Cooking time: 20 minutes

2 tablespoons extra-virgin olive oil

1 tablespoon freshly squeezed lime juice

1 teaspoon salt

½ teaspoon pepper

1 pound skinless wild caught salmon, tilapia, or mahi-mahi fillets, cut into 1-inch cubes

8 ounces uncooked medium shrimp, peeled and deveined

2 tablespoons butter or ghee

1 medium onion, diced

6 garlic cloves, minced

1 green bell pepper, seeded and diced

2 stalks celery, diced

1 teaspoon red pepper flakes

½ cup diced fresh tomatoes

½ cup unsweetened coconut milk or heavy cream

½ cup chopped fresh cilantro leaves

1 avocado, diced

In a medium bowl, combine the olive oil, lime juice, salt, pepper, fish, and shrimp and set aside.

In a medium pan, heat the butter over medium-high heat. Add the onion, garlic, bell pepper, celery, and red pepper flakes. Cook about 4 minutes, or until the onion is translucent.

Add the diced tomatoes and coconut milk. Bring to a boil, reduce to a simmer, and cook, uncovered, for 5 minutes. Stir in the fish mixture. Return to a simmer and cook 5 more minutes, or until the shrimp is opaque. Serve hot, with cilantro and avocado on the side.

Macronutrient Information

Total calories: 829
Fat: 41 grams / 369 calories

Carbs: 24 grams / 96 calories
Protein: 91 grams / 364 calories

Moroccan Lamb Stew

2 servings

The Moroccan spice combinations in this dish will make you feel like you're on a vacation adventure in North Africa. This dish is best eaten with lots of loved ones and candles—so make it for an extra-special occasion and enjoy!

Prep time: 10 minutes
Cooking time: 20 minutes

4 tablespoons butter or ghee

1 small onion, diced

1 teaspoon grated fresh ginger

6 garlic cloves, minced

1 pound ground lamb

1 teaspoon smoked paprika

2 teaspoons cumin

2 teaspoons turmeric

½ teaspoon cinnamon

2 teaspoons salt

1 teaspoon pepper

2 cups cauliflower florets, cut into bite-size pieces

8 tablespoons tomato paste

½ cup unsweetened coconut milk

1 cup beef or chicken bone broth

½ cup plain full-fat Greek yogurt

Zest and juice of ½ lemon

½ cup chopped fresh cilantro leaves

1 avocado, diced

In a medium Dutch oven over medium-high heat, melt the butter. Add the onion, ginger, and garlic. Sauté 3 minutes, then add the ground lamb, paprika, cumin, turmeric, cinnamon, salt, and pepper. Continue to sauté until the lamb is cooked through, about 5 minutes, stirring occasionally.

Add the cauliflower, tomato paste, coconut milk, and bone broth and stir to combine. Bring to a boil, then reduce to a simmer. Simmer, uncovered, for 5 minutes.

In a small bowl, whisk the yogurt with the lemon zest and juice.

To serve, top individual servings of stew with cilantro, avocado, and lemon-yogurt sauce.

Macronutrient Information

Total calories: 1,105
Fat: 81 grams / 729 calories

Carbs: 35 grams /140 calories
Protein: 59 grams / 236 calories

Beef Taco Casserole

4 servings

This casserole eschews the traditional base of white rice in favor of lighter, low-carb cauliflower rice. The cauliflower takes on the delicious flavors of all the many warm and mouthwatering spices in the sauce, so go ahead and keep a supply of cauliflower rice in your fridge or freezer so you can whip up meals like this anytime you like.

Prep time: 10 minutes
Cooking time: 25 minutes

2 tablespoons lard, divided

1 (16-ounce) bag frozen cauliflower rice, or prepare 16 ounces of chopped cauliflower in food processor

1 red or green bell pepper, seeded and diced

1 onion, diced

2 pounds ground beef

1 tablespoon cumin

1 teaspoon coriander

1 teaspoon salt

½ teaspoon pepper

1 teaspoon chili powder

1 teaspoon garlic powder

8 tablespoons tomato paste

1 cup shredded Cheddar or Colby cheese

Toppings

1 cup full-fat sour cream

2 cups shredded greens, such as romaine or cabbage

1 cup diced fresh tomatoes

½ cup diced black olives

2 avocados, sliced

1 cup chopped fresh cilantro leaves

1 jalapeño pepper, seeded and thinly sliced

1 cup prepared salsa

Preheat the oven to 425°F.

In a large skillet, heat 1 tablespoon of the lard over medium-high heat. Add the cauliflower rice and sauté until brown. Transfer to a 9- × 13-inch casserole dish and set aside.

In the same skillet over medium-high heat, melt the remaining lard. Add the bell pepper and onion. Cook until just softened, then add the ground beef. Add the cumin, coriander, salt, pepper, chili powder, and garlic powder and toss to coat, breaking up the meat as it cooks.

Just before the meat is cooked through, stir in the tomato paste and mix thoroughly. Layer the beef mixture on top of the cauliflower rice, top with shredded cheese, and bake for 12 minutes.

Remove the casserole from the oven. Spread sour cream over the top, then follow with the remaining toppings, sprinkling them over the sour cream in layers.

Macronutrient Information

Total calories: 1,090
Fat: 70 grams / 630 calories

Carbs: 39 grams / 156 calories
Protein: 76 grams / 304 calories

Beef and Broccoli

This popular ancestral staple meal is better than ever, thanks to the addition of freshly grated ginger and chopped nuts. Your mouth is going to water just thinking about it! Note: Coconut aminos is a liquid condiment similar to soy sauce, but instead of being fermented from soybeans, it's fermented from the sap of coconut palm trees and sea salt. It's gluten- and grain-free and used often in Asian cuisine. It's a great replacement in recipes calling for soy sauce or tamari.

Prep time: 5 minutes
Cooking time: 15 minutes

- 4 tablespoons extra-virgin olive oil or avocado oil, divided
- 1½ pounds sirloin steak, sliced against the grain
- 4 cups broccoli florets
- ½ cup coconut aminos
- 4 garlic cloves, minced
- ½ teaspoon red pepper flakes
- 1 teaspoon grated fresh ginger
- ½ cup chopped nuts, such as Brazil nuts, macadamia nuts, almonds, or pecans
- ½ cup thinly sliced scallions
- ¼ cup beef bone broth

Heat 2 tablespoons of the oil in a large skillet over high heat. Add the steak and brown quickly, then transfer to a plate and set aside.

Reduce the heat to medium-high, then add the remaining oil. Add the broccoli and cook 5 minutes, stirring occasionally. Return the steak to the pan, then add the coconut aminos, garlic, red pepper flakes, ginger, nuts, scallions, and bone broth. Stir to combine and cook 2 minutes to thicken slightly. Serve immediately.

Macronutrient Information

Total calories: 1,550
Fat: 106 grams / 954 calories

Carbs: 34 grams / 136 calories
Protein: 115 grams /460 calories

Chicken Thighs with Chard in Mushroom Cream Sauce

2 servings

Never underestimate how indulgent chicken thighs can taste when you roast them and add cream and mushrooms. Instead of using cans of condensed mushroom soup, opt for the real deal, with fresh mushrooms and organic heavy cream (or coconut cream if you prefer).

Prep time: 5 minutes
Cooking time: 25 minutes

1 tablespoon Italian seasoning

2 teaspoons salt

1 teaspoon pepper

4 bone-in chicken thighs

2 tablespoons extra-virgin olive oil

4 slices uncured bacon, chopped

8 ounces fresh mushrooms, chopped

3 cups chopped Swiss chard

4 garlic cloves, minced

1 cup heavy cream or unsweetened coconut cream

1 teaspoon chopped fresh thyme

Salt and pepper to taste

Preheat the oven to 375°F. Line a baking sheet with parchment paper.

In a small bowl, combine the Italian seasoning, salt, and pepper. Arrange the chicken thighs on the prepared baking sheet and cover evenly with the seasoning mixture. Bake for 20 minutes.

In a large skillet, heat the olive oil over medium heat. Add the chopped bacon and sauté until fully cooked. Using a slotted spoon, transfer to a bowl, reserving the fat in the skillet.

Increase the heat to medium-high and add the mushrooms. Cook until golden brown, then add the chopped chard, garlic, cream, and thyme. Cook to wilt the chard, about 3 minutes. Add the cooked chicken thighs and bacon and simmer for 3 minutes. Taste and adjust seasoning, then serve hot.

Macronutrient Information

Total calories: 903
Fat: 71 grams / 639 calories

Carbs: 13 grams / 52 calories
Protein: 53 grams / 212 calories

Italian Stuffed Bell Peppers

2 servings

Stuffed bell peppers are typically filled with rice, but you can do better with ground beef and Italian sausage. Top with Parmesan and broil, and you have yourself the most convenient of gourmet meals. Try it tonight!

Prep time: 10 minutes
Cooking time: 25 minutes

½ pound ground beef

½ pound bulk Italian sausage

2 tablespoons extra-virgin olive oil

1 onion, diced

2 stalks celery, sliced

6 garlic cloves, minced

1 tablespoon Italian seasoning

1 cup diced fresh tomatoes

½ cup chopped fresh parsley

2 red or green bell peppers, cored, seeded, and halved lengthwise

½ cup grated Parmesan cheese

In a large skillet over medium-high heat, cook the ground beef and sausage, breaking up the meat into bite-size pieces. When the meat is cooked through, transfer to a plate and set aside.

Heat the olive oil in the same skillet, then add the onion and celery, cooking until softened, about 3 minutes. Add the garlic, Italian seasoning, and diced tomatoes. Cook 5 minutes, then return the cooked meat to the skillet. Add fresh parsley and toss to combine. Remove from the heat.

Preheat the broiler to its highest setting. Line a baking sheet with parchment paper, then arrange the peppers on the sheet, cut side up. Using your hands, fill the pepper "boats" with the meat mixture, rounding the tops. Top with the Parmesan cheese and place on the middle shelf of the oven. Broil for 2 to 3 minutes, until the cheese is bubbly and golden. Serve hot.

Macronutrient Information

Total calories: 955
Fat: 67 grams / 603 calories

Carbs: 27 grams / 108 calories
Protein: 61 grams / 244 calories

Mediterranean Stuffed Bell Peppers

Mediterranean flavors, such as olive, lemon, artichoke, and feta, always make for an intense and satisfying meal. Naturally salty, these peppers will taste delicious after you have ditched processed foods and your body is craving a healthy dose of sodium.

Prep time: 10 minutes
Cooking time: 25 minutes

½ pound ground lamb

1 tablespoon butter

1 tablespoon avocado oil

½ pound bulk Italian sausage

1 onion, diced

4 garlic cloves, minced

1 teaspoon Italian seasoning

1 teaspoon dried oregano

¼ cup chopped kalamata olives

½ cup drained and chopped marinated artichoke hearts

½ cup diced fresh tomatoes

¼ cup chopped fresh parsley

Zest of 1 lemon

2 red or green bell peppers, cored, seeded, and halved lengthwise

¼ cup crumbled feta cheese

In a large skillet over medium-high heat, cook the lamb and sausage in one tablespoon of butter, breaking the meat into bite-size pieces. Sauté until cooked through, then transfer to a plate with a slotted spoon.

To the fat remaining in the skillet, add a tablespoon of avocado oil and onion and cook until translucent, about 3 minutes. Add the garlic, Italian seasoning, oregano, olives, artichoke hearts, and diced tomatoes. Cook 5 minutes more, then return the cooked meat to the skillet. Add the parsley and lemon zest and toss to combine. Remove from the heat.

Preheat the broiler to its highest setting. Line a baking sheet with parchment paper, then arrange the peppers on the sheet, cut side up. Using your hands, fill the pepper "boats" with the meat mixture, rounding the tops. Top with the feta cheese and place on the middle shelf of the oven. Broil for 2 to 3 minutes, until the cheese is bubbly and golden. Serve hot.

Macronutrient Information

Total calories: 875
Fat: 63 grams / 567 calories

Carbs: 23 grams / 92 calories
Protein: 54 grams / 216 calories

Spiced Fish Taco Bowl with Avocado-Lime Crema

2 servings

Any meal featuring this exotic creation is sure to be a hit. The macadamia nut topping will make you the star of any potluck gathering.

Prep time: 10 minutes
Cooking time: 10 minutes

2 large fillets (about 14 ounces each) halibut or cod, chopped into bite-size pieces

1 teaspoon salt

½ teaspoon pepper

1 teaspoon cumin

½ teaspoon chili powder

2 tablespoons extra-virgin olive oil or avocado oil

2 cups fresh or frozen cauliflower rice

2 cups shredded green cabbage or coleslaw mix

4 radishes, thinly sliced

¼ cup chopped macadamia nuts

For the dressing

1 avocado

1 bunch fresh cilantro leaves

½ cup avocado oil–based mayonnaise, such as Primal Kitchen Mayo

Zest and juice of 2 limes

1 garlic clove

1 teaspoon salt

Pat the fish dry with paper towels and season with salt, pepper, cumin, and chili powder.

Heat the oil in a large skillet over medium-high heat. Cook the fish until fork-tender, 6 to 8 minutes total, turning halfway through. Add the cauliflower rice, toss, and remove from the heat.

To make the dressing, combine the avocado, cilantro, mayonnaise, lime zest and juice, garlic, and salt in a blender. Blend until smooth.

Spread the cabbage at the bottom of a large bowl, then layer the fish mixture over it. Top with the dressing, radishes, and macadamia nuts.

Macronutrient Information

Total calories: 1,866
Fat: 106 grams / 954 calories

Carbs: 68 grams / 272 calories
Protein: 160 grams / 640 calories

Dill Pickle Super Burgers

2 servings

Classic dill pickle is paired with pepperoncini, cream cheese, and fresh dill and finished with a healthy scoop of gut-healing sauerkraut. The satiety score is off the charts. Are you salivating yet?

Prep time: 10 minutes
Cooking time: 12 minutes

1 pound ground bison or beef

1 teaspoon salt

½ teaspoon pepper

1½ teaspoons garlic powder, divided

1 teaspoon onion powder

1 tablespoon lard or beef tallow

8 slices uncured bacon, diced

4 ounces full-fat cream cheese, softened

½ cup diced dill pickles

1 tablespoon dill pickle juice

¼ cup diced pepperoncini

1 tablespoon chopped fresh dill

¼ cup thinly sliced scallions

2 large romaine or Bibb lettuce leaves

½ cup drained sauerkraut

In a medium bowl, combine the ground meat with the salt, pepper, 1 teaspoon garlic powder, and onion powder.

In a large skillet, heat the lard over medium-high heat. Fry the bacon pieces until just crisp. Remove with a slotted spoon, reserving the fat in the pan.

Shape the meat mixture into two oval patties. Sauté in the remaining fat over medium-high heat for 3 minutes per side.

In a small bowl, combine the cream cheese, dill pickles, pickle juice, pepperoncini, remaining garlic powder, dill, and scallions. Arrange each meat patty on a lettuce leaf and top with a generous dollop of the cream cheese mixture and sauerkraut.

Macronutrient Information

Total calories: 857
Fat: 57 grams / 513 calories

Carbs: 12 grams / 48 calories
Protein: 74 grams / 296 calories

Lemony Tuna Casserole

Put a creative spin on an all-American classic by using cabbage or spaghetti squash instead of pasta.

Prep time: 10 minutes
Cooking time: 15 minutes

1 stick butter

1 large onion, diced small

4 stalks celery, diced

1 small or medium head green cabbage, cut into ½-inch strips, or 4 cups cooked spaghetti squash (see note below)

12–15 ounces sustainably harvested canned tuna packed in water, drained

6 garlic cloves, minced

Zest of 1 lemon

Juice of ½ lemon

¼ cup chopped fresh parsley

½ teaspoon salt

½ teaspoon pepper

¼ teaspoon red pepper flakes

½ cup frozen green peas, thawed (optional)

In a large skillet, melt the butter over medium heat. Sauté the onion and celery until translucent, about three minutes. Add the cabbage, then increase the heat to medium-high. Toss frequently and cook until softened.

Add the tuna, garlic, lemon zest and juice, parsley, salt, pepper, red pepper flakes, and peas if desired. Remove from the heat and toss to coat. Adjust seasoning, then serve hot.

To roast spaghetti squash, preheat the oven to 450°F. Line a baking sheet with parchment paper. Cut a small spaghetti squash in half lengthwise, scoop out the seeds, and season generously with olive oil, salt, and pepper. Place the halves cut side down on the prepared baking sheet and roast until fork-tender and slightly golden, about 25 minutes.

Macronutrient Information

Total calories: 1,052
Fat: 64 grams / 576 calories

Carbs: 49 grams / 196 calories
Protein: 70 grams / 280 calories

Spring Vegetable and Chicken Carbonara Skillet

2 servings

Use asparagus in the spring, brussels sprouts in the fall, and cabbage in the winter—or choose from among other fresh seasonal options at your local farmer's market.

Prep time: 10 minutes
Cooking time: 20 minutes

8 slices uncured bacon, diced

1 small onion, diced small

4 boneless, skinless chicken thighs, cut into 1-inch cubes

1 teaspoon salt

½ teaspoon pepper

1 small bunch asparagus, trimmed and cut into bite-size chunks

¼ cup frozen green peas, thawed (optional)

4 garlic cloves, minced

Zest of 1 lemon

Juice of ½ lemon

¼ cup chopped fresh basil

¼ cup chopped fresh parsley

1 stick butter

½ cup heavy cream

½ cup grated Parmesan cheese

In a large skillet, cook the bacon pieces over medium-high heat until crisp. Using a slotted spoon, transfer the pieces to a plate and set aside, reserving the fat in the skillet.

Add the onion to the skillet and cook until translucent, about 5 minutes. Add the chicken thighs, salt, and pepper. Just before the meat is cooked through, add the asparagus, peas (if desired), garlic, and lemon zest and juice. Sauté for 2 minutes, then add the basil, parsley, butter, cream, and Parmesan.

Stir to combine. Bring to a boil, then reduce the heat and simmer for 3 minutes. Adjust seasoning, then serve hot.

Macronutrient Information

Total calories: 1,150
Fat: 94 grams / 846 calories

Carbs: 15 grams / 60 calories
Protein: 61 grams / 244 calories

Roasted Crowns Casserole

2 servings

Cruciferous vegetables such as cauliflower and broccoli pair beautifully with healthful mayonnaise and melted cheese. Italian sausage rounds out this dish with a big dose of protein and nutritious fat. Once you've made this a couple of times, you'll have it committed to memory and be able to whip it up in no time.

Prep time: 10 minutes
Cooking time: 15 minutes

2 cups fresh cauliflower florets

2 cups fresh broccoli florets

¼ cup extra-virgin olive oil

1 teaspoon salt

1 teaspoon pepper, divided

1½ pounds bulk Italian pork sausage

4 garlic cloves, minced

Zest of 1 lemon

1 tablespoon freshly squeezed lemon juice

½ cup avocado oil–based mayonnaise, such as Primal Kitchen Mayo

½ cup shredded sharp Cheddar cheese

1 bunch scallions, thinly sliced, divided

Preheat the broiler to its highest setting. Line two baking sheets with parchment paper. Arrange the broccoli and cauliflower florets in a single layer on the baking sheet and season with olive oil, salt, and ½ teaspoon pepper. Place the pan on the top shelf of the oven and broil for 3 to 5 minutes, or until the florets begin to char slightly. Remove from the oven and set aside.

Reduce the broiler heat to its lowest setting and place a shelf in the bottom half of the oven. In a large, ovenproof skillet over medium-high heat, cook the sausage, breaking it into bite-size pieces.

Meanwhile, in a small bowl, combine the garlic, lemon zest and juice, mayonnaise, cheese, half the scallions, and remaining ½ teaspoon pepper. Once the sausage is cooked through, add the broiled broccoli and cauliflower to the skillet and toss to combine. Top with the seasoned mayonnaise mixture, then place the pan on the low shelf and broil until the top is golden and bubbly, about 3 minutes. Sprinkle with the remaining scallions and serve hot.

Macronutrient Information

Total calories: 1,692
Fat: 140 grams /1,260 calories

Carbs: 33 grams / 132 calories
Protein: 75 grams / 300 calories

Sheet-Pan Sausage and Cabbage

2 servings

This German-inspired dish is naturally low in carbohydrates, easy to prepare, and absolutely delicious.

Prep time: 5 minutes
Cooking time: 20 minutes

4 cooked sausage links of your choice

1 small head green cabbage, cut into 8 wedges

4 tablespoons extra-virgin olive oil

1 teaspoon salt

½ teaspoon pepper

1 teaspoon garlic powder

1 teaspoon onion powder

French Whole Grain Old Fashioned Mustard (sugar-free brand) for serving (1–2 tablespoons to preference)

Preheat the oven to 450°F. Line a baking sheet with parchment paper.

Arrange the sausages and cabbage wedges on the prepared baking sheet. Drizzle the cabbage with olive oil.

In a small bowl, combine the salt, pepper, garlic powder, and onion powder. Sprinkle the seasoning mixture generously over the cabbage. Roast for 20 minutes and serve hot with whole-grain mustard.

Macronutrient Information

Total calories: 677
Fat: 49 grams / 441 calories

Carbs: 26 grams / 104 calories
Protein: 33 grams / 132 calories

Shepherd's Pie

Ground lamb and yellow curry powder combine with fresh vegetables and healthful fats, butter, and Parmesan cheese to bring you comfort in every bite. This is wonderful any time of year, because the vegetables can be sourced year-round. Fresh ground lamb is in peak season in the United States from March to October but can generally be found frozen during the winter.

Prep time: 15 minutes
Cooking time: 25 minutes

1 medium head cauliflower, cut into large florets

2 garlic cloves

1 tablespoon plus 1 teaspoon salt, divided

2 tablespoons lard or beef tallow

1 medium onion, diced

2 celery stalks, thinly sliced

2 carrots, diced

4 ounces fresh mushrooms, diced

2 pounds ground lamb

1 teaspoon pepper, divided

½ teaspoon yellow curry powder

1 teaspoon smoked paprika

6 garlic cloves, minced

1 stick butter, melted

½ cup grated Parmesan cheese

¼ cup chopped fresh parsley

Preheat the broiler to its lowest setting.

Place florets, whole garlic cloves, and 1 teaspoon salt in a medium pot. Add just enough water to cover. Bring to a boil, reduce heat, and simmer for 12 to 15 minutes, until florets are fork-tender.

Meanwhile, in a large ovenproof skillet, melt the lard over medium-high heat. Add the onion, celery, carrots, and mushrooms. Cook 3 minutes. Add the lamb and season with 1 tablespoon salt, ½ teaspoon pepper, curry powder, paprika, and minced garlic. Cook, stirring occasionally, until lamb is cooked through.

When the cauliflower is fork-tender, drain well and transfer to the bowl of a food processor. Add the melted butter, Parmesan, and the remaining ½ teaspoon pepper. Puree until smooth. Taste and adjust seasoning.

Top the meat mixture in the skillet with the cauliflower mash and broil in the oven for about 6 to 8 minutes, or until warmed through and slightly golden. Serve hot, garnished with chopped parsley.

Macronutrient Information

Total calories: 1,027
Fat: 79 grams / 711 calories

Carbs: 19 grams / 76 calories
Protein: 60 grams / 240 calories

Asian Lettuce Cups

2 servings

It's amazing how fresh herbs and spices and good-quality cooking oils can transform your meals. Ginger, sesame oil, and chili garlic sauce make these Asian lettuce wraps extra mouthwatering without leaving you feeling stuffed or bloated. Warning: restaurant versions of this dish will pale in comparison to your creation forevermore!

Prep time: 10 minutes
Cooking time: 15 minutes

2 tablespoons lard

1 small onion, minced

1½ pounds ground turkey or chicken

4 garlic cloves, minced

1 teaspoon grated fresh ginger

1 carrot, shredded

2 stalks celery, thinly sliced

¼ cup coconut aminos

1 tablespoon toasted sesame oil

1 tablespoon prepared Yai's Thai Chili Garlic Sauce (sugar-free brand)

1 head Bibb lettuce

1 cup chopped fresh cilantro leaves

½ cup chopped nuts, such as macadamia nuts or almonds

Melt the lard in a large skillet over medium-high heat. Add the onion and sauté for 2 minutes, then add the ground meat. Cook through, stirring occasionally to break up the meat, about 10 minutes.

Add the garlic, ginger, carrot, celery, coconut aminos, sesame oil, and chili garlic sauce. Cook for 2 minutes, stirring to combine well.

Divide the mixture between the two lettuce cups and top with cilantro and chopped nuts.

Macronutrient Information

Total calories: 1,372
Fat: 100 grams / 900 calories

Carbs: 26 grams / 104 calories
Protein: 92 grams / 368 calories

Instant Pot Pulled Pork and Coleslaw

4 servings

Have you tried cooking pork in the Instant Pot electric pressure cooker? Every tender and juicy bite will taste just as if it's been slow-cooking all day. After you make it this way, you won't want to cook it any other way. Enjoy this throughout the week over a big pile of leafy greens, in a bowl with cauliflower rice, or just by itself—it's that good!

Prep time: 8 minutes
Cooking time: 30 minutes

2 tablespoons lard

1 large onion, cut into large dice

8 garlic cloves, minced

3 tablespoons cumin

1 tablespoon coriander

1 tablespoon paprika

1 tablespoon oregano

1 teaspoon powdered mustard

½ cup coconut aminos

1½ teaspoons salt, divided

1½ teaspoons pepper, divided

3 pounds pork shoulder or sirloin roast, cut into 2-inch cubes

½ cup bone broth

1 cup avocado oil–based mayonnaise, such as Primal Kitchen Mayo

¼ cup apple cider vinegar

2 bags coleslaw mix (11 ounce/240 gram bags or 8 cups total)

Combine the lard and onion in the bottom of an Instant Pot and cook on the sauté setting for 2 minutes. Then add the garlic, cumin, coriander, paprika, oregano, mustard, coconut aminos, 1 teaspoon salt, 1 teaspoon pepper, and pork. Stir to coat, then add the bone broth. Cover and cook on the meat setting for 20 minutes.

Meanwhile, combine the mayonnaise, vinegar, remaining ½ teaspoon salt, and remaining ½ teaspoon pepper in a large bowl. Add the coleslaw mix and toss thoroughly to combine.

When the pork is done, remove it from the pot, shred or chop it, then return it to the pot so it can soak up the juices.

Serve hot, spooning the pork over the coleslaw mixture or serving coleslaw on the side.

Macronutrient Information

Total calories: 1,285
Fat: 85 grams / 765 calories

Carbs: 45 grams / 180 calories
Protein: 85 grams / 340 calories

Skillet Reuben

2 servings

Salty corned beef broiled with sweet Swiss cheese captures hearts every single time, so make this when you need a little extra self-love or when you're wanting to share that love with a friend.

Prep time: 5 minutes
Cooking time: 15 minutes

3 tablespoons butter

1½ pounds corned beef, coarsely chopped

1 large bag coleslaw mix (11-ounce/240-gram bag or 4 cups total)

1 bunch scallions, thinly sliced

4 slices Swiss cheese

1 cup sauerkraut

For the dressing

1 cup avocado oil–based mayonnaise, such as Primal Kitchen Mayo

1 tablespoon tomato paste

1 tablespoon prepared horseradish

1 teaspoon apple cider vinegar

½ teaspoon salt

½ teaspoon pepper

Preheat the broiler to its highest setting.

In a large ovenproof skillet over medium-high heat, melt the butter. Add the corned beef and sauté for 3 minutes. Add the coleslaw mix and sauté for 5 minutes, stirring occasionally. Top with scallions, then cheese slices, and place under the broiler for 2 to 3 minutes, or until cheese is bubbly and golden.

In a small bowl, whisk together the mayonnaise, tomato paste, horseradish, vinegar, salt, and pepper.

Remove the skillet from the broiler and serve with the sauce drizzled over the top and the sauerkraut on the side.

Macronutrient Information

Total calories: 1,245
Fat: 77 grams / 693 calories

Carbs: 50 grams / 200 calories
Protein: 88 grams / 352 calories

Lemon and Herb Pork Tenderloins with Broiled Broccoli

4 servings

Adding lemon zest to a warm recipe like this gives it a special burst of flavor, so try to keep fresh lemons in your kitchen at all times. Get comfortable using your broiler by watching the pan carefully and pulling it out when the meat and vegetables are perfectly bronze and crispy but not burned. Adjust the cooking times based on your experience, because ovens can vary a bit.

Prep time: 15 minutes, plus 30 or more minutes of marinating time
Cooking time: 20 minutes

Zest and juice of 4 lemons

1 cup extra-virgin olive oil

8 garlic cloves, minced

1 tablespoon French Whole Grain Old Fashioned Mustard

1 tablespoon chopped fresh rosemary

1 tablespoon chopped fresh parsley

1 teaspoon chopped fresh thyme

1–2 tablespoons salt, or more or less to taste

1 teaspoon pepper

2 pork tenderloins, about 1 pound each

For the broccoli

5 cups fresh broccoli florets

¼ cup extra-virgin olive oil

1 tablespoon salt

1 teaspoon pepper

Combine lemon zest and juice, olive oil, garlic, mustard, rosemary, parsley, thyme, salt, and pepper in a large nonreactive bowl, glass baking dish, or gallon-size resealable plastic bag. Add the pork tenderloins and marinate at least 30 minutes or overnight.

Preheat the broiler to its highest setting and heat a grill to medium-high. Line a baking sheet with parchment paper and arrange the broccoli on it in a single layer. Season with the olive oil, salt, and pepper and set aside.

Place the tenderloins on the grill, reserving the marinade. Cook for 6 to 8 minutes on each side, until the internal temperature reaches 140°F. Remove from the heat and let rest for 10 minutes before cutting.

Meanwhile, place the broccoli pan in the top third of the oven and broil for about 6 minutes, or until the florets are crisp-tender and beginning to char.

Transfer the remaining meat marinade to a small saucepan. Bring to a boil, then boil for 3 minutes. Remove from the heat.

Slice the tenderloins into one-inch rounds and serve with broccoli and warm marinade drizzled over the top.

Macronutrient Information

Total calories: 1,065
Fat: 81 grams / 729 calories

Carbs: 15 grams / 60 calories
Protein: 69 grams / 276 calories

Chaffle BLTs with Avocado and Lemon-Garlic Aioli

2 servings

Remember my brilliant suggestion to make chaffles in advance so you can have them ready in the freezer when you need them (page 226)? Well, now's the time to haul those chaffles out and whip up these open-faced sammies with mouthwatering lemon-garlic aioli. The savory taste will make them a favorite as soon as you take your first bite!

Prep time: 5 minutes
Cooking time: 15 minutes

2 large pastured eggs

1 cup shredded cheese, such as Cheddar or a mixture of half Parmesan and half mozzarella

½ teaspoon pepper

1 scallion, thinly sliced

4 large romaine or Bibb lettuce leaves

8 slices uncured bacon, cooked

1 avocado, sliced

1 large fresh tomato, sliced

For the aioli

½ cup avocado oil–based mayonnaise, such as Primal Kitchen Mayo

1 large garlic clove, minced

Zest and juice of ½ lemon

¼ teaspoon pepper

In a medium bowl, combine the eggs, shredded cheese, pepper, and scallion. Pour the batter into a waffle maker and cook according to the manufacturer's directions—in two batches if necessary—until golden brown. Transfer to a wire rack.

While the chaffles are cooking, make the aioli: in a small bowl, whisk together the mayonnaise, garlic, lemon zest and juice, and pepper.

Onto each chaffle, layer a lettuce leaf, followed by two slices of bacon, some avocado slices, and some tomato slices. Drizzle the sandwiches with aioli and serve.

Macronutrient Information

Total calories: 763
Fat: 59 grams /531 calories

Carbs: 25 grams / 100 calories
Protein: 33 grams / 132 calories

Quick Butter Chicken and Cauliflower Rice

2 servings

If you're tired of plain old chicken, reinvigorate your taste buds with this preparation of cubed meat simmered in butter with diced tomatoes and fresh herbs and spices.

Prep time: 10 minutes
Cooking time: 30 minutes

4 tablespoons butter or ghee, divided

4 boneless, skinless chicken thighs, cut into 1-inch cubes

1 small onion, minced

4 cloves garlic, minced

1 teaspoon grated fresh ginger

1 teaspoon turmeric

2 teaspoons garam masala

1½ teaspoons salt, divided

¾ teaspoon pepper, divided

½ teaspoon smoked paprika

1 teaspoon cumin

1 teaspoon coriander

½ teaspoon cayenne pepper

1 (14-ounce) can diced tomatoes

½ cup heavy cream or unsweetened coconut cream

3 cups fresh or frozen cauliflower rice

1 tablespoon freshly squeezed lemon juice

½ cup chopped fresh cilantro leaves

In a large pot or Dutch oven, melt 2 tablespoons butter over medium-high heat. Add the chicken and sauté until almost cooked through, about 8 minutes. Transfer to a plate and set aside.

Add the onion to the pot and cook until translucent, about 3 minutes, stirring occasionally to scrape up brown bits from the bottom. Add the garlic, ginger, turmeric, garam masala, 1 teaspoon salt, ½ teaspoon pepper, paprika, cumin, coriander, and cayenne. Stir and cook until fragrant, about 30 seconds. Add the diced tomatoes and simmer for 10 minutes. Using an immersion blender, blend mixture until smooth. (Alternatively, transfer the mixture to a blender, blend until smooth, then return to the pot.)

Add the cream and stir to combine. Return the chicken and its juices to the pot. Bring to a simmer, then simmer for 5 minutes.

Meanwhile, melt the remaining 2 tablespoons butter in a medium saucepan over medium-high heat. Add the cauliflower rice and the remaining ½ teaspoon salt and ¼ teaspoon pepper. Cook until the rice is heated through and begins to brown slightly.

Divide the cauliflower rice between two serving plates. Top with the chicken and garnish with the lemon juice and cilantro.

Macronutrient Information

Total calories: 1,311
Fat: 99 grams / 891 calories

Carbs: 51 grams / 204 calories
Protein: 54 grams / 216 calories

Dry-Rubbed Chicken Thighs with Broiled Zucchini

2 servings

Summer, when zucchini is at its best, is the perfect time to put this recipe on Repeat. A little Parmesan cheese goes a long way, heightening this dish's naturally sweet and salty flavors.

Prep time: 5 minutes
Cooking time: 25 minutes

4 boneless, skinless chicken thighs

4 small zucchini, cut in half lengthwise

1 teaspoon salt

½ teaspoon garlic powder

½ teaspoon onion powder

½ teaspoon paprika

½ teaspoon Italian seasoning

1 teaspoon pepper, divided

1 tablespoon extra-virgin olive oil or avocado oil

2 tablespoons grated Parmesan cheese

Preheat the oven to 425°F. Line two baking sheets with parchment paper. Arrange the chicken thighs on one and the zucchini halves on the other.

In a small bowl, combine the salt, garlic powder, onion powder, paprika, Italian seasoning, and ½ teaspoon pepper. Rub the seasoning mixture into the chicken thighs with your fingers. Put the chicken in the oven and bake for 20 minutes.

Meanwhile, drizzle the zucchini halves with the olive oil and sprinkle with Parmesan and the remaining ½ teaspoon pepper.

Turn the oven to its lowest broiler setting and move the chicken to the bottom rack. Place the zucchini pan in the top third of the oven and broil for about 5 minutes, or until zucchini is fork-tender and the cheese is bubbly.

Once the chicken thighs reach an internal temperature of 160°F., remove them from the oven and serve with the zucchini immediately.

Macronutrient Information

Total calories: 756
Fat: 36 grams / 324 calories

Carbs: 20 grams / 80 calories
Protein: 88 grams / 352 calories

Broiled Salmon and Asparagus

Freshly broiled salmon served with seasonal vegetables is one of the greatest culinary pairings known to humankind. Keep a supply of frozen wild-caught salmon fillets in your freezer so you can whip up this dish anytime, along with the freshest vegetables of the season.

Prep time: 5 minutes
Cooking time: 10 minutes

2 garlic cloves, minced

½ teaspoon minced fresh rosemary

½ teaspoon minced fresh thyme

1 tablespoon prepared whole-grain mustard

¼ cup plus 1 tablespoon extra-virgin olive oil, divided

1 teaspoon salt, plus more to taste

½ teaspoon pepper, plus more to taste

Zest of 1 lemon

Juice of ½ lemon

2 salmon fillets, about 8 ounces each

1 bunch fresh asparagus, ends trimmed

Preheat the broiler to its highest setting. Line a sheet pan with parchment paper.

In a small bowl, combine the garlic, rosemary, thyme, mustard, ¼ cup olive oil, 1 teaspoon salt, ½ teaspoon pepper, and lemon zest and juice.

Arrange the salmon fillets and asparagus on the prepared sheet pan. Drizzle the asparagus with 1 tablespoon olive oil and season with salt and pepper. Broil on the middle rack of the oven for 2 minutes, then cover the salmon fillets with the mustard-herb sauce and broil until flaky and just cooked through, about 5 minutes. Remove from the oven and serve immediately.

Macronutrient Information

Total calories: 1,009
Fat: 53 grams / 477 calories

Carbs: 12 grams / 48 calories
Protein: 121 grams / 484 calories

Asian Turkey Meatballs with Roasted Spaghetti Squash

2 servings

Anyone who takes the leap and replaces grain-based pasta with spaghetti squash knows the truth: not only is spaghetti squash much more healthful, it also tastes much better! If you have an Instant Pot, your squash cooking time will be reduced dramatically, giving you more time to play outside.

Prep time: 10 minutes
Cooking time: 25 minutes

1 small spaghetti squash

2 tablespoons extra-virgin olive oil

Salt and pepper to taste

1 pound ground turkey

1 cup chopped fresh cilantro leaves, divided

1 cup chopped scallions, divided

1 tablespoon Yai's Thai Chili Garlic Hot Sauce, plus more for serving if desired

2 tablespoons coconut aminos

3 garlic cloves, minced

1 teaspoon grated fresh ginger

1 large egg

1 teaspoon sesame oil

1 teaspoon sesame seeds (raw or roasted at 350°F for 12 to 15 minutes on parchment paper, tossing every 5 minutes; stored in airtight container after completely cooled)

Preheat the oven to 450°F. Line two baking sheets with parchment paper.

Cut the spaghetti squash in half lengthwise. Scoop out the seeds, then season the inside of both halves with olive oil, salt, and pepper. Place the halves cut side down on one of the sheet pans and bake for 25 minutes.

Meanwhile, combine the turkey, ½ cup cilantro, ½ cup scallions, 1 tablespoon chili garlic sauce, coconut aminos, garlic, ginger, egg, and sesame oil in a medium bowl. Roll into balls about 2 inches in diameter and arrange them on the second sheet pan.

When the squash is done, set it aside to cool, then preheat the broiler to its highest setting. Place the meatballs in the bottom third of the oven and broil for 13 minutes.

While the meatballs cook, scoop out the spaghetti squash flesh with a large fork and divide it between two serving plates. Serve the hot meatballs over the spaghetti squash and garnish with the remaining cilantro and scallions, the sesame seeds, and additional chili sauce if desired.

Macronutrient Information

Total calories: 746
Fat: 46 grams / 414 calories

Carbs: 20 grams / 80 calories
Protein: 63 grams / 252 calories

Grilled Cilantro-Lime Flank Steak with Spiced Sesame Green Beans

4 servings

The fresh flavor of lime pairs with the warm and grounding flavors of coconut aminos and sesame oil for a delicious and memorable combination. Flank steak marinates in just thirty minutes, making this recipe a great choice when you're pressed for time.

Prep time: 10 minutes, plus 30 or more minutes of marinating time
Cooking time: 15 minutes

1 cup extra-virgin olive oil

2 bunches cilantro leaves

2 bunches scallions (white and tender green parts only)

8 garlic cloves

Zest and juice of 6 limes

1 tablespoon salt

1 teaspoon pepper

2 pounds flank steak

2 tablespoons butter

1 tablespoon sesame oil

2 tablespoons coconut aminos

1 tablespoon Yai's Thai Chili Garlic Hot Sauce

2 pounds fresh green beans

¼ cup water

In a blender, combine the olive oil, cilantro, scallions, garlic, lime zest and juice, salt, and pepper. Blend until smooth. Pour half the sauce into a large nonreactive baking dish or a resealable plastic bag. Add the flank steak and massage to coat. Marinate at least 30 minutes or overnight.

Heat a grill to medium-high. Place the marinated flank steak on the grill and cook for about 5 minutes per side. Remove when the internal temperature reaches 125°F. Place the meat on a cutting board and tent with foil to finish the cooking process.

In a large pan, melt the butter over medium-high heat. Add the sesame oil, coconut aminos, and chili garlic sauce. Stir together, then add the green beans, tossing to coat. Cook, stirring occasionally, for 5 minutes. Add water and continue to cook, stirring, until the liquid evaporates and the beans are tender.

Slice the steak against the grain and serve it alongside the green beans, drizzled with the remaining herb sauce.

Macronutrient Information

Total calories: 1,176
Fat: 84 grams / 756 calories

Carbs: 30 grams / 120 calories
Protein: 75 grams / 300 calories

Chicken Divan

4 servings

Creamy chicken with broccoli and mushrooms gets even more comforting and pleasurable with the addition of shredded Cheddar cheese.

Prep time: 15 minutes
Cooking time: 30 minutes

1 stick butter, divided

8 boneless, skinless chicken thighs, cut into 1-inch cubes

3 ½ teaspoons salt, divided

1 ¾ teaspoons pepper, divided

3 cups broccoli florets, cut into bite-size pieces

8 ounces fresh mushrooms, diced

1 small onion, diced

6 garlic cloves, minced

1 cup heavy cream or unsweetened coconut cream

½ cup chopped fresh parsley

2 cups shredded Cheddar cheese

Preheat the oven to 425°F.

In a large skillet over medium heat, melt 4 tablespoons butter. Add the chicken pieces, season with 1 teaspoon salt and ½ teaspoon pepper, and sauté until cooked through, about 5 minutes. Transfer to the bottom of a 9- × 13-inch casserole dish and set aside.

Increase the heat under the skillet to medium-high and melt the remaining butter. Add the broccoli, season with ½ teaspoon salt and ¼ teaspoon pepper, and cook until crisp-tender, about 5 minutes. Layer the broccoli over the chicken.

Add the mushrooms, onion, and garlic to the skillet and sauté for 5 minutes. Add the heavy cream, parsley, 2 teaspoons salt, and 1 teaspoon pepper and stir to combine. Pour the cream mixture over the chicken and broccoli, then top with the shredded cheese.

Bake on the middle rack of the oven until the cheese is bubbly and golden, about 15 minutes. Serve immediately.

Macronutrient Information

Total calories: 714
Fat: 54 grams / 486 calories

Carbs: 12 grams / 48 calories
Protein: 45 grams / 180 calories

Cauliflower Fried Rice with Eggs

2 servings

As you experience the bold flavors of fresh ginger, sesame oil, coconut aminos, and cilantro, you won't be missing regular old rice (and its blood-sugar spike!) for one second.

Prep time: 10 minutes
Cooking time: 15 minutes

4 tablespoons butter, divided

2 ounces fresh mushrooms, diced

1 small onion, diced

2 garlic cloves, minced

1 teaspoon grated fresh ginger

1 carrot, diced

1 cup fresh broccoli florets, cut into small pieces

4 large pastured eggs, beaten

Salt and pepper to taste

1 (16-ounce) bag frozen cauliflower rice

1 tablespoon toasted sesame oil

2 tablespoons coconut aminos

1 teaspoon everything bagel seasoning

½ cup chopped fresh cilantro leaves

¼ cup thinly sliced scallions

Chili garlic sauce for serving

In a large skillet, melt 2 tablespoons of the butter. Add the mushrooms and cook over medium heat until golden brown. Add the onion, garlic, ginger, carrot, and broccoli. Increase the heat to medium-high and sauté until the vegetables are crisp-tender, about 4 minutes.

Make a well in the middle of the vegetables and add the remaining 2 tablespoons butter. Pour the eggs into the well, season with salt and pepper, and cook until the eggs are scrambled, stirring occasionally.

Add the cauliflower rice, sesame oil, coconut aminos, and bagel seasoning. Toss to combine. Taste and adjust seasoning, then garnish with the cilantro and scallions and serve with chili garlic sauce.

Macronutrient Information

Total calories: 540
Fat: 40 grams / 360 calories

Carbs: 26 grams / 104 calories
Protein: 19 grams / 76 calories

Meat Lover's Pizza Skillet

The big, bold flavors of Italian sausage and pepperoni are topped with sweet and creamy mozzarella cheese and vegetables. Enjoy the distinct flavors of your favorite veggie pizza, but without the bloating and sugar crash!

Prep time: 8 minutes
Cooking time: 20 minutes

1 pound bulk Italian sausage

¼ cup extra-virgin olive oil

2 cups fresh cauliflower florets

1 green bell pepper, seeded and cut into large dice

8 tablespoons tomato paste

4 ounces fresh mushrooms, sliced

½ small red onion, thinly sliced

2 garlic cloves, minced

1 teaspoon Italian seasoning

½ teaspoon salt

½ teaspoon pepper

4 ounces uncured pepperoni

1 cup shredded mozzarella cheese

¼ cup grated Parmesan cheese

¼ cup chopped fresh basil

Preheat the broiler to its highest setting.

In a large ovenproof skillet over medium-high heat, sauté the sausage until cooked through, then transfer to a bowl.

In the same skillet, heat the olive oil over medium-high heat, then add the cauliflower, bell pepper, tomato paste, mushrooms, red onion, garlic, Italian seasoning, salt, and pepper. Cook for 6 minutes, then add the cooked sausage and pepperoni. Top with the mozzarella and Parmesan.

Transfer the skillet to the middle rack of the oven and broil until the cheese is bubbly and golden, about 5 minutes. Remove from the oven, garnish with the basil, and serve hot.

Macronutrient Information

Total calories: 1,367
Fat: 111 grams / 999 calories

Carbs: 30 grams / 120 calories
Protein: 62 grams / 248 calories

Broccoli and Bacon Slaw

2 servings

Slaw doesn't have to mean just cabbage. This recipe uses broccoli and packs a big nutritional punch. Combined with fatty, salty bacon and bright lemon and apple cider vinegar, this dish is a flavor odyssey in your mouth.

Prep time: 5 minutes
Cooking time: 10 minutes

1 cup avocado oil–based mayonnaise, such as Primal Kitchen Mayo

1 tablespoon minced red onion

Zest and juice of ½ lemon

¼ cup apple cider vinegar

1 teaspoon salt

½ teaspoon pepper

4 cups fresh broccoli florets, cut into bite-size pieces

8 slices uncured bacon, cooked and chopped

½ cup roasted pepitas

In a large bowl, whisk together the mayonnaise, onion, lemon zest and juice, vinegar, salt, and pepper. Add the broccoli, chopped bacon, and pepitas and combine thoroughly. Chill or serve at room temperature.

Macronutrient Information

Total calories: 1,270
Fat: 122 grams / 1,098 calories

Carbs: 19 grams / 76 calories
Protein: 24 grams / 96 calories

Sesame-Ginger Chicken and Vegetable Stir-Fry

2 servings

Want a super-satisfying meal super fast? Try this stir-fry with a bunch of green vegetables, fatty chicken thighs, and Asian-inspired seasonings. This is wonderful enjoyed on its own as well as on a bed of cauliflower rice.

Prep time: 10 minutes
Cooking time: 15 minutes

2 tablespoons butter or ghee

4 boneless, skinless chicken thighs, cut into 1-inch cubes

2 tablespoons avocado oil

1 small onion, diced

4 garlic cloves, minced

2 teaspoons grated fresh ginger

1 cup fresh broccoli florets, cut into bite-size pieces

1 carrot, cut into 1/4-inch slices

2 stalks celery, cut into bite-size pieces

1/2 small head green cabbage, chopped

1/4 cup coconut aminos

1 tablespoon toasted sesame oil

1 teaspoon Yai's Thai Chili Garlic Hot Sauce

1 teaspoon sesame seeds

1/2 cup chopped fresh cilantro leaves

1/2 cup thinly sliced scallions

In a large skillet over medium heat, melt the butter. Sauté the chicken until cooked through. Transfer to a plate and set aside.

In the same skillet, heat the avocado oil over medium-high heat. Add the onion, garlic, ginger, broccoli, carrot, celery, and cabbage and cook for 4 minutes, stirring occasionally. Return the chicken to the skillet, then add the coconut aminos, sesame oil, chili garlic sauce, and sesame seeds. Toss to coat and cook 2 more minutes.

Serve garnished with cilantro and scallions and additional spice on the side, if desired.

Macronutrient Information

Total calories: 682
Fat: 42 grams / 378 calories

Carbs: 32 grams / 128 calories
Protein: 44 grams / 176 calories

Jalapeño Chicken Bake

2 servings

This adds a new dimension of flavor to an old favorite with the creative combination of chicken thighs, bacon, vegetables, and cream cheese. If you want the poppers to be less spicy, simply use jarred pickled jalapeños instead of fresh.

Prep time: 10 minutes
Cooking time: 20 minutes

2 cups fresh spinach leaves

4 boneless, skinless chicken thighs, cut into 1-inch cubes

4 ounces fresh mushrooms, diced

1 small zucchini, diced

8 ounces uncured bacon, cooked and chopped

1 teaspoon salt

½ teaspoon pepper

4 ounces full-fat cream cheese, softened

4 ounces goat cheese, crumbled

2 jalapeño peppers, seeded and minced

1 teaspoon minced garlic

2 scallions, thinly sliced

Preheat the oven to 425°F.

In an 8- × 8-inch baking dish, layer the spinach, followed by the chicken, mushrooms, zucchini, and bacon. Season with salt and pepper.

In a medium bowl, combine the cream cheese, goat cheese, jalapeños, garlic, and scallions. Drop the cheese mixture in small dollops over the chicken and vegetables and bake for 20 minutes, or until lightly browned. Serve hot.

Macronutrient Information

Total calories: 643
Fat: 35 grams / 315 calories

Carbs: 12 grams / 48 calories
Protein: 70 grams / 280 calories

Acknowledgments

Today, our constant access to information can be overwhelming and confusing, often catering to short attention spans and featuring salacious, lowest-common-denominator messaging. These days, a book is a special production, requiring an incredible level of research, strategic planning, team contribution, and methodical revision and fine-tuning. This end product is designed to stand proudly on your bookshelf as a helpful resource for years to come. Thanks are due to everyone on the team who contributed to it, but I also want to acknowledge you, the reader, for your commitment to healthful living. We wish you the best in your pursuit of living awesome!

Resources and Suggested Reading

Books

8 Steps to a Pain-Free Back, by Esther Gokhale, LAc

Adrenaline Dominance, by Michael E. Platt, MD

The Art and Science of Low Carbohydrate Performance, by Jeff Volek, PhD, and Stephen D. Phinney, MD, PhD

Becoming Supernatural, by Dr. Joe Dispenza

Becoming a Supple Leopard, by Dr. Kelly Starrett

The Big Book of Endurance Training and Racing, by Dr. Philip Maffetone

The Big Leap, by Gay Hendricks

The Biology of Belief, by Bruce H. Lipton, PhD

The Bordeaux Kitchen, by Tania Teschke

The Carnivore Code, by Paul Saladino, MD

Carnivore Cooking for Cool Dudes, by Brad Kearns, Brian McAndrew, and William Shewfelt

The Carnivore Diet, by Shawn Baker, MD

The Case Against Sugar, by Gary Taubes

Chicken Soup for the Soul, by Jack Canfield

The Circadian Code, by Satchin Panda, PhD

Death by Food Pyramid, by Denise Minger

Deep Nutrition, by Catherine Shanahan, MD

The Diabetes Code, by Jason Fung, MD

Don't Just Sit There, by Katy Bowman

Eat to Live, by Joel Fuhrman, MD

Everything is F*cked, by Mark Manson

Fast Food Nation, by Eric Schlosser

Fat Chance, by Robert H. Lustig, MD

Fat for Fuel, by Dr. Joseph Mercola

The Fatburn Fix, by Catherine Shanahan, MD

Food Politics, by Marion Nestle

Good Calories, Bad Calories, by Gary Taubes

Grain Brain, by David Perlmutter, MD

Gratitude Works!, by Robert A. Emmons

The Hacking of the American Mind, by Robert H. Lustig, MD

The Harvard Medical School Guide to Tai Chi, by Peter M. Wayne, PhD

The Hidden Plague, by Tara Grant

The Imperative Habit, by Dave Rossi

Keto Cooking for Cool Dudes, by Brad Kearns and Brian McAndrew

Keto Diet, by Dr. Josh Axe

Keto for Women, by Leanne Vogel

The Keto Reset Diet, by Mark Sisson with Brad Kearns

The Keto Reset Diet Cookbook, by Mark Sisson with Lindsay Taylor, PhD

The Keto Reset Instant Pot Cookbook, by Mark Sisson with Lindsay Taylor, PhD, and Layla McGowan

Lights Out, by T. S. Wiley with Bent Formby, PhD

The Longevity Paradox, by Steven R. Gundry, MD

Lore of Nutrition, by Tim Noakes and Marika Sboros

Lore of Running, by Tim Noakes, MD

Men Are from Mars, Women Are from Venus, by John Gray, PhD

Move Your DNA, by Katy Bowman

The New Evolution Diet, by Arthur De Vany, PhD

NurtureShock, by Po Bronson and Ashley Merryman

The Obesity Code, by Jason Fung, MD

The Overfat Pandemic, by Dr. Philip Maffetone

The Paleo Diet, by Loren Cordain, PhD

Paleo Happy Hour, by Kelly Milton

Perfect Health Diet, by Paul Jaminet, PhD, and Shou-Ching Jaminet, PhD

The Plant Paradox, by Steven R. Gundry, MD

The Primal Blueprint, by Mark Sisson

The Real Meal Revolution, by Professor Tim Noakes, Jonno Proudfoot, and Sally-Ann Creed

The Sleep Revolution, by Arianna Huffington

The South Asian Health Solution, by Ronesh Sinha, MD

The Subtle Art of Not Giving a F*ck, by Mark Manson

Take a Nap! Change Your Life, by Sara C. Mednick, PhD

Wanderlust, by Rebecca Solnit

Way of the Peaceful Warrior, by Dan Millman

Wheat Belly, by William Davis, MD

Why We Get Fat, by Gary Taubes

You: The Owner's Manual, by Michael F. Roizen, MD, and Mehmet C. Oz, MD

Websites

TwoMealsADayBook.com (contains hyperlinks for all the books, websites, videos, and shopping resources mentioned here; a comprehensive list of research links, including videos, interviews, health journalism, news reports, and scholarly articles; plus bonus content and e-book downloads)

8WeeksOut.com (Joel Jamieson—MMA trainer, recovery, and HRV expert)

AncestralSupplements.com/about-us (Brian "Liver King" Johnson—ancestral living tips and inspiration)

AndreObradovic.com (Australian life and endurance training coach)

BenGreenfieldFitness.com (biohacker, podcast host, elite adventure athlete, and bestselling author of *Boundless*)

BradKearns.com (*Two Meals a Day* coauthor, podcast host, elite athlete)

CarnivoreMD.com (Dr. Paul Saladino, carnivore leader and author of *The Carnivore Code*)

ClevelandClinic.org/Roizen (Dr. Michael Roizen, coauthor of *You: The Owner's Manual*)

CraigMarker.com (strength and conditioning coach and antianxiety expert)

CulturalHealthSolutions.com (Dr. Ronesh Sinha, author of *The South Asian Health Solution*)

DeepakChopra.com (physician and megabestselling author of *Ageless Body, Timeless Mind*)

DeniseMinger.com (blogger, author, conventional wisdom skeptic)

DietDoctor.com (Dr. Jason Fung—insulin, obesity, and diabetes expert)

DoctorJKrauseND.com (Dr. Jannine Krause—naturopathic doctor, acupuncturist, podcast host)

DoctorOz.com (Dr. Mehmet Oz, bestselling author and TV personality)

DrAxe.com (Dr. Josh Axe, health author, natural medicine physician)

DrCate.com (Dr. Catherine Shanahan, NBA diet consultant and bestselling author of *Deep Nutrition*)

DrDaphne.com (Dr. Daphne Miller, integrative physician and advocate of nature-based healing)

DrFuhrman.com (Dr. Joel Fuhrman, bestselling author of *Eat to Live)*

DrGundry.com (Dr. Steven Gundry, bestselling author of *The Plant Paradox*)

DrJoeDispenza.com (neuroscientist, author, peak-performance expert)

DrPerlmutter.com (Dr. David Perlmutter, bestselling author of *Grain Brain*)

DrRagnar.com (Dr. Tommy Ragnar Wood, ancestral health expert and pediatrics researcher)

DrWeil.com (Dr. Andrew Weil, bestselling author and natural-medicine expert)

ElleRuss.com (podcast host and bestselling author of *The Paleo Thyroid Solution*)

EvolutionaryAnthropology.duke.edu/people/Herman-Pontzer (Dr. Herman Pontzer, TEE expert)

FacultativeCarnivore.com (Amber O'Hearn, carnivore-diet advocate)

FoodPolitics.com (Dr. Marion Nestle—bestselling author, researcher, and antipropaganda advocate)

GaryTaubes.com (science journalist and bestselling author of *Good Calories, Bad Calories, Why We Get Fat*, and *The Case Against Sugar*)

GokhaleMethod.com (Esther Gokhale—bestselling author of *8 Steps to a Pain-Free Back*; posture correction and back-pain-relief expert)

Gottman.com (Dr. John Gottman, relationship expert and bestselling author of *The Seven Principles for Making Marriage Work*)

HealthfulPursuit.com (Leanne Vogel, podcast host and bestselling author of *The Keto Diet*)

Instagram.com/TheUsefulDish (Dr. Lindsay Taylor, social psychologist and coauthor of *The Keto Reset Diet Cookbook* and *Keto Passport*)

JackCanfield.com (bestselling author of the Chicken Soup franchise; peak-performance and self-empowerment expert)

JackKruse.com (neurosurgeon, biohacker, and expert in circadian rhythms)

KetoGains.com (Luis Villasenor—bodybuilder; founder of ketogenic-diet and coaching service)

MarksDailyApple.com (my number-one-ranked ancestral-living blog, home of the Primal Blueprint lifestyle; contains extensive library of articles, success stories, and free e-book downloads)

MarksDailyApple.com/keto/keto-results/Brian-McAndrew (Brian McAndrew's body-transformation story)

MarksDailyApple.com/ancestral-resting-positions (contains my research with Matt Wallden)

Mercola.com (Dr. Joe Mercola, alternative-health leader and bestselling author of *Fat for Fuel*)

MichaelMerzenich.com (brain plasticity expert and author of *Soft-Wired*)

MichaelPollan.com (health journalist and bestselling author of *The Omnivore's Dilemma*)

MyCircadianClock.org (Dr. Satchin Panda's time-restricted feeding app and research)

PaulJaminet.com (astrophysicist and ancestral diet expert, coauthor of *Perfect Health Diet*)

PerfectHealthDiet.com (Shou-Ching Jaminet—molecular biologist, cancer researcher, coauthor of *Perfect Health Diet*)

PeterAttiaMD.com (surgeon, podcast host, longevity expert, biohacker, self-experimenter, and extreme endurance athlete)

PhilMaffetone.com (chiropractor, endurance-training expert, bestselling author of *The Big Book of Endurance Training and Racing*)

PlattWellness.com (Dr. Michael Platt, expert in bioidentical hormone therapy and author of *Adrenaline Dominance*)

RobertLustig.com (antisugar crusader and bestselling author of *The Hacking of the American Mind*)

SaraMednick.com (University of California at Riverside psychology professor and author of *Take a Nap! Change Your Life*)

Shawn-Baker.com (orthopedic surgeon, carnivore-diet leader, world-record-setting masters rowing athlete, founder of MeatRx.com)

TheNoakesFoundation.org (Dr. Timothy Noakes, preeminent endurance exercise physiologist, bestselling author of *Lore of Running* and *Lore of Nutrition*)

ThePaleoDiet.com (Dr. Loren Cordain, health and exercise science professor, Paleo researcher, bestselling author of *The Paleo Diet*)

TheReadyState.com (Dr. Kelly Starrett, CrossFit coach, physical therapist, bestselling author of *Becoming a Supple Leopard*)

TonyRobbins.com (motivational speaker, peak-performance expert, bestselling author of *Awaken the Giant Within*)

UsainBolt.com (retired Jamaican world champion, Olympic gold medalist, and world-record sprinter)

Verkhoshansky.com (the late Dr. Yuri Verkoshansky, Russian-American plyometric training expert)

VirtaHealth.com (Dr. Jeff Volek, ketogenic-diet researcher and bestselling author of *The Art and Science of Low Carbohydrate Living*)

WestonAPrice.org (Weston A. Price Foundation, a leading resource for the global study of the diet and health habits of indigenous peoples)

WheatBelly.com (Dr. William Davis, cardiologist and bestselling author of *Wheat Belly*)

WimHofMethod.com (Wim Hof, a.k.a. the Iceman, Dutch record-setting endurance and cold-exposure athlete)

ZachBitter.com (podcast host, endurance coach, and world-record one-hundred-mile ultramarathon runner)

YouTube Videos

Use these search terms:

Brad Kearns—Chest Freezer Cold Water Therapy

Brad Kearns—Dynamic Stretching Routine to Start Your Day

Brad Kearns—How to Do a Sprint Workout the Right Way

Brad Kearns—Morning Routine

Brad Kearns—Preworkout Dynamic Stretching Routine

Brad Kearns—Running Form: Correct Technique and Tips to Avoid Injury

Brad Kearns—Running Technique Drills: Beginners

Brad Kearns—Running Technique Drills: Advanced

Fillet-Oh!-Fish [fish farm industry exposé]

Get Over Yourself Podcast—Dude Spellings

Get Over Yourself Podcast—The Ultimate Mark Sisson Interview

Hatha Yoga for Beginners

The Great Dance—A Hunter's Story [!Kung bush people persistence hunt]

Jeanne Calment Interview [world's longest-lived human at 122 years]

Joe Rogan—Mark Sisson Interview

Mark Sisson—Amazing Keto and Fasting Facts

Mark Sisson—Archetypal Rest Postures

Mark Sisson—BASS (Bigass Steak Salad)

Mark Sisson—A Day in the Life

Mark Sisson—Keto Roundtable: Metabolic Flexibility and the Human "Closed Loop" System

Mark Sisson—Micro Workouts How-To and Benefits

Mark Sisson on Health Theory [why the keto diet will change your life]

Mark Sisson—Primal Essential Movements

Mark Sisson—Sprinting Workout

Mark Sisson—What Is Intermittent Fasting?

Pilates at Home for Beginners

Restorative Yoga for Beginners

Tai Chi for Beginners

Yoga Sun Salutations

Internet Shopping Resources

AncestralSupplements.com (100 percent grass-fed animal organ supplements)

Askinosie.com (dark chocolate)

ButcherBox.com (sustainable animal foods; home delivery club)

ChiliTechnology.com (chiliPAD mattress cooler)

CoracaoConfections.com (dark chocolate)

CreoChocolate.com (dark chocolate)

DryFarmWines.com (sugar-free, chemical-free wines; home delivery club)

Evolution-Athletic.com (resistance bands)

HuKitchen.com (dark chocolate)

IrisTech.co (screen color-temperature-optimizing software)

JaquishBiomedical.com (X3 Bar home strength-training device)

JustGetFlux.com (screen color-temperature-optimizing software)

KellerManniChocolate.com (dark chocolate)

LillieBelleFarms.com (dark chocolate)

LoneMountainWagyu.com (100 percent purebred, grass-fed Wagyu beef)

MeatRx.com (carnivore diet community and educational programming)

NzCordz.com (StretchCordz and other resistance-training bands)

PerformBetter.com (mini bands)

RAOptics.com (fashionable blue light–blocking eyewear)

TazaChocolate.com (dark chocolate)

ThriveMarket.com (healthful organic foods with online discount)

VariDesk.com (stand-up desks and creative office furniture)

VitalChoice.com (wild-caught seafood with home delivery)

WildIdeaBuffalo.com (grass-fed, naturally raised buffalo from the Great Plains)

Index

About the Authors

Mark Sisson is widely regarded as a founding father of the ancestral health movement. A former world-class athlete in the marathon and the Ironman Triathlon, he presides over a wide-ranging Primal enterprise, featuring the Primal Kitchen line of healthy condiments, dressings, and sauces, the Primal Health Coach Institute, a line of premium performance and nutritional supplements, and numerous books and online educational courses. He publishes daily tips and inspiration at MarksDailyApple.com, the top-ranked blog in its category for the past fifteen years. Mark lives in Miami Beach, Florida, with his wife, Carrie, where he standup paddleboards the inland waterways, plays Ultimate Frisbee against hotshots half his age, and enjoys his new role as a grandfather.

Brad Kearns is Mark Sisson's longtime coauthor, host of the B.rad podcast, and an elite masters athlete. He broke the Guinness World Record in Speedgolf at age 53, is a #1 USA–ranked age 55-59 high jumper and a former US national champion and #3 world–ranked professional triathlete. Brad lives in Lake Tahoe, Nevada, with his wife, Elizabeth, and enjoys a daily cold plunge in the lake year-round.

NATURE'S KEEPERS

NATURE'S KEEPERS

On the Front Lines of the Fight to Save Wildlife in America

MICHAEL TOBIAS

John Wiley & Sons, Inc.

New York · Chichester · Weinheim · Brisbane · Singapore · Toronto

Published by John Wiley & Sons, Inc.
Published simultaneously in Canada.

Library of Congress Cataloging-in-Publication Data:
Tobias, Michael.
    Nature's keepers : on the front lines of the fight to save
wildlife in America / Michael Tobias.
      p. cm.
    Includes bibliographical references (p. 217) and index.
    ISBN 0-471-15728-7 (cloth : alk. paper)
    1. Undercover wildlife agents—United States. 2. Game wardens—
United States. 3. Poaching—United States—Prevention. 4. Wild
animal trade—United States. 5. Wildlife conservation—United
States. 6. Endangered species—United States. I. Title.
HV7959.T63 1998
364.16'2—dc21   98-24395

Printed in the United States of America
10 9 8 7 6 5 4 3 2 1

To Jane Gray Morrison,
A great artist and animal rights activist,
who has helped me to more passionately see,
and persistently love, the Creation.

CONTENTS

PREFACE

Nearly 30 years ago we placed men on the barren desert surface of the moon, at great cost. The effort required a national
consensus that held that the benefits outweighed the public
expenditure. This euphoric and idealistic event occurred at
the height of the Cold War, and several years prior to the creation of the U.S. Environmental Protection Agency. At the
time, it would have been unthinkable to consider the ethical
consequences of introducing foreign life-forms on the lunar
surface. Yet this is precisely the kind of debate that later entered the mainstream of scientific discussion with regard to a
manned mission to Mars. Such ecological concerns are new to
our thinking.

The very notion of assessing our impact on the environment at every juncture—whether in space, during the construction of a new housing project, in a chemical laboratory,
or at a car dealership—suggests that we are maturing as a
species, more aware of our biological responsibilities and in-
terrelatedness than ever before. Our laws have changed rapidly
to reflect this newfound "religion" of ecology. Many international treaties have placed environmental obligations at the
forefront of their legalese. The public in nearly every country
has been increasingly sensitized to the plight of many animal
species by the media. Vegetarianism is on the rise, and there
are more nongovernmental organizations focused on the protection and restoration of natural habitat than ever before.

These generalities are all cause for good cheer and opti-
mism. But they are surface observations that fail dismally to
detect other truths and trends which have cast serious doubt

on our ability as a human collective to restrain our destructive tendencies. Yes, we placed men on the moon. No, we have not evidenced sufficient will to fully protect songbirds in Los Angeles or panthers in Florida, any more than we have figured out how to save children from abuse, or women from rapists. This particular analogy with human victims may be apt. Too often, fear and trauma prevent these latter individuals from speaking up or identifying their assailants. Nonhuman animals have no voice to do so. Who speaks on their behalf?

Relative to the known number of committed crimes—as defined by law—there are few Americans directly involved in the many battles to protect wildlife. Those individuals find themselves confronted by daunting odds. Wildlife crime is at epidemic proportions and seriously threatens the very existence of thousands of species worldwide. Americans have been shown to be involved in such crimes more than any other national group. Hence, despite this country's supposedly enlightened concerns about the environment (relative to many other countries) and its unprecedented wealth (which should argue for an ecological trickle-down theory), the United States remains overwhelmed by environmental problems and disappearing wildlife.

This book sets out to chronicle the efforts of several people who are indeed fighting to save wildlife, and to highlight certain cases and actions that are representative of the arena of wildlife protection in the United States. It is by no means intended as a comprehensive examination of the subject. For one thing, the book has narrowed its consideration to "wildlife," a word whose meaning may be ethically arbitrary. From the crucial perspectives of animal rights and spiritual ecology, we should treat all living beings with equal respect. Hence, our behavior toward a mountain lion, a rattlesnake, a pigeon, a fox, an armadillo, or a rat should be no different than our treatment of (domesticated) cows, chickens, or pet dogs and cats.

Extending the circle of compassion beyond the human community to include all other species represents a huge leap for many people. English philosopher Jeremy Bentham spoke of an "insuperable line" when it came to humans granting nonhumans any moral rights.

Granted, there are other community standards regarding animal rights that have been legally and ethically agreed upon for millennia by some other cultures. While animal (and plant) rights has entered much mainstream thinking in the West, it is, admittedly, still viewed by many as a fringe philosophy. And while it is my deeply held belief that animal rights, animal welfare, and animal liberation are ultimately central to humanity's own dignity and survival, this book does not enter into that fray. That is another book.

What concerns me here are contemporary wildlife laws in America and how they are being enforced. It must also be stated, however, that the wildlife protection efforts described herein all stem from the same animal rights impulse: to moderate humankind's behavior towards kindred life-forms. Because the field of wildlife protection is so broad, I have necessarily focused on a narrow range of concerns in this book. They include some discussion of poaching in America's national parks, and the hunting ethos that is so widespread; U.S. Fish and Wildlife investigators, wildlife law, wildlife forensics, and certain controversial activities within the U.S. Department of Agriculture; and some mention of the ethics, psychology, and spirituality of our relationships with other species.

This book is primarily concerned with Americans, and American wildlife, though certain wildlife smuggling cases involving international conspiracies are treated. Greatest emphasis is placed on cases involving crimes and crime-busting in Alaska, Oregon, North Carolina, Georgia, Florida, New Mexico, California, Texas, Wyoming, Missouri, Montana, and a few other states.

It is my hope that this book will help better inform those who may be unaware of the extent and nature of crimes involving wildlife in this country, and suggest certain practical and ethical avenues for those wishing to be part of the solution, rather than the problem.

It is also my intention to suggest that our behavior toward other species is not merely a function of law, but of morality. Hence, this book is ultimately about our capacity—and choice—to be decent, generous, and compassionate.

ACKNOWLEDGMENTS

I wish first to thank Jane Morrison, my partner on all projects.

I am indebted to Carol Gold, whose strong belief in this book was key to its origination.

To my editor at John Wiley, Emily Loose, I have only profound thanks and admiration for her sensitive and intelligent work on behalf of this publication. I wish in addition to thank the copyeditor, Jim Gullickson; the book's text designer, David denBoer of Nighthawk Design; and the book's jacket designer, José Almaguer of Wiley.

I am especially indebted to a number of individuals and organizations, many chronicled in this book. Those include: Ruth Musgrave of the Center for Wildlife Law at the University of New Mexico; Jim Hannah of the Wrangell–Saint Elias National Park and Preserve; Ken Goddard of the Clark Bavin National Fish and Wildlife Forensics Laboratory; Ranger John Garrison of the Great Smoky Mountains National Park; Dennis Burnett of the National Park Service; Terry Grosz of the U.S. Fish and Wildlife Service (USF&W); John Doggett, formerly of the USF&W; Anne-Berry Wade, formerly a public affairs specialist with USF&W; Special Agent Doug Goessman of the USF&W and the many new agents of SABS 22; Sergio Acosta, a deputy chief with the U.S. Attorney's Office; Peter J. Murtha, trial attorney, Wildlife and Marine Resources Section, U.S. Justice Department; Robert Anderson, a senior trial counsel with the U.S. Department of Justice; Special Agent Dan Burleson and his USF&W colleagues in Missouri; Kathryn Love and the Missouri Department of Conservation; Ranger Tom May; the many good people of Van Buren, Missouri;

Acknowledgments

Edward L. Dowd Jr., U.S. attorney, and Curtis O. Poore, assistant U.S. attorney, both with the U.S. Attorney's Office, Eastern District of Missouri; Larry Keck of the Missouri USF&W; Daniel Goodman, assistant U.S. attorney in Los Angeles; Professor Marc Bekoff of the University of Colorado; Pat Wolff; the publishers and associates of the Wildlife Damage Review in Tucson, Arizona; Tom Skeele and his colleagues at the Predator Project; the work of Dr. Michael Wells; Dr. Con Slobodchikoff at Northern Arizona University; Professor William F. Andelt of Colorado State University in Fort Collins; Bob Crabtree; Dick Randall; Peter Matthiessen; Peter Singer; William Russell and Rex Burch; Paul and Anne Ehrlich at Stanford University; E. O. Wilson of Harvard University; Michael Fox; Susan Hagood and the Humane Society of the United States; Special Agent Lucinda Schroeder of the USF&W in New Mexico; Tom Smith of the General Social Survey of the National Opinion Research Center at the University of Chicago; Peter D. Hart Research Associates; Professor Stephen R. Kellert of Yale University; and Jane Goodall.

In addition, I want to thank those many others who graciously allowed me to interview them, but whose extraordinary efforts to protect animals—both domestic and wild—could not be chronicled in this particular volume. Hopefully, that material will be incorporated into a future work. Those people include: Ingrid Newkirk, Mary Beth Sweetland, and Zoe Rappoport of People for the Ethical Treatment of Animals (PETA); Randy Coronado; Gene and Lorri Bauston of Farm Animal Sanctuary; and Christine Stevens of the Animal Welfare Institute in Washington, D.C.

NATURE'S KEEPERS

PROLOGUE

Confronting the Crisis

American history can be read in many ways, and one is as the record of a people who have continually strived to efficiently commandeer the vast natural resources of a perpetually changing frontier. That has unfortunately all too often involved the systematic manipulation and exploitation of the environment. This was one of Alexis de Tocqueville's hardest-hitting critiques of American culture: its appetite for destroying nature in pursuit of the maximal extraction of profits from the land.

In pursuit of expansion and progress, wild animals have consistently been branded as dangerous or as nuisances, in one form or another: blackbirds to be poisoned, coyotes to be shot, wild beasts to be bountied and put down—the bane of farmers and ranchers and a threat to early settlers. Note the many myths surrounding wolf attacks, which first gained notoriety with the printing of Charles Perrault's "Little Red Riding Hood" in Paris in 1697. The very word "wilderness" stems etymologically from the Old English pejorative term *wilddeoren,* a place of wild beasts, best suited for purposes of hunting.

Predators and other potentially lethal animals can evoke a fear and hatred out of all proportion to the actual threat they pose. The fear of poisonous snakes, for example, is a reflex reaction for many. And farmers and ranchers in particular can be heard to express intense loathing for a number of predators, most notably coyotes, but also, in no particular order of disdain, foxes, ferrets, prairie dogs, mountain lions, badgers,

wolverines, bears, and wolves. Americans are certainly not alone in this animus. "In southern Norway," comments writer Andrew Rowan, "the traditional wolf range now carries millions of sheep, millions of people, and five to ten wolves. It would seem that so few wolves should not disturb people, but the recent sighting of a wolf in southern Norway sparked a frenzied wolf hunt and a lucrative tourist trade in wolf artifacts that did not end until a wolf was shot dead, doused with champagne, and dragged off first to a school, then to an old people's home, and finally to the steps of the national parliament."[1] Wolves, which have almost never attacked humans, and many other wild animals have been marginalized in the natural world to such an extent that they can only be found today in the most inaccessible regions of America, or any other country. At one time in American history the value of a wolf was exactly one penny—the price paid to bounty hunters for killing them.

It is today sadly uncommon for people to come in contact with wild animals other than birds or squirrels, chipmunks, and deer. The upshot of this is that the endangered status of many wild animals is not well understood or appreciated by most people, be they urban or rural. Lack of exposure to the wild has desensitized the vast majority of us. The irony is that there is a rich tradition of reverence for the wild in American culture. Much of America's early infatuation with pastoral settings— the romantic wilderness depicted in the popular writings of Wordsworth, Longfellow, Chateaubriand, Byron, Shelley, and others—grew up in the cities, as historian Roderick Nash has pointed out, fueled by literary armchair wanderers. That romance was galvanized by painters such as Albert Bierstadt and Frederick Church, studio photographers like Carleton Watkins, and, in this century, Ansel Adams and the Kolb brothers, who established an industry of picture postcard imagery, inviting curiosity seekers into havens like Yosemite, Yellowstone, and the Grand Canyon.

Today's urban majority pays tens of millions of annual visits to the national parks each year, and yet despite such popularity, Americans are tasting a sense of true wildness less and less. A study carried out on tourists to the Grand Canyon showed that the average visit (as defined by the amount of time that the tourist actually left the seat of his or her tour bus or automobile, walked across a tarmac parking lot, and stood outside and admired the distant view) was nineteen minutes. Such a visit affords very little, if any, actual interaction with wildlife. Yellowstone's Lamar Valley exposes tourists, from the safety of their automobiles, to the sight of wild bison, elk, and the very rare grizzly bear or red fox. But Yellowstone is unique anywhere in the lower forty-eight states for its remaining mixed concentration of wild animals.

All over the country—and the rest of the world—habitat is vanishing, its integrity being impinged upon on all sides. When habitat is lost, species extinction soon follows. Consider the list of human activities (as drawn up by the California Department of Fish and Game) that are deemed detrimental to wildlife in America: development; livestock grazing; off-road vehicles; agriculture; the introduction of other exotic plants and animals; water projects; human and equestrian trampling; fire management; mining; landfills and garbage dumping; logging; flood control activities; energy development with its associated pipelines and power lines and discharges and leaks—10,000 oil and chemical spills each year just in Alaska and New York states; water quality degradation; vandalism; newly introduced predators; pesticides and other poisons from the nearly 300,000 new chemical compounds released by the chemical industry each year. Add to that an astonishing 60,000 square miles of road surface throughout the United States, an area the size of Georgia that has been rendered totally dead and which contributes to hundreds of millions of roadside killings each year; tens of thousands of miles of railroad tracks, also implicated in a serious death toll, particularly of larger

animals, like bears in Montana; a strip of land the equivalent of eleven miles wide spanning the entire United States, owned and operated by the U.S. military and strictly off-limits to any conservation laws; tens of thousands of miles of fencing, usually barbwire fencing; human recreation—from boating, which kills the endangered manatees in Florida, to hiking that can cause serious disruptions for animals attempting to hunt, or breed, or simply relax; ground ozone pollution that kills trees, acid rain that kills lakes and fish, the greenhouse effect with its deleterious impact on balanced growth; and that vast assemblage of hunters, both legal and illegal. And the myriad swaths of human expansion broadly described as "demographic pressure" that increasingly threaten, undermine, or directly extirpate other species. Together, these many intrusions constitute an overwhelming assault on America's plant and animal populations.

More than 900 plants and animals in the United States are seriously endangered.[2] In some instances, populations are down to a few dozen, as in the case of the California condor. Red wolves number fewer than 300, grizzlies—which each need up to 100 square miles of feeding range—number less than 1,000 in the lower forty-eight states. Fewer than 50 Florida panthers remain. As for its magnificent cousin, the jaguarundi, the last ever seen in the wild was run over in Texas in 1986. It may be extinct in the wild. From exotic Oahu tree snails and green pitcher plants to red-legged frogs, the reclusive Hawaiian 'alae'ula waterbird, and the nearly extinct ocelot, America's wildlife are in grave danger.

One of the most troubling threats comes from illegal trade in wild plants and animals—both live animals and their body parts, which are sold as pets, as trophies, or as exotic food types, amulets, leather goods and countless other "luxury" items, as delicacies, or for use in medicinal products. As Glen Kaye, head of the interpretive division of the National Park Service in Santa Fe, New Mexico, recently told me, "The vandals are

in the temple." Hides, teeth, claws, pads, gallbladders, horns, testicles, fur—they are all avidly pursued by poachers. Take just one of countless cases concluded recently along the eastern seaboard. In August 1995, a joint task force of rangers, investigators, Virginia game wardens, sheriff's deputies, and U.S. marshals from Shenandoah National Park and the Blue Ridge Parkway arrested eleven men for wildlife offenses that occurred during the previous three years in and around Shenandoah National Park. In all, sixty-one federal and seventy-five state charges were lodged, including the "commercialization of deer, bear and reptile products."[3]

The herbal medicine market is booming. The rage for rare cactus, mushrooms, and orchids is increasing. As the prices keep escalating, the poachers push biological reserves closer and closer to extinction. Biologists have determined that at least 105 species of wildlife have been systematically poached in America's national parks in the last few years, comprising 48 species of mammals including black bear, grizzly bear, polar bear, wolf, moose, bobcat, mountain lion, bighorn sheep, antelope, bison, caribou, lynx, musk ox, harbor seal, sea otter, and sea lion. In addition, 27 avian species have been poached. Of these, at least 12 species were listed as threatened and endangered.

In the United States, "the level of poaching has reached a crisis," says Ruth Musgrave, founder of the Center for Wildlife Law at the School of Public Law of the University of New Mexico in Albuquerque. Consider that there are some 250 million animals killed by hunters every year in this country. At least 14 million of those die slowly in traps. Much of that suffering is technically legal, but much of it is not. Most people not involved in the direct carnage will never experience that toll firsthand. In absence of the visceral truth, the horrifying reality of such biological attrition inevitably recedes from daily human lives. Only upon closer or dedicated inspection, often with the eyes of a biologist, a crimebuster, an environmental

lawyer, or simply the sheer stamina of someone with a diligent conscience (and sturdy stomach), are the signs of this professionally hidden warfare revealed. In America's most populous state, California, where the annual wildlife protection budget has dropped in recent years to approximately $22 million (a small sum for the eighth largest economy, and one of the most biodiverse regions, in the world), poachers are cashing in on what's left, and there isn't a lot. They clandestinely lay miles of drift lines studded with thousands of hooks in protected marine areas just offshore, by dark. And, as one investigator has reported for the *Los Angeles Times*, the poachers "mow down elk, including their calves, with AK-47 assault rifles. Or run over wounded deer when bullets run out. They harvest organs and paws from bears and leave the carcasses to rot. They bring to this war forged permits, spotlights, diving gear to take lobster and abalone from protected areas, off-road vehicles, police radio scanners, infrared spotting scopes, military weapons, illegal lines that fish a mile of ocean. . . . And, an understaffed and outgunned state Department of Fish and Game can't slow the slaughter."[4]

Already, the U.S. Fish and Wildlife service has set a conservative estimate of $200 million for the paid market value of illegally caught domestic animal by-products, and at least an additional $1 billion paid out by Americans to smugglers of wildlife from abroad. Worldwide, figures for illegally caught wildlife are estimated at between $10 and $30 billion, and the United States is the worst offender. Some investigators have come up with a price tag of $3 billion or more that Americans spend each year on illegally caught wildlife and wildlife by-products. Wildlife crime is underworld crime, and often involves countless middlemen and hard-to-trace transactions. The illegal products include everything from snow leopard pelts to turtle shells, from seal penises, eagle feathers, and bear paws and gallbladders to walrus tusks. The types of species are bewildering. In one year, at over 25 cities in the United

States (ports for smugglers), U.S. Fish and Wildlife agents confiscated over 1,000 bear carcasses and body parts of 11 different species, most of them endangered; rare mules, woodpeckers, orangutans, Mongolian Bactrian camels, Indochinese hogs, 5 species of endangered sheep, and over 1,200 rare deer from Mexico to North China were recovered. But the numbers do not even intimate the wider carnage occurring. At least 95 percent of all those engaged in illegal kills get away, time after time. And for those few hunting guides and their clients, single-minded poachers, illegal occasional hunters, and weekend opportunists who do get caught, fines and/or sentencing are often so trivial as to have little ascertainable impact on the trends. Each year tens of millions of containers are shipped in and out of the United States. Only a minute percentage of those shipments can be scrutinized by the 72 full-time U.S. wildlife inspectors and 235 field operatives.

Logic suggests that as the depletion of the wilderness experience verges towards extinction for an increasingly large segment of the population, America's capacity to be moved emotionally by the plight of wild animals will correspondingly diminish, an "extinction of experience" to use a phrase coined by ecologist Robert Michael Pyle. The majority of this generation of Americans (as distinct from our great-grandparents, who grew up in a largely rural world) are almost entirely divorced from the raw materials of their biological being, from the origins of the products they consume. These products exert a heavy burden on the environment—they pollute soil, streams, and the air we breathe—and such impact cannot be dissociated from its effects on wild animals, whose habitats are being squeezed out of existence. Our lack of contact with the wild is a precondition for much of the violence against nature we inflict, however unwittingly, in a vicious cycle of psychic numbing that only innovative and outspoken education and direct experience can reverse. When excesses of destruction are brought to the public's attention, however, we have shown

7

that we are capable of making inspired choices to diminish the damage done. Our uses of biological bounty can be tempered, our excesses modified. There are numerous champions of that reasoning, some of whom are profiled in this book.

Outmaneuvered, outgunned, and vastly outnumbered, a few thousand women and men across America are fighting a war to save our wildlife. Some are with the government, some in university teaching, others running private nonprofit foundations or for-profit organizations; and still others are simply out there, on their own, independently trying to make a difference the best way they know how.

This book highlights a few of the thorniest problems involved in the fight to preserve and protect what's left of the wild animals in the United States and, by implication, throughout the world. For many animals, the battle has already been lost. What I am principally focused on here are those animals whose future can still be preserved.

The subject of animal preservation is enormous, and has preoccupied scholars, activists, and experts in dozens of fields for countless decades, if not centuries. Comprised largely of key interviews from specialists involved in animal issues from around the country, I hope that this report from the front lines might contribute some modest reckonings to a hotly debated field. Ethology (the study of animal communications), animal preservation, animal rights, animal welfare, animal liberation, conservation biology, systematology—are all treating a similar phenomenon: the nature of our relationship to other species. It is an arena loaded with ethical and practical considerations applicable to the end of the millennium; to a time worthy of our taking stock of our animal selves. We share the planet with tens of millions of other species—hundreds of billions of individual animal lives. How we behave towards them has importance, not only to them, but to us. This obvious biological interconnectedness (obvious to many, not all) is replete with ethical dimensions and particulars that must evoke a continu-

ous reassessment of the laws governing our actions toward other species.

Summary of the Chapters

Chapter 1 introduces several facets of wildlife law enforcement, and looks particularly at a case in Alaska and a government undercover operation in Great Smoky Mountains National Park. It describes the one animal forensics laboratory in the United States, in Ashland, Oregon, and considers some of the challenges to lawmakers whose regional statutes are often at variance from state to state.

Chapter 2 examines the world of the U.S. Fish and Wildlife Service law enforcement branch, as seen through the eyes of young cadets at FLETC, the Federal Law Enforcement Training Center just outside Brunswick, Georgia. USF&W agents are rigorously trained there, then go out into the field to pursue poachers, among other things.

Chapter 3 provides an in-depth portrayal of one particular USF&W case, Operation Renegade, involving the illegal smuggling into the United States of wild-caught parrots from Africa, Australia, and South America. The Lacey Act, applicable to Operation Renegade, and the strongest piece of wildlife legislation in the United States, is analyzed through the eyes of a senior trial counsel for the U.S. Justice Department, one of the government prosecutors in the Renegade case.

Chapter 4 looks into the mind-set of hunters in America, by examining a particularly disturbing case in southern Missouri involving a father and son who were charged with wildlife infractions under both federal and state laws. The culture of hunting in Missouri, and the many points of view exhibited by all those involved in the case, is illustrative of the complexity of the ethical values concerning wildlife that lawmen must confront. Those values are particularly strong in rural America,

9

where many have grown up sharing a set of perceptions about hunting that are not easily tampered with.

In chapter 5, I examine the activities of an agency within the U.S. Department of Agriculture known as Animal Damage Control, or ADC, whose mandate is the control of wildlife (ostensibly predators) for the protection of human health and property. There are staunch critics of this program, and the outspoken views of three in particular form the basis for an examination of America's attitude towards predators in general and the problems the USDA must confront in convincing taxpayers that what they're doing by killing off millions of animals is justified.

All these explorations form the basis for the concluding chapter, which seeks to understand past trends while probing future possibilities for animal protection. Do wild animals stand a chance in a world of 12 or 15 billion human consumers? What about the crisis of shrinking wildlife preserves and populations? Is it our right and responsibility to legally protect every species, or is ecological triage fundamental to evolution? Can we intervene to make amends? Does bioengineering offer the possibility for preserving endangered species?

These questions, and many others, form the backdrop for an embrace of the challenges confronting those concerned about animal protection in the twenty-first century.

1

On the Front Lines of Battle

Jim Hannah is a ranger (official title: resource protection/ pilot) who patrols one of the world's largest natural protected areas, the Wrangell–Saint Elias National Park and Preserve in south-central Alaska. The Wrangells are the name of the mountain range—America's most rugged—and Mount Saint Elias is the highest peak there. At 18,008 feet, it is the second highest peak in the United States, after Alaska's Denali, also called Mount McKinley (20,320 ft.). On this day Hannah and his partner board their government aircraft, a 1,900-pound Arctic Tern. He revs up the single engine, files a flight plan, and heads off down the tarmac beyond the little hangar near his office in the town of Gulkana. Hannah swings a U-turn, stares down the runway, then advances the throttle. The engines grind and howl. They have lift-off at forty-five miles an hour, and soon they are but an indistinguishable aerial mote amid prodigious wilderness. His partner checks radio and video scanners to make sure they're operational. Hannah cleans off his sunglasses, crouches comfortably in his pilot's seat, and admires the rugged terrain all around him.

Anyone who's ever flown up to Anchorage from Seattle on a clear day has probably gaped at the Wrangells. Erupting precipitously out of the Pacific to over 18,000 feet, their brilliantly glazed walls—sheer ice the color of azure in sunlight—constitute the highest vertical rises in the world, more monstrous, even, than Mount Everest. Like some fabled, prehistoric

labyrinth, these mountains block entrance to a lost world populated by wolverines, black bears and grizzlies, wolves, and caribou, the 12,000 to 15,000 Dall (white) sheep, bison and moose, and countless other native wildlife. Glaciers pour forth furiously into an even more furious ocean of gigantic swells and whitecaps. Trees are routinely torn from their roots and funneled down raging rivers and spat like toothpicks onto the five-mile-deep windswept beaches, where they weather quickly into misshapen giants and sculptured flotsam. Sea foam, hurtled by the perennial winds, plasters their twisted, tawny hulks. Handsome cinnamon-hued grizzly bears, their paws the size of large pizzas, scavenge the interiors. The coastal griz, which wander along the tortuous shores, may weigh up to 1,200 pounds—graceful behemoths. Only rarely can one catch the glimpse of a human being in this wilderness—a specter of a figure huddled beneath an enormous parka, usually carrying a rifle, and searching for something, or waiting. No more than a few hundred people inhabit these wild margins of life.

Among those residents are Jim Hannah and his wife, Shirley. Jim used to teach high school biology in Vernal, Utah. A dedicated outdoorsman who loves to fish, he decided to join the park service in 1969 and began working at Dinosaur National Monument, along the Colorado-Utah border. It was at a time when the first major battles between developers and conservationists were gaining public notoriety. Paul Simon and Art Garfunkel were singing such memorable verses as "I'd rather be a forest than a street" and Supreme Court justice William O. Douglas was proposing a "wilderness bill of rights." Hannah rose through the ranks of the park service, honing in on his convictions and gaining skills that would later distinguish him among his peers. Now, at age fifty-two, he's at the top of his pay scale, a GS-12, with a base salary of $42,000 plus a nontaxable 25 percent cost-of-living allowance that makes it possible for him to live in Alaska, an expensive state. In addition, Shirley works for their local school district and takes

home $45,000 a year. Between them—a park ranger and school office manager—they're quite comfortable, which certainly commends the system. "I'm happy," says Hannah.

The Wrangell–Saint Elias National Park and Preserve, which extends up to the Canadian border, comprises 9 million acres of park and an additional 4 million acres of preserve. It is certainly one of the most beautiful protected areas in the world, equivalent in grandeur and biological significance to parts of Antarctica, East Africa, Indonesia, and the Amazon. But "protected" is a word fraught with ambiguity, because it offers certain exclusions unique to Alaska that are seldom allowed in the lower forty-eight: namely, registered commercial hunting in the preserve and subsistence hunting within the parks. In this respect, the conservationist elements at work are less sophisticated or effective than those, say, in Kenya's Amboseli National Park, where no hunting whatsoever is allowed, even by the local cattle-herding Masai tribes. Here in Alaska, hunting guides charge clients about $6,000 for a ten-day hunt, and are only allowed to do their commercial killing in the various preserves, including the Wrangells, though not in the national parks. The parks were made inviolate by Congress on December 2, 1980, as part of the Alaska National Interest Conservation Act (ANICA).

There is a chilling catch, however. The licensed guides may go into Alaskan parks if they are "subsistence users." Such grammatical provisions were hammered into law after substantial pressure from locals. According to Hannah, such hedging makes it tough for rangers to distinguish users from abusers. Most subsistence hunters will eat their dinner off the land. But some may use the subsistence definition as a license to kill for other purposes, thus compromising the ability of government biologists to monitor and conserve healthy populations. The law against killing in excess is very logical. Kill too much, and a species goes extinct.

The subsistence ruling is meant to continue "traditional

and customary use" claims by local residents, not merely Native Alaskans, but nonnatives as well, both old timers and newcomers to Alaska. The ruling is quite specific with regard to established seasons and bag limits. The laws were predicated on the assumption that subsistence users would be voluntarily restrained in their killing of animals, taking only what they needed. There are plentiful examples of such indigenous modesty. Anthropologists have long pointed out sustainable habits of hunting among tribes like the Kayapo in Brazil, or the Semai in Malaysia, or the Hadza in Tanzania. But in Alaska, where big money often is involved, confusion may reign between what is bona fide subsistence hunting versus sport hunting. As a result, any self-enforcing sustainable quota concept is rather fragile. While trapping is allowed, it is controlled through season and bag limitations. Yet at least one trapper is known to have killed an entire wolf pack and the state was helpless to stop him. The trapper was even allowed to sell the furs because his income was defined by state law as subsistence income.

Only grizzlies and goats are excluded from what is deemed customary and traditional kill animals in the park. They are thus off-limits to subsistence hunters. Yet commercial hunters can kill them in the preserves, and they can also kill them in the national park if they claim that it was self-defense or defense of property. In such instances, the hunter by law is supposed to turn in the head and hide of the bear within fifteen days. But usually, says Hannah, the hunter hides the carcasses to avoid questioning. Moreover, some locals have always complained about predators and will not hesitate to kill a wolf or bear or wolverine on the spot. It's tradition.

What has legally come to be known as multiple use management is an approach to hunting that is laced with contradictory inclusions. There are those who view subsistence hunting as a necessary way of life for some in Alaska, and federal areas are managed to continue such practices. But this continua-

tion can give rise to legal entanglements as a result of actions perpetrated by those few who would abuse the system and use subsistence as a defense where profit and trophy motives may have been involved.

People in the surrounding eighteen communities are allowed to subsistence hunt within park boundaries, Hannah says. In the preserve, there are an additional 300 sheep hunters and 17 registered hunting guides. Hannah believes that, in addition to all these hunters, there are probably 10 serious poachers who are getting in and getting out with major kills, and so far, Hannah and his team have not been able to catch most of them.

When does subsistence hunting become sport hunting, and then illegal commerce? One photographer took a photo of a record sheep and was offered $10,000 for information on its location. He stayed within the spirit, if not the letter, of the law and turned down the offer. But that's how badly trophy hunters are willing to pay. World record animals—animals like a trophy Dall sheep—are going for $100,000. So the financial temptations are very real. Sometimes a registered hunting guide who normally works out of a place like Anchorage will enter the region with a "friend" who is actually a client. But the law is very clear: no commercial hunting in the park, only in the preserve. However, subsistence users can harvest in the park, though not outsiders. Moreover, subsistence trappers can legally sell furs caught inside the park. From the standpoint of conservation biology, which is concerned with overall protection, the lawmakers' attempt to delineate users invites blurred boundaries, compromise, and infractions. Some critics question the wisdom of allowing the killing of any animal within a national park.

Abusers of the system will adamantly claim that Alaska is free and wild, wide open. That's why they came here. There is a grassroots "Robin Hood" philosophy some hunters espouse that dates to early periods in American history. The

first colonists were unhappy that they could not enjoy the same license to harvest animals as the representatives of the British Crown, who laid claim to ownership over all the wildlife in this country. As a form of rebellion locals in Massachusetts would go out to kill deer. Two hundred years later, the tradition of unlimited hunting collided head on with the first ecological realizations that biological bounty was not infinite. The Lacey Act was enacted in the year 1900 to deal with the disastrous overhunting of ducks. It was the first such federal law protecting game under the jurisdiction of the U.S. Department of Interior, and with it, American sportsmen were put on notice. But the Robin Hood syndrome prevails in many areas of the country; it merely disguises a very proprietary, profit-driven motive.

Today, there are still hunters who blatantly defy the Lacey Act and who poach avidly in the national parks and preserves. And they can do so largely with impunity, relying on the fact that it is so difficult for the government to stop them. Certainly that is so in a place like Alaska, a state which writer John McPhee once said was so big you could hide Italy in it.

Even if abusers do get caught, and even if the full force of the Lacey Act is thrown at them, at worst, they can expect a $250,000 fine and five years in jail. There are thousands of poachers, but few ever bear the full brunt of the Lacey Act. More typical for major offenders are fines of a few thousand dollars, and, occasionally, the forfeiture of an aircraft (worth, on average, $50,000) or a land vehicle, possibly a hunting license for two to five years, and a $1,000 hunting rifle. Often, offenders get immediate probation, trivial fees are imposed, and a judge chides.

If distinguishing one kind of hunter (and his impact) from another seems problematic, consider, says Hannah, the bigger problem—the very vastness of the Wrangells. How does one even begin to patrol such an area?

There are only five law enforcement rangers in the entire

Wrangell–Saint Elias National Park and Preserve region. They are based in small towns that come close to ranking as mere villages: Yakatat, Chitina, Slana, and Gulkana. The rangers' annual budget is a mere $250,000, which includes salaries, maintenance of aircraft, operating expenses, office costs, and anything else you can imagine. Hannah's GS-12 salary alone, modest though it is, constitutes nearly 20 percent of that total. Each ranger has 2.5 million acres to cover—nearly 4,000 square miles. That's an equivalent ratio to five men trying to protect a country the combined size of Switzerland and El Salvador; or all of Costa Rica; or both the Netherlands and Haiti. If that isn't enough to sear the left brain, think of it like this: one person responsible for protecting an area larger than Lebanon, twenty times larger than Singapore. Or try Belgium and Albania combined; or Kuwait, Singapore, Bahrain, Fiji, Malta, Luxembourg, and Barbados. Five guys with a couple of small planes and a few handguns who are in charge of protecting all of Rwanda and Israel, or Denmark and Cyprus. At least in such countries there tend to be paved roads and easy access, easy backup. In the Wrangells, it's more difficult. Access is by aircraft—when the weather permits—or two lonely roads, or by horseback.

There are five radio repeaters for relaying in-flight communiqués in the park/preserve, but as Hannah's aircraft slips and wends through gigantic valleys, passing those steep, snow- and ice-covered granite walls of Mount Saint Elias, he stays well below the incoming cloud line, temporarily losing all contact with the outside world. The radio goes static. That's normal. Suddenly, down below, his partner catches a glimpse of two airplanes and three guys on the ground. "That must be them," both men concur.

Hannah had received a tip that a group was heading out of Valdez by aircraft and that they were going after wolves. They were not sport hunters, but poachers.

Going after poachers was nothing new for Hannah. Once,

he and his partner had watched ("monitored") sport hunters for three days, traveling by foot to a log cabin in the middle of the national park. They expected there to be three people in the log structure. Instead, as they approached, eleven people stepped outside. Hannah was carrying a mere revolver, hardly the way to subdue so large a group, only two of whom had a permit to shoot bear. Hannah and his partner were nonetheless up-front with the eleven individuals, conducting interviews, though not without fear. It turned out that one of the hunters had downed a grizzly. The gallbladder, thought by some to be the ultimate aphrodisiac, and a cure-all for everything from impotency to aging, had evidently been removed.

As Hannah flies in low, he can see that the three men on the ground have laid facedown in the snow in an attempt to avoid being detected by the aircraft camera. But their efforts are in vain. With a video camera and zoom capability, Hannah's partner has made out the registration numbers on their C-185 aircraft. He does two flybys but does not land, not today. The Arctic Tern needs more landing area in the snow. Most hunters, however, are now using Supercubs, Piper PA-18s with 180 horsepower and huge, soft tires. They know they've got to get in and get out, fast. But they're able to do that because they started flying before they started driving, as teenagers. They handle their aircraft like skateboards, landing on a dime and giving you nine cents change. Some can land in 50 feet, take off in 100. The Supercubs are under a thousand pounds. They carry no heavy batteries because the pilots handstart them. They've got no special radio or survival gear. "They're unafraid. And they'll land anywhere—on a glacier, tundra, gravel bars. They're good. And there's money in it. Lots of money," says Hannah.

The rangers cut a wide arc in the increasingly cloudy sky. A heavily glaciated mountain range like the Wrangells creates its own weather in spades. Put such mountains against an ocean and you have a recipe for meteorological chaos. It can

be sunny one moment, and blizzarding the next. Hannah flies without benefit of radar or control towers. You're on your own up there. Gusts can be hurricane force. Wind sheer factors on the wing are elusive and can be fatal. More Alaskan bush pilots get killed than any other pilots in the world. Hannah avoids flying in the mountains, if possible, during turbulence.

The Crime Lab

As Hannah comes back around, both planes have taken off, one disappearing into clouds. They're gone. With his scanners running, Hannah and his partner search the sky. Five miles away they detect one of the aircraft. And then the scanners suddenly pick up the radio frequencies and they are able to eavesdrop on the conversation between the two escaping pilots. The conversation is recorded for evidence.

The next day, Hannah lands at the site in a different aircraft, hoping to obtain additional evidence that can be used against the three men. He knows from their behavior and the overheard conversation that they killed an animal. But he has to prove illegal activity. He needs hard evidence, as in any homicide case. With the help of a state fish and wildlife protection officer, they run a "crime scene" at the location. They find blood and hair fiber, bag them carefully, and then recover the stashed rifle. The blood and fibers are sent to the Clark Bavin National Fish and Wildlife Forensics Laboratory in Ashland, Oregon, to determine the type of species (they would be determined to have been wolf and wolverine). Later that week, a search warrant is served in Valdez on the three individuals. There, Hannah finds the planes and the state lab technician recovers additional blood and hair fragments, as well as aeronautical maps on which park boundaries are coded in color. The poachers knew where they were. They had the maps. They have no excuses.

The Ashland laboratory was set up in 1988. The only wild-life crime lab in the world, it serves the Fish and Wildlife agents, U.S. Forest and National Park services, and fifty state fish and game agencies. In addition, the 120 national signatories to the 1975 CITES (Convention on International Trade in Endangered Species of Wild Fauna and Flora) have access to it when necessary. The crime lab already possesses nearly 300,000 forfeited body parts from confiscated, illegally caught wildlife. Ken Goddard, a top administrator and investigator at the lab, used to work forensics for a police department. Today, he has seventeen scientific and fourteen support personnel working with him in Ashland. Their annual budget is $2.2 million. According to many in the anti-poaching world, Goddard and crew work miracles.

For example, when federal agents sent a dead spotted owl and surrounding evidence from the kill sight to the lab—evidence that included "two beer cans, a Band-Aid, the nail [which had been driven through the bird's neck], a match and the typewritten note [which read, 'If you think your parks and wilderness don't have enough of these suckers, plant this one']"—the lab was able to determine precisely what had happened, and how long before.[1] Goddard and his team have found ways to distinguish ancient from modern ivory, quite a task considering there is a known 13 million pounds of 20,000-year-old mastodon ivory in the marketplace. They were able to accomplish this task with a $250,000 scanning electron microscope and a $0.25 protractor. Moreover, Goddard's people were able to establish DNA profiles down to one in four million for a poached walrus. Such databases enable scientists to better gauge the genetic drift, as it's called, of isolated species and subspecies and determine whether their populations are healthy, or inbreeding (like the African cheetah), or vanishing. Being able to distinguish new from old ivory is crucial in any court of law because of the amount of marine mammal poaching going on. In February 1992, the U.S. Fish and

Wildlife undercover unit (known as special ops) concluded its Operation Whiteout, a net of Alaskan infiltrations that resulted in the arrests of twenty-five people for head-hunting—that is, the killing of walruses for their heads, and the taking of their ivory. Had investigators been unable to prove that the ivory was new, defendants could have insisted before a jury that the ivory belonged to long-dead mastodons. There's nothing illegal about salvaging it.

The Ashland crime lab does significant DNA blood and tissue matching. They have been able to identify the blood of bears, wolves, parrots, and deer. The first such DNA case occurred in Pennsylvania. The blood on a knife with which a man had poached a doe out of season was proven to be that of deer, not goat, as the man insisted. The evidence in court was so compelling that the defendant got up and openly confessed. In another instance, Goddard and his team were able to determine that the minute blood sample from a baby Amazon macaw's feather showed the bird had been captured in the wild and illegally smuggled into the United States, rather than sired in domestic captivity. The findings were the result of an extensive computer matchup of DNA with 900 blood samples from 900 macaws—450 males, 450 females. Says Goddard, "My team got covered in shit and urine. It was one of the less dignified but most satisfying of all cases." Because macaws are endangered, penalties are in the $10,000 range. They managed to pull in more key evidence than you see in most murder trials. Thus far, Goddard and his coworkers have looked at nearly 900 cases, of which Hannah's is one.

Hannah waits. The judicial process is slower than he'd like. It takes a year, but the case is successfully prosecuted. The three poachers plead guilty. Each will pay $5,000 and have their hunting privileges taken away for two years. They did not have to give up their planes, as part of their plea bargaining. Nor did it ever go to trial. The poachers were using a .308 Savage lever-action rifle. They described how they had wounded

a wolf and had been tracking it in deep snow, past rivers and sandbars, following the trail of blood, before finishing it off and returning to their planes, when Hannah's aircraft flew overhead. They did not know it was a park ranger but nonetheless dove for cover.

By his estimate, Hannah has successfully stopped about twenty-five poachers. He knows, and his wife knows, that what he does is dangerous. But, he says, "we all have missions in life. Mine is to be a park ranger. I love the outdoors. I hunt, I fish. But we all have to abide by the rules or the resources will suffer for future generations. It's that simple."

The Odds against Protecting Wildlife

With well over 20 million hunters in the United States, and untold buyers throughout the world, wildlife law enforcement has become dominated by tactics, strategy, and duress. Hunters outnumber conservation officers by nearly 10,000 to 1. Because of the odds against catching poachers—not just in vast spaces like those of the Wrangells, but in crowded areas like Yosemite, or Yellowstone, or the Great Smoky Mountains National Park— and the restricted budgets, law enforcers tend to focus on the bigger cases and the largest commercial poaching rings. This means that the smaller hunters are more likely to get away, and they are the ones who are wreaking havoc with so-called endemic clusters of local species, whittling away wildlife. You add up tens of thousands of such clusters, and the biologically fragmented world in which we now live surfaces in the imagination like so many local Armageddons.

Wildlife law enforcers cannot begin to keep up with all the infringements. One of the most revealing compromises in wildlife law that makes their job even harder can be found in the very language of the 1966 Endangered Species Act (ESA), described in the literature as "a landmark decision." Under its

provisions it is legal to "take" a species, even if that species is listed as endangered or threatened. What does "take" mean? The actual text of the act is striking, both for its candor and for lurking ambiguities. It means that one can "harass, harm, pursue, hunt, shoot, wound, kill, trap, capture, or collect, or attempt to engage" if the harmful action is "incidental to a legal activity." In other words, if the killing is not the primary intent, but somehow a secondary action, it is lawful. The burden of proof—was the animal slaughter primary or secondary, voluntary or involuntary—falls upon the courts, which in turn must rely on the Jim Hannahs of the world for making determinations in the field and collecting evidence. Those determinations can be logical, or gut instinct. But the odds against success are disturbing. Consider that as many as 59 percent of all species allegedly protected under the Endangered Species Act in the United States are declining in number. Only 25 species (out of more than 700 on the endangered list) have made any kind of recovery.

When Jim Hannah catches three wolf poachers in central Alaska, after their damage has been wreaked, that might not seem earth-shattering. But even in the face of such glaring limitations, wildlife enforcers know that the law's the law, paradoxes and all. Those same poachers will possibly think twice before next time committing a crime—perhaps. The goal of enforcement is to maintain healthy genetic stocks and whole ecosystems. Sometimes the practical contradictions and legal loopholes are daunting, even absurd. Frequently the greatest benchmarks of conservation are scarcely visible. Too often, the process fails. But the work of individual rangers, however much against the odds they are working, is a crucial component of the overall preservation fight. Incremental change. Individual lives saved.

John Garrison is a ranger at Great Smoky. Like Jim Hannah, his job is to combat illegal hunting. But he—and the thirty-three other rangers there—must also contend with fire

suppression, search and rescue, emergency medical care, drug enforcement, park management, traffic jams, theft, homicide, rape, and the like. They double up on everything. Unlike the situation up in the Wrangell–Saint Elias National Park and Preserve, with its 13 million acres and relative inaccessibility, Great Smoky hosts a mere half a million acres. Even at that, it is the second largest national park in the East after the Everglades. It's in demand, and because the park sits within one day's drive of two-thirds of the nation's total population, it is no surprise that over 9 million restless visitors come there each year. Says Garrison, "Every morning I have to tell myself, I still like people." Whatever conflicts are likely to arise between humans and other life-forms, rangers like Garrison will probably have to go out and deal with them.

Of those thirty-four rangers in the district (including the park), only six are designated for animals, plants, and habitat. And of those six, only one, at best two, are ever in the backcountry at any one time during the poaching season. In winter, they're able to let four or five rangers get back there. Most of the half-million acres of Great Smoky Mountains National Park are backcountry. But most of the 9 million people who visit come to what's called "front country," which you can get to by car, and that's why the rangers have to spend their time in front country. With so much of the park rangers' time committed to the more crowded zones, poachers feel emboldened in the backcountry. According to Dennis Burnett, a regulations program manager in the Ranger Activities Division of the National Park Service, for every known poacher, there are thought to be at least thirty others who will never get caught. "I think our biggest problem is we don't know how bad the problem is," Burnett told me. He attributes this, in part, to the ratios: the sheer size of the national park system and the breakdown of square miles versus number of visitors versus number of rangers. There is one ranger for every 300,000 visits. One ranger for every 80,000 acres. And they are the same ranger. In southern

California the Department of Fish and Game finds that it cannot even manage to get an agent out to any one holding even once a year. The staff is just spread way, way too thin.[2] Moreover, says Burnett, the technology of the poachers has gotten to be highly sophisticated. Poachers in Shenandoah National Park and the Great Smokies are running their dogs with electronic collars, which means that the poachers can wait outside the park. When they monitor the fact that their dogs have stopped moving, it probably means they've treed a bear. The poachers can then move in quickly and get their prey. Burnett and his colleagues are currently rewriting part two of their general park regulations book to insert control of electronic devices.

Rangers estimate that there has been a big increase in summertime poaching in recent years. So huge, adds Garrison, reflecting Burnett's own fears, that he and his cohorts have "no sense of just how many poachers there are. The scope is too big."

Garrison is a district ranger. He wears a gun and a uniform most of the time. He's been at Great Smoky for thirteen years. He's a local boy, born in Franklin, North Carolina, just twenty-five miles from where he now sits in his office. He loves this area, and because he grew up here he's always had an uncanny feel for what's going on. He knows too many of the opportunists who tear into the park in pickup trucks with their dogs, a rifle, and a spotlight on Saturday nights. They impact heavily on endemic species. And he's also met his share of those who have made a career of crime, of systematically going after natural resources for their commercial value.

Occasionally, park rangers will slip into blue jeans and boots, and adopt an undercover look. But, as Garrison insists, "our undercover work involves no magic, no hocus pocus. We simply engage the groups." That can mean many things. The key is to observe and document illegal activities with enough punch to get convictions in a court of law. That's where the crime lab in Ashland keeps cropping up. The rangers are not

allowed to "create a market" for illegal animal parts. That would be entrapment. They have to engage the bad guys honestly, buying and selling from them. The lines of offense are easily blurred, but never the intent. They want to stop the illegal killing.

"Amazingly," says Garrison, "some of the poachers are decent people, if you can say that. Families in the region have been hunting animals for multiple generations. They see nothing wrong with it and do not take kindly to a ranger telling them to stop." Especially one like Garrison, who was born and raised among them. He waves to old acquaintances on the streets, friends who might just turn around and go poaching later that day. And because the rangers can put them behind bars, Garrison has witnessed open hostility toward himself and other rangers, their families and property. "You run a high risk. It is certainly dangerous," Garrison says, echoing the concerns of wildlife enforcers in more than half of America's 366 national parks that poachers have targeted. Part of that risk comes not so much from hot-tempered locals whom you may have known all your life, but from outsiders. You also get a wide range of personalities. Some are hiding out from child support. Many are drug dealers, or addicts looking for quick dollars to get their next fix. They're desperate and they see that old black bear's gallbladder as the key to their next six months' worth of highs.

But Garrison is particularly concerned by what he describes as the ignorance of people in land management positions. By and large, he says, the managers simply feel "these boys [referring to the poachers] need to have their hands slapped. It's only a little problem. The BIG problem is people breaking into cars in our parks." Sighing, he adds, "People don't realize what we [the nation] are dealing with."

Garrison would like to see an "avenue of discussion between hunters and animal rights people and the general public. They all need to form a united front to help. I wanna grab

them all by the neck and tell them that commercial hunting and loss of habitat are wake-up calls. We can argue philosophy over coffee, later. But we need help. If the majority of people don't help us, then we're in trouble." He's referring to informants. The park rangers need local people to give them tips. That's how Jim Hannah knew that three poachers were coming into the Wrangells in search of wolf. Without that tip, those guys would have gotten away with it. Without the informants, there is no hope, Garrison says. "People must become involved in the parks. They have to think, 'Next time I see them I'm going to turn them in.' There must be a united front." The good news is that informants can make tens of thousands of dollars for tipping off agents to wildlife infringements. It's a great incentive. Eleven states have statutes providing citizen informants with generous rewards. In Hawaii, informants get half of all recovered fines. In many states, anonymous toll-free hotlines have facilitated reporting of violations. In Missouri, citizen informants were responsible for nearly 84 percent of all successful poaching arrests.

The rangers haven't a chance of succeeding unless two things are assured: a concerned public that elects representatives who will, in turn, maintain essential conservation budgets; and a legal and judicial system that can be strengthened so as to effectively combat and deter illegal encroachment upon wildlife. Because the public is oftentimes fickle about nature (note the famed conservationist Aldo Leopold's pointed statement, "There are some who can live without wild things, and some who cannot . . . "), much of the fight to save U.S. wildlife depends upon lawyers whose hearts are in the right place.

The Legal Battle to Save Wildlife

That's where Ruth Musgrave comes into powerful play. As a child growing up watching giant snapping turtles on the

Chattahoochee River in Georgia, Musgrave would explore tide pools and feed the wild animals. Later, in high school, she would care for a tank of dolphins at a marine park. These experiences stirred her love of animals. After completing law school in 1979, she went to work with a team of biologists at Shark Bay, north of Perth in Australia. At night she'd go down to the water and the dolphins would let her rub their backs. By that time, she knew she had to use her legal talents to help such animals. This was at a time when environmental law was becoming a major topic of interest on campuses. Superfund litigation was fanning out into communities around the country. Hundreds of lawyers were getting jobs fighting polluting industries. There was no end to the prospects for a young and talented lawyer with an environmental calling. Famed legal minds like Christopher Stone at the University of Southern California were publishing books that asked such questions as, "Shouldn't trees have legal standing?" As one national park ranger put it, "A black bear can't write its congressman when a family member gets killed."

After fifteen months of difficult fund-raising, with a desk and a telephone given to her, Ruth Musgrave founded the Center for Wildlife Law at the School of Public Law of the University of New Mexico in Albuquerque in 1990. While wildlife law is now taught in at least ten universities in the United States, Musgrave's center is the only one in the world devoted solely to the cause. Her uncommon command of state laws enables her to enlist at any one time a dozen state and federal agencies, citing every legal precedent relevant to a case, and pushing for consistent nationwide legislation. With her shaggy blond hair, striking eyes, and athletic physique, she is a charismatic blend of youthful idealism and tough legal acumen. In five years' time she has raised more than $1 million for her center, published a wildlife law newsletter, and is engaged in dozens of battlegrounds across the country, all the while schooling a new generation of tough, empathetic legal minds

at the university. She also receives the occasional ominous warning from ranchers who are irritated by her ecological altruism. Musgrave brushes such threats aside. Her ecological loyalties may be a passion, but they are grounded in her respect for the letter of the law.

Musgrave has adopted a systems approach to conflict resolution that began with her center's 840-page *State Wildlife Laws Handbook,* the first comprehensive tome to list all laws affecting wildlife and habitat in every state, and to point out problematic discrepancies, like the above-cited ambiguities in the Endangered Species Act. Many of the laws date to the last century (no herding of rabbits allowed in downtown Denver, for example) and remain unchanged, out of touch with twentieth-century ecological literacy. What's legal in one state may be illegal in another.

Those discrepancies, says Musgrave, include the fact that poaching in some states barely gets noticed, while in others it is a minor misdemeanor, and in still others a felony. Regulations from state to state are a miscellany of inconsistencies that work against the goal of national biological conservation. Musgrave, and most biologists, know that wise land use cannot be segregated by the arbitrary borders of individual state customs, history, predilections, and political or economic determinations. Like the weather, watersheds, rivers, and airborne pollutants, animals migrate. Their habitat corridors and populations require protection wherever they lie, even over multiple state lines. To Musgrave's mind, that means that threats to wildlife from state to state must invite a unison of combative legislation.

In many states, Musgrave has learned, parking tickets are more expensive than the fines for illegally slaughtering animals. Fines for poaching can be as little as $10, and the judicial system exerts virtually no deterrent to poachers in most places. In North Carolina, if a poacher is caught using spotlights at night to kill animals, the fine is as low as $25. Musgrave has

edited a volume written by Sara Parker and Mimi Wolok for the University of New Mexico's Center for Wildlife Law in which many of the economic factors influencing poaching, and the discrepancies between laws in different states, have been compellingly highlighted.[3] Incredibly, thirty-one states still do not prosecute hunting guides if their party illegally hunts, or if they aid poachers. With such open-door options, poachers are free to view the United States as one enormous butcher shop, with no guards, no burglar alarms, and no police for hundreds of miles around. A single U.S. Fish and Wildlife operation recovered 17,500 illegal furs worth $1.2 million. One wildlife investigator in New York saw 2,000 bear gallbladders for sale in Chinatown, at $800 per gram. A single gallbladder recently sold in South Korea for $64,000. A motorist in South Dakota stepped out of his car on a freeway, aimed his rifle, and blew a bald eagle to smithereens. Nothing but feathers were left. But a single feather is worth $100. They are especially valuable to certain Indian tribes. In 1993, for example, the U.S. Fish and Wildlife Service received 1,854 individual requests for eagle feathers and other eagle parts from Native Americans. Suitable eagle carcasses could not be located and 90 percent of those requests have been "backlogged." The bottom line: eagles are scarce. An elk's antlers are worth $140 a pound. The horns of a Rocky Mountain bighorn go for $1,000 an inch. Those of a desert bighorn command upward of $100,000.

A market now exists for teeth of nearly any wild animal. Coyote teeth are $2 apiece. And big game ranches have sprung up throughout the West offering "canned hunts" to poachers who can't aim straight. The hunting guide will go out and trap a bear or a mountain lion, cut their feet, use a razor blade to slow them down, or merely put the animals in leg snares or cages and then let their clients come and blow them away at a few paces distance. In China and Taiwan they are doing the same thing with tigers, Asiatic black bear, and other rare specimens. The 486 elk confiscated by U.S. Fish and Wildlife au-

thorities during the past decade scarcely touches the problem. Twenty years ago, a U.S. Fish and Wildlife survey of 3,600 waterfowl hunters revealed that 70 percent of them openly admitted to poaching.

Oddly enough, nearly half the states in this country still allow hunters to use machine guns, poison, explosives, and nearly any other kind of deadly device, as long as the killing is in season, within the right boundaries, and/or within the allowable quota.

When Ruth Musgrave confronts such statistics, and plots a strategy that will, perhaps, exert a persuasive force of change on the legal thinking in this country, she must focus like a dentist on the teeth of existing laws in both state and federal spheres. The regulatory framework fits within a dozen federal laws: the Lacey Act, the ESA and accompanying provisions of the CITES convention (1975), the Marine Mammal Protection Act (1972), the Eagle Protection Act (1972), the Migratory Bird Treaty Act (1918, 1960, and 1972), the Migratory Bird Hunting and Conservation Stamp Act (1934), the Bald and Golden Eagle Protection Act (1962), the Airborne Hunting Act (1971), the National Wildlife Refuge System Administration Act of 1966, the Antarctic Conservation Act of 1978, the African Elephant Conservation Act (1988), and the Wild Bird Conservation Act of 1992. The Department of Interior's Fish and Wildlife Service Division of Law Enforcement is the primary agency charged with policing those laws. Then there is the National Park Service, which is responsible for maintaining law and order within its precincts. In addition, each state has its own fish and game departments with law enforcement personnel. The Department of Agriculture is responsible for monitoring the Animal Welfare Act, which carries over into industrial, agricultural, and biomedical uses of animals. The Federal Bureau of Investigation (FBI), local sheriff's departments, and police will occasionally get involved in wildlife issues. Ultimately, the judicial system must make sense of it all,

as persuaded one way or the other by the increasing numbers of wildlife lawyers, and the men and women who bring in the cases to begin with.

Special Operations

People like Terry Grosz. He is a no-nonsense U.S. Fish and Wildlife law enforcement officer based in Denver who says he's never seen a worse poaching situation in all his thirty years working in the field. Grosz is an urgent person. There is a kinetic gravity about him which reflects the fact he has seen too much killing. He seems beleaguered and impatient. Most of his colleagues are subsurface, undercover. They come up for air every month or so. Currently, USF&W hires centrally (out of Arlington, Virginia), filling about ten jobs a year from an application pool of some two thousand. "We pick survivalists," Grosz warns. "Compared with other agencies, we're peanuts. The money is always the problem. We don't have staying power. No time for long surveillance. We have a total of two hundred thirty-five agents around the country and an annual budget of about thirty-five million. And with that we have to fight people who will pay a dollar per square inch for polar bear fur; who are marketing bear claws like they were some unique Winchester rifle. The profits are unreal. Nobody says anything. It's all underground."

Unlike, say, Jim Hannah's job—going after a few illegal intruders in the park and hoping you can find them through the cloud layers—Grosz and his colleagues are engaged in broader thrusts of high-risk special operations. At any given time, there are between eight and ten USF&W undercover agents assigned to the special ops branch. They are the Green Berets of anti-poaching, cloaked in near total secrecy. In the early 1990s their Operation Brooks Range resulted in the arrest of twelve hunting guides. The sting involved the booking of illegal hunts on

the North Slope of Alaska by special agents posing as good ole boys in New York and Wisconsin.

Sometimes their efforts make the news, as in the case of Operation Trophy Kill at Yellowstone back in the 1980s. There, the media seized upon the crimes because the USF&W had uncovered a home video shot by the poachers themselves to document their own "courageous" acts of slaughter—men shooting arrows through the faces of black bear cubs, and countless other horrors.

In 1988, Operation Smoky was launched, involving six undercover operatives from the National Park Service and U.S. Fish and Wildlife, in North Carolina, Georgia and Tennessee. John Garrison, who was not an operative at the time and had only a small role in the takedown, nonetheless remembers it well. The operatives went after twelve target groups suspected to be poaching in Great Smoky Mountains National Park. What they uncovered was a Pandora's box of killing, much of it of black bears whose gallbladders and other parts were being sold on the international market. But the agents also stumbled into a wide net of other killings: of turkeys, wild boar, fish, plants, deer, birds, and medicinal herbs, all within park boundaries, and often in the company of professional hunting guides, mercenary types who knew exactly where to go within the half million acres of Great Smoky. In just one year, one of the twelve targeted groups was discovered to have killed twenty-eight bears, cut open their insides, removed the gallbladders, and left the corpses to rot. Young bears, old bears, cubs. It didn't matter.

Operation Smoky lasted about three years. The number of offenses was skyrocketing and the six agents were unprepared for such complexity, nor did they have the funding to pursue it. Yet, the money spent was a bargain compared with, say, drug operations. Thirty poachers were convicted at the end of Operation Smoky, and the fines levied exceeded $100,000.

But that operation was the tip of the iceberg, says Garrison.

At Great Smoky, twenty different animal species continue to be illegally killed. And the park is losing so many plants that it's impossible to know the long-term biological consequences, except to say they're very, very serious. Countless flowering plants and herbs are exploited for the floral industry: orchids, ginseng, goldenseal, and bloodroot. Whole species of orchids have been wiped out there in one season, each individual flowering plant selling for $35. Ironically, the survival rate is very low because the transport of illegal live plants through the underground pipeline is brutal. The poachers dig up the plants, hustle them to a buyer, and then split. There is no concern about longevity.

"Folks," says Garrison, "if you have natural resources where you live, then you have a poaching problem. It's there. It's growing, all over the country. And it's because of money. It'll make people do anything. It could be in your very backyard. And believe me, folks, if we keep going like this the pressure on those species will threaten their very existence. Remember the passenger pigeon."

He refers to the most historic example of an extinction in the United States. According to biologists Paul and Anne Ehrlich, "the passenger pigeon may have been the most abundant bird ever to exist." An observer for the Audubon Society estimated that during a three-day period in the mid 1870s, near the Petoskey Point, Michigan, nesting site, 300 million birds passed overhead in one hour. The collective roar of their wings could be heard six miles away. One individual flock in the East numbered 2 billion birds. Their droppings were one of the greatest sources of fertilizers in North America. Americans began eating the birds, sporting with them, devising ever more heinous ways to exterminate them. The term "stool pigeon" entered our vocabulary as the result of one of the countless trapping decoys devised to kill them. These docile birds with blue backs and pink breasts were burned alive, their heads crushed by pincers, and actually used in shooting gal-

leries. Any child could pay a penny to have a go at blasting them away. Americans went on a killing spree and there were no laws at the time to prevent it. In 1878, a single hunter in Michigan reportedly killed and sold 3 million passenger pigeons. Such massacres, in addition to the rapid deforestation by the lumber trade of the birds' favored oak and beech forests, led to their sudden dwindling in number. By the 1890s the birds were gone. The Lacey Act of 1900 came around too late to save them. As famed nature writer Peter Matthiessen describes in his devastating, must-read classic, *Wildlife in America* (1957), the last one, named Martha by her captors, took her last breath at the Cincinnati Zoo in 1914.

It is a sobering reminder that if the largest wildlife population in North America can be rapidly driven to extinction, then the thousand remaining grizzly bears and the fifty surviving Florida panthers are almost surely doomed. Unless society sees fit to authorize lawmakers and law enforcers with the means and the mandate to save them. Current efforts to push the legal understanding of biodiversity principles into the courts in tougher and more enlightened ways, state by state, are key to envisioning any kind of future for U.S. wildlife.

How ecologists and conservation biologists can cope with government downsizing and the loss of funding at the very moment that human demographic pressure and poaching are at an all-time high will determine their ability to undertake ambitious inventories of wildlife—to know just what's out there, what's left—and to appropriately recommend where priority conservation status must be applied.

Ultimately, wildlife will be saved by committed individuals—people like Jim Hannah, John Garrison, Ken Goddard, Ruth Musgrave, and Terry Grosz. They wake up every day and go off into the trenches, one step at a time, to face up to the many challenges: poachers discharging automatic weapons into innocent creatures; laws that need reforming or implementing; societal trends and ethics that require discussion

and reshaping. The challenge underlying the battle to save wildlife is the moral and pragmatic calling that confronts those who would strive to make a difference amid the rough seas of consumption patterns and stubborn comfort, of strange obsessions and deeply ingrained habits that translate into a wide range of beliefs and practices—all of which must be respected, considered, understood, and worked with if any lasting change is to come about.

Such individuals fighting to save America's wildlife marshal a special grace, if you will, in the face of terrible crimes and near overwhelming adversity. They are remarkable not because they are necessarily so courageous, but because their common sense is in tune with their conscience. As Vice President Al Gore has said, such conscience for other life-forms must surely dictate the terms of the twenty-first century by which we all live.

2

Handcuffs and Aikido

I pull into a large parking lot beside a multistory office building in an easy-to-miss complex of other commercial buildings
in a nondescript section of Arlington, Virginia, twenty minutes from downtown Washington, D.C. I've come to spend the
morning with John Doggett, chief of law enforcement for the
U.S. Fish and Wildlife Service (USF&W). One would hardly
detect that the personnel housed in this building were charged
with protecting over 90 million acres of land and water. They
control the third most sizable chunk of real estate in America,
after the Bureau of Land Management, which controls a whopping 340 million acres, and the Forest Service, with its own
300,000 square miles, or 192 million acres. The National Park
Service ranks fourth with 80 million acres. But there is a huge
difference between the types of management exerted across
the more than 400 National Wildlife Refuges by USF&W agents,
and those charged with overseeing these other properties.[1] The
difference is in the quality control. BLM lands, for example,
require management, in its most mundane and bureaucratic
sense. There is seldom anything too obvious, or particularly
emotional, at work. Whereas Fish and Wildlife agents are emphatic shepherds, charged with express guardianship, the last
stand between a species' right to exist unmolested and possible extinction, if not in total, then certainly within a specific
region. And to hear those guardians speak of it, the countless
refuges are being gutted by overzealous hunters, and by

poachers, as well as all those who benefit from the unspeakable actions of poachers: the buyers and sellers, the collaborators, and indirect marketeers. In previous times, it was the sheepherders, miners, timbermen, and mountainmen who posed problems of wildlife attrition. Today, it is the sophisticated criminal that keeps the USF&W severely overtaxed.

It is here, in Arlington, where the special agents are hired and from whence all oversight of operations is conducted. Those protective endeavors frequently include a collaborative stakeout or legal offensives in concert with the attorney general's office, the Forest Service, and National Park Service, with the BLM, Interpol, the Bureau of Alcohol, Tobacco, and Firearms (ATF), the FBI, U.S. Customs, the State Department, and the CIA. Wildlife cases can be congested. A single offense might break a dozen laws. Doggett, who was directly in charge of the Special Operations Branch, which had just successfully winded down the international, multijurisdictional Operation Renegade, was himself to retire this week, after five years at the helm.

"There's an extremely high incidence of assault with firearms, as you might imagine, because most of the people that we run up against in field situations are armed," he starts off, laying out the bottom line immediately. "The damage done by poaching is just exponentially increasing. Public education, understanding, and support for the protection and conservation of wildlife resources is critical to the success of our mission. There's just a huge commercial drain on wildlife. We have to pick and choose and try to make the most impact we can with our enforcement activities because we're just spread thin and there's such a vast area of activity."

The first guardian of a protected area in the United States— possibly in the world—was a fifty-two-year-old explorer named Galen Clark, who became a ranger in Yosemite in 1866. Fourteen years later, Harry Young took over the task of enforcing quotas on hunting in Yellowstone National Park. There were 150 cavalry troops on permanent patrol to help him. In 1905,

a plume hunter killed an Audubon game warden named Guy Bradley at Oyster Key, Florida, and was freed by a local jury. On March 12, 1927, a park ranger was killed on the job; according to historian Paul Berkowitz, it happened to be the first time in his career that Ranger James Carey of Hot Springs National Park had ever gone out on his rounds without wearing his .38 caliber sidearm.[2] Since that time, both in the national parks and refuges, there have been gun battles, and numerous other rangers have been shot and/or killed in the line of duty. And while Bureau of Land Management undercover agents began armed patrols following passage of the Wild Free-Roaming Horse and Burro Act of 1971 (each agent covering an implausible one to five million acres of terrain), it was not until 1976 that the secretary of the interior was empowered to officially designate certain officers with the right to carry firearms—to make it a policy of the Department of the Interior (DOI), though many had been doing so long before to protect themselves. But there was some controversy surrounding the notion of the benign Ranger Rick as being armed and dangerous. Indeed, as late as 1978 the superintendent at Yellowstone prohibited rangers from carrying guns during the day. "If someone shoots at you, run back to your car and call the highway patrol or the sheriff's department," Yellowstone's chief had advised.[3]

John Doggett has never been fired at in the field (that he knows of), but, by his own description, he's had plenty of "excitement"—major arrest situations, execution of warrants, delicate infiltrations. For all the admitted stress, he calls it "a beautiful job" and waxes enthusiastically at how you're out there on a hunting violation, a stakeout, and as you're watching this gorgeous sunrise you're thinking, "They're actually paying me to do this!" Doggett views U.S. Fish and Wildlife as "the embodiment of the public conscience. If people won't obey the law out of their own conscience, and desire for doing what's right, then we have to make them. We have to force

them to do so through the threat of prosecution and arrest." Doggett believes his agents are possibly more mature than many others in different branches of government. Perhaps, he says, because they're thinking very clearly about future generations. About what it means when something goes extinct. He also points out that because U.S. attorneys' offices are so political—"They're political animals, fighting for dollars"—wildlife cases are competing for their understaffed time with bank robbers, rapists, and murderers. Here is someone killing geese, and here is someone killing children. Who do you think the U.S. attorney is likely to be more concerned about?

Children, I reply.

Maybe, says Doggett, maybe not. "More and more, senior U.S. attorneys want our wildlife cases because of the way they're presented, the professionalism, the details with which they're brought forth." He reminds me that USF&W agents are among the very best. They've got the best and most diverse training, and they love their jobs. There's something inimitable about a person who loves his job. Moreover, he points out the public relations possibilities of going after someone who has been poaching Smoky the Bear, or America's national bird. An attorney gets a lot of mileage out of that.

Doggett's jurisdiction is comprised of three primary areas: interstate commerce and transport, poaching or removal of species from federal lands, and impact on species federally protected. It constitutes an enormous realm of possible violations—the primary crime topography involving wildlife—and Doggett is quick to point out that his agency could easily double the size of its force, if only Congress would see the light. He cites with some envy U.S. Customs with its nearly 3,000 agents, compared with his 235.

During Doggett's time as chief, U.S. Fish and Wildlife criminal investigators managed to pull in significant jail time for those involved in organized smuggling activities. The service does not have the means of tracking the actual man-hours

behind bars because of the migratory nature of prisoners within the system, but they do know that hundreds of people have been arrested, and the figures are way up from previous years. So are the offenses. It's no longer simple citations for killing one too many ducks. The crimes are international, and USF&W cases have included sawed-off walrus husks in Alaska (Operation Whiteout); illegally imported African parrots, leopard skins, and rhino horns; eagle feathers from Mexico; live primates from the Philippines, turtles from India, snakes from Indonesia, felines from South America, and butterflies from New Guinea. Often, drugs are involved, the animals being force-fed small baggies filled with cocaine or heroin, to cite but one form of the relationship. To catch domestic infractions, USF&W agents will often establish bogus businesses. They'll work with Dun & Bradstreet, engender elaborate covers, obtain false social security numbers or driver's licenses, and do whatever they need for elaborately constructing an undercover identity. Doggett says it is increasingly challenging because the bad guys are wise to these undercover operations and are using their profits for overhead to investigate people they're doing business with. The stakes are high because so many species are going extinct. Says Doggett, "It's Economics 101—as the supply goes down, demand goes up."

As I head out of Doggett's office, he shows me a grizzly bear at the elevators. It was killed by George Abrams in 1986. Abrams was an agent on a sting operation in which hunters were illegally leading clients. To maintain his cover, the agent had to kill the magnificent bear, which must have stood nearly nine feet tall, otherwise the poachers would have smelled a rat and probably left him for dead out there in the Alaskan wilds.

The explanation leaves me queasy—ethical choices and the best available tactical strategies spinning in my brain—but I have no immediate response. "We're very proud of our agents, and of their successes," Doggett affirms, as I shake his hand beside the waiting elevator. But he strikes a dour note which

must come from his nearly retired status, a kind of philosophical window on the service. "When you have congressmen on the hill that come out and want to downsize government and take away law enforcement vehicles from us; and when you have residents from out in Idaho that don't want any government interference and try to get legislatures to take away our law enforcement authority or restrict officers from carrying firearms, well, all these things are just harassment that interfere with the effectiveness of the officer in performing his duties. We've got some of the most professional law enforcement people in the world working for this department and for somebody to come in and say, 'Well, we think we ought to take away their guns,' or say they can only carry firearms if they get a permit from the sheriff of the county, that's bullshit. Such stuff is demoralizing to professional law enforcement people who are doing a good job."

Doggett then suggests I go down to FLETC—the Federal Law Enforcement Training Center. His office would get me clearance and I could check out the quality of the agents for myself.

In the Land of Armadillos

In the early spring of 1997 I took up Doggett's offer and headed up the coastal route past the offshore Barrier Islands of Georgia into the old town of Brunswick. Ten miles out across the embayment, like a shimmering oasis low to the waves, Jekyll Island once played host to America's exclusive club of late-nineteenth-century billionaires—the Morgans, Rockefellers, and Pulitzers. The island's glorious beaches also happened to be the site for the last illegal arrival of a slave ship from Africa. These days, its fame is largely confined to tourist haunts, the odd historical relic and easygoing hotel, as well as the shy armadillos, who live among the thick canopies of forest and too

frequently step out into the way of oncoming traffic. I pass two of them foraging in the predawn hours, an omen for the good, it seems in retrospect. Their gentleness has come about over millions of years of evolution; two creatures moving silently through the undergrowth without the slightest concern for their own safety, though wary of headlights. Several miles away, millions of dollars have been invested by a very different kind of species to protect those armadillos, and what their wildness stands for across America.

My destination this day was FLETC, a few miles up the road from Brunswick, and into the scattered dry pines. SABS 22 (Special Agent Basic School, twenty-second session) was in its final week, and I was keen to meet this year's new crop of U.S. Fish and Wildlife special agents. Though their modesty would preclude superlatives, it would become clear to this observer that these young people (all under thirty-five, all of them with various college or graduate school degrees from all over the country) were, in fact, for wildlife protection the equivalent of U.S. Marines. They were game wardens, special operations experts, weapons-trained environmental managers often coming from previous state wildlife refuge or U.S. Customs positions, field-hardened conservation biologists, adept in the labyrinths of environmental law, highly sophisticated policemen, and—first and foremost—ecological activists all rolled into one. They are the elite force and they all concur that (1) they love what they do and (2) to keep up with the out-of-control spate of crimes against wildlife, there should be thousands of them, not on average between 230 and 235. "Talk to your congressman," I would hear repeatedly. "The service [Fish and Wildlife] needs more support, more staff, more money, and we're not even allowed to mention it."

By now, this year's new group of nine prospects—seven males, two females—would have spent eighteen intensive weeks together. For their instructor, Special Agent Doug Goessman, this was to be his last stint at FLETC. He was restless and had

decided to go back out into the wilds of Montana and catch bad guys.

FLETC has the appearance of a sprawling college campus, beautifully ensconced, in many ways quite mellow. But there are immediate differences that accost the visitor. First, the entrance gate, awash in security clearance protocols. And second, the fact that *everybody* seems to be carrying. A gun, that is. Over 2,000 adrenalin-thick students dressed in the regalia of their respective agencies, divisions, departments, and bureaus, from across almost the entire spectrum of government law enforcement come here for their training. FLETC is the consolidated hub for legal studies: the place to learn the legal codes, arrest procedure, search and seizure, the fine points of self-incrimination, weapons use, hand-to-hand combat, and the planning and execution of raids, investigations, and takedowns. All the federal agencies use FLETC, with the exception of the Justice Department, which operates programs out of Quantico, Virginia, for FBI and DEA agents. But it is here at FLETC that every other special agent comes for an intense schooling, whether Customs, Secret Service, U.S. Marshal, or Fish and Wildlife. They go through a nine-week Criminal Investigator Training Program and then, when they graduate from that, each agency runs its own extended specialty program lasting from between six and fourteen weeks. It is one vast boot camp, and by 7:30 A.M. the myriad corridors and buildings are alive with the plaintive grunts and stamina-building groans and hoots of various workout routines.

Doug and I stop at a convenience store on the way to class. Standing in line to get a caffe latte and doughnuts, everyone around me is armed with heavy weapons, muscles tight and flexing. Anyone remotely paranoid about anything—a string of unpaid parking tickets, or worse—might well sweat it out at FLETC.

As we walk to the classroom, someone in front of us emits noisy flatulence. A young, armed U.S. Marshal walking briskly

to his own tune, and to his own class, turns, points at the offender, and says with a straight face, "I heard that. Put a lid on it."

We've got time before the class starts in a large room with blue mats extending wall to yellow-striped wall. So Doug gets me up to speed on what the training has thus far consisted of. Initially, the agents are required to attend the nine-week Criminal Investigator Training Program, where they'll actually write and execute search warrants, do vehicle surveillance, go before a magistrate or judge, have a mock trial, do fingerprinting and scores of other tasks. Then they come over to Doug's care for another ten weeks, which is the real specialty training for Fish and Wildlife agents.

A week of orientation—during which time they're issued their laptop computers—is followed by the real thing, the practical training. They go into depth on areas of federal wildlife law, including the dozen primary legal codes protecting plants and animals and habitat. They are graded after several weeks. They have to maintain a minimum score of 70 percent. On the firearms it's 80 percent. If they flunk one test, they get a retry. If they flunk the second, they go home. Their career with USF&W is over. But those who do make the grade then go on to learn comprehensive identification skills and spend a full seven days in a classroom where they are required to maintain an 80 percent level of accuracy on all waterfowl identification. They have several hundred study skins from throughout North America, along with carcasses, wings, and other body parts, for examination. They also have live eagles and other raptors, and learn falconry. This year the training included cooperative red-shouldered, Harris, and kestrel sparrow hawks. The agents spend forty hours just on CITES (the Convention on International Trade in Endangered Species, of which, of course, the United States is a signatory), and another forty hours studying the Migratory Bird Treaty Act. They do twenty hours of interview and interrogation, with content analysis based upon the

Israeli Secret Police model. They explore Native American law, and bring in an Indian who works for the service to discuss the full range of legal precedents and sensitivities pertaining to Native American culture. They study wilderness survival, the Asian medicinal trade, survey antigovernment organizations, set up raid houses, practice at indoor firing ranges, learn how to put out boat fires, and examine a few major cases anatomically, including those coming out of the Special Operations branch.

One of those study cases concerned a collaborative undercover investigation involving Canada, Native Americans, and three states. Fish and Wildlife agents opened up an undercover storefront to buy and sell illegal takes from the Great Lakes, Ontario, and two tribal lakes protected under Indian law. A number of people went to prison for literally decimating perch populations. Major players were bootlegging walleyed pike off two Indian reservations. A large number of defendants were apprehended in Wisconsin, Minnesota, and Illinois. This was probably the first time that Fish and Wildlife agents worked hand in hand with the tribal folks to get a handle on protecting tribal wildlife. The reservations are given the same status as a foreign country, which means if you kill an animal on a reservation and transport it off the reservation, it comes under the provisions of the Lacey Act (see chapter 3).

Fish and Wildlife agents, working with the Indians, went after the larger buyers, not the small-time dealers on the corner. They needed to find the next rung up—the wholesalers, basically—and the restaurants that were creating the market in the first place. It was identical to investigating an organized crime syndicate. There were all of two undercover agents handling the case. They examined all their own records and did their own subpoenas. The operation was laid out start to finish for the SABS initiates. Doug says that some of the agents had assumed it was a matter of somebody killing a few fish over the limit. But the days of tramping around in the boondocks and

checking every two-bit hunter is pretty much over. Wildlife crime has become big business.

In the last eight weeks, Doug has also led the new agents through various import-export scenarios, including the creation of a border port and mock customs facility. There, cadets learn how to detect fraudulent documents. The trainees got their own aircraft for navigation scenarios and had to respond to a fabricated complaint of illegal activity. They had to come up with a plan, fly to the area of suspected illegal activity, photograph it, come back, develop their film, and go back in at night on the ground to document and gather evidence. Then they'd write their reports.

In this case the complaint involved illegal baiting. Evidence is placed: a fifty-pound sack of corn spread across a waterfowl area forty miles north of FLETC. Agents flew in amphibious aircraft to document from above the telltale signs. "It's not as hard as you might think," Doug tells me. I am perplexed, trying to imagine seeing corn spread across a marsh from high up in the air. But Doug insists it is visible. His staff have gone in and spread the corn out for the ducks. Fish and Wildlife often receives anonymous tips referring them to a baited area. It's usually one hunter who is pissed off at another for doing it. Agents have to determine, in the real world, whether the tips are factual or not. At SABS, it is real corn that is baited, and it is real birds that come at it. But then, there is no hunting. I ask him if, by total coincidence, a poacher has ever had the ill fortune to try his luck on these particular marshes in question, the ones utilized by FLETC.

"You know," he says, "I'm waiting for that to happen."

Once the agents have come back and developed the photographs, they plan their expedition by foot into the marshes at night, usually commencing just after dark. Doug walks in with the first group. They're out by midnight.

Following the corn caper, the agents were on pirogues and motorboats for three days getting certified. Their firearms

qualification tests encompassed pistols, shotguns, as well as mini .14 rifles. They were also required to complete a pursuit and emergency response driving program. In addition, during the last couple of years Doug has been having his students look at contaminants, which are taking an increasingly serious toll on plants and animals. The incoming agents study oil pits, heap leach mining, and the use of pesticides to kill predators—which has, inevitably, quantifiable nontarget impact on migratory birds and bald and golden eagles.

It seems like an impossibly heavy dosage for nine weeks, I point out. Doug does not disagree. Four hundred hours crammed into a nine-week program. Several Ph.D. preparations all in one, along with a bit of Outward Bound, Israeli Ulpan (rapid language acquisition) and police academy. But Doug reminds me that that's only the beginning. Once the agents leave FLETC, they'll be graded by training officers throughout the United States—in Sacramento, Jacksonville, JFK International Airport up in New York, wherever the agent is going—and at the end of their first year, they'll be given a graded report that they send down to FLETC for analysis. There is a broad checklist of things that the agents need to accomplish within their first year: writing search warrants, executing the arrests, meeting with U.S. attorneys, and so on. The bottom line, says Doug, is that old Chinese proverb: Tell me and I'll forget. Show me and I'll remember. But let me do it for myself, and I'll understand.

Doug finishes his coffee and the day's session begins. The agent trainees have assembled. Doug, whom I guess to be just under six feet tall, in his mid-forties, a rugged outdoorsman sort of guy, stands before the group.

"Right!" begins Goessman. After a few minutes of joking around he launches into it. "Motor skills decrease during a chase situation. Under high stress encounters—when the heartbeat exceeds 145 beats per minute—you get this inverted V hypothesis. What is it? Well, there's an increase of stress and a

simultaneous decrease in motor performance. Now, let's examine Hick's law. You decrease your opponent's reaction time, and thus increase your options. You've got to decide: penetrate or disengage. And what do you have—you have your baton, OC-10 pepper spray, your angle kick and lethal force. Now I don't want to see any of that embarrassing 'Cops' stuff where the big woman is complying and the arresting officer is still going crazy trying to get the cuffs on her. We're going to stand, eyes closed, and do twenty-five repetitions. This is the speed cuffing method. Now let's pair up."

The agents form five one-on-one teams and spread out. They're barefoot or in socks.

"It's real life. This is good," says a trainee.

The students stand, their eyes closed, trying time after time to get the handcuffs in proper position, to rotate the ratchet and get them open. One of the two female agents laughs, and her face turns red as the cuffs fall down her pants. She collects them at her feet. "Now that would be funny on 'Cops,'" she says.

"Seventy percent of all assaults on officers come from intoxicated assailants," Doug reminds his charges, before recommending toothpaste or baking soda for working through any "cavities" in the ratchets to speed up the handcuffing procedure. "The handcuff is the number one defensive tactic a special agent will ever use."

They will spend much of the morning doing nothing but handcuffing. Trainees have to be sure to double cuff to avoid swelling and the possibility of lawsuits.

"Ambush the hand," Doug demands with a jolting gusto. "Do not come from way out here, do not hit the ulnar bone. Target areas on a small portion of the, say, between the glove and the coat. Always use the top cuff first. It is imperative that the top cuff goes on first. Ask them a distracting question: Do you work out, are you married, do you do needle point? That'll get a chuckle, then have them spread their legs, arms back, now ambush the hand with the top cuff. Do it fifty times."

Doug glares at one of the less agile of his students. "I'm not saying it was slow, it's just that everybody's clothes went out of style while you were doing it."

For the next eight hours this room, and one down the hall which we would move into later in the day, resounds with the hand-to-hand combat, arresting commands, and loud threats of the training. "Sir, you're under arrest, for your safety and mine, bend over at the waist, put your arms behind your back, spread em' like airplane wings, higher, spread your fingers, look forward, palms up, spread your legs, d'you do needle pointing?"

"Come in from your strong hand side! Bladed stance! If it goes to crap, push off, get both hands free, ready yourself for action!" Doug orders.

"Roll that thumb forward and lift up on the handcuff, step and drag back at the same time; loud verbal command—'Get down on the ground!' Keep your extended arm six to eight inches up, iron wristlock, spread your legs, ankles on the ground, palms up, sir, are you married? Do not go on your knees, get on to the balls of your feet, always stay above him. Fingers pointed to the top of his head. Knees to his back, weak knee to the top of his butt, double lock, roll him over, frisk him, stand him up. Now you're ready to transport him."

The Supreme Court in several cases has determined guidelines for the arresting officer that are basic to all law enforcement, but it comes down to a few seconds in the field where officers have to make their own decisions. For two of the agents, this is the first time they've ever used cuffs. But by the end of the day, they are doing it in less than a second.

"What's this pile of skin on the mat?" Doug says, referring to some torn skin from a badly maneuvered pair of cuffs, a shit-eating grin forming, while an agent holds his hand and bites down on his teeth to conceal the pain.

"Now we're going for speed. We're going on the clock now," Doug says.

It's all right out of the Defensive Tactics Instruction Manual. Doug stands with a stopwatch, peering at his class like a rancher watching his boys roping cattle—1.36 seconds, 1.01 seconds, 0.77 seconds, 0.76 seconds.

"South of the border, you run, they shoot. Civil liberties is an American thing," says Doug. "In Mexico they tortured a DEA agent by aspirating a twelve-ounce bottle of carbonated pop up his nose. Anticipate the fears of other cultures and ethnic groups. In the real world it's not a big mat. There's gravel parking lots in places like Mesa, Arizona. Hundred thirty degrees." He's goading the young agents. He knows what it's like out there, where fancy terms like motor dysfunction, temporary muscle paralysis, methods of controlling resistance, and all the other stuff described under the general heading of PPCT—pressure point control training—don't mean squat.

Doug leads them through the ropes, beginning with verbal noncompliance; passive resistance; deadweight—going limp; defensive resistance; active aggression—punching, kicking, biting; aggravated active aggression; and finally, lethal force. These are the stages of combat. He punctuates his discourse with charming anecdotes, like the one about the game warden in northern Minnesota who was run over by a snowmobile as the poachers got away.

"Stimulus response. Take your positions," says Doug.

The five paired teams reverse roles. The good guys and bad guys switch. A real fight erupts, someone gets away, the good guy goes after his neck. Now the escort position. Bad guys pull away. I recognize, by now, the C clamp just above the elbow. Doug butts in: "You want to hit the common peroneal, never on the thigh. Put their palm on your pelvis, push them down. Fingers extended above the head. Elementary aikido. Straight arm bar. Remember, some of the criminals haven't been to FLETC and don't know what to do." He laughs.

And then he comes up to me and—taking my hand—shows me a neat little trick. "Your wrist is not supposed to turn that way." I lurch in pain. He proves his point: the bad guy will be down faster than he ever imagined possible.

Later the group is into digital (as in thumb and index finger) manipulation of the hypoglossal (the lower neck region), the infraorbital (the nose), and the mandibular (that region just under the jawbone). These are three highly sensitive parts of the body, and if you happen to be fighting hand-to-hand with a poacher out in the wild, it's good to know about them.

The agents are instructed in ways of distracting their opponent with a good devastating kick to the thigh or to the inside of the knee. "Get a warrior mind-set," Doug tells them. "There are a few of you who have probably never been in a fight, never even smacked a person." And he's right. The two women admit it. "Well, you must become the hunger. You are mine," Doug says, more Zen master than Rambo at this point. They take out minimats which can be affixed to each other's thighs and Doug walks them through the shin kicks at right angles to the peroneal nerve.

"You're mine, homeboy," one of the students says to his paired opponent, with a burst of karate-like kicking.

"Why not go for the groin?" asks one of the ladies.

"Because a well-placed groin kick can be fatal," Doug quickly responds. "This is not Hollywood. Also, don't forget, you might miss. The groin is a relatively small area. Your kick might be ineffective. The femoral nerve below the groin is better, it's a larger area. First blast the femoral, then the common peroneal nerve."

We break up for lunch, convening over a table in the cafeteria with slabs of cafeteria food at government prices—$1.89 for a vast quantity of greens and french fries. Cokes all around, and a few thousand armed law enforcement rookies and veterans.

A Special Job

The conversation at once leads to the unanimous feeling among the new cadet agents that this is "a special job." These candidates were chosen on a ratio of one acceptee per hundred applicants. And most of those applicants—a pool this year of over 1,500—were top notch. So these chosen ones already know they're the best. But it has not gone to anybody's head. The work is still before them. They've all dreamed of outdoor jobs. And they share a sense of pride about their mission.

Doug had characterized it this way for me, when I first spoke to him about this year's SABS: "This is all you want to do twenty-four hours a day. I mean you cannot believe that you are having so much fun conducting investigations and catching poachers, catching commercial wildlife violators. There is something to be said for sitting in federal district court when the judge looks down at the defendant and says, 'I therefore remand you to the custody of the attorney general of the United States. That means you're going to jail now, we're done playing. The American people and the federal government take wildlife crime seriously.'"

Doug is not with us at lunch, however. The chain of command is such that he has generously advised me that if he's around, the agents won't say much. They'll defer to him. So, in the interest of candor, I tell Doug to eat his lunch at another table. He smiles and takes a hike.

One of the new agents, a former wildlife inspector from Boston named Ellen, will be going to Albany, New York. She has a degree in criminal justice, though she started out as a biology major. When she first got on with Fish and Wildlife five years before she says there were only sixty-five wildlife inspectors nationwide. At that time, there were as many customs inspectors just in Boston. In fact, she says, she was shocked by the discrepancy in human resources, given the fact that the trade in illegal wildlife was, even then, second only to drugs.

"When you look at our manpower to combat the [illegal wildlife trade], which is so low, it's almost like the American taxpayer doesn't want us to succeed."

Ellen went on to work border patrol in parts of Michigan, where she saw an abundance of live reptiles being smuggled out. Canadians routinely come across the border in hopes of picking up cheap domestic shipments from Florida or California and simply driving the animals back across the border. When they'd get to the Canadian side, says Ellen, they would just declare them as tropical fish or something. The Canadian customs officials really weren't concerned; they'd just wave the shipments through. According to Ellen, Canadian customs hadn't a clue about international trading at that time.

Kate has an environmental biology degree and began in the service as a typist, then got assigned to the migratory bird management office as an intern. She managed to get her so-called biologist rating and worked in the ecological services office doing endangered species biology and a lot of contaminants work. From there, she was assigned to the Port of Los Angeles for fourteen months as an inspector before making it as an agent. Los Angeles frustrated her, she says. "The amount of stuff [smuggled wildlife] that gets through. The legal paperwork alone is unbelievable. We don't really have an idea of all the illegal stuff that's coming in. My first time walking into a warehouse, going to inspect fish, there was over five hundred boxes of fish. My mouth just dropped."

Kate explains how the Endangered Species Act (ESA) is broken down into several sections. The part that she had worked was Section 7, federal agency consultation. If any federal agency was working on a project, then the service had to scrutinize it and give it their endangered species impact assessment. For her, the amount of paperwork was frustrating. She wanted to get out into the field. She was working in North Carolina, where there are considerable numbers of freshwater mussels that are endangered. And she would be working with

the same engineering firm for four years going. "'Okay, you guys. Just like last time. Keep your pipes out of the water, attach them to the bridge.' It was the same thing all the time and you have to go through the same process, the same process. And I wanted to be able to say, 'No, you can't do that.' Instead, I had to say, 'If you're really nice, the service highly recommends that you attach these pipes to the bridges, or whatever.'"

I spoke with Rich, a gentle giant, serious athlete type, whose father was an active agent, and a legendary one at that. His father was a game warden when Rich was growing up. He used to go out with him and ride shotgun in the field.

"Ever since I was knee-high to a grasshopper I've been in his shadow following him. And I quickly realized as a kid that that's what I wanted to do." His dual major was in criminal justice and biology. He then obtained his masters in wildlife management and in 1991 ended up, like Kate, at the Port of Los Angeles, where he worked as a wildlife inspector.

His wife got pregnant and they decided they didn't want to raise a kid in Los Angeles. He moved on to the Rocky Mountain Arsenal National Wildlife Refuge as a collateral duty officer. Finally, he got his dream: special agent. He says it was admiration for his old man, and just feeling at home out of doors, and feeling that he could benefit the resource (read wildlife) most by being in law enforcement as opposed to doing biological research.

"I love animals, but I also love law enforcement," says Rich. "It kind of makes you feel good when you ruin someone's day who's been out there doing something that they know they shouldn't have been doing."

But there are some negatives, he adds. He remembers that when he was a kid, his dad was gone so much. He came home once after months in the field, had grown a beard and a mustache and Rich—well-trained to suspect potential bad guys—slammed the door in his face because he didn't recognize him.

"He was just always on the move," Rich recalls.

His father has been shot twice in the line of duty that Rich knows about, with a shotgun. "One time he didn't even tell my mother until after it started to heal up. It's a crazy situation. You kind of have to be a little, you have to be cut from a different cloth to really get into this job, the long hours, adverse weather, crappy lodging, low per diems. When you take on this career, you kind of sign your name, just like a priest. If you're doing it for the money, you're in it for the wrong reason." And, he adds, "There are situations that will raise the hair on the back of my neck and I've already been in a couple of them."

"Like what? What kind of things?" I ask.

"Well, takedowns. The last individual that I helped take down was going through a divorce. He didn't have a whole lot of money, but he was guiding illegally, was known to lose his temper, gotten in fights, gone to jail, so I knew I was dealing with someone who could go off like a firecracker. I was one of the two people who had to go in to neutralize him if the situation got out of hand. We aren't a big agency like the FBI or DEA, where they go in packs. Working big game, you routinely run into camps or you run into blinds where maybe it's five, six, seven, eight to one. You're outnumbered all the time, that's almost a rule of thumb. You don't try to come into a situation blind. If they're drinking and whooping it up and everything else, well, tonight's probably not the best night to come in. Maybe in the morning. Our backup, if we have backup, might be a sheriff, and they're usually not very many per county, or you might have a state game warden. Well, they may be off with their family, you may not even be able to get radio contact. You can't count on backup."

Dan, who comes from a small working station in Texas, turned down a job offer with the Secret Service to come to Fish and Wildlife because, he says, "I hunt, I fish, I fit right in, you know. I like being outdoors, the freedom. No other agency offers you the freedom. I'm never going to get rich being a cop. But it's the freedom that really counts."

Where Dan has worked, along the border, the backup issue was less critical. In fact, backup is authorized given the high drama of both mass illegal migration and drug smuggling along the Texas border. Wildlife smuggling is nearly as endemic. Dan relishes the fact that USF&W agents can choose their weapons. No other agency offers that. He insists that heavy firepower is important. He carries a .45 and keeps a 9-millimeter Smith & Wesson in his truck. The choices seem to be limited to a .40 or .45 caliber or a 9 millimeter. Officers have different preferences. It's the do you want a Chevy, an Olds, or a Ford. Dan's job provides him with a boat, a truck, two Jeeps, and an undercover Camaro. His boss is 100 miles away. "There's a lot of room for creativity," he says.

With his cost of living allowance he makes $62,000 a year. Somehow the discussion goes to lunch. I'm the odd man out—vegetarian. I'm told with grins all around that nobody will hold that against me and if I were an agent, they'd still back me up 100 percent in a life-and-death situation. In fact, there are a few vegetarians among the USF&W agents, just none present. But just a few: most of them hunt and I would learn that this is considered basic to the job.

"The difference is, we're doing it legally," says Dan. "You know what I'm saying?"

Recently, Dan's been up to his eyebrows working on an illegal jaguar hunt out of Mexico and dealing with the proverbial sixteen-year-old teenagers who go off half-cocked with assault weapons and start shooting at anything that moves in the lower Rio Grande wildlife refuges. He's the one agent at the table who has already gone through the SABS course and is here to assist Doug. All the others are new to the job.

Dan acknowledges many politically mired headaches in Texas. "If you go up north to Maine, it's considered unethical to run deer [to chase them with dogs]. But down south, it's like a way of life, it's tradition. A couple of years ago when they outlawed it in East Texas, the people went up in arms and

burned a surrounding forest. I think they also killed a Texas game warden. Landowner's rights, you know. As far as the Commission for Texas Parks and Wildlife, they basically have a policy that state game wardens don't ride with the federal game wardens inside somebody's private property if the state game warden is the one that has the key."

Dan describes what he knows already from experience to be a truth: it's one thing for people to have personal feelings about saving wildlife, but when you're dealing with those whose livelihoods are involved, "they become a lot more dangerous. That's why we take it a little more seriously. That's why I'm a little hypersensitive. People will tell you, don't let the feds find out that you saw an ocelot on your property because they'll come seize it, under the Endangered Species Act. They don't know what they're talking about. But that's how paranoid some people—and the media—can be."

Recently, Dan has gotten heavily into the subject of contaminants. He typically works in conjunction with the Environmental Protection Agency (EPA), under whose jurisdiction contaminant cases frequently fall, as well as Fish and Wildlife. "A lot of money is involved," says Dan. "And a lot of dead animals."

Normally, oil companies are permitted to dump water-based petroleum solutions into evaporation pits. But frequently there is illegal dumping going on with nonwater-based petroleum. Uncovered, the toxic pits attract birds that get trapped and die. Dan has informants scattered throughout the Texas Railroad Commission and the State Department of Transportation. They come to Fish and Wildlife and inform Dan of exposed pits and wildlife mortality. He checks it out, and then asks to see permits, which are regulated by the Railroad Commission and the Texas Natural Resource Conservation Commission, under the EPA strictures. Often, companies have already been advised to cover their pits and they have ignored formal letters and requests. Dan goes out and physically col-

lects carcasses. He takes water samples and sends them to the lab. It's then up to the U.S. attorney.

"You start poking your nose around and they'll clam up. They'll get offended that you would even think that there is something going on politically, you know, between the railroad commission and the oil companies. To prove it is hard."

Dan does not work alone in these cases, but is in touch with the Hazardous Materials Task Force, which is run through the EPA and the Texas Natural Resource Conservation Commission. Along with U.S. Customs, they form a HAZMAT (hazardous material) team. In the wake of the North American Free Trade Agreement (NAFTA) there has been, says Dan, a discernible increase in contaminants cases, as well as hunters going down into Mexico from the United States and then trying to bring back illegal kills. Dan has tried to work with Mexican wildlife authorities but, he confesses, it can be difficult because they are paid so little. "Thirty dollars a week. So they're more susceptible to corruption and to bribes, you know. And when you understand that there's rich American doctors, lawyers, oilmen, going into Mexico to hunt, it's real easy for them to fork out bribes for the local game warden."

For all that, Dan remains optimistic. He feels people will do the right thing once they truly understand what needs to happen. He's particularly interested in public education and is hoping to find broadcast time for the USF&W on television and radio, especially just before the hunting season in Texas. He wants to do a Spanish-speaking question-and-answer program with one of the Texas game wardens that looks at bag limits, possession limits, baiting issues, and the different type of shot—lead as opposed to steel. Dan has noticed over the past several years that more and more of the wildlife offenders are young—fifteen to twenty-three. They are the ones he knows he must reach. Often, their attitude stems from a sense of private property—this is our ranch, we can hunt whatever we

want. Dan himself comes from a small ranch in Duvall County, Texas. And he had definitely noticed less and less wildlife growing up. That sense of propriety over land and over the fate of wild animals therein, coupled with bad droughts, has had the effect of "kicking them when they're already down."

The conversation over lunch veers first to Florida, where one of the cadets is headed after FLETC. There, he already knows he'll be immersed in political controversies surrounding the survival of sea turtles, who are battling for their existence against the increasing sprawl of beach developments, hotels, and apartment complexes. Moreover, he says, USF&W has "a real bad rapport with the state game and fish agency." That's due to political nepotism. The commissioners are hired by the governor and so on down the hierarchy. "So we go out and enforce a lot of controversial regulations and then that comes back to hurt us in the long run as far as just a public presence, so we're starting to get into a lot more public outreach." In other words, USF&W is now teaming up with public relations specialists, doing morning shows, as Dan down in Texas is pressing for, and issuing press releases. Image building with the American public.

Andre, a thirty-one-year-old from Kansas, sums up what all of the new corps of agents seem to be saying: You've got to have the mind-set of protecting wildlife, of risking something every time you go out because it can be dangerous. "We're a team. Biologists are usually—we're pretty liberal people. Law enforcement is very rigid. But we're all working for the same goals. It's a fight for wildlife."

In speaking with the group of cadets, it was clear that they were concerned about what they characterized as a regressive political atmosphere. All were nervous about the fact that America is the number one culprit. A lot more illegal wildlife was coming into the country than going out. At the same time, within the United States a huge amount of wildlife is vanishing—and politically, says the group, the U.S. Fish and Wildlife

Service has its hands tied. Until the public demands more appropriations through Congress, the problems will only get worse as the human population, with all of its developmental wants, increases, in opposition to disappearing habitat. Moreover, many laws are unenforceable, local political situations are making it difficult for the federal agents, money is being scaled back, commercialization of illegally caught critters is exploding, and, in some cases, the USF&W has had for lack of human resources to turn its back on important situations—broader, more effective responses to migratory bird treaty infractions, for example.

And there is another, perhaps more curious concern voiced by the agents, which pertains to lifestyle and demographic shifts across the United States. Says one particularly outspoken agent, "The hunting and fishing population in the United States is disappearing, like less than 10 percent of the population. You have so many kids living now in cities and suburbs who never go outdoors. The first time they see animals are out in the zoo, and I think Fish and Wildlife needs to start bringing hunting and fishing back. People don't have to agree with it, but we need to start teaching people that there's a sustainable use. Hunters and fishermen provide, through their duck stamps and hunting licenses, most of the money. You're also looking at an ethic. If you look back at your dad, or grandfather's time, you know, it was pretty common for people to go out and shoot a deer, turkey, or a goose. They were involved, they were tied whether directly or indirectly with the resource in one way or another. Now the push has been more toward the city. People have become detached. They're no longer in tune."

"But is hunting the only way to get them in tune?" I ask.

No, the agents unanimously reply. They suggest that it can be done through "photography, hiking, or camping—the whole nine yards." But they need more money, somehow.

Hunting or no hunting, it is clear that this crop of new

agents do not believe the Duck Stamp Act provides anywhere near enough of a revenue stream for funding wildlife protection in this country. That the American taxpayer and Congress have backed away from a sufficiently robust financial commitment to preserving the natural heritage is clear. But believing that hunters should be the ones to finance preservation of other life-forms—whatever the conservation gains accomplished by some hunting organizations—is not practical. There are not enough hunters, the revenues are too meager, and hunting trends are diminishing, not increasing. From an ethical point of view, it strikes me as rather obvious that reliance on hunters for protecting other animals is about as clever as entrusting drug rehabilitation programs to crack and heroin dealers.

Says one of the agents, "Most bird-watchers I know, and hikers, too, want to pay more than their fair share—I mean they'd love to—but there are no laws or anything saying, hey, give us your money. So we need to do more PR work."

A Sense of Proactive Hope

The afternoon session is more of the same: hand-to-hand combat, kicking styles, engagement-disengagement protocols, knowledge of where and when a bone breaks, when to let up, when to push it, handcuffing under varying circumstances, and certain techniques of aikido which Doug praises.

I then went back with Doug to his office. I particularly wanted to understand this hunting mentality from the Fish and Wildlife Service perspective. For those who do not hunt—and they are the overwhelming majority of all American taxpayers—there are serious ethical concerns that would otherwise render such hobbies obsolete, throwbacks to another era.

Doug informs me that probably 98 percent of all agents have either hunted or fished or trapped. "And that helps a great deal, to be able to communicate with people in a field

situation and talk to them on their own terms," he adds. "You have to be able to talk with them. When they talk about taking a Boone and Crockett, or a four by five elk, well, you know, what does that mean? I got a nice four point in Illinois. Well that's basically four points total. That one would be a five by five muley, depending on who counts it, or a four by four, but in Illinois that would be a ten pointer. See what I mean?"

Doug takes it even a step further. He's ticked off by the fact that as we speak politicians are considering ratifying certain baiting regulations for waterfowl. If they do so, believes Doug, they'll be turning back the clock a hundred years on waterfowl. He explains that, in his view, people came to the United States to get away from the landed gentry; to freely hunt and fish the way they felt they should. But he sees us going back to the time of the cultural elite, when people who had the money and power created their own private hunting grounds that excluded everyone else. Much like the king's private reserves in the days of Robin Hood. Today, says Doug, if you have enough money to build levees and dikes and drill wells and plant crops and then knock those crops down and flood the fields, that's where all the birds are going to be, and only a few people will get to hunt them.

"If I am an average Joe Duck hunter and I want to go hunt somewhere I will have a harder time finding the birds because they'll be pulled off to larger areas, areas that have been manipulated or flooded by people with money. Private hunting clubs. If you're a private hunting club and for damn sure if you're a commercial club, you're going to make sure your levees are up, you're going to pump your water, you're going to plant your crops first and then go in and mow down all that corn. But Joe Duck hunter has to pay five hundred dollars for a day's hunt. I can't do that. Which is getting back to the reason a lot of people came to America. We're getting away from giving the resource to everybody. I have three boys. I wanted them to experience everything from running a muskrat trapline to

duck hunting, to bass fishing to everything that I got to do. I've been taking them hunting since they were four years old and now they're a bit older. I wanted the resource to be there."

I ask him if he truly believes that by democratizing the resource for hunters everywhere it is more likely to sustain healthier populations of wildlife.

"Sure, because, well, think about it. If fewer and fewer people duck hunt—I'll use duck hunting as an example—they quit because it's all locked up for the privileged, fewer people are going to buy duck stamps, fewer people are going to buy the clothing, the shotguns, the shells, the calls, all of the things that go along with duck hunting. That money will not then go back into the resource. The duck stamps sales alone, the PR [Pittman-Robertson], the DJ [Dingell-Johnson Act, also known as the Federal Aid in Sport Fish Restoration Act of 1950] funds, the sports sales. Why should I pay for a duck stamp if I can't hunt them?"

"And that money, I presume, is critical for continued conservation?"

"Yes," he says. "Because traditionally, although there are nonhunters who buy duck stamps, for the most part, it's hunters."

"Without that duck stamp revenue, what would happen to U.S. Fish and Wildlife?"

"Well, we'd be set back quite a lot."

"Do you know for a fact, have there been studies of that?"

"I don't know." But he does mention that on the state level there have been several initiatives—in Georgia, in Illinois, in Minnesota, and elsewhere—where there are nongame fish and wildlife funds that you can support by checking off the little squares on your tax returns. In fact, thirty-three states have such a fund, usually designated as a "Nongame Wildlife Fund."[4] He also points out that there have been other proposals to actually tax hiking and bird-watching gear for purposes of conservation, which is congruent with the fact that in

America the people who utilize "the resource" are the ones paying for it.

The monies raised by the various hunter-related taxes are not inconsiderable. In fact, the Pittman-Robertson program (also known as the Federal Aid in Wildlife Restoration Act), established in 1937, took in sufficient excise taxes from hunters, fishermen, and water sport enthusiasts during 1996 to be able to distribute approximately $399 million to the state wildlife agencies across America.

I tell Doug I find it curious that he, and all of the wildlife agents that I've spoken with, refer to wildlife and nature as "the resource," which is a totally different perception or concept than the one held in, say, the animal rights or animal welfare community, who would never call them a resource. They call them animals.

"Oh, they've humanized them," Doug says matter of factly. And I realize that he is not caught up in the expressions one way or another. His heart is in it, that's all; he makes no apologies for the fact we live in an imperfect world, and he has a single, I would say noble, goal which he has worked toward his entire career. "The way I see my job and responsibility and the way I've perceived it for twenty years—this is my twentieth year as a wildlife officer—is that I have a duty and a responsibility to enforce the laws of the United States and protect wildlife for future generations. That's it, that's all. That's what Congress wants, that's what the people of the United States want. And to do it constitutionally and adhere to all federal rules of criminal procedure and evidence. It's a complex job."

"Do you ever get really depressed?" I ask him.

"Periodically, yeah," he admits. "Because, think of it, from the conceptual standpoint throughout the United States, there are only two hundred thirty-five special agents with the U.S. Fish and Wildlife Service. It's ludicrous. It's nothing at all, but I'll tell you what, the American taxpayer, and you can quote me, they're getting their money's worth out of these folks.

You've got people working seventy, eighty, ninety hours a week, spending time away from their families, traveling."

He refers to the case study which they analyzed in this SABS session, the undercover operation that unveiled, among other things, an illegal fishing operation on Lake Michigan that took out millions of pounds of perch—excesses that nearly wiped out the fish species. While a number of people worked the case, two in particular made it happen. If not for those two officers—a state warden and a federal agent—who exposed the syndicate just in time, the perch would have been finished. But, he repeats, the odds of routinely catching the bad guys are not great. Even in the case of the perch, they were a year too late. It could take decades, or longer, for Lake Michigan perch to recover.

There are approximately 7,000 wildlife officers in the United States and Canada, and that includes absolutely everybody—the 235 USF&W special agents, and all the state, federal, provincial, city, and county personnel. Some are in the field, but most of them are behind their desks, far removed from the wilds. The United States *and* Canada, he repeats. And then he reminds me that we have no way of even guessing how many infringers are out there among, for example, the millions of travelers who come through a port like Los Angeles International Airport—one of dozens of ports, where, say, one crate or piece of luggage or handbag in twenty may—may—get checked for illegal wildlife. The tens of millions of hunters, among whom some percentage is going to exceed various regulations at least some of the time, deliberately or inadvertently. The crime syndicates. The systematic poachers. The wholesalers. The buyers.

And as he expresses his concerns about current trends in wildlife protection, and the American public's responsibility, my mind races to the map, taking in the enormity of the landmass, all the mountain ranges, the hundreds of millions of acres of forest, and the vast coastal stretches, the tens of thou-

sands of lakes—four of them, in Canada, stretching over 10,000 square miles—and ponds; all that diverse romantic geography—nearly 7.5 million square miles combined—which, as children, propels our imaginations on the wings of migrating geese, perks up our senses to be alert to the cry of the wolf or the loon—creatures that have been here for over 100 million years.

And Doug brings me back: "Seven thousand wildlife officers. That's about one-fourth the size of the Chicago police department."

But I can't help thinking of a more devastating analogy, given the rate of habitat destruction, extinction, endangerment, and sheer attrition among wildlife: 7,000 officers versus 7.5 million square miles of operational territory for poachers. That translates to about one officer for every landmass the size of Yosemite National Park (which is roughly 1,200 square miles). And that one officer is doing everything: answering phones, manning the entrance, filling out forms, racing up and down trails, surveying backcountry, giving out speeding tickets, checking on fire hazards, and a hundred other things.

If that doesn't crystallize the problem, how about thinking of it in urban terms: one officer for every three cities the size of Los Angeles.

But it's not just the exasperating, denuded discrepancies of the number of good guys versus the unquantifiable proliferation of possible bad guys. "There are horrible, horrible problems with wildlife," Doug reiterates. "For example, you've got less than one thousand black palm cockatoos in Indonesia. It's an extremely rare, secretive bird. So people have a chance to make ten thousand dollars off these things. Well, they're not going to try to sell these in a Third World country. They're going to come to the United States, where somebody can write a check for thirty thousand dollars, or whatever the market will bear. And at the same time, out of the same checkbook these people are making contributions of five hundred

dollars to some conservation organization to clear their conscience. We buy our way out of it. There's going to come a point in time when you can't buy these things back. They're gone. We have some success stories, too. But for the most part, we have to understand that in the United States we're part of the problem. You have to really think, you know, What am I doing? Do I really need an ivory bracelet, the scrimshaw, especially now, when you can make it out of plastic? It just doesn't make any sense to me. If you've ever seen a carcassed-out elephant, or seen the evidence storage room in South Africa for the South African police of the ivory seizures that are smuggled in and out of the country, and the rhino horns—there's one right there." He points to horns mounted on the wall of his office from some earlier police raid. They're huge and heavy; the blood that must once have splattered them when they were sawed off had been erased. "I mean, that used to be a living animal." And he goes on, "They're just teetering."

Despite the fact, says Doug, that historically the American public has been "reactionary"—by which he means that we drive the passenger pigeon to extinction and only then enact tougher laws protecting birds; we nearly wipe out the American bison, and only then find a refuge for the remaining twenty—despite all that, he believes that "the American people have a good heart. They really do. But it takes a little bit of education and just a bit of common sense and caring and keeping abreast of what's going on throughout the world" to change things.

Doug ruminates out loud. He knows that species are going extinct. For them, it doesn't get any worse. But he also radiates a sense of proactive hope which I have felt among all the special agents of the U.S. Fish and Wildlife Service this day. For Doug Goessman, it seems to come down to one simple truth: the love of nature. He might not talk about it in such terms— I suspect he wouldn't—but to know him, and those like him,

is to catch signs of it in every aspect of their demeanor and obvious commitment.

To love something, to cherish nature, you have to have experienced it, been sensitized to it. "I'm a parent," Doug says. "And parents have a responsibility to their kids. They don't have to hunt or fish, but just get them exposed to the out-of-doors, through the Boy Scouts, through whatever means."

It's late in the day, and I'm hankering to visit one of the Barrier Islands. Doug lights up, hands me a map, and starts rattling off where I can find the most beautiful beaches, special groves of trees, and likely flocks of birds. "Get the hell outta here," he says. "Sun's going down."

3

Operation Renegade

In 1993, the U.S. Fish and Wildlife special ops branch concluded Operation Renegade. It involved a series of investigations into the underground parrot pipeline that led from Africa and the Amazon to New Zealand and Australia, Mexico, Los Angeles, Chicago, and New York. Sadistic opportunists and pet store owners had sustained a cozy little business for several years. Broadly speaking, it still persists, and 70 percent of all exotic avians are endangered. But at least one cast of these nasty characters was dismantled because a few decent people were outraged enough and called in a tip to the federal government. Operation Renegade would result in the uncovering of an elaborate laundering and smuggling scheme valued at well over a million dollars that had profited at the expense of thousands of rare birds that were savagely captured and painfully transported to buyers.

This case merits close attention, as much for the strange twists of psychopathology that would compel a bird expert to break the law, as for the law itself, whose history in terms of wildlife preservation reflects a jittery pattern of increasing sensitivity to the kinds of things people like ornithologist/philosopher Theodore Barber have been saying for generations. Wildlife law is only as good as the work of wardens, inspectors, rangers, special agents, and prosecutors fighting to enforce it. The agents deliver the evidence, but it is the prosecutor who must effectively justify the charges before a judge

and/or jury. In order to come through with convictions, agents and prosecutors must work closely together.

The prongs of Operation Renegade, as the many separate cases involved in the operation are referred to, concerned unrelated smuggling rings with conspirators operating in several countries in Africa; in Paraguay, Argentina, and Mexico; in Australia and New Zealand; and several regions across the United States. In many smuggling cases, birds are transported in tires, or drugged and stuffed in tiny containers, their wings and beaks taped so that for days, or weeks if shipments get caught up at customs, they cannot move their wings or eat or drink, thus drawing attention to themselves. More often than not, the animals will die, or are permanently maimed and traumatized, or flushed down toilets on airplanes because they may have had the bad timing to hatch while being carried in body packs. But because an exotic parrot can command $10,000 or more at your local pet store, the economics are always in the poacher's favor. He may kill 100 birds. But if he manages to get a live one to an American neighborhood, he has struck gold.

How a small team managed to infiltrate this kind of major illegal bird-smuggling ring and track down international criminals through a maze of multijurisdictional paperwork, bank accounts, false leads, local informants, and cooperating law enforcement agencies is but one of many stories at the heart of what the wildlife wars are all about. The legalities, forensics, and crime-busting techniques, as well as the overall ecological concerns, biological dynamics, and habitat issues, all came into play throughout Operation Renegade in a manner that says much about the promise of conservation, and of law-abiding citizens, when efforts to combat poaching are earnest and well-coordinated.

It is not possible to name all of the defendants, agents, prosecutors, and wrongdoings. Or to revisit the thousands of pages of particulars that came out in various testimonies. Books

could be written about Operation Renegade and all of its important implications. I have chosen to highlight a few of the cases of the multitiered investigation—in particular, one Justice Department prosecutor whose own commitment to fighting wildlife crime is especially exemplary and indicative of the high quality of his cohorts, the five or so prosecutors employed at any one time by the Wildlife and Marine Resources Section of the U.S. Justice Department for the sole purpose of prosecuting wildlife cases.

The story is best begun, perhaps, with what was to become known as the United States of America versus John Allen and Bess Kelly (I've invented the names of all those charged, out of respect for their families). This case involved a conspiracy by numerous bird traffickers who were pursued by the special ops branch and ultimately convicted on a variety of charges, including the illegal smuggling into the United States of 186 rare hyacinth macaws and countless other species from South America.

The Lives of Birds

An abundance of groundbreaking research into interspecies communication that goes by the name of cognitive ethology seems to support the contention that birds "conceptualize," possess extraordinary "navigational intelligence," "form abstract concepts," harbor an "ability to play with joy and mate erotically," and "communicate meaningfully."[1] Theodore Barber, one of the most compelling researchers in this field, writes, "The voluminous data I encountered during my six years of total immersion in avian studies and observations led to the unexpected conclusion that not only are birds able to think simple thoughts and have simple feelings, but they also are fundamentally as aware, intelligent, mindful, emotional, and individualistic as ordinary people."[2]

Having lived for some time in the immediate company of diverse parrot companions—environmental refugees that have become a major part of my family and homelife—I can attest to Barber's perceptions. To share in their majestic, evocative lives and be needed by them is to shudder with absolute horror before the all-out assault on their kinds by rapacious poachers.

It is believed that as many as 80 percent of all so-called exotic birds in the world are doomed to extinction, given the current killing taking place, largely as a function of illegal trade—the smuggling of parrots, primarily, from their jungle and rain forest homes to the United States and other countries, where they are brokered, usually, by pet store owners who knowingly collaborate with the smugglers, or acquit their hearts by simply playing dumb. An estimated 90 percent of all parrots captured in the wild for purposes of smuggling abroad die before reaching their destination. According to TRAFFIC USA, a division of the World Wildlife Fund, as of the mid-1980s, at least 800,000 wild-caught and rare birds were being imported into the United States every year. While the Wild Bird Conservation Act of 1992 appears to have reduced that overall number, there are still, for example, an estimated 50,000 rare birds being smuggled across the U.S.-Mexico border each year. Most are parrots. At least 40 species of parrot are thought to be facing extinction, probably a conservative number in light of the fact that rain forests are disappearing at an escalating rate over even a few years ago. And this despite so much alleged consciousness-raising worldwide.

Hyacinth macaws are found deep in the Brazilian Amazon and in parts of Bolivia and Paraguay, where their behavior in the wild is little known. With body lengths of 100 centimeters or more, they are the largest of all the parrots in the world. The adults are monogamous for life; their babies (which are blind and naked at birth) require three to four months in the nest before they are ready to fly away. For most of the first year, the young are still fed by their parents.

Theodore Barber has suggested that "birds are able to generalize, form abstractions and nonverbal concepts . . . they remember, or 'store' past information as proficiently as humans. At times, when it is useful in their niche, they manifest a long-term memory that is superior to that of most humans."[3] Parrots are known to be descendants of the dinosaurs. Their brain cavities are spacious. According to Joseph Forshaw, one of the world's foremost authorities on parrots, reports pertaining to extraordinary parrot intelligence began surfacing as early as the time of Aristotle and Alexander the Great.[4] A famed physician in the court of a Greek king made mention of a certain plum-headed parakeet accustomed to speaking an Indian dialect that was taught to speak Greek. Yet, it wasn't very long ago (1957) that the phrases of speech articulated by members of the family Psittacidae were declared in the *Encyclopaedia Britannica* (under the "Parrot" entry) to be inconsequential: "It must not be thought that this implies anything more than a mimetic power, or that the bird understands what it is saying."

Today there are countless celebrated parrots whose intelligence has been recognized as much more than mere mimicry. Alex, an African gray parrot, has been in captivity for nearly two decades. During that decidedly unnatural period he has accommodated himself to his human companions and learned the meaning of hundreds of English words which he speaks fluently, creatively, inventing his own original sentences, answering abstract queries, and tellingly interacting with the investigators around him.

All evidence regarding birds points overwhelmingly to their possessing powers of intellect, sensitivities, and curiosity previously reserved by humans for dolphins and chimpanzees. Like these two mammalian species, parrots engage in extensive sensuous foreplay before lovemaking. And like at least some humans, as the mother parrot feeds her young, so, too, the male parrot feeds his mate. And, also like dolphins and

chimpanzees, the parrots are distinguished by their unfortunate penchant for bonding, under some circumstances, with humans, a fact implicit in their current endangerment.

A few native species of parrots used to inhabit the United States prior to their deliberate extinction. The last of them, the Carolina parakeet, died out the same year as the last passenger pigeon, Martha, in 1914. There are still some flocks of parrots that can be seen routinely in parts of southern California and Texas, though it is believed that these are composed of birds that had been captive and escaped. Thick-billed Mexican parrots frequently cross the U.S. border. But efforts to reintroduce the once native Arizona parrot have failed dismally.

The total retail value of the 186 hyacinth macaws smuggled into the United States by those pursued as part of Operation Renegade was estimated by the courts in 1994 to be $1.3 million. Today there may be fewer than 2,000 wild hyacinths left.[5] At current trends, these long-tailed, cobalt beauties will soon be gone.

And it is not just hyacinths whose flocks were pillaged, birds yanked out of their nests, drugged, and stuffed into tiny cardboard containers, false-bottom suitcases, or plastic pipes by the thirty defendants convicted at the conclusion of the Operation Renegade investigation. Among the various cases of Renegade, other rain forest avian species were pursued along with the hyacinths. These included crimson-bellied, Queen of Bavaria, and blue-throated conures; vinaceous Amazons ("so rare they are considered priceless");[6] Cuban, yellow-shouldered, yellow-faced, lilacine, and red-browed Amazons; lesser sulphur-crested cockatoos; yellow-collared, red-fronted, Illiger's, and the nearly extinct Spix's macaws; the Chilean flamingo; the thick-billed parrot; Toco toucans; and the Mount Apo lorikeet. Exotic-sounding names, but to see them, in their audacious spectral hues, all the colors and more of the aurora borealis, coursing the winds of humid air above the forests is an unforgettable experience.

The Case Develops

John Allen, Chicago-based ringleader of his own little band of smugglers, one of the Operation Renegade prongs, knew precisely what birds he was obtaining. His knowledge stemmed from real expertise. He'd grown up with parrots and at an early age began compiling research and then publishing in magazines. In his mid-twenties at the time his illegal activities evidently began, he was already recognized for his supposed compassion for and knowledge of parrots. He had authored two noted books, *A Monograph of Endangered Parrots* and *A Monograph of Macaws and Conures.* In the first book, he had actually described the hyacinth macaw as "being worth its weight in gold." In 1989 Allen became curator of birds at Loro Parque, a bird sanctuary in the Spanish Canary Islands. Bess Kelly, his mother and codefendant, lived in Illinois. Both of them should have been aware of the fact that the birds they were importing had been deemed by the U.S. Fish and Wildlife Service—the CITES enforcement authority within the United States—as endangered species under the Endangered Species Act, Title 16, U.S. Code, Section 1537(a). Twenty-three parrot species in all are currently listed as endangered under ESA. Classified under Appendix I, these birds were known to be "threatened with extinction, unless protected by law." In fact, Allen himself had written, "Unless all of the pressures (including illegal trade) are brought under control, this species may be unable to survive in the world to greet the 21st century." And it was Allen who had helped found a Recovery Committee to save the Spix's macaw—considered to be the rarest parrot in the world—from extinction. The blatant contradictions demonstrated by this supposed lover of avians shocked many in the bird conservation community. Allen, after all, was one of them. He'd written scores of articles commending the fragility and beauty of these birds. He attended all the aviculture conferences and was something of a star. Maybe the stardom went

77

to his young head. I have spoken with numerous bird people and investigators, all of whom have their own, off-the-record perceptions of why Allen compulsively broke the law. Personal financial gain seems to have been a powerful motivation.

The details of Allen's smuggling operation have largely come to light. Their mundane particulars make for no action thriller. Allen had met one Butch Jenkins at a trade show in the fall of 1985. Jenkins was at that time an exotic bird importer, not doing very well, and seeking to establish ties with a South American vendor. Jenkins eventually agreed to let Allen use his quarantine station near O'Hare International Airport for smuggled birds, if Jenkins himself could have some of them for his own subsequent profit. While Allen was publicly advocating strict rules for the trade in exotic birds, he was secretly conducting an operation that included a thoroughly orchestrated scam at Jenkins's quarantine station. Birds arrived with forged paperwork. According to a USF&W memo, "The birds were brought inside and the back door sealed. But while [Allen] distracted the agents [a Department of Agriculture employee engaged in preparing quarantine paperwork in the front office of the station], [Butch Jenkins] unscrewed the hardware holding the seal and slipped the illegal birds out the back door. Other bird crates stored nearby were placed on the pile, so agents wouldn't notice the sleight-of-hand." The principal supplier for Allen was a woman named Monica Sánchez, who lived in Asunción, Paraguay. She was never tried because the smuggling of birds is not part of the U.S. extradition treaty with that country. However, there is an outstanding warrant out for her arrest in the United States resulting from this case.

In addition to violating the ESA and CITES, Allen also violated U.S. Department of Agriculture quarantine requirements for failing to declare the imported species and thus posing a threat to the domestic poultry industry in America. The disease most feared by the DOA is exotic Newcastle disease, caused by a virus not found in the United States and to which domes-

tic chickens and turkeys are highly susceptible. There is no known cure. All birds imported to the United States must be quarantined and checked for at least thirty days prior to their release. In the case of the psittacines smuggled in by Allen and his coconspirators, the birds were immediately transferred away from the quarantine station and sold to various pet store retailers around the country.

The Chicago quarantine station was not the only receiving port for the smuggled birds. According to the June 1994 grand jury charges, defendants Allen and Kelly received or transported birds between states from the vicinities of San Diego (where a safe house had been set up), Los Angeles, and Miami. And in at least one instance, following an advertisement Allen took out in the August 1989 issue of *American Cage Bird Magazine,* a breeding pair of Queen of Bavaria conures were sold for $5,000 to a resident of the Commonwealth of Virginia.

The conspiracy began around July 1985, and would continue until it was finally shut down one early morning when special agents entered the homes and work environments of the many coconspirators across the United States on January 17, 1992. In a taped phone conversation between Allen and an individual known to the authorities as the "Cooperator" on or about August 7, 1990, Allen dismissed the Cooperator's fears about getting caught or going to jail because, as he put it, "neither you nor I are gonna be anywhere near those birds when they land there." He was referring to the fact that others in the U.S. smuggling operation would take the heat.

The many laws broken by Allen, his colleagues, and others involved in the separate cases of Operation Renegade were not merely those of the United States, however. Wildlife protection is taken seriously in the many countries of origin that were affected—namely, Argentina, Bolivia, Brazil, Ecuador, Mexico, Paraguay, Australia, and New Zealand. But because the majority of end users were American, Operation Renegade reflects a very serious concern among law enforcers: the fact

that it is here, in the wealthiest nation in the world, that the vast majority of global wildlife crimes are consummated. The United States is the largest importer of wild-caught (illegal) birds.

In the government's proffer regarding admission of co-conspirator statements, infringements of the Endangered Species Act and the Lacey Act (for which it is a criminal wrongdoing to purchase or sell wildlife with a value of more than $350 in violation of any treaty, law, or regulation of the United States), as well as false income tax reporting and false bills of sale—tax conspiracy—were all part of the general indictment. The smuggling pipeline began with John Allen buying hyacinth macaws and other protected psittacines from a bird supplier in Argentina who had covertly obtained them from the seller in Paraguay. The live birds were shipped by air to Mexico, and transferred onto flights bound to Chicago. The smuggled birds were then commingled with legally imported birds at the Jenkins quarantine station in Rosemont, Illinois. The cover was easily maintained. In late 1987, the Argentine coconspirator was dropped from the program after many of his illegal shipments were received dead on arrival. Then Jenkins found himself overwhelmed by financial difficulties, which led him to close down his quarantine station in 1989. After that time, Jenkins ceased to commit illegal activities. But Allen and Kelly continued to search for other means to continue their profitable smuggling operation. At the same time, and based upon various statements and his own articles, one suspects that John Allen began justifying his actions to himself on the grounds that he was saving the rare parrots from other poachers in the wild. He knew how to take care of them. He loved them. And he was an expert. He knew what was best for them.

Through an intermediary, an unsuccessful attempt was made to bribe a Mexican customs official. During this period, Allen recruited another individual who agreed to assist him in

his scheme to smuggle hyacinth macaws into the United States. That individual, who was later to become a Cooperator with the U.S. government, went straightaway to the Wisconsin Department of Natural Resources, reported Allen's crimes, and then agreed to work with USF&W in an undercover capacity. Beginning in early January 1990, the Cooperator recorded many of his conversations with Allen, Kelly, and others. For two years he managed to tape 194 discussions about illegal smuggling activities. Code words were used. The hyacinths were referred to as "azules" or "blues." Eventually, a conspirator was identified in southern California who got birds across the border, delivered them to a business known as the Pet Ranch near San Diego, and then arranged to have the live animals sent via air freight to Allen in Chicago. A supplier in the Philippines was implicated. Conversations drifted to a smuggled parrot-feathered headdress, an elephant tusk, the problems at the Mexican border, and a buyer who ran an animal business called Zoological Imports in Miami. That buyer acquired 35 "azules" from Allen in one shipment. According to the government's proffer, most of these hyacinths died shortly after they were received in Miami, indicating the extent to which these birds had suffered in capture and transport. In fact, a veterinarian examined the avians and "found that the birds suffered from a variety of fungal and bacterial infections that were consistent with prolonged captivity in ground pits used to trap the birds in the wild."[7]

Part of the government's evidence against Allen and Kelly included photographs of piles of yellow-collared macaws and baby Toco toucans that had arrived at the quarantine station from Mexico dead. A note in Kelly's handwriting, also yielded up as evidence, explained: "Photos made at the moment of taking them [the birds] out of the box."

In other evidence that surfaced, it was shown that two buyers from Virginia met Allen around midnight outside Kelly's home, where Allen produced a dozen hyacinth macaws in cages

stuffed into his car. The two buyers purchased six of the birds, paid Allen $24,000 in cash, and drove back to Virginia. On paper, such machinations fail to convey the privation endured by the birds throughout all of these transactions; birds which had just survived the long flight in storage to Chicago, via Mexico, Buenos Aires, and Paraguay, smuggled under conditions in which nine out of ten typically perished, only to end up in the totally alien environment of a Chicago suburb at night, prior to being driven all the way to Virginia. Evidence shows that several of these particular Virginia-bound hyacinths died in subsequent days.

By the time of the takedown in January 1992, agents had already traced money transfers to South America, Allen's personal travel itinerary to Paraguay and back, and smuggling notes with expressions such as *"nuevo embarque"* ("a new shipment"). As early as March 2, 1989, New Zealand wildlife officials informed the USF&W that they had arrested an individual attempting to smuggle four African gray parrots into that country. A resident of New Zealand had already admitted in a recorded conversation with an undercover USF&W agent that he was to receive the parrots from that arrested individual, who had, in turn, received them from Allen.

That same month, according to a government brief, Allen directed a California bird breeder to "drive him in a pick-up truck to a residential location outside of Los Angeles where a number of Chilean Flamingos bound in nylon were tossed into the back of the truck." These rare birds were purchased by Allen for $50 apiece.

Meanwhile, Allen was continuing to be secretly taped during conversations with the undercover Cooperator. Allen acknowledged that he knew the birds were being wild-caught. In once instance he said, " . . . I mean I know like—I know the Red-vents aren't Captive-Bred . . . they've got burns . . . from mist nets on their feet."[8]

Allen and Kelly had also smuggled mammals into the

United States, including 9 golden lion tamarins (out of a total wild population on earth of 350). In addition, a dozen white-faced marmosets and one woolly spider monkey had been illegally shipped by the Argentine connection, who testified to one of the Fish and Wildlife special agents.

From records seized in the search warrants, it became clear that the coconspirators had not reported to the Internal Revenue Service gross income of at least $168,325 from the sale of these avians and mammals, representing a tax loss of $47,131 to the federal government. Some of the illegal sales were verified in an interview conducted in the United Kingdom by an agent from Scotland Yard who was able to determine that one British citizen had paid Allen $50,000 for wildlife. Other documents showed deposits and exchanges of checks through the Guarani Cambios Paraguayan currency exchange—more than $370,000 in transfers. Multiple bank accounts were utilized; cash deposits were orchestrated to avoid currency reporting requirements; cash was laundered into South America using employees of the Paraguayan national airline; checks were misdated and signatures forged; receipts were also forged and records falsified.

Four years after the sting operation began, on January 30, 1996, Allen pled guilty to two felony counts, including the broad wildlife smuggling conspiracy charge and "relevant conduct" as well as filing a false tax return. Kelly pled guilty to filing a false tax return. The government's sentencing memorandum revised its earlier estimates and now figured that the total market value of all the wildlife involved in the offenses was between $1,500,000 and $2,500,000. This value was based upon the "fair market retail price," not the "smuggler's price." The value was derived from affidavits from various expert witnesses, including a scientist at the San Diego Zoo, and from a comprehensive survey of bird prices conducted by TRAFFIC USA, an organization devoted to the monitoring of international illegal wildlife trade and part of the World Wildlife Fund in Washington, D.C.

While the government goes out of its way to be fair in such cases, ascribing an average price within a definable range of market values, in the case of the blue-throated conures, no value whatsoever was ascribed because the birds were deemed "priceless."

Pricing out birds is not as easy as it might seem, but it is crucial to sentencing. Consider the cockatoo egg-smuggling case, the so-called Australian prong of Operation Renegade. (Note that this involved an entirely separate cast of characters from those in the Allen smuggling ring.) The defense would argue that because a lot of the birds would have died in the wild had they not been spirited away by poachers, the government's figure on wildlife value was unreliable. The government's market value estimation was computed by multiplying the number of eggs of each species smuggled times the typical amount paid to the smugglers for each bird of that species raised to the age at which it could be sold. But there are many loopholes by which bird smugglers might try to lower the imputed value of the wildlife they have smuggled in hopes of reducing their fines or jail time, as determined by the judicial system of Sentencing Guidelines. A defendant might argue that he did not smuggle birds, but rather eggs; and he might add that the declared market value for the adult birds should be reduced by the amount the smuggler spent to raise those eggs. He might also point out that 90 percent of the birds hatched from those eggs had died, and hence had no value; and since biologists concur that many birds die in the wild before they reach adulthood, the smuggler should be congratulated for actually saving birds. Judges are not likely to be impressed by such circumlocutions. In the case of the cockatoo eggs, the judge had important legal precedents to assist him in his considerations. One such case was *United States* v. *Oehlenschlager* (76 Fed.3d 227), which was appealed and denied. Mr. Oehlenschlager had smuggled duck eggs from Canada to Minnesota, had raised the birds, and then had sold them.

When he was sentenced, the government prosecutors were able to point to Oehlenschlager's own price lists, which he had maintained. His sentence appeared to be a done deal. Not exactly. Oehlenschlager, incredibly, contested the market value assumptions presented by the prosecution by describing how he wasn't very good at raising wild ducks and many of them had died. Therefore, he didn't make as much as the prosecutors were claiming. Furthermore, he had his own expenses. By such logic, if he had been totally inept and had killed them all, there would be no value and therefore he should have been entitled to the benefit of being a bad husbander, analogous to the guy who kills both his parents and then pleads he's an orphan and should be treated leniently.

In the Australian prong of Operation Renegade, prosecutors added enormous credibility to their bird egg valuations by flying in expert witnesses like Joseph Forshaw, the world authority on parrots whose testimony is, to put it mildly, not easily negated. But regardless of the clarity of evidence brought before the judge, the federal Sentencing Guidelines impose a mechanism on the sentencing process that doesn't allow for arbitrary determinations of the severity of the defendant's conduct. Rather, federal judges have to employ a formulaic approach in fashioning the sentence. In wildlife cases, the jail time is determined according to a series of criteria, various offense levels (points) which translate into months behind bars or fines. The levels are computed according to whether, for example, it can be proved there was commercial conduct in the case, or a failure to quarantine, or a proven conspiracy. The offense levels rise again if there has been an obstruction of justice. If the defendant has been arrested on prior crimes, that, too, might bear upon sentencing. The judge gave the individual in question a $10,000 fine and sixty months' incarceration with no possibility of probation. There is no parole in the federal system. None. One can get a little time off for good behavior; it's called "good time" and can be up to 5 percent.

But there is no parole as there is in the state system, where, for example, a child molester might get ten years and eighteen months later be up for a parole hearing.

Indictments in the Australian prong of Operation Renegade took place in Montana, Florida, and Los Angeles. Five individuals pleaded guilty without a trial; one person went to trial and got thirty-seven months.

Meanwhile, in Chicago, Sergio Acosta, deputy chief of the U.S. Attorney's Office and lead prosecutor in the Allen affair, was wrapping up the government's case. Following his signing of the detailed plea agreement, John Allen suddenly reversed his disposition and—according to the characterization in the government's Sentencing Memorandum—alleged that he led a "fundamentally blameless existence." The memorandum went on, "[Allen] has consistently refused to accept moral responsibility for his crimes that have resulted in the plundering and suffering of wildlife—with a tenuous foothold on their very existence in the wild—in exchange for his personal profit and self-aggrandizement."[9] All of these facts combined led the court to impose a sentence for Allen of eighty-two months and a $100,000 fine. Kelly received a sentence of twenty-seven months and no fine.

Federal wildlife cases are complex and the legal aspects are handled, normally, by U.S. attorney's offices throughout the nation, often with the assistance of the Wildlife and Marine Resources Section (begun in 1979), a section within the Department of Justice's Environment and Natural Resources Division. One of the senior trial counsels of the Wildlife and Marine Resources Section is a tall, sturdy fellow in his early forties by the name of Robert Anderson. It took me many months to obtain clearance for an extended interview with him. He was graciously hesitant to speak. Sit-down interviews with senior government prosecutors are apparently rare. They are generally prohibited from doing this, often because cases that may be in the public record may also still be on appeal.

Clearly, Anderson's colleagues trust his prudence. He has a reputation for being one of the most serious, knowledgeable, persistent, and effective of the prosecutors concerned with wildlife in the United States, and he is quick to acknowledge that the information concerning encroachment upon wildlife is very important and that the public needs to understand what's going on.

Once we finally met, Anderson could not have been more cooperative and forthcoming, though he forewarned me that his comments would be measured to the extent of not giving "too much aid and comfort to the enemy by providing smugglers with inside information about how we do our jobs." His is a level of concern and professionalism that is inspiring. Anderson, I found, is also tremendously modest about his own efforts and was not keen to be singled out. He is a part of a team and has no desire for the slightest celebrity.

A graduate of the University of Montana School of Law, Anderson works out of the Denver Field Office within the Environment and Natural Resources Division. The kinds of cases his section is likely to take on range across the whole spectrum of wildlife infractions. For example, perhaps the Sierra Club decides to sue the U.S. Fish and Wildlife Service based upon its belief that a plant or animal has not been listed under the Endangered Species Act; in that case, civil lawyers in Anderson's section might represent the Fish and Wildlife Service. Or, if a lawsuit erupts over spotted owls and salvage logging in the Northwest, or the reintroduction of wolves into Yellowstone, Anderson's section may well be called upon to litigate.

Anderson prosecutes criminal federal cases involving wildlife laws. While he is an expert on the criminal provisions of the dozen primary federal wildlife statutes, like the Endangered Species Act, the Marine Mammal Protection Act, the African Elephant Conservation Act, and the Bald and Golden Eagle Protection Act, he is particularly knowledgeable about the Lacey Act, passed into law in the year 1900 and repeatedly

amended since that time, and has written one of the definitive essays on its history and legal context.[10] The Lacey Act is often characterized as the most far-reaching and effective wildlife law in any democratic country in the world. I say democratic, because in at least a few nondemocratic countries, poachers have been known, on occasion, to be executed.

The Lacey Act and American History

In Anderson's essay on the Lacey Act for the *Public Land Law Review,* he presents highlights of various cases recently prosecuted by the Department of Justice to intimate the sheer range of wildlife crimes punishable under Lacey, and to illustrate the "scope of the problem" facing wildlife enforcers in the United States. He refers to various live animals, eggs, and body parts smuggled into this country: pythons from Papua, New Guinea; "laundered" gray parrots from Africa; over 3,700 sea turtle eggs from El Salvador; a tiger skeleton, a rhino horn, and bear bile brought in by a Chinese; Alaskan protected sea duck eggs; Sonoran desert saguaro cactus; gazelles and Pakistani sheep; illegal caviar and mussels; and endangered crocodiles. Often, Anderson emphasizes, "prosecutors may also file smuggling, conspiracy, tax, and even money laundering charges against those who traffic illegally in wildlife."[11] Drugs are sometimes involved in the wildlife cases. In the period between (fiscal) 1993 and 1994, Anderson points out that "more than 700 Lacey Act criminal counts were filed in U.S. federal courts" and the resulting charges amounted to some "315 months" of jail time and over "$1 million" in criminal fines.[12] At first glance, the total seems like a lot of counts. But, after a moment's calculation, one is sadly aware of the fact that all those counts, and all that incarceration time, is short-lived in comparison, say, with the normal jail time, or, more likely, fines that would greet a corporation that has exceeded its air

pollution quota or illegally dumped toxic wastes. And yet, Lacey, which falls under the administrative duties of three departments—Interior, Commerce, and Agriculture—is the most potent and far-reaching of all wildlife laws in a country distinguished for harboring more wildlife crime than any other nation. There is no easy explanation for this seeming laxity, except to recognize that America has had a long history of minimizing the inherent value of wildlife. As author Peter Matthiessen relates, there was a time a few hundred years ago when, in Boston, you could buy six dead passenger pigeons (also known as turtledoves, or wood pigeons) for a penny—the same penny you earned from the Massachusetts Bay Company as a bounty for killing a wolf.[13] It was precisely this pattern of devastation of America's natural heritage that prompted Congressman John Lacey of Iowa to introduce the bill into the House of Representatives in the spring of 1900.[14] The congressman solemnly understated his resolve: "There is a compensation in the distribution of plants, birds, and animals by the God of nature. Man's attempt to change and interfere often leads to serious results."[15] Even with the Lacey Act affirmed, the subsequent evolution of a demonstrative concern about other species has been a sluggish and checkered one, more often marked at best by grudging acknowledgment and at worst by outright indifference. Laws, judges, and lawyers are a reflection of a society in all of its ambivalences, and American society is still far more exercised over crimes perpetrated against humans and human property than any other life-forms. The theft or destruction of a lifeless thing, should we possess it, throws us out of whack, by and large, more thoroughly than a massacre of other species. And a person who writes a few bad checks or steals a loaf of bread is likely to receive greater punishment than someone who tortures a horse or kills a chimpanzee.

When the Lacey Act came into being, America was largely in denial about its decimation of the bison and the passenger pigeon and countless other known species. In 1957, in his first

book of nonfiction, *Wildlife in America,* a work which, like Rachel Carson's subsequent *Silent Spring,* helped usher in the most recent phase of reflective, retroactive environmentalism, Peter Matthiessen cataloged the glaring litany of American wildlife exterminations. But by then, at least, there were scores of laws trying, however unavailingly, to counter the tide of biological devastation in North America. But back in 1900, when the Lacey Act was passed, our concept of extinction was primitive.

Consider just some of the species Matthiessen details that Americans drove forcibly, even deliberately in a few instances, to or near extinction: the bison, the passenger pigeon, the short-tailed albatross, the West Indian monk seal, white-tailed kites and Aplomado falcons, the masked bobwhite, the eastern gray wolf, the cougar, the heath hen and Attwater's prairie chicken, river sturgeons, the fisher, the sea mink, the Pacific right whale, Steller's sea cow, the Pallas cormorant, the Guadalupe fur seal, Brewster's linnet, the Colima and Cincinnati warblers, the ivory-billed woodpecker and the Townsend bunting, the western bighorn sheep, the Arizona and tule elks, the Dawson and woodland caribous, the Eskimo curlew, the California condor, the Everglade kit, and the Cape Sable sparrow.[16]

American legal history mostly ignored these creatures. Americans feared them, hated them, ate them, impaled them, skinned them, poisoned them, ran them off their land, and made a show of slaughtering them in numbers that defy quantification. We would like to think that decades of increased environmental consciousness have refined the public's appreciation of wildlife in this or any other country. And to a very major degree, there has been a learning and love-of-nature curve. But the ambivalence is still there.

Consider the unspectacular case of certain city prosecutors today who have endeavored to shut down the pigeon-related activities of a woman in Pasadena, California. The case has received nominal notoriety and pertains to a resident who

has been leaving birdseed and water in a little bowl every day for about fifty wild pigeons in front of her house. This practice evidently violates a Pasadena city ordinance, the maximum penalty for which is six months in jail and a $500 fine. The prosecutors say they want to keep the city streets clean and fear that the pigeons could spread salmonella and respiratory ailments. This "quiet churchgoing woman with a bag of seeds" (as she was characterized by the *Los Angeles Times*) describes the pigeons in the following way: "God created each one of them. He used his hands and his time to create them. They were here long before us, and they will be here long after us." As far as Theodore Barber's research has shown, pigeons "conceptualize at a high level of abstraction," doing things it was believed only humans or primates were capable of. They can "hold in mind" a sequential order; they can recognize one person in a crowd, as well as all "twenty-six letters of the English alphabet." They can distinguish human from nonhuman, different types of triangles, "put together a series of known elements in creative ways to solve a new problem," and perform "at least as well as mammals" on a variety of subtle psychological tests.[17] In referring to the city of Pasadena, the accused pigeon lover declares, "They are not harassing me, they are harassing God." The prosecutors say they would have no problem if she fed the birds in the city park, and her attorney has suggested a compromise whereby they leave a trail of bread crumbs from her house to the park.[18]

This incident, however innocuous on the surface, reflects an antipathy underlying America's historical perception of wildlife, the strong feelings such hostility has generated among animal lovers, and the uncertainties of the lawmakers who must steer a tenable course between perceived public need and the preservation of a natural heritage.

North Americans have never agreed on what is, biologically speaking, a tenable course. Take just one rather astonishing set of data which Peter Matthiessen graphically presented

in *Wildlife in America,* the brazen particulars of a slaughter that was totally sanctioned by lawmakers, hunters, corporate sellers and buyers, and the ordinary consumers who obliviously partook of the by-products: "A Hudson's Bay Company sale, in November 1743, disposed of 26,750 beaver pelts, as well as 14,730 martens and 1850 wolves; that these were by no means the only victims, even among their own kind, is indicated by the fact that 127,080 beaver, 30,325 martens, and 1267 wolves, as well as 12,428 otters and fishers, 110,000 raccoons, and a startling aggregation of 16,512 bears were received in the French port of Rochelle in the same year." Matthiessen adds, "People today who have no reasonable expectation of seeing even one of these creatures in the wild without considerable effort to do so might well look carefully at these figures."[19]

When Congressman Lacey put forth his act, Americans were fiercely convinced of their proprietary right to do virtually anything they wanted with the land and its nonhuman inhabitants. A Supreme Court ruling in 1896 (*Geer v. Connecticut*) reasserted that each state "owned" its wildlife, meaning neither property holders nor the federal government could intervene. In practice, ownership went with ownership of the land. If you owned your land, most Americans tended to do what they wanted with it. Further complicating such cultural norms, hunters—and hunting laws—respected no such thing as ownership. Hunters set traplines over vast terrains, ran dogs from property to property, set out on long horseback journeys over backcountry, or through rural woods, that might be held by any number of ranchers, farmers, or government agencies, in pursuit of their quarry. What made *Geer v. Connecticut* so troubling was its prioritization of legal mandates such that well-conceived national conservation strategies could exert little leverage over a multiplicity of state-run gaming commissions whose membership was comprised of hunters. (*Geer v. Connecticut* would not be overruled until 1979, at which time the

federal government claimed its rightful authority in the pursuit of national conservation.)

According to Matthiessen, the wolf vanished from the East Coast around 1900, the cougar in 1903. These animals did not just fall back to safer, wilder terrain: they were bountied, shot by hunters who earned for their troubles a few dollars each. In 1890, America and Great Britain almost went to war over England's refusal to temper the appetite of Canadian sealers in the Pribilof Islands of Alaska. Yet our own abuses sailed clear off the charts. For example, in 1900 the Alaska Company, which in the previous twenty years had managed to slay 47,482 sea otters in the American Northwest, could find only 127 animals left to kill.[20] By 1905, the Badlands bighorn sheep was extinct. In Delaware, hunters exterminated the last of the white-tailed deer by 1910, the same year emergency measures were effected to curtail the extinction of America's pronghorn antelope. Similar eleventh-hour machinations had saved the last of America's great bisons, reduced from at least 60 million just fifty years prior to a mere 20 weary, genetically starved individuals. Much has been written about the staggering hatred and near genocide unleashed upon the American bison, revisited most recently in the Montana-sponsored slaughter of 1,074 of the majestic beings.[21] Their protection came only after they, and the Native Americans who relied on them for their own sustenance, were essentially gone. As Matthiessen describes, President Ulysses S. Grant had refused to sign long-debated and delayed bison protective measures in order to better ensure the extermination of the Sioux Indians. It must be rememberd that the Indians themselves had also wantonly massacred the bison, sometimes leaving the entire animal for its evidently desirable tongue.[22] Today there are an estimated 150,000 bison in mostly private herds across the United States. This slow rejuvenation (their populations will never come close to regaining the genetic viability they enjoyed up until the

mid-nineteenth century) is the result of Theodore Roosevelt's commitment to saving them, after his having walked through deep prairie grass littered to the horizon with scattered bison bones.

Like the once abundant bison, the passenger pigeon was so numerous, even as late as 1880, that a single nesting area in Wisconsin was said to have contained 136 million birds. That's 136 million high avian IQs. No conservationist imagined that these gentle and unassuming beauties would ever require protection. But eyewitness accounts of their slaughter started making it into newspapers. When they would roost "there were literally thousands of hunters and trappers on hand, armed variously with net, fire, and shot, as well as with an assortment of homemade contrivances designed to perform the most heroic destruction in the shortest possible time."[23] Millions of birds would be killed in one long night, and shipped off at prices of about a penny to two pennies per bird. The unthinkable happened; extinction came swiftly and the last wild passenger pigeon was killed "for scientific purposes" in the spring of 1900, within days of Congressman Lacey's presentation before his peers.

Congressman Lacey was determined to inject a stringent legal regard for all that had been previously denied in American history: the recognition that other species could become extinct, and that those already pushed toward the brink must be allowed to recover, must be granted the right to exist unmolested. For many species, like those referred to above, the Lacey Act was too late, or nearly so. As Matthiessen writes, "Protection has spared not the multitudes but the stragglers."[24] The Lacey Act forbade interstate commerce involving unlawfully taken wildlife. It also manifestly rejected all imports from other lands of creatures for which there was no permit. By setting the regulatory tone for what was to become the U.S. Fish and Wildlife authority, the Lacey Act gave serious warning to all those who would profit illegally at the expense of wildlife.

Three years after Lacey, the first federal wildlife refuge was established, at Pelican Island, Florida. And within ten years of the act, three other serious national wildlife protection treaties and statutes were enacted, indicating the government's firm intention of intervening at the state level, as need be, for purposes of protecting migratory species and any seriously endangered plants and animals. This newfound interest in conservation did not encompass predators, raptors, rodents, or most "dinner" species, however. Nor were hunters easily convinced that bag limits were necessary.

While there are now eleven laws and seven international treaties that form the framework for federal wildlife protection, the Lacey Act remains the government's key mechanism for deterring crimes against wildlife and is generally considered to be the first federal law in American history to systematically attempt to protect wild species.[25] It is by far the most rigorous challenge to any lawbreaker, as it is boosted by sentencing parameters that may exact the most jail time and fines.

In trying a defendant under the Lacey Act, one important strategy among many available to government prosecutors is the matter of trying to prove that the person "knew the wildlife was, in some fashion, taken, possessed, transported, or sold illegally." The defendant did not have to know anything about the Lacey Act itself.[26] Depending on whether the "state of mind" of the defendant was "negligent" or "intentional," and whether the charges invoked were of a misdemeanor or felony type, fines and incarceration for a single individual can range up to a maximum of $250,000 and five years in prison.[27]

Every state has at least one—and usually several—U.S. attorney offices, and the prosecutors therein are typically engaged in cases across the criminal spectrum: bank robberies, drug-related crimes, white-collar fraud, crimes against federal property, and, of course, wildlife-related cases. Robert Anderson frequently serves as a resource for assistant U.S. attorneys (AUSA's) all around the country who are involved in federal

wildlife litigation and need some backup. He'll "midwife" a case, or take the lead in prosecuting it himself. His primary clients include the National Park Service, the U.S. Fish and Wildlife Service, the Forest Service, the National Marine Fisheries Service, and the Bureau of Land Management. At any given time, he calculates, he's involved to varying degrees in as many as ten wildlife cases, not necessarily as the principal prosecutor but as the "backstop." At any one time, however, he might have five to ten defendants, and they may be located all over the country. Anderson, who is married and has one child, travels, on average, about seventy-five nights a year.

Anderson's frenetic pace is not unusual for lawyers in his section. Anderson himself points out, "The colleagues that surround me continually impress me and make me proud to be a government employee. The agents particularly that I work with, work tremendous hours for low respect, certainly from the public. There's no recognition. They don't work their buns off because they're making a lot of money or they're getting a lot of benefits or they're getting a lot of strokes. These are people who are doing it for the resource." And he reiterates the lack of prestige associated with the job: the fact that it's not going to engender an automatic jump to the next level of any career; and that, as a lawyer, he's not going to be courted by the big civil law firms. "You're going to cul de sac yourself into a very narrow specialty of the law. If you don't love it, you're not going to want to do it because you're going to get no respect, you're not going to get rich, you're going to be on the road, away from your family *all* the time. There's no other way to do it well."

But Anderson also points out that wildlife law is a field sparsely occupied. "What I like about this job is that, unlike areas involving pollution crime or habitat degradation, there are very few lawyers specializing in this particular area. As a law student, and even later as a lawyer, I did not know the field existed until I had contact with the Wildlife Section attorneys."

Operation Renegade harbored precisely the kinds of cases that Anderson knows best: international illegal trade ending up in America. While destruction of habitat is considered the primary threat to many species, illegal trade is the second most devastating problem. And for some species like rhinos, Bengal tigers, the giant panda, and macaws, to name but a few, trade is the number one threat. When Anderson was called in as a prosecutor in Operation Renegade, the cases came from several different arenas, all tied together by the fact that numerous birds of various species were being smuggled out of Australia, South America, and Africa, and a tight force of special ops (the undercover agents with the USF&W) were tracking the crimes. All that paperwork would ultimately be handed over to a small team of Justice Department prosecutors. Some of the cases within Operation Renegade are still in court and Anderson was not at liberty to discuss them.

Operation Renegade comprised several ongoing investigations. John Allen and his South American coconspirators constituted one of those prongs. The smuggling of African gray parrots out of several sub-Saharan countries by a second group of culprits was another. Australia was a third prong. In this latter instance, a group of people in the United States were going to Australia every year in the fall to steal cockatoo eggs from nests they had mapped out, often in national parks. They actually hired people whom they labeled "mules," using drug dealer parlance, to carry the cockatoo eggs in concealed body vests back to this country, where the eggs were hatched, the babies reared, and then sold quite openly and fraudulently as having been captive-bred.

The poachers knew when to expect the egg-laying period, but for any pair of birds there's going to be some daily variation. This meant that the poachers could not gauge precisely the levels of maturation for any given egg they wrested from the nests. One can "candle" eggs by holding a bright light behind them and observing the stage of the embryo's

development, but that technique doesn't tell you when the egg will actually hatch. Trial testimony revealed that there were occasions in which mules would be on the plane flying back from Australia and a chick would start to hatch out inside the smuggler's hidden vest and begin to peep and cry. In such cases the hatching eggs were flushed down the toilet of the aircraft. Eggs that started to hatch out in the motel rooms in Australia were also destroyed.

Australian cockatoos are listed as CITES (Appendix II in that international treaty). Australia does not allow their export for commercial purposes, and some of the subspecies are very difficult to breed in captivity. Emotionally, physically, these birds are incredibly fragile. When you add those facts together—restricted export, difficulty in captive breeding—you get a bird that is highly sought after by collectors. Parrots caught wild, except under certain exemptions for research, cannot be legally trafficked in the United States. Captive-bred birds can, which is unfortunate: it encourages an insensitive industry of captive breeding, where only money is at issue, not the fate of the birds, who are difficult, demanding pets and find themselves frequently in transit between disgruntled owners who no longer think them "cute." Parrots form rapid emotional attachments. When these are repeatedly severed by uncaring human companions, the birds suffer. In addition, this captive breeding loophole in the law, which makes it nearly impossible to actually track the true origins of pet birds, provides a shell for smugglers who know that birds like the Australian cockatoos will command as much as $15,000 apiece in the United States.

The details surrounding the undercover work on the Australian prong of Operation Renegade are better left unrevealed. In the end, Australian customs agents were able to identify patterns of frequent travel among suspected individuals.

Of course, multiple passports had been obtained by the poachers, which made trailing them more difficult. The smug-

gling ring went on for about a ten-year period, during which time at least 860 eggs were brought into the United States. There is no way to know how many others were destroyed in the process. In some cases, the eggs were being smuggled from Australia to New Zealand, put in aviaries there and made to appear as if they were captive-bred, then exported from New Zealand to the United States. Once the birds made it to this country, the smugglers advertised in bird magazines and sold them very openly as captive-bred. In exchange, the conspirators in New Zealand were receiving smuggled eggs from the United States—especially African gray parrots and macaws. One of the defendants in the New Zealand prong was the operator of the U.S. Department of Agriculture Pet Bird Quarantine in Los Angeles, where some of the live birds from New Zealand arrived. The defendant, a woman, allegedly allowed the smugglers to evade quarantine in exchange for a few of the birds. She was, like Allen, a professed bird lover who probably felt that she was helping her friends, importers who she believed really wanted these birds, felt they were beautiful, and were going to take good care of them. But when you have a quarantine operator who's so connected to a smuggler that he or she turns a blind eye to an illegal import, the whole system breaks down because that's the first line of defense. Once the animals are in the country they're easily laundered, because there is no sort of permit system whereby the U.S. Fish and Wildlife Service continually checks every breeder to make sure that the amount of progeny match the amount of birds. The available manpower is not even close to ensuring such scrutiny.

As a rule, the fortress is weak because the job of clearing wildlife shipments is so stretched. Without the reliability of quarantine operators, the task is that much more difficult. Most of the time inspectors look at the paperwork on the shipment, not the shipment itself. If you ship in two tons of bananas from Paraguay, the inspector is not going to look at every banana,

but trust that the operators and the paperwork, in concert, are reliable indicators of a legitimate shipment.

Sometimes the inspectors conduct secondary searches and turn up people with considerable contraband in their possession; individuals at LAX with snakes wrapped around their bellies and ankles heading out to China, or coming in with bear gallbladders strapped around themselves. One man was caught with seventeen bear gallbladders attached ingeniously to his waist.

The End of Renegade

Early in the morning of January 17, 1992, the various prongs of Operation Renegade came to a head. Armed marshals, local police, and undercover agents who had worked the cases—some thirty state and federal agents in all—served search warrants and collected evidence in Florida, California, New York, and Chicago, all at the same moment. Anderson was in New Paltz, New York, handling coordination of the legal aspects of the takedown in that area for the day, and was not involved in the Los Angeles or Chicago search warrants.

The head conspirator of the Australian cockatoo egg prong was abiding in Van Nuys, California, where agents had tracked him and "freshened" (prepared) a search warrant. Meanwhile, affidavits were being prepared and reviewed by the local Los Angeles assistant U.S. attorneys.

In the case of the New Zealander, he'd been tempted back into the United States. His flight was delayed. Everyone around the country was holding off until that plane touched down.

And then the coordinated search and seizure went down as planned, coordinated with precise (and rather dramatic) simultaneity around the country. Special agents confiscated everything relevant to the cases—canceled checks, travel stubs, passports, incubators, bird feathers, ads, invoices, receipts, let-

ters from buyers, brochures for various businesses, and photographs.

After warrants were served, Anderson and his boss, John Webb (the assistant chief of the Wildlife and Marine Resources Section of the Justice Department in Washington, D.C.), were the two prosecutors most involved in the various prongs of Operation Renegade. But there were too many individual parts, too many defendants, too many thousands of pages of paperwork. Prosecutor Sergio Acosta in Chicago took the lead in the Allen case and Anderson withdrew in order to devote more time to the cockatoo case. No one person could be lead prosecutor for all of it. In fact, when Anderson got into Operation Renegade, he was still finishing up duties pertaining to the USF&W's Operation Whiteout, up in Alaska, involving drug dealers, an Eskimo community, and the slaughter of walruses for their tusks.[28] The man was stretched across numerous bloody battlefields. Despite his heavy schedule, Anderson managed to be lead prosecutor against the cockatoo egg conspirators, fifteen individuals in all.

The leader of the cockatoo egg case would go to jail on a sixty-month sentence under Lacey Act smuggling and money-laundering convictions. According to the testimony, that lead conspirator was an aviculturist with a bachelor's degree in biology and a peregrine falcon expert.

The various avian species victimized by the defendants in Operation Renegade are likely to invoke a range of sympathy from those who hear about the cases, particularly in regard to those birds that are endangered. But, as Anderson points out, "the endangered status of the species may not be relevant." And, he goes on, "we are always careful to ask the jury to judge the case on the facts and the law, not based on sympathy they may feel for the dwindling numbers of animals in a population. Of course, if the crime charged is an Endangered Species Act violation, we are required to establish that the species is threatened or endangered. However, we still can't ask the jury

to convict out of sympathy for the species or the individual animals involved in the case or out of anger at the defendant."

In an age when lawyers have been reduced, too often, to the picture of money-grubbing ambulance chasers, wildlife prosecutors certainly defy the stereotype. Not that their message is entirely comforting. As we wrap up our conversation, Anderson muses, "It seems clear that poaching and the illegal trafficking in wildlife around the world is at epidemic proportions and likely to continue as species decline and increasing rarity makes prices rise. Here in the United States we are doing a fairly good job of interdicting illegal wildlife, but it's doubtful that we're catching the majority of it. In other countries the situations are probably no better and in some places it is clearly worse. But it's a problem that people need to wake up to. Everyone has heard about saving the rain forest because the serious problem of habitat loss and degradation is well-publicized. But wildlife trafficking is also serious: it poses the most direct threat to survival for some species; it promotes the introduction of disease and pest species; and it's very often inhumane. It's not yet in the public mind, for example, to think about smuggling or poaching when they see an exotic lizard in a pet store or a parrot in a cage. Folks assume that if the animal is being sold openly, it must have a legal origin. All too often, this is not the case, and people should get in the habit of thinking twice and asking questions before they buy an exotic pet or a product made from animal parts like a dream-catcher or a reptile-skin purse or a trinket made from ivory or bone."

I tell him that I hope people will read this chapter and think, you'd have to be really dumb to try to get away with something like this when government prosecutors like Anderson and his colleagues are out there waiting to nail them. And Anderson replied, "Well, I hope our cases have a deterrent effect. Though we certainly don't catch them all we are finding that the courts, the public, and the media are starting to take

a serious interest in the cases we do bring forward, and the message should be clear: if you are caught smuggling or poaching wildlife, you may face a fairly stiff penalty."

Given the rotten odds of catching the bad guys, I asked him—as I tended to ask everyone I interviewed—what keeps him motivated.

"I'm lucky. I love my job because as a prosecutor it's my job to seek the truth and try to see that justice is done. As a Department of Justice lawyer it's my privilege to represent the people of the United States in court. And as a specialist in wildlife crime it's my pleasure to work with a truly committed group of investigators on cases that seem meaningful. And along with the day-to-day prosecutions, every now and then I get to handle a large-scale case aimed at a fairly significant wildlife trafficking problem. That's very satisfying to me."

4

Hunter and Hunted

We're winding our way along a dirt road through the Mingo Reserve, the last giant bald cypress and tupelo swamp in the state of Missouri, near mist-engulfed Lake Wappapello. We're making a slight detour on our way to Van Buren, a compact, picturesque town in the southern part of the state. The road travels through primeval mangroves that are home to the rare alligator snapping turtle (*Macroclemys temminckii*), the largest freshwater turtle in the world, with recorded weights exceeding 200 pounds; hellbenders—big aquatic salamanders worth their weight in gold throughout the Orient; endangered collared lizards; and a decreasing number of box turtles. And every December rare black-billed trumpeter swans fly through here and stay several months. There are less than 1,000 left in the lower forty-eight states.

"It always bugged me," says Dan Burleson, who holds tight to the rattling steering column, "that the crew of the starship *Enterprise* never wore seat belts." It's not that Dan is that uptight. He readily emits loud laughter and has a playful and boyish demeanor. But at forty-one years of age and seasoned in his business, Dan is an intensively dedicated, not-to-be-messed-with lawman, one of four U.S. Fish and Wildlife special agents in Missouri, a state where hunting is basic to the temperament, history, and lifestyle of many of its denizens. And many Missourians have strong feelings about hunting, as, of course, do hunters everywhere. Walt Disney grew up in

Missouri, and whatever feelings about nature might have been inculcated in the lad certainly found expression later in his film *Bambi,* a great work of art, but one reviled by many hunters in Missouri who view it as an antihunting diatribe.

The issues surrounding sport hunting are thorny and the emotions and beliefs about hunters' rights and responsibilities run deep. Though many hunters respect the letter of the law and espouse passionate views in support of a healthy environment, there are others who blatantly flaunt regulations and display only a grotesque disregard for animal life. One particularly troubling poaching case that Dan Burleson is wrapping up when I visit him reflects deeply on the nature of hunting, and the kinds of hunting-related conflicts and mind-sets that arise on either side of the law.

A recent Missouri Department of Conservation (MDC) annual poll of environmental attitudes throughout the state revealed that at least 25 percent of those surveyed were hunters and that 90 percent considered hunting for food acceptable. Nearly two-thirds of Missourians felt trapping was "okay" as long as it was regulated. A smaller majority supported hunting when "the motives for the activity were camaraderie and tradition." Most of those questioned "were opposed to hunting for an exceptional animal, or trophy hunting."

In 1996, during the statewide firearms deer season, which lasts from November 16 through November 26, Missouri hunters killed 180,395 deer. January 3, 4, and 5 are also open hunting days for antlerless deer. The autumn is for turkey hunting; in 1996, Missouri hunters harvested 13,144 birds.

Missouri's "outdoor calendar" is published by the state Department of Conservation. As in every other state, it lists the bag limit (daily possession) and open and close of every hunting season per animal. For example, hunting season on bull and green frogs begins June 30 and closes October 31. A hunter with a permit can take up to eight of them a day (or possess sixteen), using a .22 caliber rimfire rifle or pistol, pellet gun, or

longbow. Mark Twain, that famous Missourian, who celebrated the jumping frog, would probably cringe at the notion of a single hunter killing nearly 1,000 of the animals during a season—the approximate limit, albeit an extremely unlikely sum per person. Twain might also be concerned by the fact there has been a noticeable number of deformed frogs turning up in the state, which researchers are investigating. Presumably ozone is involved, or chemicals. Of course, by the end of Twain's own life, there were many other signs of wildlife attrition: much of the big game, including elk and buffalo, as well as deer—the principal diet for the native Sauk and Fox Indians—had been exterminated, along with panthers and bears. Even the wild turkeys and beavers had nearly vanished. The successor species, at least from the standpoint of Missouri hunters, comprised "possum, skunk and civet cat."[1]

There are no current limits on the number of groundhogs that can be killed in Missouri between May 6 and December 15. The restrictions are more limiting, however, for common snipe, doves, and blue, snow, Ross, Canada, and white-fronted geese; for brant and gray partridge; for quail and rabbits; for ruffed grouse, squirrels, teal, bearded turkeys, and Virginia rails. If you're trapping rather than hunting, there are no limits to the number of beavers, coyotes, or other furbearers that one can kill in the state of Missouri. Beavers, which were gone from the state by 1915, have made a spectacular comeback in recent times.

Hunting for meat is a long-standing tradition here. It is said that "an average deer yields about 8 pounds of tenderloin, 14 pounds of roasts, 18 pounds of steaks and 20 pounds of ground venison." Meat packers across Missouri charge customers who bring in their dead deer about $8 to skin the animal and around $45 to process and package the meat.[2] A resident deer-hunting permit costs $11; nonresidents spend $110. With a permit and what's called bonus permits, a person is allowed a maximum of three deer kills per season.

With one deer averaging 140 pounds, the total amount of known deer meat harvested in Missouri in 1996 was approximately 25,255,300 pounds, of which approximately 10,823,520 pounds were edible meat. Most of that meat is eaten by hunters and their families and friends. Of course, parts of the deer are also used in various industries, such as the production of buckskin clothing and deerskin rugs. So there are some economic benefits involved.

But for a large number of Missourians, hunting is valued more as a way to be in touch with nature. Missouri is a state that boasts a remarkable profusion of diverse ecosystems, from freshwater marsh and sinkhole pond swamps to bottomland prairie and forest, chert glade and savanna, and prairie fen. Grasslands, lakes, rivers, and mountains. The state has much to offer the nature enthusiast. And its flora and fauna are astonishingly diverse. But the most immediate sign of life in Missouri's forests is the deer. In the early years of modern conservation (beginning in 1946), the Missouri deer-hunting season was severely restricted to just one county and a total of three days, due to the small and delicate population of deer, who had been decimated in previous decades. But there has been a systematic comeback. Now, all of the state's 114 counties are open for at least eleven days of deer hunting, and the sport has been on the upswing. Recently, the Missouri Department of Conservation even sponsored a "Becoming an Outdoorswoman Workshop," a three-day event at a Benedictine monastery where—along with sessions on how to recognize edible plants like elderberry, sorrel, and Queen Ann's lace—the women learned about deer and turkey hunting, bait- and catfishing, shotgunning, riflery, and bowhunting.

In order to control the amount of hunting and try to prevent the decimation of the deer population, which had happened in the past, the Conservation Department issues quotas that biologists have deemed acceptable. Those quotas are divided up according to the state's fifty-seven deer management

units, and the managers figure out how many animals can be killed according to a labyrinth of data derived from computer models, hunter consensus, observations by conservation agents, and the number of deer killed in car accidents. Hunting is the primary cause of deer mortality, however, and every year between 40 and 70 percent of all antlered bucks, and about 25 percent of all does, are hunted down.[3] Because the managers try to the extent possible to keep track of rebirths in each unit, they are able to show that with this number of kills the population remains stable, more or less, from year to year.

Therefore, while there is a great deal of hunting going on, there is at the same time a strong environmental ethic at work in the state. Yet this ethic is not perceived as contradictory to the strong spirit of hunting. The fact is that many avid hunters tend to profess an avid love of wildlife. For some people who do not support hunting, this duality might seem logically untenable and disingenuous. Those who advocate a philosophy of absolute nonviolence are unlikely to find much comfort in the backwoods of Missouri. For hunters, hunting organizations, and most conservation programs, however, there is no contradiction. The conservation perspective that dominates in the hunting circles declares that humans are in a position of control and are charged with maintaining a healthy balance in the wild.

In May 1997, the Missouri Department of Conservation awarded $110,000 in grants to thirty-five elementary, middle, and high schools across the state for developing outdoor education classrooms; an effective way to put young people in closer touch with nature. Conservation agents in the state are responsible for nearly 14,000 radio programs and 4,000 articles each year, all promoting sustainable environmental protocols, an astonishing track record for any agency. Missouri is probably the only region in America where people would celebrate a giant catfish (Ol' Blue), a thirty-pound monster which, after serving seventeen years as the MDC "spokesfish" and

living out its languorous life in a 155-gallon aquarium at the Missouri State Fair, was released into the 55,600-acre Truman Lake, for purposes of "retirement." When a fisherman caught the leviathan months later, it was well on its way to weighing 100 pounds. He liberated it back into the lake. Thus, while many Missourians have a great enthusiasm for hunting (note the more than 100,000 deer killed over the first typical weekend of a hunting season), they also take much pain over the preservation of biological diversity. You can have both—controlled hunting *and* biodiversity—according to most (not all) conservationists the world over.

In the "1994–95 Wildlife Diversity Highlights" report, the Missouri Department of Conservation described its efforts to "reclaim some of what has been lost" by "dynamiting homes for rare turtles," "releasing ospreys, prairie chickens, pallid sturgeons, Niangua darters, collared lizards," and keeping tabs on a number of threatened or endangered species like gray and Indiana bats, alligator snapping turtles, peregrine falcons, freshwater mussels, Ozark cavefish, and rare pondberry plants.[4] The state is working with the national organization Partners in Flight (PIF) to find ways to better preserve habitat for the "greater prairie-chicken, loggerhead shrike, dickcissel, cerulean warbler, ovenbird, Kentucky warbler, wood thrush and tanagers," birds in need of conservation throughout Missouri.[5] The same state government that has no limits on the number of crows that can be killed also informs residents as to when and where they can best view, and play host, to the arrival of hummingbirds or eagles returning in winter, much in the same way that Californians are told about the best places to watch whales during the same season. In addition, the MDC publishes information on how to help migratory purple martins, bluebirds, chickadees, and wrens nest more easily in the state by providing nest boxes at home and controlling parasites with "a teaspoon of sulfur, cedar chips or diatomaceous earth (found at garden centers) in each compartment of a

martin house."[6] And finally, the state has begun Operation Game Thief, in which people can anonymously call a toll-free number twenty-four hours a day to report mischief. Brothers have turned in brothers, neighbors neighbors. Rewards are granted. The number is 1-800-392-1111.

According to a survey by the Humane Society of the United States, Missouri hunters kill nearly 5.5 million animals each year—a number that exceeds the total human population of the state, and is the seventh-largest number of animals killed by hunters in the United States—after California, Illinois, Louisiana, Alabama, Pennsylvania, and Texas. Missouri hunters spend approximately $339 million per year on their sport, most of which goes to private business. A little more than 1 percent of that total, $4.2 million, is collected for refuge preservation under the Pittman-Robertson Act. Nonhunters who merely enjoy wildlife without killing it contribute more to the state's economy, roughly $440 million each year.[7]

Because hunting is so common throughout Missouri, there are going to be, and there are, scores of poaching incidents. But in a region where 5.5 million animals are legally killed each year, it is not surprising to find a judicial system that is too frequently "soft" on poachers. Nine times out of ten, if you kill a deer out of season, without a license, or over your bag limit—even in a state park—all you're likely to get—assuming you get caught—is a ticket. Normally, in state court you pay the court costs and no fine. But the official maximum penalty is a $500 fine and six months in jail (unheard of). More often than not, the case will be dismissed, and all you end up paying for is the ten-minute court cost, between $50 and $100. It varies from county to county, whom you know, or whether you're a repeat offender. Dan has seen cases dismissed or fines lowered as a direct result of favoritism.

That sort of politicizing of wildlife infractions is not unique to Missouri, by any means. Dan worked for USF&W in Minnesota for two and a half years before coming to Missouri. He

once appeared before a Minnesota judge with a sixty-year-old who had pleaded guilty to shooting an eagle, an officially endangered species in that state at that time. The man informed Dan, and the judge, that he thought it was an owl. Under the Lacey Act, as a Class A misdemeanor, he stood to pay $100,000. But he was poor, on a very low, fixed income. Dan felt that $200 would be a reasonable fine, probably more than the man could pay off in a year. But the judge wanted the case thrown out entirely. That utterly surprised Dan Burleson.

"The judge had made several bad calls against us [referring to the U.S. Fish and Wildlife Service]. He didn't like us as an agency, I guess," said Dan, speculating that perhaps the judge himself had once been caught in the act and had a personal hunting violation against him. Whatever the reason, the judge actually told the defendant "I think you can beat this, so I'm not going to accept your plea." And he instructed the U.S. attorney to "find a civil remedy to take care of it." In other words, dismiss the case.

And it's not just poachers the system tends to downplay, but also the keeping and breeding, under often murky (read horrible) circumstances, of any kind of exotic wildlife. As the saying here goes, "If it ain't from Missouri, it ain't shit." The saying refers to nonnative wildlife or Class II animals—hyenas, camels, tigers, grizzly bears, aardvarks, whatever the animal—that can be sold off, auctioned, bred, walked down Main Street, kept in dreadful hellholes, without any regulations. A person can have the rarest animals or body parts on earth in Missouri, and sell them legally, even if those animals are on the endangered species list, as long as they're not taken across state lines. If I sell you a nearly extinct Siberian tiger today in Saint Louis, and you move in two months to Nevada and take it with you, the law has to prove that you intended upon purchase of the animal to deliberately and secretly transport it across state lines. Lacking proof, no crime was committed. Same with, say, hyacinth macaws. Missouri has thus become a haven for those

who profit at the expense of captive-bred exotic creatures, but the lawmakers are not particularly interested. In Missouri, there are more USDA Class A–licensed pet stores and Class B puppy mills than any other state in the union. Cage sizes are unregulated, and state cruelty laws are very hard to prosecute. Canned hunts are rumored to occur, though difficult to track. Speaking of the exotics in general, Dan calls them "a very low priority. Tigers and primates in Missouri are a dime a dozen."

Illegal hunting, however, is a whole different story. Most hunters are adamant about playing by the rules. Those who cheat, as I would frequently hear, "spoil the resource for everybody." But cheating a little bit is not entirely frowned upon. In some southern parts of the state, where Dan's current case is coming to a head, poaching is not only condoned but encouraged. "It's part of the thrill to go out and do it and not get caught," says Dan. "But they don't waste it." That is the greatest sin among hunters.

Dan hunted in high school. He grew up in Pennsylvania, where deer hunting was the rage. On the first day of buck season—the first Monday after Thanksgiving—Dan says you could not find a single male in school. Everyone, everywhere in the state, had a gun and was out searching for deer. Teenagers would go out at night in groups and turn on the headlights spotting for deer. Today, Dan no longer hunts, though on occasion his undercover work forces him to join in. But as a rule he admits to a strong preference for fishing. "My family doesn't particularly care for wild game, so there's no use killing it if we're not going to eat it."

Dan Burleson never intended to go into law enforcement. He got a degree in marine biology, and spent long hours collecting data on dolphins and whales for the National Marine Fisheries Service and documented the incidental take (killing) of dolphins by the U.S. tuna fleet. He worked as a USF&W wildlife inspector at the port of Houston, noting a daily avalanche of smuggled wildlife. He learned how to distinguish Asian

elephant ivory, eggs from the Cameroon ostrich, also endangered, and the twenty-seven endangered species of crocodile whose leather would show up as wallets. He then applied for and made it into the 1988 group of USF&W special agents. After graduating from FLETC, he was assigned to Region III, St. Paul, Minnesota. He adhered religiously, in the beginning, to anonymity; an imputed fear that the bad guys would come after him. His children did not know what their father did for a living. His phone number was unlisted. At least one person has drawn his gun on Dan, but he's never had to fight. At 6'2" and 285 pounds, he's a bruiser, and a disarming one. At his home, however, where I have briefly seen him after work, and after having driven hours on the job through hair-raising hailstorms and a tornado watch, Dan falls effortlessly into the noisy frolic of a sizable, young family, with its goldfish and a gigantic white Pyrenees.

The Case of a Father and Son

In March 1995 Dan got what he assumed was a fairly routine phone call from a Van Buren game warden by the name of Tom May. A meeting was to take place between May, a local Van Buren park ranger, and one of their colleagues, along with Burleson. As it would turn out, this was no ordinary case that May was calling about. It involved two local Van Buren hunters, a father and son, who had, by May's as yet unproven reckoning, made a mockery of hunting regulations in the region. May had long been on to them, but catching them in the act, or with the goods, was not as simple as such things might seem. May needed help. It was time to bring in the feds, which meant Dan Burleson.

To understand the intricacies of the case, one needs to understand the ins and outs of hunting and trapping in the region around Van Buren, an attractive town of some 800

pocketed away in the southwestern portion of Missouri. The small town is framed pastorally along the Current River, which runs through town and into the Ozark National Scenic River-way Big Spring Wildlife Refuge. The area is clad in a tapestry of hardwoods and shortleaf pine, home to Missouri's cele-brated pine warblers. The river is alleged to have the cleanest springwater in the world. And the fishing is considered prime, where the talk is all of gigging, In-Line Bucktail Spinners, Floater-Divers, and Jointed Wobbling Lures. A land of white bass, crayfish, crappie, and channel catfish. Heavily forested and hilly, it is a remote part of America, though all of three hours south of St. Louis, and it is also considered (along with some neighboring towns) to have one of the most endemic poaching traditions anywhere in the United States. The region lies just above the Bootheel region of Missouri (one look at a map explains the moniker), bordering up against the back-woods of Tennessee, Arkansas, and Kentucky; it is called "hill-billy" country, where people covet their private property, their guns, and their "game."

Dan and I drove into Van Buren around noon, where I was introduced to Tom May and others in the back of a café on the main street as lunch was served up. This was a café in which some food items cost under a dollar. Later, Tom and I would spend hours driving all through the Big Spring Refuge while he pointed out historic landmarks, darting herds of deer, flocks of turkey down among the dogwood (the state tree) and red-bud, numerous winter sparrows (of which there are twenty-one types in the state), as well as specific kill sites relevant to the now-concluded case I'd come to investigate. Tom showed me the spot where an albino deer—a favorite of townsfolk—had been slaughtered.

"See him?" May peers towards the crook in a high tree. "That's a bald eagle. Probably got an eight-foot wingspan." The bird perches high in a hickory tree beside a clearing with good hunting vantages. "Good eyesight," I said to Tom. "That

goes for both of you," meaning him and the bird. It was one of an estimated 2,621 eagles currently in the state. And down there below, in the meadow, he pointed to where the poachers had shot a deer at twenty yards using a six-millimeter rifle. "Pretty effective load. It'll drop him. Single hit," he added. Such a bullet explodes inside the animal after traveling between 3,000 and 4,000 feet per second. After the poachers killed it, they cut the head off, then reduced it down to antlers. Coyotes or bobcats scavenged the rest of the corpse, which had been mostly eaten when May found it one winter (on the second day of January, to be precise; he keeps track). It was one of many such corpses May would find.

A herd of several hundred white-tailed deer went bounding through the cottonwoods and sycamores, their little white tails prancing in a mirage of movement. Spring peepers were animating the forest with their rhythmic vibrations. May had driven these dirt roads thousands of times. Yet his obvious love of the land was undiminished.

Tom May is a man with a distinguished career. He embodies the best of this region. Hospitable, easygoing, respectful but tough, a connoisseur of natural beauty (he has photographed hundreds of the nearly 1,600 different flower species in the area, and gives slide presentations), he is a dedicated conservationist and a tenacious lawman.

May drives a Jeep and carries a Glock semiautomatic .40 caliber weapon with sixteen shots. He's never yet had to fire it at a human being. "Hope I never have to," he says as we bump along through the subtle but gorgeous country. May, who is fifty-nine and at the top of his pay scale (he takes home just under $40,000 a year, not much considering the risks and the fact he is on call twenty-four hours a day, seven days a week), is seriously thinking about retirement. He's been doing this for thirty-two years, but now has a hard time going after poachers by foot because he's developed circulation problems in his legs.

Born and raised in Scott County, the southeastern part of

the state, about halfway between Sikeston and Cape Girardeau, Tom May followed in his brother's footsteps to obtain a job with the Missouri Department of Conservation, Fish, and Wildlife around 1960. From the beginning, his mandate was to work with conservation groups and try to promote good hunting practices and good wildlife management. It's a broader role than is traditionally connected with a game warden. Unlike many parts of the United States, this particular region contains a vast amount of huntable land, both public and private, and this has attracted hunters from all over the country. The pressures are extreme during the actual hunting season. It's mostly about white-tailed deer, wild turkey, fox, and gray squirrels, the latter going into "hot pots"; that's gray squirrel fried with red pepper. There are probably as many recipes in the Bootheel as there are gray squirrels. As for the whitetails, the best racks, as hunters think of the animals, are developed between the ages of five and six years. But, says Tom, most deer never live past the age of five around here, either on account of the hunters, the coyotes and bobcats, or recent epidemics of hemorrhagic disease.

Every state and region across America has its own hunting regulations and bylaws that tend to reflect local conditions. Usually, government biologists provide the necessary data for determining bag limits and hunting seasons and durations. These are strict assessments that people like Tom May take very seriously. Hunters, too. But not all of them. The terms and quotas that come with a hunting license are spelled out in various forms, newsletters, postings, and, most importantly, the annually published *Wildlife Code of Missouri*. Anybody born after January 1, 1967, has to pass a ten-hour hunter education course and exam prior to getting a license. It covers everything from safe gun handling to ethics. And it plants firmly in one's head the legal requirement of obtaining permission from landowners before you can hunt on their personal property (a ruling since 1933). It also recommends (though cannot

require) that a hunter share food with someone if it is killed on his or her land.

The course clarifies precisely when, where, by what means, and which animals of which sex and at what age a hunter can kill in the wild. And it spells out facts pertaining to all the basics: the types of "center fire rifles" that are legal (this rules out the rimfire .22 and any weapon using a bullet that is not big enough to kill a deer: the goal is to kill the animal with one shot and not have it wander off bleeding to death); the number of deer or turkey that can be taken with a firearm, or a bow or crossbow; the eleven deer-hunting days in November, and the three additional days in January—two for the general public, one reserved for special hunts; the furbearer season, which begins November 20, there being no limit to the number you can kill; the fact that with the exception of bobcat, fur prices were up in 1997 for the first time in several years (a function of increasing scarcity). Bobcats are now high on the list of desirable prey, for trappers primarily. During the 1996–1997 season, trappers killed at least 1,235 of the felines. The price of pelts has dropped considerably for bobcat, from $200 to $20 per fur. But there are plenty of men who are happy to lay traplines with even a $20-per-head incentive. In the case of most other furbearers, the prices are now up at local auctions: beaver from $5 per pelt to $17.57, raccoon from $6 to $19.95, and otter pelts for $40.25. In fact, 1997 was the first year ever that trapping otters in the region was legalized. Throughout the state, 4,500 licensed trappers killed at least 1,040 otters that were presented to conservation agents for tagging.[8]

The hunter licensing course indoctrinates novitiates on the delicacies, if you will, of bringing down the three allowable wild turkeys with a bow, and another three with a firearm. It used to be a total of four, but the numbers are constantly being adjusted according to the perception of population vitality. What never changes are the hunting hours: daylight to dark-

ness. You have to be able to see a person. Hunters must wear orange, easy-to-see garb. If it's a deep fog, you're not allowed to be out there. During the season, thousands of hunters are tramping these woods. The gun blasts are heard throughout the day, and frequently, says Tom, after sunset. He'll get at least three and four calls throughout the night from residents who are upset that hunters are somewhere on their property shooting at critters. Tom has to prioritize the calls. He doesn't sleep much during those periods, staking out sites almost every night through the fall. The fact is, he acknowledges, there is a "serious poaching problem" in the area. You've got to be at least eighteen to buy a gun. But there's no minimum age for owning a gun. Even a five-year-old can have one, as potentially dangerous as that sounds.

In May's home, he introduces me to a ram curl, a set of horns that must weigh forty pounds, and a second confiscated rack mounted on a wall. It was a so-called Boon and Crockett deer that scored 178 points, referring to the various measures of the antlers, the length, the symmetry, and the overall aesthetics. "Nobody could kill one of these and not be totally thrilled with it," says May with a tone of tragic irony.

In a similar tone, May describes how he was once held at gunpoint by five poachers threatening to kill him, each with pointed gun. He was in the remote Sinking Creek area of an adjoining county, a hotbed for poaching types. He had hiked in from his vehicle, carrying a two-inch .38 caliber sidearm. He had observed the goings-on, then started issuing various violations, including citations for using double-aught buckshot in their shotguns, which is an illegal load, and hunting deer in closed season. The poachers surprised him with their fury, and would hold him for four hours. Eventually he talked his way out of being murdered, and even (incredibly) finished writing up the tickets. But the poachers were never brought to any justice. The prosecutor in the area was not supportive. In fact, he later arrested May, along with the head of the Game

Division and a professor at the University of Missouri, for confiscating a poached bear, the first one killed in Missouri in fifty years. Bears are rare in the state. May had delivered it to the university where, according to regulations, it could be used for research and educational purposes. The charges against May and the professor were frivolous and he has not been prosecuted for them, yet they've still not been dropped.

One of the real problems with poaching is that it doesn't take many poachers to alter a delicate biological balance within a region. When you get individual hunters who are each killing twenty to thirty deer a year, primarily the bucks with fine antlers, there's going to be a significant and rapid impact on the deer population. The locals, says Tom, have no problem with someone who kills a deer or two out of season each year for extra meat on their table. And they also know that Tom will eventually catch up with them, and cite them. The system generally works in their favor and there's little cause for alarm. Even if they commit a wildlife felony, as opposed to mere misdemeanors, the punishment can be as trivial as one day in jail. Nor is there normally any forfeiture of equipment, not even the gun. The majority of other states seize gun and vehicle and charge higher fines. Neighboring Arkansas, for example, has confiscation laws. But Missouri is still operating on the penalties that were fixed with the establishing of its Conservation Department in 1937.

Until recently, Tom lived nearby one Robert LaRue (his real identity being altered here out of respect to his family's privacy). May and LaRue could have shouted to one another from their respective living rooms, and at times I'm sure they wanted to. LaRue, his wife, and their boy had many years before set down roots in this quiet little Van Buren neighborhood with its finely kept, neatly arrayed homes, all originally built or purchased for $15,000 to $30,000. While poaching was commonplace in these parts, May suspected that his near neighbor, LaRue, was particularly systematic about it, but he just

couldn't prove it. For twenty years he was on his neighbor's trail. LaRue was careful to avoid getting caught in the act. May needed more evidence. The fact is that it can be very difficult to catch a poacher.

Agitating matters further, the two men had had a long-standing quarrel that stemmed from their respective dogs, both now long dead. LaRue says May's German shepherd viciously attacked and killed his son's beagle, while May watched without doing anything from his car. LaRue says that same shepherd killed other neighborhood pets as well, but May was cold and callous about the whole thing. "He's a mean, aggressive person and there's nothing people can do," laments LaRue. May denies that he ever saw the incident with the dogs, though he doesn't doubt that it might have occurred. The German shepherd was a stray his son had rescued one freezing winter night—a pretty wild creature. But May certainly took no pleasure in dogfights. As for LaRue, he was not about to let it rest. When that shepherd next ventured across his property line, possibly in an attempt to kill his pet wild turkeys, LaRue shot and killed the dog, then buried it. May learned of this, LaRue figures, prompting a vendetta—May's determination to fabricate an elaborate poaching case against him. LaRue thus denies that he was the poacher May believes him to be. LaRue alleges that "May confronted him with a pistol, shaking, out of control, like someone who has had a stroke." He adds, "May said he was going to get me if it's the last thing he ever did. He threatened to kill me here on the spot. 'I will stalk you and get even with you.'" May calls the allegation a "total fabrication."

Later on, after the takedown, LaRue was convinced that there was no point trying to describe any of this to the judge. Moreover, LaRue alleges that "the prosecutor is a cocaine addict" and in cahoots with May.

May shakes his head when I ask him about these allegations. The man is just plain dangerous, he says, and "real sneaky." He even speculates that "LaRue was the type that at some point

wouldn't be satisfied shooting animals. He'd killed so many of them and he was the type that could have been a serial killer." He uses the past tense.

And LaRue expresses similar ill will toward May. May's interest in LaRue's poaching patterns, he says, started when he began receiving reports back in the late 1960s, beginning with word out on the street that LaRue and his father had killed a mighty black bear in May 1969 in the nearby Mark Twain National Forest. LaRue was nineteen at that time. May had already arrested LaRue's father on a couple of occasions for poaching. The son, Robert, grew up in his father's footsteps, says May. And Robert's son, the same. "Killing everything they'd see. Just shooting it to shoot. For the racks." Definitely not for food, he added. LaRue "was a full-time poacher. He didn't pretend to do anything else. And a lot of times he would go out and park a vehicle or his wife would take him out and drop him off, especially if they were hunting a refuge area, and he might not come back for three or four days." May describes how LaRue would drive out of town three or four miles, then stop to see if anybody was following him, then backtrack. May worked by himself, covering a territory of 600 square miles. His office didn't (and still does not) have the budget to assign a full-time person to any one alleged poacher. That only happens during USF&W special operations, like Renegade and Whiteout.

Moreover, says May, LaRue was a real "loner," making any covert operation next to impossible. No stranger could get close to him. When LaRue left teaching and got into real estate, says May, he specialized in selling properties to hunters from out of the area and also specialized in telling them about his own hunting exploits, and showing off all the antlers he'd collected. Some of those would-be buyers came to Tom May. "Why can't you catch him?" they'd ask. "He's slaughtering everything." May estimates he received between fifty and seventy-five reports about LaRue's poaching over the years.

Then the big break came in the form of a diary (two vol-

umes) documenting kills with gruesome regularity. May says that LaRue "made enemies very frequently with his employees because from all the reports he was cheating them out of money." (LaRue, to the contrary, details the many loans, the financial gifts, the shirts off his back that he gave to staff.) But one of those employees, a disgruntled person, did, in fact, provide a copy of the diaries to Tom May, having read them and knowing what they suggested.

May describes his own reaction at first reading the two books. "It was sickening. It really was. I've been a turkey hunter, I've killed a lot of turkeys, but it was just the slaughter that was taking place by him and his son . . . "

To an outsider, it requires some speculation: the key to distinguishing between killing "a lot of turkeys" legitimately and an illegitimate "slaughter," as described above, that would be enough to sicken someone, has to do with the letter of the law. If you kill by the book, say lawmakers, fine. If not, you're in trouble. The morality is tied to the law, with its bag limits and precise seasons, and overall procedural biology for maintaining "healthy" populations, and ensuring a viable differentiation of gender and age groups within those populations, not the killing itself. And this is a fact, right or wrong, inherent in modern conservation.

Diaries of Anonymous Origin

When Tom May placed that phone call to Dan Burleson, it was because he finally had enough telling evidence to move effectively forward in his investigation: diaries that LaRue had apparently kept hidden away in his office. The two volumes appeared to be written in his own hand (though later handwriting samples produced for FBI authorities by LaRue—forty different pages worth—could not be conclusively matched to that of the diary. LaRue says it proves he did not write the

books, nor is there any name in the diary). Nevertheless, the diaries enabled May, and then Burleson, to begin putting together a sequence of events they believed linked LaRue and his son to countless acts of poaching that had thus far eluded May in his twenty-year pursuit.

Part of that sequence was substantiated by a laboratory examination report, dated April 21, 1989, referring to a December 1988 illegal hunt for mule deer. It came from the Game and Fish Department of the State of Wyoming. A forensic scientist at the state crime lab had submitted details pertaining to an illegal kill in that state by LaRue, whose travel itinerary, hotel receipts, and precise phone calls would all be unearthed for corroboration. The samples of the kill contained two swabs of blood traced to hair retrieved from a plastic bag, and bloodstains removed from a retrieved hacksaw blade. Twenty hair fragments showed characteristics similar to those present on animals in the deer family, Cervidae, including elk, moose, and white-tailed deer. It was known that LaRue had been caught in Montana in 1975 with illegal sheep, and stopped, though not cited, in 1988 with some other evidence: a dead mule deer and footprints. Other hunting jaunts at other times had taken him to Montana, Colorado, and Alaska. But the vast majority of line items in the diaries concerned hunting within Missouri, a vast litany of kills dating back nearly thirty years. In fact, May and Burleson would eventually be able to match every one of the 189 racks confiscated from LaRue's garage to specific incidents recorded in the diaries.

Even armed with the diaries, May knew that the only way to push this case toward closure was to get some additional eyewitness information, hopefully audio/video and photographs. He wanted to get inside the LaRue house, but given the longstanding enmity between May and LaRue, that was out of the question. He needed someone else, someone unknown in these parts. He needed Dan Burleson to come down from St. Louis in an undercover capacity. And because alleged

poaching in other states was involved, the multijurisdictional nature of the case required the power of the federal government. Ultimately, it would be the Missouri Department of Conservation, the Ozark National Scenic Riverway division of the National Park Service, and the U.S. Fish and Wildlife Service, working with a Carter County prosecuting attorney and the assistant U.S. attorney, that would put the case to rest.

Because LaRue ran a real estate company specializing in properties that were ideal for hunting ("damn near right out your back window," said Dan, paraphrasing LaRue), Dan, posing as an interested buyer, showed up on May 26, 1995, with a woman, his partner, and spent seven and one-half hours with LaRue. Fifteen minutes of that time was devoted to talk of real estate. For the remainder, LaRue recounted his greatest poaching stories: "I killed a deer here, a turkey there."

They were in LaRue's real estate office for approximately one and a half hours. During that time the audiotape failed. Dan kept excusing himself to use the office rest room, where he could make notes. Afterward, they all drove around for about two hours before proceeding to LaRue's home. As the three of them were driving along in the Ozarks, LaRue suddenly stopped his vehicle, jumped out, and grabbed a young poult walking along the road with her wild turkey mother and siblings. It's illegal to do that, but they don't run very fast and LaRue had the edge. He took the critter home, where he has well over a dozen domestic and a few wild turkeys fenced in to the side of the house. He then escorted Dan and his partner through his house to show off his trophies.

"My brother would love to see this stuff. Do you mind if I videotape it?" said Dan. "No, no, go right ahead," replied LaRue.

The audiotape was up and running again and the video footage was shot. But it was during that first hour, says Dan, when LaRue incriminated himself royally. The camera recorded 189 antlers mounted in the garage. Then the tape ran

out and Dan didn't have another one. He forgot to turn off the camera. It was dangling from his side, the battery running low. Two neighborhood teenagers came round, young protégés of LaRue. They paid LaRue a few bucks for some ammo that LaRue kept in his workroom. LaRue had a federal license as an arms dealer, which gave him the right to buy cartridges at bulk rates (receiving a two-thirds discount) and to conduct occasional shooting range activities in the woods behind his house using silhouettes, clay decoys, and steel targets. But it was not legal for him to be selling ammo to minors. These two boys were seventeen-year-old friends of his son. They got into the two boxes of CCI .22-caliber, rimfire rounds—100 to the box—when Dan and his partner were there and witnessed the exchange. LaRue insists this was totally trivial—indeed, the $3 amount *was* trivial—but Dan knew this might be crucial in exerting leverage in a courtroom to get LaRue on other, often too easily dismissed, charges. What Dan didn't notice was that the teenagers were wise to him, or at least sensed that something was wrong. They saw the video camera with its red tally light on. They had a hunch. They mentioned it to LaRue's wife and she to her husband. LaRue suddenly grew tense. He had long anticipated trouble in the form of a duplicitous stranger. Now, in his mind, the shakedown was unfolding.

The next day, Dan and his partner returned to resume their search for the perfect property. It was clear instantly that the terms of the greeting had changed dramatically. Something was wrong. "Our cover's been blown," Dan thought. LaRue was solemn and suspicious. He didn't say a word about hunting. They went out and looked at some land. Dan could detect that LaRue was carrying a weapon.

"Here was a man who had killed well over a thousand animals, many illegally. I felt that he was capable of anything," says Dan, reliving the edginess of the moment. Dan's partner kept her weapon within easy reach inside her purse, while Dan stayed close on LaRue's shooting arm. Then a second man

showed up. Dan didn't know if he was carrying or not. The situation now seemed very dangerous. They were tramping through a remote hunting property in the Ozarks, immersed in the pine and oak woods. Anything could have happened.

But no fight ever erupted. In fact, LaRue—for all of his hunting in days past—comes across as a very peace-loving individual. This much I can attest to, after repeated long phone conversations with him, and a meeting with him and his wife at their house, a few weeks before LaRue headed off to a federal prison.

The two days in LaRue's company gave Dan enough evidential support to generate a search warrant. It took him a week to write up and obtain that warrant (two, in fact), documenting probable cause. By then, having been spooked by the video, LaRue had hidden some of the incriminating evidence. This obstruction of justice, a felony, is what probably sent him to jail. Had he cooperated, he might have gotten off merely with fines on the wildlife misdemeanors, and the press—which had a field day with the case—might have been disinterested.

The case of LaRue and his son is not your ordinary Missouri poaching violation. Many months before actually going to Missouri to research the events in question, I'd heard about the highlights from Dan, who'd mentioned these curious, unsubstantiated, but nonetheless damning diaries. Later, both May and Burleson showed me the volumes—first xerox copies and then the originals. They were in May's possession. When I asked LaRue about the notebooks, he did not exactly deny writing them, but did not come out and admit it, either. He was testing me, I think; wanting to know my own conclusions about this whole sorry affair. But he did seem agitated by their discovery and the allegations swirling around them. However, a former friend and longtime hunting companion of LaRue's insists, without any doubt whatsoever, that LaRue wrote them, saying "it don't take no rocket scientist to figure that out!" Moreover, a former employee told me that LaRue had made

much of the fact that he wasn't worried about the diaries because the statute of limitations had run out, in his opinion, on most of the dead animals. Further proof, said the employee, that LaRue wrote them.

Whoever wrote them, and the government believes LaRue did, they are a veritable Missouri Book of the Dead. Grimly, the line items detail the animals killed, along with the day, time, and place of those kills; whether the animal was brought down with a gun or a bow, the number of shots required to effect the kill, at what spot in the animal the fatal wound was made, and the distance of the animal from the killer. The diaries enumerate the approximate weight of the animals, the number of points on the racks, and the spread measurements of the antlers. Listed in the two notebooks are 190 white-tailed deer, 275 turkeys, and a host of other animals: mule deer, groundhogs, a variety of birds, foxes, raccoons, bobcats, bears, coyotes, antelopes, prairie dogs, sage grouse, caribou, elk, bighorn sheep, and moose. It is not uncommon to find several entries for a single date.

Even the most hardened "hillbilly outlaws" in the area (as the local press referred to them) were said to have been outraged by the mountain of evidence that convicted LaRue and his boy. In Dan Burleson's hundreds of pages of investigative reports, every known detail of the forensics was set forth. Photographs documented deer hair evidence, bone fragments, stomach contents, the trash bags used. Such evidence was available wherever Dan or Tom or another member of their team were able to locate the remains of the carcass. In fact, whether it could be located or not, nearly every carcass had been left. LaRue and his son were interested in trophies, not corpses. And that violates a long-esteemed if unstated rule among hunters: you don't waste meat. You never shoot just for the hell of it.

"I think he [referring to LaRue's poaching] was proud of his accomplishments," says Dan. "I don't think he ever stopped

to consider what he was doing. He will tell you that ninety-nine percent of them [referring to all the kills] were legal. The only thing he might feel shame about is getting caught." But what he really did, says Dan, is inflict damage on the whole hunting community and its ethical standards, because most hunters do things more or less by the book. For reasons of their own, two previously close friends of LaRue decided to talk to the authorities.

One of them, a "Cooperator" who wishes to remain anonymous ("I still gotta live in this town," he reminds me—so I call him "Bud"), described LaRue's poaching as simply "a macho thing." He "just wanted to see if he could get away with it." This individual started hunting with LaRue when he was a young man of fourteen. He kept a detailed record of everything he ever did in the wild. He remembered how LaRue's son had laughed about certain kills; and how he had this bad tendency of "shooting high at everything," which meant missing the mark and invariably inflicting slow death on the animal. The goal of a hunter is to kill the animal mercifully, with one shot. That means, in the case of deer, hitting it just behind the front legs where its lungs and heart are located; and in the case of wild turkey, in the head and neck regions. If the animal is moving in thick forest, it's a difficult shot. The majority of hunters wait for the animal to stop. The son would often miss that mark because he'd shoot over his dad's shoulder, using it like a tripod. And that might have had something to do with the fact, according to Bud, that the son was forced to go hunting, in his opinion. In these parts it was "a rite of passage." Deer season comes around and everyone is talking about "who's going to kill the biggest buck." Bud bought his first deer tag when he was nine years old. But they start hunting when they're around seven in the Bootheel area of Missouri. May says Bud "saw the light before LaRue's case came down. It wasn't a matter of him getting scared" and wanting to turn evidence in order to cut a deal. He simply "saw the light."

Over coffee with Bud, a friend of his, Dan, and Tom May, the friend says that "people here think these deer are here to eat and nobody should interfere. When they want one they just go out and shoot it." Bud point outs that the Bible states that "all the animals on the earth and the fowl in the air and every living creature was put here for man's consumption." But he also adds, "The Bible says you must abide by the laws of the land."

Bud says poaching has changed now. They're out there doing it for fun. It used to be for food. "Twenty years ago, even less years than that, you didn't hear of nobody going out here and shooting a deer and cutting the head off of it. Boy, if you did, I mean, they'd look at you, why you low life . . . You didn't dare say nothing like that."

"What changed you?" I ask him. He pauses, reflectively, and declares, "I had an appendicitis attack and nearly died over that deal. And I just decided there comes a point that, you know, you just gotta do something right. I knew all these twenty years that stuff was wrong. I had to clear all that up, do something right for a change. Certain things, you know, there comes, you have to, you got to be stopped. I didn't want everybody in town to always think of me as being nothing but a desperado all my life." Bud was afraid that people would think of him the same way he says they think of LaRue. "Ninety percent of the people in town hate him, but they'd never say it to his face and you'd never get him to believe that. I told him many times, I said, 'Some day when the sun comes up, they're going to find you somewhere in some field. People say that if they ever caught you on their property they'll kill you stone dead.'"

"Because of his hunting practices?" I ask.

"Well, he cut it short for everybody. You take a small community like this and you go out here and kill twenty or twenty-five bucks in a couple of months, well, you've really took an edge off, because these old boys that live around here like my-

self, you go out here before deer season and you know about where you're going to hunt and this, that, and the other. It got to the point where nobody would say anything about seeing any deer because they knew if LaRue ever heard about it, where there was a big buck, the buck would die. You couldn't go nowhere with him. He kept me a nervous wreck all the time. I mean, you know, he had to do a little bit of something illegal in anything he done. He was obsessed with the numbers, you know. It was like, 'If I kill all these deer everybody's going to look at me like I am the greatest hunter that ever walked.'"

A former employee of LaRue says categorically, "He loved to kill. That's all he talked about was killing. Most of those pictures were plastered in his office of all the dead animals."

"He was just obsessed with the great numbers," reiterates Bud. "He enjoyed it, there's no question."

"The blood?" I ask him.

"Yeah, I think so. He just liked to kill. I mean just liked to kill things and he wanted that boost from everybody of, 'Man, you're the great hunter. I mean, man, only you could do that!' And you know, when I was younger, I wanted to be a hunter like him, you know. I wanted to kill things like he did and all that."

Bud describes how they first went out to Glacier Park in Montana together, he and LaRue. Bud was fourteen. LaRue killed a bighorn sheep and it scared Bud to death. "I was afraid we was going to get throwed in jail and he [LaRue] was pretty rough about it, you know. 'You just shut up, I'm going to do this and that's it.'" The year was 1975. They did get caught. Bud was fined $300, a fortune for a fourteen-year-old. LaRue was fined $600. Two years later, they went right back and did it again. Much later, on August 12, 1993, according to the government indictment against the father and son, the two LaRues were in Wyoming on a mule deer hunt. They had purchased hunting tags for the animals, the first time they'd ever done so in any western state. They paid $500 each, and also paid a

guide $1,400. The mule deer season closed, the guide left, and neither LaRue had gotten a deer. So they went to Yellowstone National Park after an elk "so that the trip wouldn't be a total loss," according to Burleson's Application and Affidavit for Search Warrant. The father held a light on a 6-by-6, 800-pound elk (some reports say it was a 12-point) while the son blew it away. The men cut off the antlers and drove back to Missouri. While undercover, Burleson alleges that LaRue stated "the one time they tried to hunt legally they were unsuccessful and had to resort to poaching." LaRue actually showed Burleson the 6-by-6 elk antler on a plaque hanging from the attic floor of his garage. Rangers who originally found the carcass in Wyoming in 1993 also managed to recover the bullet. It matched one of LaRue's rifles seized in 1995.

Reminiscing on earlier visits to Yellowstone prior to 1993, Bud described how they had once mingled discreetly with other campers snapping pictures in a meadow seventy-five feet away from two big bull elks. The animals were semidomesticated by all the attention over the years from tourists. LaRue, his son, and Bud watched the animals throughout the day and into the night, as the enormous elks bedded down in the timber. With a crossbow, LaRue then struck one of them near dead. The animal moved about bleeding all night. It died by morning. LaRue and the two boys went searching for it, the goal being to cut off its horns. They found the animal lying exposed atop a rock bluff out over a creek. The arrow was sticking in its side. Tourists standing there were appalled. The ranger was notified. In the meantime, LaRue and company hightailed it out of the park. That arrow can now be found at the Smithsonian Institution, where it had been kept all these years in connection with an unsolved poaching incident.

The same powerful impact LaRue had on Bud was manifest throughout Van Buren. "He was kind of a leader," says Bud, recollecting how LaRue put ideas in people's heads (mostly young boys) and got many a wanna-be poacher started.

At the same time, LaRue knew that someday he was going to get caught. But his favorite saying was, "Possession is nine-tenths of the law. If you're not standing right there with a smoking gun, you're not guilty. On a misdemeanor charge, there's not a jury in the county would put him away." He said, "It may cost one thousand dollars for the lawyer but you [I] can beat it." LaRue was particularly distinguished as a poacher, says Bud, because he talked about it so much. Other poachers never said a word about their exploits.

When the search warrants were executed, LaRue played it real cool, according to Dan. He'd already altered the racks, putting notations on the back that would have dated them to the time of his friend, the Cooperator's deceased father, who was also a poacher. It was dinnertime on June 5, 1995. Tom May, Dan Burleson, and twenty-eight other officers had divided into various teams for the purpose of descending on the LaRue home and several other relevant locations around town. Dan headed up the seizure on the house. But LaRue was undaunted and smugly blew them off. "You'd think I shot the president," LaRue says with some incredulity. He adds, "Burleson lied and laced reports with erroneous statements to the court. The feds probably spent three to five hundred thousand dollars to decipher something akin to killing a flea. It was nothing more than family hunting. In the old days you could shoot three deer tomorrow, go to the judge, insult him, and you'd probably still get a reduced ticket," he told me gamely. Dan Burleson estimates they actually spent no more than $50,000 on the case.

LaRue had already hidden much of the incriminating evidence against him at a few friends' and neighbors' places, including 248 turkey "beards," one set of bighorn ram curls (the ones I saw at Tom May's house), a set of elk antlers, photographs depicting hundreds of wildlife kills, the two diaries, a Remington .280 rifle, an H&R .30-.30 caliber rifle, a Remington 6-millimeter rifle, a bear hide, some deer meat, and written information on plaques containing deer antlers. LaRue

didn't realize at the time that two of his friends had already talked to the authorities. But LaRue was so certain of the judicial loopholes in southern Missouri that he didn't even bother calling for a lawyer. LaRue's wife insists that Dan took her aside and tried to scare her into talking and divorcing her husband. Dan denies that, explaining that what he did try to explain to the wife was how much better it would be for everyone if her husband was simply up front with the authorities. At four in the morning, the search team left LaRue's house carrying bags and boxes filled with antlers, mounts, deer meat, guns, documents, receipts from taxidermists, ledgers, records of travel to Montana and Wyoming, hotel receipts, canceled checks, maps, 6-millimeter ammunition, rifles capable of shooting 6-millimeter ammo, photographs of kills, and videotapes. They went through every scrap of paper, took out every page of the phone book, turned every page of LaRue's *World Book Encyclopedia*. LaRue, according to Dan, enjoyed every minute of it. He was convinced there was no way he was going down. "Smug as hell, like, I've got one on all of you," is how Dan characterizes him.

At 6:30 in the morning Dan returned to LaRue's place to find LaRue sleeping soundly. Dan, who had found LaRue's stashed items, went up to him and said, "LaRue, by law this property belongs to you, but since I didn't get it here I need to give you a receipt for it." That was the stuff LaRue had hidden. He couldn't believe that Dan had found it. His jaw dropped and he said, "Well, what do I do now?"

"I guess we just sit down and get your statement," Dan explained.

What would make this case particularly unusual, aside from the sheer volume of the dead, was the fact that LaRue was not selling the racks of his kills. Over the years the prosecution would admit evidence of $277,000 worth of wildlife that LaRue and his son killed. The value was an average taken from eight surrounding states. That includes 287 deer at $500 each and

300 wild turkeys at $200 each. In addition, in Wyoming, Montana, and Alaska, there were 19 antelopes, four bighorn sheep, four elks, and hosts of squirrels, prairie dogs, rabbits, and other animals. The state of Wyoming, as of this writing, is still deliberating on the likely fine for the illegal mule deer. It could theoretically be as high as $30,000. The government confiscated a video in which LaRue and his son sat in their vehicle somewhere in Wyoming blowing prairie dogs to smithereens. I've seen the video. The prairie dogs explode like puffs of smoke. There's virtually no commentary from LaRue or his son. This comes across as just routine target practice.

On October 31, 1995, the state of Missouri filed fifty-two charges against LaRue and his son. They pled not guilty to all counts and were freed on a $20,000 secured bond. Astonishingly, LaRue asked permission from the federal judge, Lewis Blanton, to hunt with either a crossbow or a normal bow during the remainder of the deer season during his arraignment in federal court. The request was denied. Within a year, both father and son entered guilty pleas in federal and state courts to the multiple game violations. In the end, LaRue would pay $20,300 to the state of Missouri, $33,000 to his lawyer, and forfeit his gun collection—nineteen rifles and five handguns—to the local Carter County Crime Reduction Fund, to be sold at public auction. The collection was worth $20,000. LaRue, who had a bachelor of science degree with a major in wildlife management from Arkansas State University, had once worked for the Park Service (there is a picture of him in uniform), and had taught science in high schools for six years, would also lose both his teaching and real estate licenses. He is now a felon. He can never own a gun, never hunt again anywhere in the United States. His son is never allowed to hunt in Missouri. But he'll be able to hunt in other states if he so chooses. LaRue complains that since the rash of press publicity surrounding the case, he has received death threats by phone.

Among the countless items confiscated in the takedown of

June 5 were photo albums of LaRue and his son's hunting exploits over the years. Leafing through them and the diaries provided a shocking view into the extreme mentality of trophy hunting. A picture of LaRue with the bear that he'd baited, then skinned. A white corpse hangs strung up. Handwritten notes read, "Friday, May 2, 1969, 8:15 p.m. 360 pound black bear. Beaver Forest Tower, 15 miles north of Poplar Bluff, Mo. Shot at once; hit in head with bolt action Rem. [Remington]; 700 in; 6mm caliber; 100 grain Nosler bullet." A photo from 1961, LaRue with his first illegal deer, his own father on the right. From 1965, a shot of a 100-pound doe killed illegally before the start of the official hunting season that year. Another one in 1969: LaRue is getting older, becoming a better and better poacher. He'd go out the night before the hunting season commenced to shoot his buck and then display the rack of a 15-pointer sitting in his Chevrolet pickup.

The photos also reveal his career as an archer, not infrequently preying across the State Management Area before the legal season. His first elk shot in Yellowstone Park in 1974; then eight pronghorn antelopes, followed by illegal bobcats, and scores of mule deer in Wyoming. Then his first illegal bighorn sheep in Colorado in 1975. And another one at Glacier National Park in Montana, in 1977—an absolutely gigantic mass of an animal. An illegal elk in Wyoming (a state where there is no statute of limitations on the charge of wanton waste, a fact that would come back to haunt LaRue) in 1986. A description of a day's hunt—twenty doves, then a deer, its head cut off. A picture of all the bloody doves on the floor. A record-size bass. A hawk. Thirty-four blackbirds in one shot. His two hundredth groundhog. A few squirrels before lunch, five to be exact, which he is holding sitting next to his car. The killing of five teal in one shot. In a single evening, ten groundhogs, two red foxes, two squirrels and a crow. Two salmon. One hundred thirty-six buffalofish. At least ten wild turkeys a year. There he is holding his trophies.

And as LaRue's son gets bigger, he, too, shoots bigger and bigger deer. At age eight the boy kills his first buck. Later, in 1991, there is a photograph of him with the famed albino deer that he killed at close range in the wildlife refuge at the Ozark National Scenic Riverway. Many of the locals used to feed this deer. It was tame. When it disappeared, the locals all knew it had been poached. There's the son posing with fifteen deer racks he took in 1992, twenty-one in 1993. And a host of images of the boy going after wild turkeys from the time he was very young, when the turkeys were nearly his own size. In 1992, the son reenacted one of his father's most notorious poaching escapades when he journeyed into Glacier National Park with his dad acting as guide and managed to slaughter his very own bighorn sheep at night several feet off a trail where they had tracked it, and actually fed it by hand earlier in the day. There are pictures of the boy killing multiple squirrels when young, using a birdcall (a little megaphone) to bring in unsuspecting crows. A kind of family vendetta against rabbits and groundhogs and prairie dogs. Later, the killing extends to large badgers and bobcats. There is an image of him holding dead coyotes, his face painted for camouflage.

The gun types are profuse: Valmets, Berrettas, Kimbers, Rugers, Remingtons, Renegade Hawkins, in addition to a high-tech crossbow. LaRue's favorite gun, according to Bud, was the Remington .700 heavy barreled varmint special 6 millimeter. He got it when he was sixteen years old. He was fond of its trigger pulls and smooth action. He also liked the Valmets.

Eighty-seven percent of all these animals, according to the prosecutors, were illegally killed. Many were unlawfully transported across federal lands, a large number of which had been killed in national wildlife refuges. At least eleven were run down with the aid of dogs. The government is uncertain about the illegality of another 12 percent of them. Only 1 percent were supposedly killed legally. LaRue argues just the opposite, continuing to insist that 99 percent were taken legally.

Regarding that 1 percent of illegal kills, he says, "I know I'm guilty. I understand. I have a conscience. I'm not arrogant. It's almost as if somebody else did it." He describes why he took his son on a big game hunt in other states without getting a license: "Permits are very restrictive and expensive." A big trophy ram—the most coveted trophy in the United States—would have cost them $30,000 to take legally. They went in ten miles by foot at night in an area of high grizzly concentration. He said "it was like pioneer days having to endure dangers." But he is very bitter about charges he insists were trumped up. He says sometimes he and his son were each charged with killing the same deer. And there's no proof that even that one deer was killed by them. Regarding the 189 racks in his garage, he insists that those were shot by his father at the rate of three or so deer a year, for fifty years, "most of it legal." The prosecution "made it look like a massacre," he says. And this particularly galls him because, as he described himself to me, he is "an environmentalist that loves animals."

As the process got under way against him, he says he "could see the charade unfolding." And he believes that the odds of what happened against him were one in a million. He is certain that had he gone to court in Van Buren, as opposed to Cape Girardeau several hours away, he and his son would have been freed. In fact, Tom May also believes that had the case gone to trial, the LaRues might well have walked away free men. A unanimous jury decision might have been hard to obtain in the area.

But the case never went to trial. The LaRues had separate attorneys, and each pled out bargains before a judge on the state level. On January 28, 1997, LaRue and his son were sentenced before U.S. District Judge Richard Webber in Cape Girardeau, Missouri. The father was found guilty on four misdemeanor and three felony counts. The state violations charged him with killing deer and turkey out of season, hunting in a wildlife refuge, and endangering the welfare of children. It

was acknowledged that he had illegally hunted and killed hundreds of animals. He violated the Lacey Act by conspiring to illegally transport antlers across state lines. He was charged with taking one bighorn sheep in Glacier National Park with intent to transport said animal to Missouri; with killing an elk in Yellowstone National Park; with violating his license as a firearms dealer for selling ammunition to minors; and with conspiring to remove property to prevent seizure. He was sentenced to twenty-one months federal confinement for the felonies and twelve months on the misdemeanors, the sentences to run concurrently. And he received two years supervised probation after his prison term, during which time he is banned from all national parks. As a felon he can never vote again, and never possess a firearm. The fines were both state and federal, and included so-called restitution payments on the charges related to the illegal killing of the elk and bighorn sheep.

In fact, the judge gave LaRue the minimum sentence. The public was not pleased. The same judge, just a week before, let walk two deer-poaching brothers who had harmed a conservation officer while he made a routine permit check for possible violations. The men hit him with a fist-size rock across the head. Bud agrees that LaRue got off easy and expresses his own belief that the laws should be tougher.

As for LaRue's son, he was found guilty of four misdemeanor counts. The son's attorney had hoped that all forty-two state and federal cases against the young man (himself a teacher now and fresh out of a local college) would be dropped and that psychological treatment instead of prosecution would be considered. The attorney claimed in court (and nobody expected this turn) that the son had suffered abuse from the father. The judge did take that into consideration. He decided against house arrest (which the prosecution had urged) and ruled instead that the son be confined for six months in a town ninety miles to the north. In addition, he was to receive psychological evaluation and treatment, if warranted. The

young LaRue is not a felon. Tom May thinks highly of the son and told me that he believes he is essentially a good person. He was a fine student and an excellent teacher, and never really enjoyed hunting in the first place, despite all the evidence to the contrary.

The killing that took place—as it was portrayed blow by blow in the diaries, and can be divined from all the photographs and associated evidence gathered prior to conviction and written up in several hundreds of pages of U.S. District Court, Eastern District of Missouri, Southeastern Division briefs, as well as Circuit Court of Carter County criminal docket sheets and scores of other documents[9]—is a very different picture from that which emerges in speaking with LaRue himself, a man of deep convictions and passions and obvious intelligence. His self-professed motives, ethical standards, and perception of events leading up to the arrest of him and his son, and his subsequent incarceration, are largely at odds with those of his accusers. LaRue likes to talk and, for someone who has been described as "sneaky," I found him extraordinarily open and trusting.

"I've always been a person with a conscience," he repeats. LaRue admits to having gotten an extra deer once in a while. That was the atmosphere he was raised in, on a farm twenty-four miles north of Van Buren. "As I got older, there was no excuse for what I did," he said. But he insists he has always "had respect for the animals" and was always the first person to declare, "You should only shoot within the limits."

LaRue believes that Dan Burleson, Tom May, and the local prosecutor, Bradshaw Smith, all "went overboard." He claims "they" (referring to Burleson and/or May and/or the government) threatened and bribed his friends, and told his son his parents didn't love him and were considering disowning him, and that the son's best bet was to testify against his father. "My only regret is that there has been so much corruption," LaRue says, likening it to the Mafia, and referring, in part, to the dog

incident with Tom May; to May's "get even attitude." He believes that if May were to undergo a psychiatric examination, he'd be dismissed as game warden. "He's a bully. He tortures you with a satisfaction that feeds his ego and he's done this for twenty-five years." He also believes that May tried to hire someone to kill him, that May spent thirty minutes providing the would-be killer with a motive, and how to make it look like a hunting accident with a 3-inch magnum 12-gauge hit to the face, like a turkey misfire. May denies such claims.

As for Burleson specifically, LaRue has no hesitation in stating he's "intelligent as far as doing his job," but he adds, "I think he's obsessed to the point of destroying a person. To wipe out the family. It's almost like a vengeance, though he had no motive, and it's not because he's concerned about wildlife."

"Everybody in the county is finishing me off," LaRue complains, referring to the financial hit he and his wife and son are taking as a result of this whole affair. Their $90,000 nest egg is gone. He'd hoped to use that to buy his son a house. As a realtor, LaRue says he could make $100,000 a year. His wife has been a science teacher in good standing for twenty-three years. She is a very lovely woman. Now she's going to have to try to work real estate as well to make up for her husband's absence. As for LaRue's son, his college teaching career could be in jeopardy given the way the rumor mill can work in small towns. Understand that father and son were splashed across the local newspapers for two years. When LaRue is released from prison, he hopes to go back to real estate, unless "they wipe me out." He believes he can be a real asset to the community. But he also sees how the government could make him into a pauper, or a pumper of gas. "I can see why people just give up." He's also concerned about having to pay additional fines out of state for the trophy kills of years before.

LaRue is upset that nobody has ever recognized his good deeds—especially the fact that he has spent thousands of dollars and dug probably fifty wells on various properties for

wildlife, pools of water to help the animals out during dry years. Nor has anybody mentioned the fact that he was a park service ranger and naturalist at the age of twenty-two, a prodigy with a dedicated interest in conservation and a deep love of the land.

LaRue insists he has shot nothing illegally and reminds me that the land and the river around Van Buren are as they were 500 years ago. There are "Buddhistic" people in the area, says LaRue, living nonmaterialistically as they did centuries ago, gigging the rivers, going after turkey in April, and deer in the fall. That's always been the life here, he says philosophically, nostalgically. But he also admits to fault. "We saw hunting as an innocent form of mischief, like a speeding ticket," he said, repeating an analogy he'd used earlier. But the analogy loses all meaning when LaRue points to the fact that "coyotes were nearly extinct in the 1960s. Now they're back and killing twice as many deer as the hunters." By LaRue's estimates, Missouri now has 20 deer per square mile, whereas there used to be a mere 5 per square mile. LaRue says any game warden will tell you where you can shoot 2,000 deer if you want to. It wouldn't "dent" the population. In fact, he has a rather elaborate biological theory which purports to have its foundation in the notion that if you don't kill them, they won't survive. It's the hunting, he insists, that has brought back the populations of deer and turkey. Not surprisingly, most conservationists would agree with that thinking. He says he has friends throughout the Ozarks for whom it is not unusual to kill 40 deer a year. That kind of thinking, however, most conservationists would condemn. Tom May knows of just such a poacher. He lives at this very moment in Winona, Missouri, not far from Van Buren. May knows who he is and is just waiting to get the goods on him and bring him in. It'll happen one of these days.

When LaRue was a boy, he had one sister for his first eleven years, along with two beagle dogs and a couple of guns. He'd hunt "varmints like crow, foxes and squirrels." At the age

of 10 he got a .22 pump and 12-gauge shotgun, a 30/30 lever-action rifle like that which John Wayne used. By the age of 12 he bagged his first 4-point buck. "I was proud," he recalls. At the end of each day he'd get off the school bus and go up some hillside or another to chase rabbits through the black-berry briers. That was his life. No one thought anything of driving the deer with beagles that can run the animals end-lessly. "We were poor farmers. Work your butt off. Earn what you can. But it was a wonderful environment," he remarks. "If you grew up on a farm with animals that got eaten—there's something about it—I don't quote scriptures but God said waste not want not. The Bible says the animals were put here to eat. If you don't eat them, they'll rot, and turn to weed. Three to four years is as old as a wild turkey gets. They repro-duce fast. Winters kill them out, or they'll overpopulate." He recalls that turkey populations in the region since about 1970 have faltered, their hatching success plummeting. But he says even most poachers have enough sense to give the animals a reprieve if the numbers get low, though he admits that "ten percent of the poachers out there are ignorant and will kill the last one." Some might take issue with LaRue's turkey data. A Missouri Conservation Commission chaired by a citizen panel conducted a recent yearlong study of the state's turkeys and concluded that Missouri's wild flock is "robust, well-managed and able to sustain an increased harvest." There was no mention of plummeting hatching success. Not that LaRue's record of dead turkeys, at least as witnessed by the di-aries, evidenced much concern about that. Adding confusion to insult, according to the commission the population of wild turkeys in the state has grown from 2,500 birds in 1952 to "a conservative estimate of 600,000 today." Moreover, the panel declared, "one thing is certain—turkey hunting in Missouri has little influence on wild turkey populations in the state."[10]

When LaRue was growing up, he says, the animals were always left alone during the spring, when they were having

143

babies. He and his friends never went hunting during those times. But in the fall, nobody really thought about it if you killed an extra animal for your table. "Of course, even back then, we didn't have to do it to eat," he points out. He says his family used to give the meat to others throughout Reynolds County. "The good old days are over. Missouri is liberal," says LaRue. In fact, Tom May also speaks of a "liberal" Missouri. For LaRue, the word seems to imply a system of laws that has become unreasonably confining and uptight, or assbackwards. For May, "liberal" refers to a state that has probably some of the least stringent fines for wildlife violators in the country. The two men are miles apart in their thinking.

LaRue believes that less than "one out of twenty folks in this community will hold it against you," referring to his kind of poaching—noncommercial poaching. He says that half the school board are poachers, and the other half simply don't care. "I went in for a trophy. It's wrong. But there was never an attempt to make one cent. It was only hunting in the pure sense. I knew it was wrong. But I wasn't arrogant about it. I went in there for the simplicity. It was a one-time deal. The punishment to me should have fit the crime. It didn't. What's happened to me could happen to you. If they want you, they'll get you," LaRue complains. In fact, all that happened, he says, was "a father and his son going hunting like two hundred years ago. They went out for the sheer father-son companionship, like fishing or baseball." LaRue says he took the plea bargain to help his son, and that most of his prison time was for giving a couple of $3-a-box shells to his young friends, when Dan Burleson just happened to be there for an hour.

I asked Bud whether he thought cases like that of LaRue's would have a therapeutic impact around here. He wasn't sure, but reckoned, if anything, it was the teenagers you'd have to reach.

"How are you going to change them?" I asked.

"I don't know, just to be real honest with you, I really

don't. The Conservation Commission [referring to the MDC] can only do so much. I mean you can't be everywhere. It's going to take help from the community." But he reminded me, pessimistically, that this was Carter County, where people have been poaching all their lives. "Very few will make that change," he said. Or call in a game warden on their friends. "That's probably not going to happen."

Bud's friend also pointed out that the two minors to whom LaRue sold ammunition joked about it at school. "They're probably worse now than ever," she said. And at that same school, everybody knew who had killed some bald eagles. But nobody would talk and there was no way to prove anything. Tom May says that many of the young poachers he's now contending with look to LaRue as their "hero." LaRue's example trained them. After all, he got away with it for thirty-six years.

Bud says he knows who those boys are. And he says, on a more upbeat note, that he was just like them, and he was able to change. He doesn't want to come off sounding, suddenly, like an "anti-hunter." He pauses, and looks me in the eye. "'Cause I'm sure not." But he thinks something good can come out of all this. That hunters will reevaluate the sportsmanship of hunting and realize that that's where it's at, not just killing for killing's sake.

"You don't have to kill nothing. Just go out there and to be there and know, I think what done me more good than anything was I could go out there and sit down with my rifle, with my bow, or just be there and see those things, deer come by, [and] I thought, I don't have to shoot them. So what if I don't?"

"Do you think you'll ever reach the place where you'll give up the gun and just use your eyes?" I ask him.

Bud is quick to declare, "Oh, yeah. In the last three years I've done that a lot, you betcha. That's what I'm saying, you know." Bud describes a hunting trip with his sixteen-year-old daughter. Early in the morning she shot at a doe, but missed

it. Later on, the same animal walked within twenty feet of them. They didn't even raise their weapons. It wasn't legal, says Bud. But more importantly, he says of his daughter, "She'd never seen a deer that close alive out in the wild. It was quite an experience for her. She really enjoyed that, you know? And it done me good to know if that would have been five years ago, I'd a been sayin,' 'Shoot it, shoot it!'"

One morning recently Bud went out into the woods and saw forty-six deer. He never fired a shot. "You know, I ain't no better than anybody else, but you can do for yourself whatever you want. You could quit anything, especially something like that. It's not a disease. It's not like there's no way, ah, you could quit it if you want to, you can."

For LaRue's part, he says he'd already decided "to clean up their act." He was basically going to voluntarily give up hunting. He'd gone beyond that, he told me with a manner of Zen stoicism. Now he just wanted companionship with his son out in the wild. "Hunters evolve to the point where they no longer need to hunt," he said with some sentiment in his voice. "When you're young you go through the phase of how many can I get? Does two rabbits sound like I succeeded? At twenty it's easy to get six squirrels. Then you end up evolving from meat to selective trophy hunter, and finally, as you get a lot of trophies, you evolve even more. I have reached a grandpa stage," he rhapsodizes in terms approaching poetry, likening himself now to a grand old "teacher." He'll be nearly fifty when he gets out of prison. He concludes, "I don't need to hunt. An inner calmness and goodness in me prevails."

As for the presiding U.S. attorney, Edward L. Dowd Jr., based in St. Louis, he had but one, unambiguous way to characterize this whole sorry affair: "This can be described simply as slaughter. This was the most extreme case of wildlife violations I have ever seen."[11] According to Gary Cravens, supervisor of the Missouri Department of Conservation Ozark Protection Region, "I have never seen such outrageous slaugh-

ter committed by one or two people. . . . Their crimes are enough to sicken anyone—hunters and non-hunters alike."[12]

And yet even in this extreme case, the charges were incredibly modest given the amount of actual damage inflicted, as indicated by the diaries and other evidence. On the federal level, the charges brought against the father refer to only two of the animals, a bighorn sheep and an elk, in addition to the auxiliary crimes, the selling of some shells to neighbor kids, the transportation of horns across state lines (Lacey Act violations), and LaRue's knowingly conspiring to hide items in order to avoid seizure. On the state level, the charges focused on LaRue's unlawful use of a weapon, his endangering the welfare of children, and twelve misdemeanor counts of taking deer in a closed season, two counts of taking deer in a wildlife refuge, one count of taking a coyote by illegal methods (shining a light in its face), and one count of exceeding the legal limit of deer killed. LaRue was also charged with three misdemeanor counts of possession of wild turkeys in closed season. The son has similar but far fewer charges.

Human beings grow up with cultural attitudes that justify their patterns of consumption, lifestyle, sense of God-given right, or sense of justice. Given the divergent points of view that emerge with such force on either side of the law regarding hunting, as happened so glaringly in the town of Van Buren, one can only express gratitude that the law is there—haphazard, imperfect, crowded with necessary paperwork and hardworking, underbudgeted lawmen, but there, nevertheless; all posited by the public in a sometimes blind but valiant effort to sustain some modicum of honor with the land and with its wide-ranging biological occupants, a tenuous balance in the fight to save America's wildlife.

5

Best-Laid Plans

According to sources at the U.S. Fish and Wildlife Service, it would prove next to impossible to estimate how many people at any one time are behind bars in the United States for crimes committed against wildlife. This is not due to the fact that there are so many, but because there is no coordination of that data. But the agents I spoke with agree that it is not a particularly impressive number versus the number of violations. As previously indicated, state and federal agents are tragically too few to counter the onrush of illegal activities, which are growing in sweeping magnitude by all accounts. More delicate, though equally chilling, is the realization that our judicial system, and a large number of prosecutors, is not yet fully attuned to an appreciation of the severity of wildlife crimes, certainly by comparison with their more habitual universe of infractions against humanity. As the multiyear case against Robert LaRue and his son illustrates, a tremendous amount of government resources, time, money, and paperwork are required in order to get a conviction of any kind.

But poaching and a sometimes desensitized legal system are not the only obstacles to enhancing the quality of life for wildlife in America. What concerns me here is the fact that the U.S. government itself, particularly our Department of Agriculture (USDA), though also the military and the Environmental Protection Agency (EPA), has been the subject of some

very serious allegations with regard to its own concerted impact on other species.

Within the USDA, by far the most controversial arena of animal policy involves the activities of the Animal Damage Control program, known as the ADC. This program has elicited strident and persistent outcries from people who are deeply distressed by what they feel they have discovered about the ADC's activities. These activities amount, in their estimation, to a massive destruction of American wildlife that has been dictated, orchestrated, and executed by the American government.

Three of those concerned citizens are the subject of this chapter: biologist Marc Bekoff, public interest investigator Pat Wolff, and ecological activist Tom Skeele. For years these three have endeavored respectively to expose the ADC for what they believe it to be—a nearly out-of-control killing machine beneath the supposedly respectable veneer of a government agency devoted to protecting the health of plants and animals. They express a view that the government's mandate to protect health has been distorted, warped by a mission long out of fashion, but not diminished in strength or financial clout: a credo that sees the systematic curtailment of predators as the government's responsibility to farmers and ranchers.

Subsumed within the Department of Agriculture, the ADC has its headquarters in Washington, D.C., a support staff in Hyattsville, Maryland, regional offices in Tennessee and in Fort Collins, Colorado, and anywhere from two to four district offices per state. The ADC funds the discouraging or killing of animals suspected to be predators (which could mean, theoretically, a rat or a seagull, a blue jay or a grizzly bear) that have elicited the ire of any citizen who qualifies for ADC backup. The conditions of qualification for ADC assistance vary from state to state, but all ADC activities are founded on the central premise that human beings have the right to control wildlife. As an ethical position, many Americans might not

have a problem with that, with a system of self-defense whose well-intended goal is the prevention of harm to people. Where many critics of the ADC do find problems is in what they see as the excesses of killing perpetrated by the agency.

In 1921, a federal Eradication Methods Laboratory in Denver, Colorado, was established for researching the most effective poisons for killing animals. Nine years later the American Society of Mammalogists condemned the government's efforts in this domain. Nonetheless, within subsequent months, President Herbert Hoover signed into law the Animal Damage Control (ADC) Act on March 2, 1931. The act was a response to a perspective held heatedly by many ranchers and farmers that predators were bad for business. In an effort to rid America of the perceived predator threat, ADC advocates lumped together grizzly bears and rabbits, owls and mountain lions as problem species. Other targets included badgers, blackbirds, crows, prairie dogs, peccaries (javelinas), gophers, marmots, deer, bobcats, foxes, lynx, martins, ferrets, fishers, raccoons, wolves, black bears, and, most of all, coyotes. All of these species (and many others—from vultures to squirrels) were said to be potentially bad for their profits, injurious to poultry, sheep, goats, cattle, tree farms, fisheries, and agriculture. The ADC Act called for the agency "to conduct campaigns for the destruction or control of such animals" on both public and privately owned lands. The ADC's supply depot, where most of the poisons and traps for killing animals are kept, is in Pocatello, Idaho. While their products can go to most anyone, the Pocatello Supply Depot (or PSD, as it's known) provides its products only through the various ADC offices.

In referring to those "campaigns" for destruction the ADC was sanctioned to carry out, biologist Marc Bekoff describes the government's "long history of controlling and managing animals by killing them, often indiscriminately, and also for supporting research that involves a good deal of pain and suffering for the animals involved."[1] The ADC dispatches agents

into the field. An estimated 80 percent of their overall activities occur in the western states. These agents kill targeted predators, in addition to working on general animal control. Among the tools they use are snares and leghold traps, aerial gunning, traplines, denning (in which pups are killed in the den), spring-loaded cyanide devices that blow up in the animal's face, and sheep collars containing compound 1080, a poison so toxic that one pound of it can kill one million pounds of animal life. By such strategies, and others, ADC hunters have killed an estimated average of more than 3 million animals each year, though a precise numeric count is hotly debated. While the agents are supposed to treat predators implicated in killing livestock by first seeking to remedy the situation through nonviolent means, in practice, by many accounts, both targeted and nontargeted animals are killed, with apparently little thought given to nonlethal intervention. The killing is done with highly dangerous poisons, as well as with primitive traps—traps that can kill any animal, human or otherwise.

Such traps include the leghold or steel-jaw, a razor sharp steel clutch that slams shut on a leg or paw; the Conibear, which slams around the animal's throat, face, or torso; and the wire snare, which strangles the animal. These are crude devices. Animals die slowly and painfully, often trying to eat away at their paws or legs to escape. In the case of the snare, the more desperately the animal tries to free itself, the tighter the snare closes. An animal will starve or die of thirst or suffocate. A three-in-one.

Such actions constitute a grotesque chronicle of wildlife slaughtered in the United States in the name of ranchers and farmers (many of them quite wealthy) whose claims, on biological grounds, are suspect. Consider the reported death toll by ADC agents for fiscal year 1989–1990: 3,283,883 animals, including (but not limited to) 11 alligators, 1,756,775 blackbirds, 1,050 prairie dogs, 1,310 peccaries, 550 rabbits, 12,302 herons and egrets, 9,899 seagulls, 2,532 marmots, 22 owls, 484

mountain lions, 15,781 doves, 10 woodpeckers and flickers, 756 deer, 14 geese, 2,298 bobcats, 1,126 squirrels, 43 rattlesnakes, 15,804 foxes, 39 ducks, 3,517 porcupines, 1 eagle, 175 wolves, 147 minks, 347 turtles, 460 black bears, 2,531 badgers, and 177,721 coyotes. All of this slaughter is deemed by the ADC to be an acceptable response to the alleged predator impact on domestic livestock, as well as its impact on other resources like crops and human health or safety. Ignoring the ethics of such carnage, if that is possible, there is, in addition, an enormous scientific literature that refutes the claim that any of the above-mentioned species have ever exerted a serious impact on domestic-bred herds—meaning "serious" relative to the far more extensive syndromes of animal morbidity and mortality.

Not until 1963 were ADC policies, actions, and results scrutinized by an independent committee, appointed by Interior Secretary Stewart Udall. That group of conservationists severely criticized the ADC, finding the agency to be excessive and indiscriminate in its killings. Again, in 1971, the ADC was tongue-lashed by an advisory committee selected from President Richard Nixon's Council on Environmental Quality. This time, the ADC was accused of using nonselective toxins that were dangerous to the general public. A year later, Nixon banned the use of such toxicants for predator control by any federal agencies. The EPA then banned compound 1080, a predator control mixture (still in prolific use in places like New Zealand) that combines strychnine, sodium cyanide, and thallium sulfate. There is no known antidote, and it is lethal.

A year after the Nixon/EPA ban, President Gerald Ford reinstated the use of sodium cyanide in the spring-loaded killing device known as M-44, yielding to pressure from western livestock interests that wanted coyotes on the open range eradicated. Ranchers still insist it is the coyote that has maximized their losses. In 1974 the ADC's staff was expanded to more than 900 people, and its budget topped $46 million. In 1978, Interior Secretary Cecil Andrus appointed an ADC

review committee. Again, as in every previous investigation, the committee report was highly critical of the agency. Andrus responded by putting an end to denning (the clubbing to death and/or asphyxiating and burning alive of coyote pups while they nestled in their dens) and a halt to research on compound 1080 at the Denver research facility. As one ADC western states director described the agency's methodology, "It's like sausage making. . . . You don't really want to know what goes into it."[2] The Denver site was recently moved to the huge agricultural research complex at Colorado State University in Fort Collins.

During the Reagan presidency, Interior Secretary James Watt reinstated denning. President Reagan then lifted the previous ban restricting the use of compound 1080 out in the wild despite EPA administrator William Ruckelshaus calling it "one of the most dangerous toxics known to man." One-five-hundredth of an ounce of the odorless, sugarlike substance is fatal to humans. Thought of differently, one teaspoon will kill up to 100 adult human males. Its half-life in the wild, like DDT and other perdurable toxins, means it easily enters the food chain and remains there for many years. The USF&W has found that 1080 "possesses a high degree of secondary hazard. A single mouse killed with the water solution may contain enough poison to kill a full-grown dog." Throughout the 1960s and '70s, ADC agents spread 1.3 million pounds of grain spiked with 1080 across millions of acres of land, in addition to more than 7 million strychnine tallow pellets. Compound 1080 and strychnine are not the only poisons implemented under ADC guidelines. Others include the slow-acting avicide DRC-1339, a variety of rodenticides, zinc phosphide, den and burrow fumigants containing carbon and sodium nitrate, and the horrible M-44 sodium cyanide capsules. In 1986, at the written request of nineteen western senators, Reagan transferred the ADC from the Department of the Interior to the Department of Agriculture, where the ADC's budget nearly doubled. President

George Bush, late in his second term, tried to diminish the ADC funds, which his staff believed contradicted the logic of the Endangered Species Act. Congress overturned his request. But with public scrutiny increasing, the agency tried to sanitize its image and referred to itself as simply "Wildlife Services." It was too late. The information had already leaked from whistle-blowers within the ADC, and the public was beginning to learn of the disquieting truths behind the agency's work. To some critics, that systematic slaughter represents the breaking of our contract with nature. It also highlights the uncomfortable truth of the American dread of wild beasts.

As outlined in the Wildlife Damage Review, published in Tucson, Arizona,[3] the early states and territories offered boun-ties on most of America's charismatic megafauna in response to demands by the westward-moving cattle industry. By 1886, most predators—and that included many species of birds—had been officially deemed "bothersome" by the newly formed Division of Economic Ornithology and Mammalogy, which in 1905 would become the Bureau of Biological Survey. Con-gress subsequently appropriated $125,000 for the bureau to control large predators.

By the late 1920s, grizzly bears and wolves had essentially disappeared from the lower forty-eight states. The last grizzly bear was killed in California (whose state mascot is the grizzly) in 1922 in the mountains of Tulare County. Today, there are a smattering of grizzly populations left below Canada. The largest numbers exist in the Glacier/Bob Marshall ecosystem and the Greater Yellowstone ecosystem, and lesser numbers are to be found in the Cabinet-Yaak, Selkirk, and North Cas-cade ecosystems of the U.S.-Canadian border area. There is recent evidence that a few grizzlies also exist in central Idaho, and possibly the San Juan Mountains of Colorado. In all, it is estimated that less than 1,000 grizzlies can be found in the lower forty-eight states. Louisa L. Wilcox, director of Wild For-ever, a grizzly bear collaborative project involving the Greater

Yellowstone Coalition, the Great Bear Foundation, the Sierra Club, and the Wilderness Society, estimates that prior to their systematic decimation, there was probably a population of over 100,000 grizzlies in the lower forty-eight. The last wolf was killed in the Yellowstone region in 1926; against a backdrop of controversy, wolves were reintroduced from Canada only in 1995. As of late 1998 there were over 100 wolves in Yellowstone, and they are beginning to thrive. But a local judge has pressed to have the wolves removed. Ranchers outside the park are afraid of them, though such fears are built of utter myth, not reality.

Eagles were only recently taken off the endangered species list in some states. California condors are nearly extinct. And while the black bear population exceeds 600,000 and is said to be very healthy, once there were probably millions of black bears throughout this country, not remotely as numerous as the herbivorous North American bison, but far more multitudinous than today's surviving populations.

Many have pointed out the terrible irony whirling around the ADC: on the one hand, the U.S. government claims to honor the principles of conservation and ecological stewardship. It has erected a fairly impressive wildlife law enforcement system for the purpose of preserving biodiversity and arresting those who would illegally breach the codified terms of hunting decorum. Why has it not recognized and stopped the activities of an internal government branch that may be directly responsible for killing more wildlife than all the domestic poachers combined?

Moreover, ADC agents themselves have been implicated in other expressly illegal activities. For years, information had circulated throughout the environmental communities that thousands of bald and golden eagles were dying from consuming carcasses that had been laced with poisons, a practice that is strictly illegal. On September 5, 1991, government agents from the U.S. Fish and Wildlife Service, the Environ-

ment and Natural Resources Division of the U.S. Justice Department, and the EPA raided an ADC lab in Wyoming that had been at the center of an illegal poisons ring. The USF&W regional director stated that poison sufficient "to kill every man, woman, child and mammal in the western United States" had been seized, in the form of cyanide, thallium, strychnine, and compound 1080. That lab had been selling the poisons to ranchers. According to one undercover agent for USF&W, when he presented incriminating evidence "on the Commissioner of Agriculture and most every ADC supervisor in the state of Wyoming for which they could have been prosecuted," he was told "to leave the state and keep (his) mouth shut."[4]

There are legal ambiguities that buffer the ADC from widespread public censure. While President Nixon had signed an executive order outlawing the use of chemical toxicants as so-called predacides in February 1972, a decade later President Reagan, under pressure from the livestock industry lobby, rescinded the order, a prelude to the EPA approving compound 1080 for killing wildlife. It is easy to see how ADC officials might reasonably slip between the legal cracks, which would explain why nobody went to jail in the Wyoming sting operation. Compound 1080 is used now in what the industry calls LPCs—livestock protection collars—worn by sheep and cattle in six states. In a sense, the message a "protection collar" sends to the public is one of positive mediation—the protection of animal life. It is the sort of message the ADC, in general, promotes about its activities. The collar is, according to the ADC, "an inflatable bladder that is placed under the throat of a sheep or goat and is held in place with Velcro straps." What is not widely disseminated is the fact that should a hapless coyote, a dog, or anyone else for that matter (a child playing with a sheep) come in contact with that collar, puncturing it, the substance gets released and the unlucky recipient is likely to die after a few hours of cardiac, central nervous system, and respiratory failure. There is no antidote. A carcass containing

the compound, fed upon by other predators, spreads its deadly potion to other scavengers.

Marc Bekoff and the Mind of the Coyote

Dr. Marc Bekoff has studied predator behavior for two decades and is one of the foremost authorities on coyotes in the world. He loves and respects the animal and is devastated and perplexed that so many people who should know better, continue to think of it as "vermin." Based at the University of Colorado in Boulder, Bekoff is a somewhat celebrated professor in the Department of Environmental, Population, and Organismic Biology. He lives in a wild canyon above town and is something of a wild thinker. He has made at least one radical turnabout in his life: early in his career he went from partaking in biomedical research on animals to a thorough rejection of it. As a graduate student, Bekoff had been doing research involving the killing of cats, but he became morally and scientifically repulsed by such research. His work now takes him out into the wild to try to gain some insight into the behavior of predators, in hopes of persuading those who are quick to kill them that predators are, first and foremost, magnificent creatures, and second, that they are essential for any healthy ecosystem.

Bekoff has written:

The deepest problem with wildlife management may involve the tendency to confuse scientific ideas with philosophical ones. When managers argue that a population should be "culled" or otherwise managed and controlled . . . this is often viewed as a scientific recommendation. . . . However, the models that are used are often simplistic . . . and estimates of the actual numbers of supposed problem predators can be inaccurate. . . . It is also possible that only

a small percentage of people living in a given area actually want to control predators such as wolves . . . and the arguments put forth for doing so can be self-serving . . . most importantly recommendations about population control presuppose various philosophical positions with ethical dimensions and assumptions.[5]

Bekoff is a skeptic when it comes to making policy that entails setting any limits or numbers for management by hunting or culling. He insists that "killing is ethically indefensible." That's where he begins. And he believes that for the most part few management programs have ever worked. More than management, it's the "anthropocentric" nature of human manipulation, of human-specific goals and aspirations that bothers him and gets in the way of sound biological science. He knows very well that there are other types of interventions that do not involve killing. Most managers operate, he says, with a "lack of care and understanding and compassion."[6]

Bekoff's style of questioning has gained considerable currency in the animal rights movements since 1975, when Australian philosopher Peter Singer's book *Animal Liberation* was published. But it runs counter to the prevailing doctrines of nearly all government agencies in the world concerned with maximizing agricultural and ranching profits, which often occurs at the direct expense of wildlands and wild animals. Among wildlife managers, the human population control of animals is generally deemed a human right and a responsibility. But those in Bekoff's camp take a very different position.

Bekoff believes that predator control, certainly in the case of coyotes, has only fortified the animals' determination, in so many words, to live long and prosper. The greater the stress and introduced (human) threat, the more likely coyotes are to disperse and repopulate. From a systems point of view, killing random individuals, even random future generations (i.e., denning), will not curtail coyote populations. What works, says

Bekoff, is ranchers and farmers cleaning up their ranches and farms—putting in fences and guard dogs. It's not so complicated.

Bekoff not only questions the tactics, but the ethics, of predator control and nearly all human exploitation of other species. He is confident that the wide-ranging data available to the public is more than enough to prove that animals have strong feelings. In summarizing a long debate concerning non-human animal consciousness and the huge variety of perceptual acuities and capacities, Bekoff points to a famous statement by eighteenth-century philosopher Jeremy Bentham, who declared that the issue "is not Can they reason? nor Can they talk? but, Can they suffer?"[7] and concludes that "there are many good reasons for adopting Bentham's position."[8] From his knowledge of the scientific literature, he is confident that many animals share with humans not only a similar neurological organization, an extreme vulnerability to pain, but subjective worlds, emotions, dreams, feelings, and stunning intellectual capabilities, all of which compounds the human situation vis-à-vis our management of other populations and our intervention to conserve species.

Bekoff is a specialist in coyote behavior, and when it comes to coyotes, there are few scientists who have his field experience.[9] Coyotes, *Canis latrans,* along with thirty-six other species, are members of the family Canidae, order Carnivora. Along with coyotes, the *Canis* genus includes eight other species—wolves, domestic dogs *(Canis familiaris),* dingoes, Simien foxes, and three types of jackals.[10] Bekoff's work has brought him into contact with the practices of the ADC because coyotes (and after coyotes, dogs) have been implicated in the majority of sheep and calf predation on ranches. The coyote is, therefore, the primary target species for ADC agents.

In one long research project, Bekoff and his postdoctoral student, Michael Wells, studied a population of coyotes in the southeast corner of the Grand Teton National Park, near Jack-

son, Wyoming, at a place called Blacktail Butte, collecting data almost every day between September 1977 and February 1983. Direct observation was integrated with some radio tracking. Fifty-six coyotes were tagged, forty-three fitted with radio collars. The researchers found that the coyotes were a "close-knit, cohesive social unit." The animals employed "extensive greeting ceremonies" and engaged in much "play." "Clear-cut dominance relationships could not be detected" and "possession of a piece of food was rarely contested."[11] Courtship occurred during the harshest winter months, and gestation was approximately sixty-three days, the pups being born around May in dens often appropriated from other species, such as badgers or squirrels. By fall the young adults—nine to ten months of age—had spread out, more than half of the pack dispersing to new areas. Bekoff and Wells called them "roamers," whereas those who would stay with the pack were designated as "helpers," because these nonmating animals would help raise pups. Those that dispersed suffered high mortality, and the reasons for dispersal seemed to correlate with stress to the core pack, usually brought on by human predation or hunger.

Trying to divine hidden communication signals among the coyotes of one pack, and among outside visiting animals, the researchers made note of several primary positions used by the coyotes for urinating and eliminating—RLU (raised-leg urination), SQU (squat urination), and so forth—that seemed significant as means of communicating the demarcation of their territory. Monthly marking rates were graphed and three-dimensional diagrams showing the distribution of urine were also fashioned by the researchers, all in an effort to better grasp the nature of marking and to answer questions concerning territoriality. Those questions remain unanswered to this day. Indeed, coyotes, despite a good deal of research, are among the most mysterious of animals in the wild. Though Bekoff and Wells could not produce definitive results to prove their communication theory, they believe that "coyotes communicate

using a rich repertoire of olfactory, tactile, vocal, and visual signals."[12]

They also assert that coyotes pose little threat to cattle and other livestock. The coyotes studied by Bekoff and Wells showed that "it is not obvious that coyotes hunt cooperatively on any regular basis, even for prey larger than themselves."[13] Of the approximately 930 grams of food consumed per day per coyote, 90 percent was observed to be mammalian flesh, the vast majority of which consisted of small rodents, voles, ground squirrels, and remains of human kills, primarily elk.[14] Large prey animals, such as sheep, were rarely brought down, as it could take a full hour to accomplish such a task, a heavy energy burden on the predator. What Bekoff and Wells established— and it is very significant—is the "difficulty of distinguishing 'coyote kills' from those of other predators, including domestic dogs" and the fact that "large ungulates are typically consumed by coyotes as carrion," meaning that the coyotes were not responsible for actually killing them. Interesting support for their findings comes from a study of captive coyotes which showed that not all individuals were interested in killing. Some preferred play. Nor was blood an apparent stimulant to consumption.[15]

The researchers found that coyotes "appear to be monogamous"; that "a prolonged association and an essentially exclusive mating relationship is established between one male and a single female. Furthermore, only one pair per pack typically mates in a given year." Pups are blind and helpless at birth; they stay in the den for about three weeks, where they are loved intensively (about twenty-two hours per day by one or both parents), and require nearly 5 months to achieve their independence.[16]

In the book *When Elephants Weep: The Emotional Lives of Animals,* by Jeffrey Moussaieff Masson and Susan McCarthy,[17] Bekoff summarized some of his experiences with coyotes, describing a female who started out alone more and more often,

and was increasingly missed by the pack. They would follow her, howl after her, and wait for her. When she left for good, Bekoff noted that "some spark, something, seemed to have gone out of them. They missed her. I know," writes Bekoff, "that sounds anthropomorphic, and that's just fine. I also know, as sure as I know that I am attached to this world, that those coyotes have deep and complicated feelings."

This is all an uneasy but fitting prelude to the fact that U.S. taxpayers' money is being used to support the systematic killing of coyotes and many other animals that are deemed threats or nuisances. Bekoff is candid in his displeasure with the U.S. Department of Agriculture's Animal Damage Control program. He says outright, "ADC tortures and kills animals." As early as 1979 Bekoff had published his own statistical analysis of sheep kills by coyotes, as reported by the U.S. Fish and Wildlife Service, and showed that losses due to coyotes in many Western states were typically less than attrition from other known causes.[18] The fact is that the vast majority of cattle mortality comes from dehydration and starvation—rancher abuse, in other words. In fact, in a study released in 1992 by the National Agricultural Statistics Service of the USDA, of the 4,370,400 cattle lost in the United States the previous year, predators accounted for only 2.4 percent. Nearly one-third of those 4.3 million deaths resulted from "respiratory problems," and another 20.6 percent from "digestive problems." In a study by statistician Jack Spence of the ADC's effectiveness in Utah's Dixie National Forest (1981–1992) and a Bureau of Land Management district (1983–1990), he found that "in both cases there is no evidence that a single sheep, lamb or cow has been protected by the ADC lethal control program."[19]

Familiarity cannot only breed contempt, but also compassion. This certainly seems to be true for many field biologists who study animals up close in the wild. Consider the case of the eminent Dr. Con Slobodchikoff, professor of biology at Northern Arizona University and one of the world's leading

authorities on the five species of prairie dogs, which are crucial to prairie and grassland ecology. Like Bekoff and his respect
for the coyote, Slobodchikoff has acquired a deep appreciation for an animal that has, like the coyote, been viewed as
nothing more than vermin. After years of labor, he believes he
has begun to detect clear linguistic patterns among prairie dogs
and has ascertained some aspects of their complex communication skills. He asserts that prairie dogs have a "sophisticated
animal language" that comprises elements of both semantics
and syntax. While others in the ethological community have
focused on the language of parrots, chimpanzees, gorillas, and
dolphins, for ten years Slobodchikoff and his students have
been working to decode the language of prairie dogs. Yet, by
his own admission, they are "only beginning to scratch the surface of what the prairie dogs are probably actually able to communicate to one another."

Much of what the prairie dogs seem to be speaking of concerns coyotes—their primary predator, other than man. So far,
Con and his colleagues have discerned at least nine different
"words" that prairie dogs utilize "just like words in a human
sentence." Furthermore, the researchers discovered that prairie
dogs could produce different alarm calls for a hawk, a human,
a coyote, and a domestic dog. They could even differentiate in
their communications between individuals of the same species.
Con knows of only one other similar species with such a vocal
system: the vervet monkey of East Africa. When people dressed
in jeans and dark glasses but different colored T-shirts approached the prairie dog colony being studied, Con and his
colleagues noticed that the prairie dog alerts varied from individual to individual. "The prairie dogs could tell the individual humans apart," writes Con.

Con has shown that prairie dog grasslands contain higher
biodiversity than grasslands without prairie dogs. Prairie dog
habitats (or towns) have been likened by ecologists to coral
reefs. In fact, other studies in Montana and South Dakota of

prairie dog colonies have revealed associated vertebrate species numbering 163 and 134, respectively. The colonies are critical food sources for coyotes, swift foxes, and the black-footed ferret, now included on the endangered species list. In fact, the ferret is an obligate species with the prairie dog, meaning that it cannot survive without it. Hawks, eagles, and bobcats also depend to varying degrees on prairie dogs. And because prairie dogs tend to clip the vegetation, they induce a wave of fresh, nutritious shoots that both wild and domestic ungulates (i.e., bison, elk, and cows) have shown a demonstrated preference for. Yet, as researchers are beginning to understand just how critical prairie dogs are to the short and mixed grasslands, Con and his students are faced with the fact that ranchers and the U.S. government are waging a veritable war of extermination on one colony after another. The livestock industry has lobbied to have them eliminated as predators. One species of prairie dog was refused candidacy on the endangered species list, probably, many believe, because of political pressure from special interest lobbies. Writes Con, "An animal that has one of the most sophisticated vocal languages known to science and is an important component of grassland ecosystems might soon go the way of the passenger pigeon—extinct."[20]

Con Slobodchikoff asks for tolerance and understanding of the prairie dog. And by his own impressive example, Marc Bekoff advocates a radical rethinking of scientific and management hubris that would realign its perspectives and goals to be in much greater harmony with other life-forms, not least of which is the coyote. Such realignment would include granting some degree of moral status to other animals. But the wisdom of biologists is only part of the story. Another part concerns the ability of all citizens, and their political representatives, to mount effective campaigns to rethink and eventually halt the killing.

A December 1993 cover story on ADC in *Sierra,* the

magazine of the Sierra Club, entitled "War on Wildlife: When 'Control' Means Slaughter," was one of the first in a national mainstream periodical to spell out the grisly particulars of the ADC. The article inventoried ADC agents' extermination of a reported 2.2 million wild animals from 140 different species for the year 1992. The article contained a photograph, taken by an Arizona Fish and Game employee who wanted to expose the ADC's work, in 1990. The image showed thirteen severed Arizona mountain lion heads stacked atop each other. ADC agents had conducted the massacre. Western-based environmentalists had been outraged, and two ardent activists in particular: New Mexican Pat Wolff (whose work was profiled in journalist Donald Schueler's *Sierra* piece)[21] and Tom Skeele of Bozeman, Montana. Both Wolff and Skeele had been fighting for years to concentrate the public floodlights on the ADC and effect the first real public exposure.

Tom Skeele in a Land of Predators

Skeele, now in his late thirties, came from a suburban Connecticut environment and had his first—and most lasting—revelation about the human relationship to wildlife while trekking for six weeks along the northern portions of the Appalachian Trail. He woke up during one brilliant sunrise amid a bevy of wild animal sights and sounds and thought about what his siblings were doing back in urban America during those moments—taking the kids to school, setting off amid rush hour traffic for work in the computer industry. . . . He concluded how critical it was for people to understand and experience firsthand the spiritual significance of wilderness.

Tom devoted himself to outdoor education and earned his degree in that field from the University of Oregon. He would spend long months talking about natural systems to groups, working in Yosemite, the Everglades, and elsewhere. He also

did a lot of juvenile delinquent experiential educational work, again outdoors.

Tom's initial experience with wild predators was in northern Minnesota in 1980, where he got his first penetrating glimpses of predation and recognized something incredibly key to the health of an ecosystem through the eyes of wolves. While in Minnesota, he was just starting to pursue his dream of being an educator, wanting to teach people about the importance of wild things and wild places. But after eight years of seed planting in young minds, he realized that, for himself, the reaping of rewards solely through the educational process was too long a road. He wanted to find an approach that might provide him with results in a shorter time frame—a longing that led him to environmental activism. Tom went on to become an integral part of the efforts to successfully stop government wolf controls in British Columbia in the winter of 1987–1988. But his greatest interest was in the wolf controversies throughout the northern Rockies, and eventually he moved to Bozeman, Montana, with his wife, an interpreter for the National Park Service. Along with a friend, Tom and his wife then started their nonprofit Predator Project, which today has some 800 subscription members, and an annual budget— used for purposes of education—just shy of $200,000. Their goal, says Tom, is "to save a place for America's predators; both out on the land, and in the hearts and minds of the public, through reacquainting Americans with the majesty and ecological importance of predators."

Though he is not a biologist, Tom has, by now, studied predator-prey relationships for well over a decade, and has seen with his own eyes the complexity of those myriad associations. When a kill occurs, for example, Tom explains that there is an important ecological ripple effect, with food parts being left over for ravens and magpies, for vultures and insects, as well as for the grass and the microorganisms. Ethically, philosophically, and spiritually, Tom goes on, the predators provide

us with mirrors and lessons for looking at ourselves. "We are predators, too," he points out. Tom believes that predators should be regarded as "umbrella species." Save the predator, and the vast habitats they require, and you save countless other species. Predators are superb ecological rallying points for generating effective, long-range, long-term strategies for conservation, says Tom.

Much of Tom's impetus came from his five-year affiliation with EarthFirst!, during the late 1980s. What impresses him about that lightly orchestrated organization, he muses, is that for all of its supposed "radicalness," it adheres to a rigorously democratic bearing. The EarthFirst! movement is superb at empowering individuals, letting them know that they can make a difference. Speaking of the country as a whole, Tom points out that "for all of our democracy, it's incredible how democratic we're not." He refers to the unfortunate fact that some conservation organizations with great publications and superb articles do not necessarily provide very many avenues—other than sending in a check for $25—for people to get actively involved in the issues.

The Predator Project has been pushing for some very big changes in the attitudes toward and treatment of predators in the United States, and more and more consumers (though few ranchers or congressmen) seem to be listening. Tom knows some livestock ranchers who don't like the ADC, but the ones who actively oppose it are rare, he says, even though, ironically, most ranchers want government off their backs. The first and biggest bitter pill that both ranchers and farmers, and also consumers, have to swallow, says Tom, is the philosophical fact that ranching and farming entail certain losses that are inherent in the activities and must be incorporated in the price. Killing wild animals is not an acceptable substitute, he argues, for passing along financial losses to customers. There is a cost of doing business on the open range, in the wide-open prairies, in the forests. You cannot manipulate nature with impunity,

says Tom. The real problem with management by the ADC, he argues, is that because it is a federal program, those private individuals who benefit from it are not required to pay anything. What they do pay as taxpayers is only a small percentage of the total cost of the ADC program that they directly benefit from. They only need pick up the phone, call in a complaint, and sign a contract. They don't first have to use any nonlethal means of solving the problem themselves. They don't have to accept any threshold of loss before qualifying for assistance. Recognizing that predators are here to stay—and it's not likely that ranchers and farmers and city types will embrace them anytime soon—at least, Tom argues, let's insist that businessmen accept and take responsibility for the risks they themselves have incurred, rather than foisting those business liabilities on the taxpayer.

In at least one other country, New Zealand, where there is a perception of a "pest" problem in the form of possums and ferrets, the New Zealand Biosecurity Act of 1993 makes landowners responsible for their own management of pests and the related costs. When the government does aerial spraying of the poison 1080, the beneficiaries of such spraying (beef, dairy, and deer farmers) pay for it themselves. There are estimated to be 70 million possums in the country, 20 possums for every New Zealander, and it is claimed that they destroy forests. While it is unlikely that the massive spreading of poisoned baits will be phased out anytime soon, the government has, at least, begun genetic research on the possibilities for fertility intervention and reproductive control. Most New Zealanders do not have much hope for nonlethal approaches being implemented in the near future, however.[22] But at least there is an example of a democratic government placing the cost burden associated with doing business on the businesses themselves.

Here in the United States some have proposed a concept by which the ADC would not be allowed to come in and conduct

lethal control (at least on National Forest lands) until at least 5 percent of the permittee's herd had been killed by predators. Prior to that time, the owner of the livestock would be responsible for conducting his or her own control. This might encourage owners of livestock to apply nonlethal (less expensive) approaches. It's also worth pointing out that if the 5 percent threshold concept were adopted, the ADC would probably be out of the business of predator control, inasmuch as it is very rare for predators to inflict that much damage on any herd.

Tom has joined people from various conservation sectors, wool growers, biologists, a clothing designer, a community organizer, and others who have together created an organization they term Predator Friendly, Inc. PFI has initiated a certification program that says to the rancher, if you use only nonlethal methods of protecting your sheep or your lambs in the production of wool, PFI will certify your product as "predator friendly"—which, on the green market, can double the value of your return. There are predator friendly hats, coats, and blankets, and soon there will be PFI-certified slippers and sweaters. It's a beginning, says Tom.

Tom admits that he is no lover of ranching, and would like to see the whole livestock industry disappear. "They are nonnative and they ought not to be here because of the ecological havoc that they are wreaking on natural boundaries." Ranchers will say to him, "And when are you going back to Europe, too, Tom?" He is familiar with the argument. But he is passionate about reminding ranchers that "grazing on public lands is a privilege and not a right, and that the federal policies which direct the public lands grazing program should benefit the land and the American public over and above the western livestock bloc." Moreover, says Tom, the National Environmental Policy Act (NEPA) requires site-specific assessment or impact statements for any "major federal action significantly affecting the quality of the human environment." The Predator Project has been calling for public participation and full discussion of

the alternatives to those many irreversible ADC decisions affecting wildlife, under NEPA guidelines.

But Tom does not easily foresee a time when states will prohibit ranchers from shooting as many coyotes as they like—or any other predator—as a normal, accepted corollary of doing business. So what Tom is doing in the meantime is providing alternative concepts. When the ADC says to the Predator Project, well you know, we're just an unfortunate part of wildlife management, a necessary evil, Tom can reply, "No, you're not. We have alternatives and the PFI program is one of them." Unfortunately, says Tom, at the moment the livestock industry hates his ideas.

But even from within the ranks of the ADC, there have been suggested alternatives. William F. Andelt, a professor at Colorado State University, is the author of numerous articles on predation. He did his dissertation on coyotes. It was Andelt whose economic analysis of the beef industry, in relation to predators, showed that when producers lost $20 million to predators, they gained by $61 million to consumers. The financial loss to consumers was embedded, of course, in the price of beef. But poll after poll, worldwide, has shown consumers willing to pay more to save wildlife. In one such poll, cited by Andelt, some 70 percent of the American public expressed a "humanistic orientation toward animals." Ninety percent of those polled expressed their opposition to the use of poisons and their preference for strictly nonlethal means of dealing with predators. Of greater consequence to the discussion of ADC nonlethal alternatives was Andelt's enumeration of logical, benign antidotes to predation: livestock-guarding dogs, particularly the Great Pyrenees, komondor, Akbash, and other mixed breeds, as well as donkeys and gelded male llamas; seven-strand electric fences; confinement sheds for lambs; siren-strobe devices for frightening predators; the bonding of sheep and goats to cattle; the playing of a radio; strong emetics; antifertility agents; and last, but surely not least, human

herders. Why, one wonders, haven't twentieth-century ranchers implemented these methods? They are aware of alternative control methods, of course, but why pay a full-time ranch hand to protect animals nonviolently when you can call the government and have it come kill every suspect predator for free? But even that argument ultimately falters. In one study in Montana, Andelt notes that while a variety of lethal methods were used to stop predators, only nonlethal guard dogs actually succeeded.[23] In fact, across the board, lethal methods have been shown to be almost useless from a strictly practical standpoint.

Furthermore, biologist Bob Crabtree's research on coyote demographics in Yellowstone has conclusively shown that when you kill members of a coyote population, surviving coyotes tend to respond in a number of ways that suggest similarities with, for example, the constantly evolving capabilities among insects to habituate to every pesticide thrown at them. First, the coyotes may have litters more often. Second, the litters are larger. And third, the survival rate of those litters goes up. Bekoff's own research confirms this.

Crabtree points out another revealing fact. Let's say you have a six-year-old female coyote living on a large ranch. She's never attacked livestock. Didn't need to. There were plenty of rabbits. She's had a litter, she's been living out her life with no problems. Some other juvenile comes in and makes the break on her territory and attacks a sheep before the female can chase it off. The rancher calls in the ADC, and the ADC happens to catch both the rogue juvenile and the innocent adult female. Now, all the immature coyotes who had been hovering on the female's (their mother's) territory may start to wander in, without contest. They are the ones who have not yet learned to stay away from cattle. Suddenly, the ranchers have a minor war on their hands. This scenario demonstrates the illogic of the ADC's methods of control.

Ever since Tom, his wife, and a friend began the Predator

Project in 1991, they have been struggling to get congressmen to realize that (1) the ADC exists, (2) why it is that so many people have a serious problem with it, and (3) what the real alternatives are: the many methods for saving the taxpayer between $40 and $50 million each year ($41,244,708 for fiscal year 1995), while committing ranchers to becoming responsible for their businesses and themselves, and for taking every possible precaution necessary to save lives. To that end, Tom has five staffers working with him. As part of their overall concern for biodiversity and predator-prey ecology, Tom and his colleagues are also focusing on prairie dog–black-footed ferret ecosystems, as well as the lynx, wolverine, fisher, and martin, the barometers of habitat destruction in the northern Rockies. There are petitions out to get three out of four of these animals listed under the Endangered Species Act. The Predator Project is also concerned with the impact of roads on the acceleration of habitat destruction within the five national forests it focuses on in the northern Rockies. But it's the fragmentation of previously cohesive habitat and genetic corridors that has Tom particularly nervous. Moreover, roads serve as open invitations to outside exotics—grasses, seeds, birds, and other nonnative species that move right in, make themselves at home, and sometimes do considerable damage to indigenous flora and fauna. Recent American biological history is littered with examples.

Ultimately, says Tom, "the government sanction of predator control represents a whole attitude toward wildlife that is a threat to biodiversity." The Predator Project provides interested people with names and addresses of congressmen at the Rayburn, Cannon, and Longworth buildings on Capitol Hill, so that they can canvass members of the House and Senate subcommittees that are responsible for proposing to the full House and Senate what the ADC's federal appropriations should be as part of the overall Department of Agriculture's annual appropriations. In all of this Tom, his wife, and his colleagues are

173

seeking avenues for dialogue and conflict resolution. "Here's a time in our culture's history when everybody is seeking common ground. This is a rhetorical question, but I think it's an important question: are we seeking common ground with wildness? ADC represents as clear as you can the notion that we are not seeking a common ground. A resounding no."

Pat Wolff and the Enumeration of Atrocities

It is a small community of activists who are fighting the ADC. Each rooted to a particular location, a state, a history, a set of opponents, they gain strength from one another. The communal bonds are tenuous: there aren't that many of them, it's an obscure battleground (certainly not glamorous, like saving Antarctic blue whales), and the public knows next to nothing about it all.

Pat Wolff, like Tom Skeele, has tried hard to change all that. In 1994 she ran for state land commissioner of New Mexico on the Green Party ticket. She lost, but only after having garnered 12 percent of the state vote, the highest total a third-party candidate running for a state office had ever received in the history of New Mexico. Then, in September 1995, a Tucson-based watchdog group, Wildlife Damage Review, published the second edition of a special report written by Pat entitled "Waste, Fraud and Abuse in the U.S. Animal Damage Control Program."[24] In this twenty-three-page document, Wolff and WDR editors brought together a vast array of data attacking the ADC. Amplified by horrifying black-and-white photographs, the essay sets forth a coherent, credible, and devastating counterargument to the practices of the ADC. If any single piece of writing can reveal a window on a person's soul, then this is the one for Pat Wolff. The gut-wrenching accounts of wildlife body counts and methods of destruction are deeply disturbing to read.

Wolff is relentless in her enumeration of atrocities and

betrayal. The ADC now operates under the auspices of the U.S. Department of Agriculture Animal and Plant Health Inspection Service (APHIS). That the ADC should have come under APHIS is perversely ironic in terms of the public's perception of what's actually been going on for sixty-five years. One might naively assume that the service was actually intended to protect the health of plants and animals. That may be true in a very limited sense. Its official mission is "to provide leadership in wildlife damage control to protect America's agricultural, industrial, and natural resources and to safeguard public health and safety." The ADC makes much of the fact that they are not just doing predator control but are out there saving human health and safety by killing birds that are getting sucked into aircraft at John F. Kennedy International Airport or down at LAX, for example. But Pat, as well as those working with Tom Skeele's Predator Project, have examined the actual data. From 1991 to 1994, the ADC killed over 30,000 laughing gulls at JFK, which adjoins the Jamaica Bay Wildlife Refuge, to protect commercial aircraft. The refuge happens to be home to the only viable laughing gull colony in the whole state of New York. It is believed that 104 people worldwide have died since 1914 as a result of collisions between birds and aircraft. At JFK, between 1979 and 1993, there were 4.2 million takeoffs and landings. Of that number there were 340 reported bird strikes. No people were injured. The odds of a serious incident do not justify the killing of 30,000 birds, according to the ecologists who have studied the matter. There is, if not a happy ending, at least a meaningful change brought about expressly by environmentalists: the ADC responded to a lawsuit filed by the Fund for Animals with an environmental impact statement, which in turn triggered some precautionary improvements for the birds under the Migratory Bird Treaty Act.[25] These include the airport authorities using noninvasive methods to discourage the birds from parking on the runways, or flocking in the immediate vicinity of takeoff and landing paths.

In fiscal year 1994 (the year Wolff wrote the first edition of her report), the ADC killed, by her estimates, 160,000 mammals, 620,000 birds, and "harassed, displaced, and injured untold numbers more, at a cost of 37.5 million federal dollars and 19.2 million more from state, county and private sources." And she added, "Eighty-five percent of ADC's field expenditures are used to subsidize private agricultural enterprises and over half of those are livestock operations."[26] Among those killed were coyotes, red foxes, gray foxes, feral dogs, raccoons, Virginia opossums, striped skunks, kit foxes, feral hogs, squirrels, ringtails, deer, elk, black bears, badgers, house cats, crows, javelinas, ravens, vultures, and grizzly bears. In a "biological opinion" the USF&W concluded that certain very rare species could be jeopardized by ADC activities, and, in a few instances, had already been accidentally killed by the ADC. These include the San Joaquin kit fox, black-footed ferrets, Mississippi sandhill cranes, California condors, and bald eagles. The majority of creatures killed by the ADC are birds, and given the fact that many birds die after having flown off with poison-laced food in their beaks, we'll never know exactly how many birds die each year, or the secondary morbidity and mortality to other species picking up avian remains or feces. According to an ADC interoffice memo, 35 million animals are relocated or dispersed by ADC agents each year.

Dick Randall worked for the ADC as a field agent until one day in 1974, when he'd had enough and "jumped the fence." Today he is a consultant with the Humane Society of the United States and he argues that nothing has changed in 20 years at the ADC. Wolff quotes him as saying that it took him "a long, long time to back off, stand on the hill and ask myself if what I was doing was legitimate." He decided it was not. Randall's photographs are unbearable to look at, the kinds of things most people can simply not deal with. Randall states that "if you have read the propaganda recently generated by ADC, you might believe that the agency practices selective control

of predatory wildlife and champions the use of guard dogs, aversives, electric fencing, and better animal husbandry, rather than the slaughter of predators to protect livestock. If so, you've been had. To this day, predator control remains nothing more than a war on whole species, and success is measured largely by the body count."[27]

The actual numbers of animals killed by the ADC and the effects of these killings are impossible to prove. This is in part due to the fact that environmentalists have not been allowed to closely assess ADC activities. When the four women founders of Wildlife Damage Review tried to set up a public oversight campaign (which they called "100 Women Bearing Witness") in which pairs of women would request permission from their local ADC office to accompany agents into the field, they were put off and put off and eventually rebuffed by the government. Simply put, ADC—"the death squad of the livestock industry," as many critics label it—does not welcome any kind of scrutiny, anymore than the biomedical establishment invites outsiders to witness its routine maiming and killing of millions of animals.[28] Finally, two Witness meetings did occur: one in March 1996 in Arizona, and one on July 23, 1996, at the new research facility on the Colorado State University campus. But these were not the hoped-for field surveys. What the women did see was a demonstration of "control methods," including shotgun killings, neck and foot snares, quick-kill, leghold, and cage traps, an M-44, and various tracking and restraining devices, as well as avian aversion tools—propane cannons, an eagle kite, strobe lights, and noisemakers.

Among methods the ADC uses, the steel-jaw leghold trap is particularly heinous. When caught in these traps, animals often chew their own limbs off in an attempt to escape. The steel-jaw leghold trap is banned in at least seventy countries, and the American Veterinary Medical Association calls it "inhumane." Rather than suffering quick deaths, the animals caught in these traps starve to death, or die of thirst, or are

strangled, often dying over a period of days or even weeks. Wolff quotes Charles Darwin, who wrote in 1863, "Few men could endure to watch for five minutes an animal struggling in a trap with a crushed and torn limb. . . . Some who reflect upon this subject for the first time will wonder how such cruelty can have been permitted to continue in these days of civilization."

I met forty-four-year-old Pat Wolff at her home, which is tucked away in the fringes of Santa Fe. Her thirteen-year-old daughter, Justine, is equally committed to the issues her mother has been fighting for. Raised in Worthington, Minnesota, Pat has been fighting for animal rights for her entire adult life. Today, some people might ask, what does she have to show for it? No health insurance, and, in the best of years, a patched-together income of about $20,000 from odd environmental service jobs and journalism. She has a total of $10,000 saved for her retirement.

Pat's dad worked in a slaughterhouse, which initially transformed the Wolff family from extreme poverty to economic respectability. It meant the purchase of a new Chevy Caprice station wagon and a family outing to Disneyland, all in the same year. The father was a mechanic in the plant, and thus spared the paralyzing truth of the actual assembly line on a daily basis. But for twenty years he would wade in "hip-deep blood" to fix machines. Says Wolff, "It was like living next to Auschwitz." Her father was an avid hunter. "Wild animals were either things to be killed or to be afraid of," Pat remembers.

She edited her school paper, graduated from Mankato State University in Minnesota with a degree in journalism, and got married in 1979. Ten years later, she and her husband divorced shortly after moving out to New Mexico. Pat got a job with Lighthawk, the environmental air force, volunteer pilots who fly people around the state to provide bird's-eye views of environmental devastation going on at clear-cut and open pit mining sites. She later worked for Forest Guardians, a leading environ-

mental forest protection group in the southwest. One day, a Lighthawk coworker named Katherine Buehler showed her a copy of the EarthFirst! journal, in which she noticed an article pertaining to some agency called the "ADC." That was in 1989.

"I was shocked," Pat reminisces. She decided on the spot that she would take it upon herself to do whatever was needed to shut down "the horrible program." She initially thought of it in terms of saving wasted taxpayer dollars because she felt that would have more of an impact on people than talking about brutality to animals. She sent out scores of letters to congressmen, only to learn that many of them supported, or said they supported, the ADC. The letters were a dead end. So she started a one-woman op-ed campaign targeted at newspapers throughout New Mexico. She staged protests at the state capitol in Santa Fe. And she became a member of the New Mexico State Game Commission's Habitat Advisory Council.

One day during a break in a commission meeting she found herself surrounded by ADC agents and trappers, who she says made threatening remarks to her. The chairman of the commission was in the room and hastened to Pat's defense, shouting at the men to leave her alone. When the meeting reconvened, and commission members came back from their break, the chairman remarked that he would not tolerate the harassment or intimidation of any member of the council. All well and good, but later an ADC employee showed up at Pat's office. He knocked, and when she opened the door he just glowered at her and said, "I just wanted to see what you look like." The threat was clear.

Then she received her first death threat in the mail. It had been postmarked Tinnie, New Mexico. In the letter she was called a "witch who worships animals"; that "she deserved to be shot"; and that "they were putting out the word that she had to be quieted." The letter also stated that her house would be surrounded by livestock, and predators would come to get her.

Pat was concerned about the ADC operating on state trust

land, of which New Mexico has about 9 million acres. The land commissioner then was Jim Baca, and Pat went to him and lobbied to close down the ADC. Baca looked into her allegations, only to discover that, in fact, the ADC lacked any kind of operating agreement or memorandum of understanding with the state land office. He enacted a moratorium on all ADC activities on state trust lands until a proper agreement could be worked out. The ADC refused to sign any such agreement, which would have included their checking their traps every forty-eight hours to lessen the duration of suffering of animals caught in those traps. After several months, Baca banned the ADC from state trust land. In so doing, he was the first government land manager in the country to intervene with ADC activities in this way. In a news release, Baca stated, "It has become apparent that ADC has outlived its usefulness as a federal agency. This agency, which uses public funds to destroy wildlife for private industry, has shown it is nothing more than an anachronism in this day and age. On the one hand, we're trying to protect wildlife, and on the other we have an agency of the government which is indiscriminately harming wildlife. It's similar to the government's efforts to educate the public on the dangers of smoking while paying subsidies to tobacco farmers."[29]

This was Pat Wolff's first taste of victory, and it was short-lived. When Baca eventually left office, his replacement, a Democrat named Ray Powell Jr., invited the ADC back onto state trust lands. It was Powell's action that prompted Wolff to run for state land commissioner in 1994.

In February 1996, when Wolff discovered that the ADC was going to be conducting an illegal poisoning campaign throughout the Gila National Forest, she and six others organized a sit-in at the ADC office in Albuquerque. The ADC was planning to spread poisonous M-44 canisters throughout the national forest in an effort to wipe out coyotes at the behest of three welfare ranchers (ranchers who fully exploit the next-to-

nothing public land grazing fees). In New Mexico alone, between 1985 and 1992 there had been a known twenty-one reported accidents involving humans and ADC-placed M-44s. Unable to stop it legally, with no time left, Pat and her colleagues decided to stage the nonviolent sit-in as a means of calling media attention to the serious situation. At 10:00 A.M. the seven animal rights activists (three men, four women) strode through the agency's revolving door, called the press on a cellular phone, went into the ADC regional director's office carrying signs, holding metal traps in their arms, sat down on the floor, and handed him their list of demands. These included an immediate end to all operations in the Gila National Forest and a public hearing. The director, who had been reading a newspaper, his feet propped on his desk, was stunned, shocked, and confused, says Pat. The first thing he did was run to the fax machine and send off the protesters' demands to ADC headquarters in Hyattsville, Maryland. As Pat and her colleagues sat peacefully on the floor, a crowd of journalists and policemen converged. In the end, the protesters' demands were not met, though the ADC people agreed at some later date to sit down and talk with them. Pat said no. Not good enough. Everyone was handcuffed and arrested, though not put in jail. A judge dropped all charges on condition that the activists behave themselves for six months. The protesters—annoyed but undiminished in their ardor—agreed as a practical course.

In the meantime, M-44 canisters were spread across the Gila, illegally as it later turned out. These spiked and covered six-inch-long pipes contain cyanide and are baited at the top with rotten meat or Limburger cheese, then pounded into the ground. When an animal comes to pull it out the spring-loaded plunger explodes, spraying granules of sodium cyanide into the animal's mouth and nose and eyes. The granules combine with saliva to kill them within five agonizing minutes. The ADC agents spreading the poison in this instance were

found to have no licenses to do so under EPA pesticide regulations. In fact, in the state of New Mexico 120 ranchers were illegally issued licenses to set such traps, which could be purchased from the government for $15 each. The ADC was reprimanded, but the damage had been done.

Trying to find out just what the ADC is up to, since it keeps a tight lid on public exposure, has proven very difficult for Pat and her colleagues. She has been repeatedly frustrated under Freedom of Information Act requests. In New Mexico, there are some 9,000 corporations and individuals holding public land grazing permits—either state or federal, sometimes both. According to Pat, these individuals are the most pampered, subsidized group in the state. Their below-cost grazing fees are $1.60 per AUM (animal/unit/month), which actually breaks down to between ten and twenty cents to graze a cow or cowcalf pair per month per acre. They get an agricultural exemption that allows large landholders to virtually eliminate their property taxes if they have livestock grazing the land. One prominent multimillionaire, a former New Mexico politician, paid less than $24 in property taxes on a $2.8 million parcel of land in Santa Fe County in 1997 because he allowed a neighbor to occasionally graze a few cows there.

It takes, on average, 100 acres of western semiarid land to feed one cow. This is because most western habitat is not suitable land for grazing large numbers of heavy herbivores. Yet this total misuse of land and animals has formed the basis for much of the cattle industry, and the history of the West in the United States. It will not be simple to turn back the clock. Settlement of the early territories and newly created states often occurred when grazing rights, along with homesteading provisions, were used as incentives for newcomers to help build an economic base. Predator control was written into the laws of every state. Today, such statutes are anachronisms.

CONCLUSION

The Future of Animal Protection

There exists a global black market for plants and animals worth between $10 and $30 billion.[1] Between 70 and 800 species are going extinct, or are being pushed to the brink, every day throughout the world. Add to that the tens of billions of animals consumed by humans every year. The scope of damage is escalating, and the budgets to conserve, monitor, and protect such species are shrinking. And yet, an increasingly critical mass of individuals have dedicated a great deal of their time, if not their entire lives, to helping preserve biodiversity.

Simple facts suggest that Americans, like people of every nationality or other affiliation, can effect significant political and social change if they rally around a cause, an ideal, a basic moral impulse, and resolve to do so. One American who has played an important role in raising public consciousness about the threat to wildlife is the celebrated author and world-class conservationist Peter Matthiessen. In 1959, at the age of thirty-two, he published his groundbreaking book *Wildlife in America*.[2] Since that time many other important environmental works have flowed from his quill, including *The Tree Where Man Was Born, The Snow Leopard, The Cloud Forest, Sand Rivers,* and *African Silences.* For over forty years Matthiessen has kept a running log on the changing attitudes and practices of Americans, as

well as people from many other cultures, toward nature and wildlife, and he has stoked impassioned responses from a wide sector of readers and conservationists. From his own home on Long Island, Matthiessen's expeditions have taken him—well, nearly everywhere, from New Guinea to the Himalayas, from Siberia to West Africa. In his early days he ran a fishing boat, and hunted from the time he was eight years old. But in 1977, while hunting pheasants in Sagaponack, New York, he and a local man shared a strong, unspoken moment: "Even though pheasants are not endangered," he told me, "we both kind of knew it was time to stop." What struck him harder than ever before was the sheer preponderance of compromised habitat all around him, the relentless destruction of wetlands, the omnipresence of sinister chemicals in the soil and water, all culminating in a stark void of animal life, right in his own backyard.

Reflecting on ecological awareness and action in the United States in the twentieth century, Matthiessen is quick to recognize both many contradictions and opportunities. "We have an enormously powerful green lobby, a tradition of wildlife conservation stemming from people like [Theodore] Roosevelt and Gifford Pinchot. They thought they'd done it, though the only true wildlife sanctuary was Yellowstone. But they didn't really face up to the severity of the situation."

Matthiessen remembers how Rachel Carson's "one metaphor [from her book *Silent Spring*] struck everyone. Birds were disappearing. Since that time, an enormous amount of legwork has been accomplished, fueled by whole new concepts concerning total ecosystems and biodiversity; environmental justice; the fragility of nature and her interdependencies." While conservation science has improved, there are more "demons" out there, to use Matthiessen's term: "international corporations, NAFTA, GATT." He admits that he finds it very difficult to be optimistic. "I hope we haven't lost too much. I'm going to keep hammering away. The public wants a clean

environment, but the public is also lazy and does not make sure that support for the environment is carried through into legislation. There is not enough heat on the politicians, who still take very good care of the corporations."

He is firm in his recommended reforms. He says, "There has to be public education, not just cocktail parties. We must save habitat. We have to be tougher and deeper. Cesar Chavez taught me what can be done by one ordinary person. People can do a great deal even with every power base aligned against them. He even had his own Catholic Church against him. If we all do one thing, educate ourselves and our kids, start with a little, some small thing, then we can turn it around. Put people in office who know."

The same year Matthiessen's *Wildlife in America* came out, two scientists in England, William Russell and Rex Burch, published another seminal work sensitizing the public to animal issues, *The Principles of Humane Experimental Technique*.[3] The effects of this book demonstrate the remarkable capacity to change the way we view other species and our responsibilities to them. The book fundamentally challenged the traditional paradigm by which scientists justified experimentation on animals. The challenge went far beyond the cold analysis of methodologies in the research lab. Russell and Burch were seeking the humanity in science, as it might be applied to other species. Once again flexibility proved a crucial precursor of genuine, lasting change. For deep ethologists like Marc Bekoff, that would include granting moral status to other animals, a necessary prelude to nonviolent research.[4] This orientation has picked up considerable currency. According to a recent *Scientific American* issue devoted to the animal research debate, "the number of animals used in laboratory experiments is going down. In the U.K., the Netherlands, Germany and several other European countries, the total has fallen by half since the 1970s."[5] In Europe, polls have shown that the more knowledgeable people become about science, the more

likely they are to reject invasive animal research. Reduction of redundant experiments, research into alternative methods (i.e., in vitro, or using statistical or computer replacement), and a focus on reducing pain in experiments has become the goal of many, though by no means all, researchers. More money is being spent abroad to explore nonviolent alternatives, and in several countries outside the United States, including Australia, Germany and the United Kingdom, a cost-benefit analysis of any vivisection is now required prior to an experiment being permitted in the lab. Moreover, many of these same countries have developed a well-intended, albeit imprecise, pain scale to assist in better gauging the impact of research on animals' lives.

While a similar barometer of animal suffering was vehemently rejected by U.S. medical researchers, recent polls conducted by Psychologists for the Ethical Treatment of Animals (PSYETA) showed that the overwhelming majority of all American psychologists believe animal research unnecessary for their profession. And outside the laboratory, where field biologists like Marc Bekoff have spent so many days and nights among animals, other ethical protocols have recently emerged that uphold observation of animals and animal communities, while rejecting any and all invasiveness.

Methodological changes among scientists are one thing, but altering the very nature and purpose of investigations into the lives of other species is quite another. Tens of millions of privileged pets aside, most animals remain locked out of the intimate circle of human companionship or care, subject instead to indifference at best, or a range of hostilities that can be direct or indirect. Most wild animals, dangerous or not, that come into contact with *Homo sapiens* do so at extreme peril, and despite twentieth-century conservation and activism, the age-old conditioned antipathy towards wildness persists. It was Aristotle—a biologist, among many other things—who first stated that "since nature makes nothing purposeless or in

vain, it is undeniably true that she has made all animals for the sake of man."[6] While it is true that many marvel at a redwood, or a lovely rose garden, or television documentary critters like giant pandas and snow leopards, the greater truth is revealed by the silent, terrible story of the animal lives extinguished on the altar of our species' extraordinary self-interest over many thousands of years.

The list of endangered species in America provides some inkling of the loss of experience with the wild that this history of extinction will have on the next generation of children. They will grow up in a country bereft of Florida panthers (30 to 50 left at this time), Hawaiian monk seals (population less than 1,500), Schaus swallowtail butterflies (less than 100 holding on), the Eastern indigo snake (the largest benign snake in North America, number unknown), the rare Hawaiian Cooke's kokio tree (less than 50 still standing), the enormously personable Laysan duck (population 500), the red wolf (population 300), the Wyoming toad (less than 50 surviving), the elegiac whooping crane (their numbers down to 175 in the wild), and many, many others.[7]

In 1994, over 1,000 scientists from fifty countries authored the "Global Biodiversity Assessment," in which they concluded that the future of evolution, "the ability of ecological communities to resist or recover from environmental change," is imperiled like never before. They admitted that at least 4,000 plant and 5,400 animal species are threatened with extinction.[8] Two years prior to the "Global Biodiversity Assessment," the Union of Concerned Scientists (1,575 researchers in sixty-nine countries, including nearly every Nobel Prize–winning scientist alive) released a statement entitled "Warning to Humanity," which listed biodiversity loss, along with population growth, resource depletion, and climate change, as grave threats to the future of human civilization.

That's the broad picture, and one in which the upper ceiling for projected extinctions continues to rise, almost on an

hourly basis. But "God is in the details," and that means that we must continue to fight all the smaller battles that make up the war. We must continue to strive to illuminate the issues so that the greatest number of people can understand them, confront opposition, embrace discussion, make an intelligent stand, resolve differences, and determine a viable course as quickly as possible. There's very little time left, certainly for those 9,400 species referred to above.

So what are the range of "details"? This book has endeavored to reveal just a few of them, but for every chapter, and mention of an issue, there are countless others. As India's first prime minister, Jawaharlal Nehru, once remarked in a different context, "We don't have a population problem. We have 300 million population problems."

Consider the following sampling of problems, new precedents, and good reasons for insomnia, as of late 1997. These are randomly described situations, events, patterns, judicial or other government decisions, that are typical of the daily gusher of perplexing trends and/or bad news (depending on which side of the issue you stand) assailing those concerned about wildlife in America.

1. During the last decade American trophy hunters have increased their rapaciousness by 71 percent. And many of the imported trophy heads belong to endangered or threatened species.[9] Of peculiar note, women are among the fastest-growing groups of hunters in America.

2. Nearly 33 percent of all frogs and toads across the United States are now threatened with extinction.[10]

3. It is believed that "of the roughly 672 million birds annually exposed to pesticides in the United States, 10 percent—67 million—are killed." And, says Cornell ecologist David Pimentel, that estimate is "extremely conservative."[11] In addition, according to recent EPA tests at 21,000 sites, toxic chemicals have infiltrated marine sediments across America's

coastlines to the extent that "three out of every four targeted for testing contain sediment likely to injure marine life or human health." Such injuries refer to the entire vast marine ecosystem, as well as to the seabirds feeding on that biological web.[12]

4. Though the slaughter of baby harp and hooded seals was temporarily halted in 1989, it has now resumed with a vengeance off the coast of North America, quotas having been set by the Canadian government at 250,000 for baby harps and 8,000 for hooded. In 1995, 250,000 seals were killed; in 1996, 266,000.[13]

5. According to a Government Accounting Office report, a wildlife smuggler "was caught 14 times over four years but 'received no penalties or fines.'"[14] This tendency among more than a few American judges to downplay or dismiss wildlife crimes has been the bane of special agents with Fish and Wildlife. Take a recent example involving a Native American caught brutally killing bald eagles in New Mexico for alleged religious rites. One of thirty-five individuals charged with a total of 106 counts (33 felonies and 73 misdemeanors), this individual might have received two years in prison and a $250,000 fine under the Migratory Bird Treaty Act provisions, a $100,000 fine and a one-year imprisonment under the Bald and Golden Eagle Protection Act, and five years' imprisonment and a $250,000 fine under the Lacey Act, all laws which took conscientious Americans 250 years to engender. Instead, the judge in the case ordered the twenty-seven-year-old Indian to pay a mere $3,736 in restitution (no criminal fine whatsoever) and gave him two years' probation with no jail time. The man, caught in what USF&W is dubbing their Operation 4-Corners, was part of a recent phenomenon occurring among Native Americans throughout the country, the revival of "contest powwows." Among the many tribes partaking of these events are dance troupes bedecked in traditional outfits, including the adornments of endangered bald and golden eagle headdresses. In

one pueblo in New Mexico "more than 60 eagles were intentionally killed"[15] and would be sold for upwards of $800 to $1,000 per bird. The poachers would fresh-bait leghold traps, used more commonly on large mammals, and then stick their fingers down the beaks to suffocate the already weakened, suffering birds. The court in this case held that the government's rules for access to eagles for religious purposes were "unjustifiably intrusive of Native American religion"[16] and thus fell under First Amendment rights.[17] The attorney for the Native American referred to the fact that "Fish and Wildlife [Service] makes concessions to hunters and falconers—even arranges so falconers can take fledglings out of the nest in the wild and raise them for sporting birds. There ought to be the same kind of flexibility and sensitivity to the needs here."[18] According to the U.S. attorney's office, in the American Southwest, there have been more than 6,000 Native American applications that would allow them to "take" eagles. All of them now have a legal precedent which, according to senior Fish and Wildlife agent Lucinda Schroeder of Albuquerque, will work much like a blank check. "These dirtballs need to go to jail," she told me, referring to the poachers. "The judge went nuts." The pretrial proceedings were so embroiled, she explained, that the biologist who was actually a witness to one of the killings was not even allowed to bring forth indisputable evidence. In fact, there are only 4,000 breeding pairs of bald eagles left in the lower forty-eight states. If all applicants—Native Americans or otherwise—are allowed to kill eagles, the animal will become extinct. And this ruling will hasten that.

6. In late June 1997, world environmental leaders relaxed the ban on trade in African elephant ivory, after a seven-year moratorium. Poachers have now been granted an open-door policy on the world's largest endangered terrestrial species. Members of Zimbabwe's National Parks Department were seen celebrating the vote ecstatically. "This is a triumph for sanity, objectivity and for recognizing developing countries'

ability to make their own decisions on nature resource management," said one member of the Zambezi Society in Zimbabwe.[19]

7. In July, 1997, just off the coast of Los Angeles, park authorities authorized the yearlong roundup and dispersal to the mainland of all of the wild merino sheep on Santa Cruz Island, as well as the removal of the last herd of wild island horses in the western United States. Santa Cruz is part of the Channel Islands National Park. Many, if not most, of the sheep captured and removed will probably be slaughtered. Why, one wonders, would the Park Service do such a thing? Because the sheep, which have lived on the island for a century and a half, are considered less important by a few park supervisors than ironwood trees and Bishop pines, which have been more or less denuded by the sheep. The question, then, is this: how is it that a few bureaucrats have assumed the ethical responsibility, on behalf of all American taxpayers, for determining that unborn tree seedlings are more important than mammals— 2,000 feral sheep, to be precise—not to mention the unique group of horses (which give birth in the winter, rather than the spring)? In one further twist, in regard to wild horses, it was recently discovered that many of the horses supposedly protected under the U.S. Wild Horse and Burro Program, instituted by Congress in 1972, have been purchased at auction by Bureau of Land Management employees and sold for slaughter. American taxpayers have spent approximately $250 million on wild horse and burro protection in the last twenty-five years. Now, an Associated Press investigation has discovered that as many as 90 percent of those supposedly being protected are being slaughtered.[20]

8. A new gimmick has infiltrated America's back-to-nature myth: a company proposing a new shopping mall novelty comprised of an enclosed, simulated wilderness experience that will commence operation at eight sites, beginning with a mall in San Bernardino, California. Each such circumscribed wildland,

costing about $10 million, will act like a zoo, incorporating five biomes (biological zones) populated by some sixty species of creatures. Habitats are being simulated with as much authenticity as possible, considering the malls are indoors, of course. Visitors will wander through the ecosystems, feast at a nature grill (meat-eater's fare primarily), partake of interactive exhibits, and go on rides. The estimated duration of a visit is one hour, versus the average visit to the Grand Canyon, which is said to be under twenty minutes. The cost, to begin with, will be $9.95. While there is a very critical value to exposing shoppers to the American outback, other questions beg answering: will such arcades not merely reinforce the commercialization of life, providing children, particularly, with the belief that animals are best experienced in a shopping mall, rather than in their natural habitat? The company's vice president of conservation and science was quoted as saying, "Whether they [the animals] think they are outside or not, I don't know if they have that capability."[21]

9. In 1996, the U.S. Forest Service rejected a winning bid by an environmental organization on 275 acres of Okanogan National Forest in Washington State because the group had no intention of logging the trees. Instead, it preferred to protect them, and the biodiversity therein. The Forest Service went on to sell the trees to the second highest bidder, a logging company.

10. In 1996 the Humane Society of the United States (HSUS), based in Washington, D.C., requested each state game agency to provide data relating to "kill estimates" by hunters per annum. The Humane Society summarized the responses: "Well over one hundred million animals are legally killed each year by hunters and trappers for the fun of it. And for their own good, according to the wildlife departments, which sanction the killing while relying on it for their existence."[22] A host of other disquieting facts emerged from the HSUS study by author Susan Hagood, all pertaining to the dependency wild-

life agencies have on hunters, and vice versa. Money dictates the local politics in wildlife management, as in most other arenas; money spread generously around by hunting interest groups. Aside from the fact that the majority of Americans do not hunt, and do not approve of hunting, hunters nonetheless effectively bully most government wildlife agencies into submission. But what is most disturbing is the response of those state Fish and Game agencies as they witness ever-declining numbers of hunters and more and more nonconsumptive users of the outdoors. Writes Hagood, "Instead of seriously seeking alternative sources of funding, ways to include the non-consumptive public, and management that emphasizes non-hunted species, they are trying to increase hunter numbers so that they don't have to change."[23] Among the many new tactics being applied by the states is an emphasis on initiating children into the hunting culture. Montana, for example, will now sell a trapping license for $3 to any six-year-old. In North Dakota, the state has adopted a "Pathway to Hunting" charade by which a fourteen-year-old is guaranteed a license to go out and kill a deer or a Canada goose. New Jersey's Fish and Game Department has a "youth-only pheasant hunt" for kids ten to fifteen. And in Pennsylvania, the state encourages twelve-year-olds to kill deer and geese during Christmas breaks by deliberately timing the release of those animals into specified areas where the children will be sure to slaughter them.[24]

Now, to be sure, for all of the troubled waters above, there are more than a few notes of positive change. An equally random sampling suggests that Peter Matthiessen's notions of flexibility, of what he refers to as a "scraping away" of the old habits of mind, hold the keys to some kind of resurrection in the wilderness, the logical outgrowth of a human awakening.

The hundreds of nongovernmental organizations (NGOs) that have passionately rallied in defense of other species in

nearly every country gives some clue to the ecological renaissance occurring in our time. The World Wildlife Fund, for example, now works in more than 100 countries. An equally impressive and action-oriented organization whose battlefields are closer to home is the Sierra Club Legal Defense Fund. A recent overview of the Defense Fund's 1997 agenda, concerning wildlife, includes lawsuits and actions designed to help the California Endangered Species Act, coho salmon and steelhead trout, the desert tortoise, grizzly bears, critical habitat in Hawaii, Maine's Penobscot River, whales and bison, Virgin River fish in Utah, endangered forest birds in Hawaii, and countless other species and ecosystems. This is one nonprofit organization, among hundreds in the United States.

But the awakening is, perhaps, most profoundly sensed not within the large machinery of organizations, but out on the fringes where individuals work, and dream, and hope. Take the hunting issue. Since the early 1990s, states throughout the country have witnessed popular upheavals. Citizens are bypassing negotiations with the traditionally hunter-controlled state game commissions and taking their ethics and their grievances directly to the body politic by creating ballot initiatives. The results have been striking, though not unexpected: by broad strokes and incremental adjustments, the public is demanding an end to the era of hunting. Bear baiting and the use of hounds has been outlawed in Colorado and Oregon. In Arizona, voters have banned trapping on public lands. Colorado voters have said "never again" to leghold and body-gripping traps, and to poisons on both public and private lands.[25] From Massachusetts to Idaho to Alaska, voters are demanding changes that just might ultimately spell the demise of the popular culture of hunting.

In April 1997, Secretary of the Interior Bruce Babbitt set an important precedent for wildlife by dispensing with long, arduous debate and simply declaring, "These studies can't possibly yield a conclusion which will be satisfactory to me. It

isn't going to happen." He was referring to a proposal by E. I. du Pont de Nemours and Company that would permit it to mine for titanium ore on the edge of Florida's Okefenokee National Wildlife Refuge. "You can study this, you can write all the documents in the world, but they are not going to prove beyond a reasonable doubt that there will be no impact," Babbitt concluded.[26]

On the forest issue, while environmentalists lost in Washington State, they gained in New Mexico when local environmentalists outbid local ranchers for prime grazing rights along the Rio Puerco. However, the environmentalists had no intention of ever placing cattle along that already damaged riverbank. Their sole aim was to use the free-market instrument as a means of acquiring land, and then restoring it ecologically. It is a powerful idea. And there is no reason why it can't work throughout the United States and the rest of the world. Environmentalists need only put their money where their philosophies are, and this challenge may have recently been abetted by some extraordinary new bioeconomic research. In May 1997, a group of scientists published a financial breakdown of nature's free services. Insects, bats, and birds that pollinate food crops were said to be worth $117 billion; tropical forests that regulate global climate, $3.8 trillion; coral reefs that protect coasts from storms, $375 billion; and animals and insects that buffer the damage inflicted on crops by various "pests," $417 billion. The total sum, says University of Maryland ecological economist Robert Costanza, is $33 trillion that nature provides in services. If, as many argue, the figure grossly *underestimates* the true value, it is nonetheless a first draft, a fiscal "state of the union" of ecology, that suggests powerful tools for influencing long-range public policy that should better translate the importance of wildlife to the business world. Placing a few critters in a shopping mall for profit is something else entirely.

What is at issue in the fight to save wildlife is the nature of human commitment, the direction toward which consensus

about right and wrong can be mounted. There is an ecology of conscience at work in the human spirit; an instinct, at times blind and groping, to leave as gentle and light a footprint as possible on this Earth.

It has been said that nothing can be protected that is not sacred. Inviolability of habitat has always proven the key to sustainability. Animals inhabiting a particular ecosystem, if exploited or utilized by humans in moderation, will not suffer serious population declines. And this is how the world's indigenous human communities managed, with some notable exceptions, to live in relative harmony with their surroundings for probably 100,000 years.

Anthropologists who have studied the impact of other species on human culture have noted any number of emphatic enrichments incorporated into the oral folklore, the art, the social hierarchy, and religious symbolism, ritual, and self-esteem of different peoples. Claude Lévi-Strauss saw the relationship of humans to other species as key to all totemism, or primary worship. Whether animals were viewed as living deities, reincarnate ancestral spirits, souls, equals, or resources to be harvested and nurtured, the key to ecological harmony and nonviolence has always hinged upon human respect for other species and their habitat. Remarkable contemporary examples include the pro-animal life communities of the Toda tribe of the Nilgiri Massif in India's Tamil Nadu state; the Bishnoi of Rajasthan (also in India); the more than 7 million Jains worldwide; the Drukpa of Bhutan; the Karen tribe of Thailand and Myanmar; the Tasaday of the Philippines; and the Inner Badui of western Java.

Such contemplations might seem remote from postindustrial, consumerist cultures, but in fact American spiritual and ecological traditions have their historical roots in such tribal wisdoms. There are some traditional Christian expressions, for example, of respect for the rights of animals, such as in the book of Job (12:7–8): "Ask now the beasts and they shall teach

thee; and the fowls of the air, and they shall teach thee. Or speak to the earth, and it shall teach thee, and the fishes of the earth shall declare unto thee." The Palestinian Essenes, living above the Dead Sea in the caves of Qumran at the time of Christ, adhered to a nonviolent, vegetarian diet based upon their own response to the Creation as evidently bespoken by the Prince of Peace. During the fourth-century "Era of Retreat," as it was called, Christian monks and ascetics who inhabited the caves and cloisters at St. Catherine's Monastery beneath Mount Sinai helped inspire a tradition marked by Greek and Latin love poems about nature (the hexaemeron), and a penchant for cohabiting with the wild animals of the Sinai Peninsula, including hyenas, lions, and gazelles. The great ascetic Agathonicus is said to have warmed himself during snowy winters in the desert by actually joining a herd of ungulates (hoofed animals) and sleeping among them.

Distinguished by the writings of Ambrose, Basil, Augustine, Anthony, Benedict, and John Climacus, these wilderness ascetics enshrined the first "back to nature" philosophy in Western tradition, though it was not entirely original. It had been borrowed from earlier philosophies, probably dating to Thales and Pythagoras in Greece (eighth and fifth centuries B.C.), Parshvanath, Mahavira, and Buddha in India and Nepal (ninth and fifth centuries B.C.), and Lao Tzu in China (fifth century B.C.). As for Saint Augustine, nature had to be viewed in the context of itself, according to God's standards—not according to human standards.

Augustine's insight served as a fitting ideological prelude to the spectacular personage of Saint Francis of Assisi (1182–1226), who is best remembered by many as the first Western "patron saint of ecology" and proactive Catholicism (so proclaimed by Pope John Paul II in 1980). Saint Francis's love of all plants and animals was the very summation of 1,000 years of Christian compassion towards nature.[27] In his *Canticle of the Creatures* (also known as *The Canticle of Brother Sun*), written in

1225, Saint Francis expressed his love of God through his love of other life-forms. He is said to have carried on substantial conversations with animals, which attended many of his sermons. His pantheistic appreciation embraced the whole world, without division or distinction between humans and other creatures.

In 1817, the Episcopal Church of America condemned "cruelty to the brute creation" and, by implication, according to Andrew Linzey, "hunting" as well.[28] Many modern-day Christian theologians, spiritualists, and animal rights activists like Teilhard de Chardin, Paul Tillich, and Albert Schweitzer have furthered this deeply spiritual orientation to nature as fundamental to their faith. At the 1993 Parliament of World Religions in Chicago, the great Catholic scholar Hans Küng drafted the Global Declaration—signed by all those representing hundreds of spiritual traditions from throughout the world—avowing human responsibility for sustaining a healthy, humane, moral environment for all living beings. The message was clear: no religion or ethical tradition must fail to acknowledge the importance of animal rights. Christians, Jews, Taoists, Buddhists, Muslims, Zoroastrians, Sufis, Sikhs, Hindus, Jains, Native Americans, and countless other religious and indigenous emissaries from throughout the United States and the rest of the world have all acknowledged this important ecological resolution: people do not have the God-given right to harm other life-forms. To the contrary, God—the Creation—is variously believed to inhere within those other life-forms, just as God may dwell within ourselves. In late 1997, even Bartholomew I, leader of nearly 300 million of the world's Orthodox Christians, declared that "to commit a crime against the natural world is a sin." He clarified this point by adding that "to destroy the biological diversity of God's Creation" was sin—the first linking by any church of that powerful word with human behavior towards nature. Nature and our spiritual selves are reciprocal, mutually dependent. Whether one believes in God or not, this

Age of Ecology provides the greatest opportunity in human history for spiritually redressing our exploitation of the natural world.[29]

I know a certain individual, who cherishes anonymity, who has followed this path toward care and respect for animals, much in the manner of the Jains. (This community, largely to be found within India, where Jain traditions originated, may well be the ultimate exemplar of compassion toward other species, magnified by an entire people devoted to nonviolence and vegetarianism, and a long history—several thousand years old—of such consistent behavior.) This person has taken nearly 800 acres of prime West Coast real estate and converted them to an animal refuge, an oasis of sanity that resembles a kind of American Serengeti, where cows and pigs rescued from slaughterhouses, racehorses rescued from race tracks, wild Mojave burros rescued from the gunsights of government-paid bounty hunters, and dogs, cats, turkeys, sheep, and goats otherwise abandoned and in pain have been given their lives back. They live free to roam the hilly estate, and a staff of paid individuals see to their needs. These animals wander together, exuding a collective peace and love that is astounding to all who visit. The experience of being licked and addressed by hundreds of such animals in outdoor communion is a startling reminder of the possibilities of true and lasting peace on earth. Of that condition in which we, as human beings, might be unburdened of our colossal guilt for the agony we have perpetrated against other species since time immemorial. Many have commented on the cleansing spiritual energies and exhilaration that come from swimming with marine mammals. Similarly, to experience up close and personal huge meandering cows and lazing foxes that are no longer afraid of humans, and no longer have a need to be afraid; to relish the humor, silence, and fond solicitudes of burros, and partake of the eternal mystery of the family Suidae (pigs), for which no fossil relics have ever been discovered in

America, whose intelligence is beyond ordinary measure, and whose feisty communicative skills are equal to their love of pleasure, is to look into the eyes of forgiving gods. All these wondrous beings and many more have taken over my friend's 800 acres and welcome any visitor like a family member who has been away for years. In a profound sense, that is the possibility of animal rights.

Recognizing the legal, conceptual, and emotional rights of other life-forms as the next great extension of the human community suggests both a spiritual and political transformation—ungainly, facile injunctions, granted. But more specifically, it means a revolution in animal rights, welfare, and protection, or whatever one chooses to call it; an evolutionary development of respect and love for animals and their habitat (also known as biophilia) that finds its way into the laws we lay down, the judges and politicians we elect to office, and the pressure we are prepared to exert in Congress, on ballots, in local referendums, in every vote, in our purchases, consumption, diet, and integrity, on the job, off the job, around the dinner table. It portends of a necessary change from mere consumers who expect entitlements, into environmental citizens, whose rights hinge upon responsibilities from one generation to the next. It means behaving in accordance with one's deeply considered and practiced ethical convictions; convictions that have allowed for a world of harmony populated by all species, great and small.

This caretaker of 800 acres is just one of the many committed individuals who are turning up everywhere these days. I have referred to some of them in this book: people, young and old, trained and untrained, who are the true emissaries of compassion in today's world. They stand at different points of the compass, but all are marked by integrity and vision and zeal; by professionalism and deep concern; by a methodical purpose and a hope to heal—not the world, per se, but small

pockets of pain. They believe in the law, in the right of all creatures to live out their lives. They believe in this deeply, and
they know with a profound feeling in the center of themselves
some version of the truth that life, if given half a chance, will
prosper. That biology is stubborn. But they also recognize that
pain is endemic, and that human beings have needlessly caused
an enormity of that suffering. It is in our power to turn this situation around.

It is the individual who will and must effect the crucial
revolutions in the collective conscience. A ten-year-old at the
helm of his skateboard has a far greater reflex action—a flexibility—than a captain on the bow of an oil supertanker. The
tanker may require eight miles to make a change in direction, whereas that skateboard will revolve on a dime. Economic, political, and moral systems tend to behave more like
the supertanker, with rare exceptions (i.e., the ecologically
focused new African nation of Eritrea, or Bhutan in the Himalayas). Consensus building in government takes months,
years, whole political administrations, decades—whereas individuals can resolve to do things differently starting right
now. Change is not only possible, but essential, because it is
unlikely that the human species will do anything differently
vis-à-vis the imperiled cornucopia of other species with whom
we share this planet until a critical mass of dedicated individuals lead the way.

There are obstacles along that path. There always are. According to Tom W. Smith, director of the General Social Survey of the National Opinion Research Center at the University
of Chicago, the level of environmental knowledge in this country is "quite low." On college campuses professors are referring to this situation as a crisis of ecological illiteracy. Students
can identify thousands of brand names and labels, but are
largely in the dark when it comes to naming other species. In
a 1994 survey (ninety-minute personal interviews with 1,500

adult Americans throughout the country, the most thorough-going survey of its kind), respondents answered twelve ecologically and scientifically related questions. Their average score was 65 percent, an F by most collegiate standards.

A few years ago, in a poll concerning the extinction of species conducted by Peter D. Hart Research Associates and Professor Stephen R. Kellert of Yale University, 70 percent of those questioned had never heard of "biodiversity loss," and only 50 percent of those claiming to be environmentalists knew much, if anything, about it. However, once those same respondents underwent a workshop to help explain the intricacies of biodiversity, 80 percent subsequently proclaimed human obligations to protect flora and fauna. In fact, when informed of basic ecological systems, 46 percent suddenly supported legislation to protect insects. A little information, if it is correct, and to restate an old aphorism, can surely be put to good use.

Beyond the numbing and forlorn sense that individuals are irrelevant to global forces of doom and gloom, millions of nongovernmental individuals (NGIs) are fighting in unpleasant trenches to elevate the numerous mandates and mottoes of environmentalism—Animal Rights; Recycle, Reuse; Small Is Beautiful; Every Child a Wanted Child; Plant a Tree Today—phrases whose poignancy is their simple honesty; messages that are all tied to the basic and irrefutable premise of ecology: the sound, sustainable maintenance of a biological world in which and by which we solely live.

What is best for all animals is not necessarily going to happen. Not after decades and centuries of ecological vandalism in the name of profit, progress, and civilization. "Sustainability" is an ambiguous, slippery slope, hard to envision in a world of 6, let alone 12 billion human consumers. But "rebirth," in the sense of regenerating, replanting, and conserving what's left, should still be within reach, given sufficient social and legislative interest. We cannot save every species, but surely it

is our right and responsibility to intervene on behalf of as many as humanly possible. The jury is out, but ecologists may well discover that bioengineering is not simply about making bigger tomatoes, disease-free humans, and more "perfect" sheep and cows for factory farms, where their engineered and manipulated lives are a living hell, but also preserving otherwise extinct species. We have already, as a species, intervened in nature's master plan with adamantine ferocity, for thousands of years. Hence, there might well be a valid argument for genetically attempting, when possible, to redress those wrongs. Resurrection is a concept not unfamiliar to most people, and biotechnology might well be viewed as one approach to saving habitat, species, and whole lineages that we have destroyed, or nearly so.

Scientific nightmare or godsend? Ethical convictions evolve. In eighteenth-century Paris, displays of public mutilation and dismemberment of cats was called entertainment, much in the manner of the Roman circuses, which thought nothing of slaughtering hundreds of lions, camels, bears, and Christians for the bemusement of the emperor's invited guests. Descartes thought animals mere machines incapable of feeling pain. For years scientists scorned their fellow researchers if emotional bonds were developed in the laboratory between the investigator and the subject of his research. Now, as Roger Fouts and Stephen Mills recently described in their book about chimpanzee research, "When I played with Washoe [a chimp] I felt like I was with one of my brothers again." We are maturing as a species, and there is no telling how far our empathetic response is likely to travel as we become more and more accustomed to the Creation. Familiarity breeds love, not contempt.[30]

A 1988 United Nations poll found that environmentalism now numbers among its adherents more followers than any religion in human history. Environmentalism means many things to many people, but—in the end—it means nothing if

203

we are not willing to endow the concept and its myriad realizations with the broadest and most compassionate of biological possibilities.

I believe the individual is capable of that. This power is the moral and ecological bottom line, the true hope for the future of all animal life.

NOTES

Prologue: Confronting the Crisis

1. Andrew N. Rowan, ed., *Animals and People Sharing the World* (Hanover and London: University Press of New England for Tufts University, 1988), 4.

2. William K. Stevens, "Lush Life—But As Species Vanish, What Will We Lose?" *New York Times,* June 2, 1998, D8. In April 1998, the World Conservation Union in Switzerland updated its "Red List" of species threatened with extinction. Some 34,000 plants were added to the list—one out of every three plant species in America.

3. National Park Service Morning Report, "Shenandoah (Virginia)—Illegal Hunting Arrests," August 31, 1995.

4. Paul Dean, "To Catch a Thief," *Los Angeles Times,* January 10, 1993, E2.

1 On the Front Lines of Battle

1. Kim Murphy, "Shielded Species Get High-Tech Lab Help," *Los Angeles Times,* December 29, 1996, A1, A21.

2. Paul Jacobs, "Boom in Holdings Puts Wildlife Agency to Test," *Los Angeles Times,* April 28, 1997, A1.

3. Sara Parker and Mimi Wolok, "The Status of Poaching in the U.S.—Are We Protecting Our Wildlife?", ed. Ruth S. Musgrave, (Albuquerque: Center for Wildlife Law, Institute of Public Law, University of New Mexico, 1992).

2 Handcuffs and Aikido

1. The U.S. Fish and Wildlife Service came into being in 1940 when Congress merged two existing divisions, the Department of Agriculture's Bureau of Biological Survey and the Department of Commerce's Bureau of Fisheries, into one agency within the U.S. Department of the Interior, which had been created in 1849. Paul D. Berkowitz, *U.S. Rangers: The Law of the Land* (Fancy Gap, Va.: CT Publishing and Fraternal Order of Police, National Park Rangers' Eastern Lodge, 1995), 11.

2. Ibid., 27.

3. Ibid., 50.

4. The states that have such funds are: Alabama, Arizona, Colorado, Connecticut, Delaware, Georgia, Idaho, Illinois, Iowa, Kansas, Kentucky, Maine, Maryland, Massachusetts, Michigan, Minnesota, Mississippi, Montana, Nebraska, New Jersey, New Mexico, New York, North Carolina, North Dakota, Ohio, Oklahoma, Oregon, Pennsylvania, Rhode Island, South Carolina, Utah, Vermont, and Virginia. Research conducted by Barry Silvestain, CPA, Wenner, Silvestain and Company, Englewood, Colorado.

3 Operation Renegade

1. See Theodore Xenophon Barber, *The Human Nature of Birds: A Scientific Discovery with Startling Implications* (New York: St. Martin's, 1993), 3.

2. Ibid., 163. For other material on the minds of animals, see *Animal Consciousness and Animal Ethics: Perspectives from the Netherlands,* ed. Marcel Dol, Soemini Kasanmoentalib, Susanne Lijmback, Esteban Rivas, and Ruud van den Bos (Assen, The Netherlands: Van Gorcum Publishers, 1997). See also Michael Tobias and Kate Solisti Mattelon, eds., *Kinship with the Animals* (Hillsboro, Ore.: Beyond Word Publishers, 1998); originally published as *Ich spürte die Seele der Tiere* (Stuttgart: Kosmos, 1997).

3. Barber, *The Human Nature of Birds,* 99.

4. Joseph M. Forshaw, *Parrots of the World,* illus. William T. Cooper (Garden City, N.Y.: Doubleday, 1973), 27.

5. U.S. Department of Justice, U.S. Attorney Northern District of Illinois, Information Release, December 13, 1994, 2.

6. Ibid.

7. Government's proffer regarding admission of coconspirator statements, No. 94 CR 760, Judge Elaine E. Bucklo, *United States of America* v. *Tony Silva and Gila Daoud,* United States District Court, Northern District of Illinois, Eastern Division, United States Attorney James B. Burns, Assistant United States Attorneys Sergio Acosta and John J. Tharp, Jr., Special Assistant United States Attorney Peter J. Murtha, 19.

8. Government's Sentencing Memorandum, No. 94, CR 760, *United States of America* v. *Tony Silva and Gila Daoud,* 18.

9. Ibid., 54–55.

10. Robert S. Anderson, "The Lacey Act: America's Premier Weapon in the Fight Against Unlawful Wildlife Trafficking," *Public Land Law Review,* 16 (1995): 27–85.

11. Ibid., 36.

12. Ibid.

13. Peter Matthiessen, *Wildlife in America* (New York: Penguin Books, 1959), 57.

14. Anderson, "The Lacey Act," 36.

15. Ibid., 85, as quoted in 33 Cong. Rec. 4871 (1900) (statement of Rep. John Lacey).

16. Matthiessen, *Wildlife in America.*

17. Barber, *The Human Nature of Birds,* 8–9.

18. Peter Y. Hong, "Pigeon-Feeding Flap Pits City Against a Woman on a Mission," *Los Angeles Times,* Metro Section, Saturday, May 24, 1997, 7B1, B3.

19. Peter Matthiessen, *Wildlife in America,* 81.

20. Ibid., 105, 107.

21. See Doug Peacock, "The Bison Massacre: A Report from Yellowstone," *Audubon* 99, no. 3 (May–June 1997).

22. Ibid., 148.

23. Matthiessen, *Wildlife in America,* 159.

24. Ibid., 76.

25. In its trafficking prohibitions, the Lacey Act is most decisive. It reads, "It is unlawful for any person: (1) to import, export, transport, sell, receive, acquire, or purchase any fish or wildlife or plant taken, possessed, transported, or sold in violation of any law, treaty, or regulation of the United States or in violation of any Indian tribal law; (2) to import, export, transport, sell, receive, acquire, or purchase in interstate or foreign commerce -(A) any fish or wildlife taken, possessed, transported, or sold in violation of any law or regulation of any State or in violation of any foreign law, or (B) any plant taken, possessed, transported, or sold in violation of any law or regulation of any State; (3) within the special maritime and territorial jurisdiction of the United States (as defined in section 7 of Title 18)- (A) to possess any fish or wildlife taken, possessed, transported, or sold in violation of any law or regulation of any State or in violation of any foreign law or Indian tribal law, or (B) to possess any plant taken, possessed, transported, or sold in violation of any law or regulation of any State; [or] (4) to attempt to commit any act described in paragraphs (1) through [3]."

Marking and false labeling offenses are also delineated, furthering the scope of the law. See Anderson, "The Lacey Act," 30.

26. Ibid., 62.

27. Ibid., 71.

28. In discussing Operation Whiteout, Anderson referred to the fact that some people might think that spending limited money and manpower on the protection of walruses, which are not on the endangered and threatened list, is a waste of money and time. Says Anderson, "It's smart, I think, to pay attention not only to species which are officially designated as endangered, but also to those whose populations may appear healthy today but which are facing a problem, like walrus head-hunting, that needs to be kept in check in order to prevent them from becoming depleted or endangered. Congress recognized this need in the Endangered Species Act and in other laws like the Marine Mammal Protection Act. To anyone who says we should not work on such cases or worry about poach-

ing of relatively healthy populations I would say think again: think of the passenger pigeon whose flocks were vast until one day, they were just gone. Think of the millions of bison hunted almost to extinction. Examples like this abound, in America and throughout the world."

4 Hunter and Hunted

1. Jim H. Wilson, "The Hills of Home," *Missouri Conservationist* 48, no. 7 (July 1987): 15.

2. *Dateline . . . All Outdoors,* November 22, 1996, 5.

3. Lonnie Hansen and Jeff Beringer, "The Key to Larger Bucks," *Missouri Conservationist* 56, no. 11 (November 1995): 4.

4. *Dateline . . . All Outdoors,* November 15, 1996, 5.

5. "Migratory Birds Get Their Day in Missouri," *Dateline . . . All Outdoors,* April 2, 1997, 9.

6. *Dateline . . . All Outdoors,* February 7, 1997, 2.

7. Susan Hagood, "State Wildlife Management: The Pervasive Influence of Hunters, Hunting, Culture and Money" (Washington, D.C.: The Humane Society of the United States, 1997), 14, 21, 27.

8. *Dateline . . . All Outdoors,* February 21, 1997, 2.

9. In addition to numerous phone and in-person interviews with Dan Burleson, an extended in-person interview with Tom May, and three lengthy interviews with Robert LaRue (one in person at his home and two by phone), as well as in-person interviews with associates of May and Burleson, I have relied on dozens of court documents and other data provided me by the U.S. Fish and Wildlife Service, Dan Burleson, and Tom May. They include the following:

    a. "Report and Recommendation and Order," February 15, 1996;

    b. Department of Justice Press Release, "Father and Son Indicted for Violating Federal and State Hunting Laws," October 18, 1995;

c. News Release, United States Attorney, Eastern District of Missouri, "Father and Son Plead Guilty to Violating Hunting Laws and Illegally Transporting Horns and Antlers," August 19, 1996;

d. The complete itemized diaries, indicating diary entry number, seizure tag number, time of kill, date of kill, type of weapon used, legality or illegality of kill and associated facts thereof, i.e., method, season, time, check, killed on federal land or not;

e. Printed data pertaining to credit cards used, motel receipts, trailer park receipts, testimony, video footage, and diary entries for various western state trips;

f. Application and Affidavit for Search Warrant, written by Special Agent Dan Burleson to the U.S. District Court, Eastern District of Missouri;

g. Search Warrants, issued by Judicial Officer Lewis M. Blanton, U.S. Magistrate Judge, on June 5, 1995;

h. The complete "Report of Investigation," dated March 24, 1997, Department of the Interior, U.S. Fish and Wildlife Service, Division of Law Enforcement, by Dan Burleson;

i. The indictment by the Grand Jury in the United States District Court, Eastern District of Missouri Southeastern Division;

j. "Stipulation of Facts Relative to Sentencing," U.S. District Court, Eastern District of Missouri;

k. "Plea Agreement and Stipulation of Facts Relative to Sentencing," U.S. District Court, Eastern District of Missouri;

l. Thirteen separate criminal docket sheets;

m. "Plea Agreement" in the Circuit Court of Carter County, Missouri Associate Division, September 4, 1996;

n. Three documents of "Information" in the Circuit Court of Carter County, Missouri Associate Division, September 19, 1995; October 17, 1995; and November 14, 1995;

o. Extensive audiotapes from the undercover work of Dan Burleson;

p. The confiscated videos shot by the LaRues;

q.   The confiscated photo albums of the LaRues;

r.   Site surveys of some of the suspected killing areas in company with Tom May;

s.   News Release, United States Attorney, Eastern District of Missouri, "Father and Son Guilty Pleas in Poaching Case Leads to Gun Auction," September 30, 1996;

t.   "National Park Service Morning Report—Ozark, Missouri—Poaching Indictments," October 20, 1995.

10. "Blue-Ribbon" Turkey Panel Reports to Commission, *Dateline . . . All Outdoors,* March 21, 1997, 1–7.

11. Quoted in Joel Vance, "Poaching Suspects Arrested," *Field & Stream* (June 1996): 69.

12. Jim Low, "Outrageous Poaching Draws Heavy Penalties," *Dateline . . . All Outdoors,* February 7, 1997, 8.

5 Best-Laid Plans

1. Marc Bekoff, "Marking, Trapping, and Manipulating Animals: Some Methodological and Ethical Considerations," presented at the seminar "Wildlife Mammals as Research Models: In the Laboratory and in the Field," annual meeting of the American Veterinary Medical Association (AVMA), July 12, 1994, 37.

2. Pat Wolff, *Waste, Fraud and Abuse in the U.S. Animal Damage Control Program,* 2nd ed. rev. by Julie St. John (Tucson, Ariz.: Wildlife Damage Review, 1996), 6.

3. Ibid., 3.

4. Ibid., 13.

5. Bekoff, "Marking, Trapping, and Manipulating Animals," 33.

6. Personal communication with Marc Bekoff, February 12, 1997.

7. Jeremy Bentham, *An Introduction to the Principles of Morals and Legislation* (1780; reprint, New York: Hafner, 1948), 310–311. Bentham's statement came at the end of a famed footnote entitled "Interests of the inferior animals improperly neglected in legislation

by the insensibility of the ancient jurists." For a discussion of the context of Bentham's thinking, see the introduction by Emily Steward Leavitt in *Animals and Their Legal Rights,* 4th ed. (Washington, D.C.: Animal Welfare Institute, 1990).

8. Marc Bekoff, "Naturalizing and Individualizing Animal Well-Being and Animal Minds: An Ethologist's Naivete Exposed?" in "Wildlife Conservation, Zoos and Animal Protection: A Strategic Analysis," ed. Andrew N. Rowan, White Oak Conservation Center Workshop, Yulee, Florida, April 21–24, 1995, 89.

9. See Bekoff's groundbreaking study, "Social Ecology and Behavior of Coyotes," written with Michael C. Wells, in *Advances in the Study of Behavior* 16 (1986) 251–338.

10. Ibid., 252–253.

11. Ibid., 262–263.

12. Marc Bekoff, "Coyotes: Victims of Their Own Success, *Canid News,* no. 3 (August 1995): 39.

13. Bekoff and Wells, "Social Ecology and Behavior of Coyotes," 280.

14. Ibid., 289–290.

15. Ibid., 281–283.

16. Ibid., 313.

17. Jeffrey Moussaieff Masson and Susan McCarthy, *When Elephants Weep: The Emotional Lives of Animals* (London: Johnathan Cape, 1994), 221.

18. Marc Bekoff, "Coyote Damage Assessment in the West: Review of a Report," *BioScience* 29, no. 12: 754.

19. Wolff, *Waste, Fraud and Abuse in the U.S. Animal Damage Control Program,* 17. In 1992, the ADC killed approximately 100,000 coyotes nationwide. That figure was down to 82,000 by 1996. In that year, coyotes were alleged to have killed $43 million worth of livestock, according to a manager with the U.S. Department of Agriculture. See Martha L. Willman, "Crash Probed in Coyote Program," *Los Angeles Times,* April 1, 1998, A3, A16. While critics like Bekoff and Spence have questioned the effectiveness of the predator control programs, according to an American Sheep Industry Association spokesperson, other data have shown that America's

nearly 80,000 sheepherders lose nearly one million lambs and ewes each year, allegedly to predators, and that stopping the program would be "absolutely devastating" to ranchers. See Martha L. Willman, "Humane Society Decries Aerial Hunt," *Los Angeles Times,* April 12, 1998, A1, A25. It should be pointed out, however, that still other critics have reported that for every sheep or cow killed by predators, seven range animals die from bad weather (and hence, rancher neglect), eleven from illness (also attributable to rancher neglect) and five from "unknown" causes. See Scott McMillion, "Coyote Bait? Big Bucks Go Toward Predator Control, but Disease and Weather Take Much Higher Toll on Stock," *Predator Project Newsletter* (Summer 1996): 8.

20. See C. N. Slobodchikoff, "The Language of Prairie Dogs," in *Kinship with the Animals,* ed. Michael Tobias and Kate Solisti Mattelon (Hillsboro, Ore.: Beyond Word Publishers, 1998); originally published as *Ich spürte die Seele der Tiere* (Stuttgart: Kosmos, 1997).

21. Donald G. Schueler, "Contract Killers," *Sierra* 78, no. 6 (November/December 1993): 70–77.

22. See Covenor Dr. D. E. Wright, "Report from the Possum and Bovine Tuberculosis Control National Science Strategy Committee," September 1996, Wellington, New Zealand, 27.

23. William F. Andelt, "Carnivores," Denver: Society for Range Management, 1991. See the multiple references to the effectiveness of guard dogs, 139–141.

24. Wolff, *Waste, Fraud and Abuse in the U.S. Animal Damage Control Program.*

25. D. J. Schubert, "Skies a Little More Friendly for Laughing Gulls at JFK," *Predator Project Newsletter* (Summer 1994): 5.

26. Wolff, *Waste, Fraud and Abuse in the U.S. Animal Damage Control Program,* 5.

27. Ibid., 7.

28. Karen Coulter, "ADC and FBI Team up to Quell Public Scrutiny," *Predator Project Newsletter* (Fall 1993): 31.

29. "ADC Foe Nominated to Head BLM!" *Predator Project Newsletter* (Spring 1993): 13.

Conclusion: The Future of Animal Protection

1. Donovan Webster, "The Looting and Smuggling and Fencing and Hoarding of Impossibly Precious, Feathered and Scaly Wild Things," *New York Times Magazine*, February 16, 1997, 28.

2. Peter Matthiessen, *Wildlife in America* (New York: Viking, 1959).

3. William Russell and Rex Burch, *The Principles of Humane Experimental Technique* (London: Methuen, 1959).

4. See Marc Bekoff, "Marking, Trapping, and Manipulating Animals: Some Methodological and Ethical Considerations," presented at the seminar "Wildlife Mammals as Research Models: In the Laboratory and in the Field," annual meeting of the American Veterinary Medical Association (AVMA), July 12, 1994.

5. The author goes on to say, "In Canada, mammals [previously used for research] have largely been replaced by fish. The figures for the U.S. are unclear. The U.S. uses between 18 and 22 million animals a year, but exact numbers are unknown for roughly 85 percent of these—rats, mice and birds. Primate use has stayed constant, whereas the use of dogs and cats is down by half since the 1970s." See Madhusree Mukerjee, "Trends in Animal Research," *Scientific American* 276, no. 2 (February 1997).

6. See Bruce Fogle, "Summation: People, Animals, and the Environment," in *Animals and People Sharing the World*, ed. Andrew N. Rowan (Hanover and London: University Press of New England for Tufts University, 1988).

7. "The Endangered 100," *Life Magazine* (September 1994): 50; excerpted from *Witness: Endangered Species of North America*, by Susan Middleton, David Littschwager, and the California Academy of Sciences (San Francisco: Chronicle, 1994).

8. The project was headed by Dr. Robert T. Watson of the White House Office of Science and Technology Policy. The report was later published by Cambridge University Press.

9. Teresa M. Telecky and Doris Lin, "Trophy of Death," *HSUS News* (Fall 1995): 27.

10. See Jon R. Luoma, "Vanishing Frogs," photography by John Netherton, *Audubon* (May–June 1997): 60–69.

11. Ted Williams, "Silent Scourge," *Audubon* (January–February 1997): 29.

12. Marla Cone, "Solutions to This Puzzle Are Clear as Mud," *Los Angeles Times,* March 26, 1997, A1.

13. Barry Kent MacKay, "Blood and Retribution on Ice: The 1996 Canadian Seal Hunt," *Mainstream* 27, no. 3 (Fall 1996): 12–15. Read also Brian Davies, *Red Ice: My Fight to Save the Seals* (Fredericton, New Brunswick, and Yarmouth Port, Mass.: International Fund for Animal Welfare, 1997).

14 Michael J. Goodman, "It's a Jungle out There," *Los Angeles Times Magazine,* October 15, 1995, 16.

15. Anne-Berry Wade and Lucinda Schroeder, "Eagles Are Being Killed for Profit: U.S. Fish and Wildlife Service Agents Uncover Illegal Market," *News from the U.S. Fish and Wildlife Service,* November 21, 1996.

16. U.S. Department of Justice, U.S. Attorney District of New Mexico release, May 29, 1997.

17. U.S. District Court, Albuquerque, New Mexico, "Order" filing, No. CR 95-438 JP, September 17, 1996.

18. Scott Sandlin, "Dismissal of Eagle Killing Case to Stand," *Albuquerque Journal,* May 30, 1997, B3.

19. Marla Cone, "Environmental Officials Relax Ban on Ivory," *Los Angeles Times,* June 20, 1997, A9.

20. Martha Mendoza, "Trail's End for Horses: Slaughter," *Los Angeles Times,* January 5, 1997, A4.

21. Laura Bird, "Move over Mall Rats, Wild Beasts Are Taking Your Turf," *Wall Street Journal,* July 8, 1997, B1, B8.

22. Susan Hagood, "State Wildlife Management: The Pervasive Influence of Hunters, Hunting, Culture and Money" (Washington, D.C.: Humane Society of the United States, 1997), 10.

23. Ibid., 8.

24. Ibid.

25. Ibid., 12.

26. John H. Cushman Jr., "Official Attacks Plan for Mining Project," *New York Times,* April 4, 1997, A9.

27. See Michael W. Fox, *The Boundless Circle: Caring for Creatures and Creation* (Wheaton, Ill.: Quest, 1996), 68.

28. See Andrew Linzey, *Christianity and the Rights of Animals* (New York: Crossroad, 1991), 107.

29. For works that examine metaphors for this eco-spiritual renascence, see: Fox, *The Boundless Circle;* S. F. Sapontzis, *Morals, Reason, and Animals* (Philadelphia: Temple University Press, 1987); Christopher Key Chapple, *Nonviolence to Animals, Earth, and Self in Asian Traditions* (Albany: State University of New York Press, 1993); Harriet Ritvo, *The Animal Estate: The English and Other Creatures in the Victorian Age* (Cambridge, Mass.: Harvard University Press, 1987); Acarya Nagarjuna, *The Precious Garland: An Epistle to a King,* trans. by John Dunne and Sara McClintock (Boston: Wisdom Publications, 1997); Gordon H. Orians, Gardner M. Brown Jr., William E. Kunin, and Joseph E. Swierzbinski, eds., *The Preservation and Valuation of Biological Resources* (Seattle: University of Washington Press, 1990).

30. See Roger Fouts, *Next of Kin: What Chimpanzees Have Taught Me About Who We Are,* with Stephen Tukel Mills (New York: Morrow, 1997). See also Stephen R. Kellert and Edward O. Wilson, *The Biophilia Hypothesis* (Washington, D.C.: Island Press/Shearwater Books, 1993).

SELECTED BIBLIOGRAPHY

Abram, David. *The Spell of the Sensuous: Perception and Language in a More-Than-Human World.* New York: Pantheon Books, 1996.

Action Line. Darien, Conn.: Friends of Animals.

Andelt, William F. "Carnivores." Denver: Society for Range Management, 1991.

Anderson, Robert S. "The Lacey Act: America's Premier Weapon in the Fight Against Unlawful Wildlife Trafficking." *Public Land Law Review* 16 (1995).

Barber, Theodore Xenophon. *The Human Nature of Birds: A Scientific Discovery with Startling Implications.* New York: St. Martin's, 1993.

Bauston, Gene. *Battered Birds, Crated Herds: How We Treat the Animals We Eat.* Watkins Glen, N.Y., and Orland, Calif.: Farm Sanctuary.

Bekoff, Marc. "Marking, Trapping, and Manipulating Animals; Some Methodological and Ethical Considerations." Presented at the seminar "Wildlife Mammals as Research Models: In the Laboratory and in the Field." Annual meeting of the American Veterinary Medical Association (AVMA), July 12, 1994.

———. "Naturalizing and Individualizing Animal Well-Being and Animal Minds: An Ethologist's Naivete Exposed?" In "Wildlife Conservation, Zoos and Animal Protection: A Strategic Analysis," edited by Andrew N. Rowan. White Oak Conservation Center Workshop, Yulee, Florida, April 21–24, 1995.

Bekoff, Marc, and Michael C. Wells. "Social Ecology and Behavior of Coyotes." *Advances in the Study of Behavior* 16 (1986).

Bentham, Jeremy. *An Introduction to the Principles of Morals and Legislation.* 1780. Reprint, New York: Hafner, 1948.

Berkowitz, Paul D. *U.S. Rangers: The Law of the Land.* Fancy Gap, Va.: CT Publishing and Fraternal Order of Police, National Park Ranger's Eastern Lodge, 1995.

Callicott, J. Baird, and Roger T. Ames, ed. *Nature in Asian Traditions of Thought: Essays in Environmental Philosophy.* Albany, N.Y.: State University of New York Press, 1989.

Chapple, Christopher Key. *Nonviolence to Animals, Earth, and Self in Asian Traditions.* Albany, N.Y.: State University of New York Press, 1993.

Davies, Brian. *Red Ice: My Fight to Save the Seals.* Fredericton, New Brunswick, and Yarmouth Port, Mass.: International Fund for Animal Welfare, 1997.

Department of the Interior News Releases. Washington, D.C.: U.S. Fish and Wildlife Service.

Dol, Marcel, Soemini Kasanmoentalib, Susanne Lijmback, Esteban Rivas, and Ruud van den Bos, eds. *Animal Consciousness and Animal Ethics: Perspectives from the Netherlands.* Assen, The Netherlands: Van Gorcum Publishers, 1997.

Ehrlich, Paul R., and Anne H. Ehrlich. *Healing the Planet: Strategies for Resolving the Environmental Crisis.* Reading, Mass.: Addison-Wesley, 1991.

Ehrlich, Paul R., and Edward O. Wilson. "Biodiversity Studies: Science and Policy." *Science* 253 (August 16, 1991).

Ehrlich, Paul R., Anne H. Ehrlich, and Gretchen C. Daily. *The Stork and the Plow: The Equity Answer to the Human Dilemma.* New York: G. P. Putnam's Sons, 1995.

Ehrlich, Paul R., Anne H. Ehrlich, and J. P. Holdren. *Ecoscience: Population, Resources, Environment.* San Francisco: W. H. Freeman, 1977.

Forshaw, Joseph M. *Parrots of the World.* Illustrated by William T. Cooper. Garden City, N.Y.: Doubleday, 1973.

218

Fouts, Roger, with Stephen Tukel Mills. *Next of Kin: What Chimpanzees Have Taught Me About Who We Are*. New York: Morrow, 1997.

Fox, Michael. *The Boundless Circle: Caring for Creatures and Creation*. Wheaton, Ill.: Quest, 1996.

French, Hilary. *After the Earth Summit: The Future of Environmental Governance*. Worldwatch Paper no. 107. Washington, D.C.: Worldwatch Institute, March 1992.

Glacken, Clarence J. *Traces on the Rhodian Shore: Nature and Culture in Western Thought from Ancient Times to the End of the Eighteenth Century*. Berkeley: University of California Press, 1967.

Goodman, Michael J. "It's a Jungle out There." *Los Angeles Times Magazine*, October 15, 1995.

Hagood, Susan. "State Wildlife Management: The Pervasive Influence of Hunters, Hunting, Culture and Money." Washington, D.C.: Humane Society of the United States, 1997.

HSUS News. Washington, D.C.: Humane Society of the United States.

Kellert, Stephen R., and Edward O. Wilson, eds. *The Biophilia Hypothesis*. Washington, D.C.: Island Press/Shearwater Books, 1993.

Knights, Peter, and Sue Fisher. *From Forest to Pharmacy: Canada's Underground Trade in Bear Parts*. A report by the Investigative Network for the Humane Society of the United States/Humane Society International and the Humane Society of Canada, November 1995.

Lao Tzu. *Tao Te Ching*. Translated by D. C. Lau. Baltimore: Penguin, 1963.

Leavitt, Emily Steward. Introduction to *Animals and Their Rights*. 4th ed. Washington, D.C.: Animal Welfare Institute, 1990.

Linzey, Andrew. *Christianity and the Rights of Animals*. New York: Crossroad, 1991.

Luoma, Jon R. "Vanishing Frogs." Photography by John Netherton. *Audubon* (May–June 1997).

Mahavira, Sramana Bhagavan. *The Akaranga Sutra: Book 1, Lecture 1, Lesson 3*. In *Jaina Sutras*. Translated by Herman Jacobi. New Delhi: Motilal Banarsidass, n.d.

Matthiessen, Peter. *Wildlife in America*. New York: Viking Press, 1959.

Middleton, Susan, David Littschwager, and the California Academy of Sciences. *Witness: Endangered Species of North America*. San Francisco: Chronicle, 1994.

Missouri Department of Conservation. *Dateline . . . All Outdoors*. Jefferson City, Mo.

————. *Missouri Conservationist*. Jefferson City, Mo.

Montalbano, William D. "McDonald's Libel Win Is No Golden Victory." *Los Angeles Times,* June 20, 1997, A1.

Mukerjee, Madhusree. "Trends in Animal Research." *Scientific American* 276, no. 2 (February 1997).

Musgrave, Ruth S., et al. *State Wildlife Laws Handbook*. Center for Wildlife Law at the Institute of Public Laws, University of New Mexico. Rockville, Md.: Government Institutes, 1993.

NAAG National Environmental Enforcement Journal. Published by the National Association of Attorneys General and Office of Enforcement and Compliance Assurance of the U.S. Environmental Protection Agency, Washington, D.C.

Nagarjuna, Acarya. *The Precious Garland: An Epistle to a King*. Translated by John Dunne and Sara McClintock. Boston: Wisdom, 1997.

Nance, John. *Discovery of the Tasaday, A Photo Novel: The Stone Age Meets the Space Age in the Philippine Rain Forest*. Manila: Vera-Reys, 1981.

Nash, Roderick. *Wilderness and the American Mind*. 3rd ed. New Haven, Conn.: Yale University Press, 1982.

Newkirk, Ingrid. *Free the Animals! The Untold Story of the U.S. Animal Liberation Front and Its Founder, "Valerie."* Chicago: Noble Press, 1992.

————. *Save the Animals! 101 Easy Things You Can Do*. New York: Warner, 1990.

Orians, Gordon H., Gardner M. Brown Jr., William E. Kunin, and Joseph E. Swierzbinski, eds. *The Preservation and Valuation of Biological Resources*. Seattle: University of Washington Press, 1990.

Parker, Sara, and Mimi Wolok. "The Status of Poaching in the U.S.—Are We Protecting Our Wildlife?" Edited by Ruth S. Musgrave. Albuquerque: Center for Wildlife Law, Institute of Public Law, University of New Mexico, 1992.

Peacock, Doug. "The Bison Massacre: A Report from Yellowstone." *Audubon* 99, no. 3 (May–June 1997).

Rifkin, Jeremy. *Beyond Beef: The Rise and Fall of the Cattle Culture*. New York: Dutton, 1992.

Ritvo, Harriet. *The Animal Estate: The English and Other Creatures in the Victorian Age*. Cambridge, Mass.: Harvard University Press, 1987.

Robbins, John. *Diet for a New America*. Walpole, N.H.: Stillpoint, 1987.

Rowan, Andrew N., ed. *Animals and People Sharing the World*. Hanover and London: University Press of New England for Tufts University, 1988.

Sapontzis, S. F. *Morals, Reason and Animals*. Philadelphia: Temple University Press, 1987.

Schaller, G. B. *The Serengeti Lion: A Study of Predator-Prey Relations*. Chicago: University of Chicago Press, 1972.

Shepard, Paul. *Nature and Madness*. San Francisco: Sierra Club, 1982.

Singer, Peter. "The PETA Guide to Animal Liberations." Washington, D.C.: People for the Ethical Treatment of Animals, 1993.

Skeele, Tom. *Predator Project Newsletter*. Bozeman, Mont.: Fall 1991–Summer 1996.

Soule, Michael. "A Vision for the Meantime." The Wildlands Project, *Wild Earth—Special Issue.* Cenozoic Society, 1992.

Spencer, Colin. *The Heretic's Feast: A History of Vegetarianism.* London: Fourth Estate, 1993.

Stone, Christopher D. *The Gnat Is Older than Man: Global Environment and Human Agenda.* Princeton, N.J.: Princeton University Press, 1993.

Telecky, Teresa M., and Doris Lin. "Trophy of Death." *HSUS News* (Fall 1995).

Thomas, Keith. *Man and the Natural World: A History of the Modern Sensibility.* New York: Pantheon, 1983.

Tobias, Michael. *Life Force: The World of Jainism.* 2nd ed. Berkeley, Calif.: Asian Humanities Press, 1998.

———. *Rage and Reason.* 2nd ed. Edinburgh, London, and San Francisco: AK Press, 1998.

———. *A Vision of Nature: Traces of the Original World.* Kent, Ohio: Kent State University Press, 1995.

———. *Voice of the Planet.* New York: Bantam Books, 1990.

———. *World War III: Population and the Biosphere at the End of the Millennium.* New York: Continuum, 1998.

Tobias, Michael, and Kate Solisti Mattelon, eds. *Kinship with the Animals.* Hillsboro, Ore.: Beyond Word Publishers, 1998. Originally published as *Ich spürte die Seele der Tiere* (Stuttgart: Kosmos, 1997).

Tobias, Michael, Jane Gray Morrison, and Bettina Gray. *A Parliament of Souls: In Search of Global Spirituality.* San Francisco: KQED Books and Tapes, 1995.

TRAFFIC USA: A Newsletter on International Trade in Wildlife Products. Washingotn, D.C.: World Wildlife Fund.

U.S. Fish and Wildlife Service Division of Law Enforcement. *Annual Briefing Materials.* Washington, D.C.: U.S. Department of the Interior.

————. *Annual Review.* Washington, D.C.: U.S. Department of the Interior.

Verney, Peter. *Animals in Peril: Man's War Against Wildlife.* Provo, Utah: Brigham Young University Press, 1979.

Wagenaar, Hinne. Introduction to *Agriculture and Spirituality: Essays from the Crossroads Conference at Wageningen Agricultural University.* Utrecht: International Books, 1995.

Walker, Anthony R. *The Toda of South India: A New Look.* New Delhi: Hindustan Publishing Corp., 1986.

Webster, Donovan. "The Looting and Smuggling and Fencing and Hoarding of Impossibly Precious, Feathered and Scaly Wild Things." *New York Times Magazine,* February 16, 1997.

Williams, Ted. "Silent Scourge." *Audubon* (January–February 1997).

Wilson, Edward O. *Biophilia: The Human Bond with Other Species.* Cambridge, Mass.: Harvard University Press, 1984.

————. *The Diversity of Life.* Cambridge, Mass.: Belknap Press, 1993.

Wolff, Pat. *Waste, Fraud and Abuse in the U.S. Animal Damage Control Program.* 2nd ed. Revised by Julie St. John. Tucson, Ariz.: Wildlife Damage Review, 1996.

INDEX

ACKNOWLEDGMENTS

We would like to express our sincere appreciation for the assistance we received in writing both the first edition and now the second edition of this book. For over a decade, we have been refining our approach to understanding the industry as well as our strategies for obtaining consulting assignments. We have taught and lectured to thousands of students and career-changing professionals, receiving valuable feedback that helped us further refine our message and adapt to a continuously changing environment. We reviewed resumes and interviewed more job candidates than we can count. The contact we had with each individual contributed to the lessons and advice we have included in this book. We thank all those who have contributed to the development of our concepts: practicing consultants and leaders of firms, business academics, professional recruiters, industry thought-leaders, and undergraduate and graduate students at Brown University, Yale School of Management, Cornell Johnson School, Wharton, and the University of Pennsylvania.

In particular, we are grateful for the assistance of the following people: Lisa Adams, president of The Garamond Agency in Boston; Barry Nalebuff, Milton Steinbach Professor at Yale School of Management in New Haven; Rena Henderson, editor; and the editors at John Wiley & Sons, Inc. We would also like to thank the consultants who contributed original essays to Chapter 4, "Perspectives on Consulting."

ACKNOWLEDGMENTS

Each of the following consultants provided us with a rare insider's view of his or her own consulting career, offering insight into their personal choices to enter, remain with, and even move on from the consulting profession: Gary Neilson, Booz•Allen & Hamilton; Bill Matassoni, McKinsey & Company; Barry Nalebuff, Yale School of Management; George Stalk Jr., The Boston Consulting Group; Charles P. Hoban, Mercer Management Consulting; Paul Smith, Bain & Company; Ellen McGeeney, Braun Consulting; Catherine Arnold, Sanford C. Bernstein; Arun Maira, Arthur D. Little; Rudy Puryear, Accenture; Bruce Kelley, Watson Wyatt Worldwide; Laura Freebairn-Smith, Good Work Associates; Brian Murrow, PricewaterhouseCoopers; Joseph B. Fuller, Monitor Company; Glenn Cornett, Razorfish (emeritus); Andrew L. Busser and Jeffrey S. Edelman, Wilkerson Partners LLC; and Eileen M. Serra, McKinsey & Company (emeritus).

Finally, we extend a special acknowledgment to the Kennedy Information Research Group in Fitzwilliam, New Hampshire. The generosity of Wayne Cooper, president, CEO, and publisher of *Consultants News,* enabled us to incorporate the latest and most accurate data on the consulting industry into this book. By granting us access to their consulting industry data not just once in 1999 but also a second time in 2001, we have been able to gain insights into the evolution and continued growth of the industry that might otherwise have remained hidden. Kennedy Information is the leading information provider on the management consulting profession, with more than 25 years of experience in this role. Through its two flagship publications, *Consultants News* and *The Directory of Management Consultants,* Kennedy maintains an extensive database of the most up-to-date and comprehensive information available on management consulting.

A great deal of collective effort and intellectual thought has gone into the production of this book. We thank all of those who were involved in both the first edition and now the second edition of *Management Consulting: A Complete Guide to the Industry.*

CONTENTS

CONTENTS

Chapter 7
NEGOTIATING YOUR OFFER   193

Appendix I
FIFTEEN ESSENTIAL FRAMEWORKS   209

Appendix II
ONE HUNDRED CASE QUESTIONS
AND TEN SAMPLE ANSWERS   239

Appendix III
DIRECTORY OF ONE HUNDRED
CONSULTING FIRMS   299

INTRODUCTION

$\mathbf{A}$s someone interested in the field of management consulting, you probably already know that it is one of the most popular career choices for today's graduating students and career-changing professionals. Especially now with the decline in popularity of Internet-related and technology start-up companies, consulting has regained its position as one of the top, if not the top, career choice at many undergraduate and business schools in the United States as well as abroad. The industry is growing quickly, both in the demand from organizations seeking consulting services and in the supply of candidates seeking a consulting position. Although thousands of individuals receive offers every year, tens of thousands compete for those offers. In the face of such intense competition, applicants need all the help they can get.

Students, who especially like the accelerated professional track of consulting, have turned the field into one of the hottest choices for entry-level professionals. Approximately 40 percent of graduates in each MBA class attempt to enter the consulting industry, and between 30 and 35 percent of these candidates get an offer. Undergraduates, too, find the field incredibly attractive and often face the same intense competition to land a consulting job offer. Intrigued by the doors that consulting can open, even graduating JDs, MAs, MSs, PhDs, MPPs, MIAs, and MDs, to name but a few other degrees, have been applying for positions in increasing numbers. And even professionals with established careers look toward consulting for opportunities to accelerate their professional development, or to switch career directions entirely. As management consulting firms multiply and grow, the demand for experienced hires who can establish and build new practices will likewise grow. But once again, the number of candidates exceeds the available positions, making the competition fierce.

Firms, literally buried in resumes, have developed a highly stylized and occasionally mysterious tool to select the top candidates from the masses: the case interview. The most challenging hurdle to clear in the job search process is the abstract and often technical case question. Even if you are fortunate enough to be invited to interview, you might be quickly eliminated by a single case question such as "How much does a Boeing 747 jumbo jet weigh?" or, "How does Amtrak price a rail ticket from Boston to Washington, D.C.?"[1]

And even if you make it through the first case interview, you typically have to survive three to five more. The process closely resembles the old carrot and stick maneuver: As you successfully navigate each case interview, you feel another step closer to that elusive offer. Guess again. Yet another savvy consultant stands ready to challenge you with an additional case interview. Any one of these interviews has the power to eliminate you, even if you impressed the firm in previous interviews. Only those candidates who maintain the stamina and drive to succeed in each and every case interview will ultimately receive an offer.

The competition has become so severe that candidates now have to invest considerable time in researching firms and practicing cases. Just as test prep courses for standardized tests like the SAT or GMAT have helped people get higher scores, so too has interview training become the key to a successful consulting job search. You need all the help you can get to remain competitive with your peers, who are preparing for interviews at the same set of leading management consulting firms. Everything counts: knowing the firms in detail; understanding one's strengths and weaknesses and how to position them to a firm; being comfortable with the language of consulting and being able to think on one's feet; and appreciating the importance of organizational culture and "fit."

Are you completely discouraged? Don't be. By simply reading this far, you have already started your preparation and are that much ahead of your peers. *Management Consulting: A Complete Guide to the Industry* is the first consolidated resource containing information on every step of the management consulting job search. From the initial introspective stage of considering consulting as a career, to learning about the work and lifestyle from those who experience it every day, to interviewing and, finally, negotiating among offers, this book will help you stand apart from your competition. The chapters that follow cover each step of the consulting job search process in detail, providing valuable insider information on the work and lifestyle of the profession, as well as tools and techniques for successfully landing a job offer.

Chapters 1 through 4, by painting an objective, candid picture of the industry, will help you decide whether management consulting is the career for you. After you have evaluated your interest in consulting and are ready to begin the job search, continue with Chapter 5 and learn how to get your foot in the door. Chapter 6 then teaches you a proven step-by-step method for successfully navigating case interviews, as you work your way to an offer. And finally, Chapter 7 teaches you how to negotiate among your offers for the most attractive package.

In addition, three unique appendixes provide critical information for a successful consulting job search. Appendix I lists 15 of the most common case frameworks to draw on when answering case questions. Even if you have a prior academic or professional business background, you can benefit from reviewing these business topics and learn to use them effectively during case interviews. When you are ready to practice interviewing, turn to Appendix II, where you will find 100 case questions and 10 sample answers. And for easy reference, Appendix III provides a directory of 100 consulting firms.

By arming yourself with knowledge of the industry and its firms, and by mastering your interview skills, you will be prepared to successfully navigate the consulting job search process. We believe you will find this book an invaluable investment in your future career as a management consultant.

CHAPTER 1

THE MANAGEMENT CONSULTING INDUSTRY

Management consultants directly out of business school can earn over $150,000 a year. You can too, if you are able to estimate how many gas stations are in the United States.

Starting salaries in management consulting are among the highest available for entry-level professionals, rivaling the traditionally high earnings potential of jobs in investment banking, venture capital, and law. Whether changing career paths or graduating from school, candidates are inundating firms across the country with applications for a relatively few coveted jobs. The recent softening of demand for talent in the technology sector has resulted in a flood of talent seeking to enter the consulting industry. This increased demand coupled with the general downturn in the economy has resulted in a more competitive environment for the prospective consultant. In 1998, top business school graduates fortunate enough to land a management consulting job received starting salaries of approximately $95,000[1] plus signing bonuses up to $40,000, while undergraduates received base salaries of $40,000 to $45,000 plus a bonus of around $5,000.

But the potential to earn stratospheric salaries is only one of the attractions of consulting; candidates also recognize its power to accelerate a career. Former consultants are valued for their carefully trained analytical minds and for their presumed expertise at solving business problems. As a result, many who leave consulting are likely to enter companies at higher levels than their peers who have worked the same number of years, but in other fields. There is a strong and arguably justified perception that a stint as a management consultant is the key to future professional success.

Sounds great, but is the occupation right for you? Are you ready and willing to jump on the consulting bandwagon? With the information in this chapter, you can begin to develop a complete and candid picture of management consulting. We introduce you to the profession that has attracted such high interest and help you answer these and other questions as you explore your career goals. We describe several kinds of management consultants and what they do. We then examine the consulting product and explain some of the popular theories of strategy. We show you how to segment the wide range of consulting practices into categories to obtain a broad view of the industry. And finally, we look at the origins and development of the profession, and offer some perspectives on emerging trends in the industry. The rich and multifaceted story of management consulting is entertaining as well as helpful as you move toward becoming an industry expert.

THE ROLE OF A MANAGEMENT CONSULTANT

The traditional professional titles of "lawyer," "architect," or "medical doctor" have widely recognized definitions. But when people hear the title "management consultant," they tend to define it either as (1) an extremely important, impressively bright individual, who deals only with the top management of large companies on critical matters; or (2) simply an unemployed individual who has resorted to selling time for a fee until a real job comes along. Neither description is entirely accurate.

To truly understand what a management consultant does, we need to analyze the role of a "consultant," a universal term for any professional who provides assistance to others, usually for a fee. Under this definition, we can imagine consultants operating in just about any industry—and indeed they do. Graphic design consultants,

6

wedding consultants, fashion consultants, and career consultants are recognizable consulting roles, but other consultants with whom we deal all the time are college advisers, headhunters, travel agents, and even realtors. The list is almost infinite. Simply select an industry name or practice area, add the word "consulting," and you have identified yet another type. Management consulting is but one kind of consulting in the marketplace, and it is by no means the only trade referred to in that sense.

What, exactly, do management consultants do? Of their many responsibilities, perhaps the most common is the identification, diagnosis, and resolution of business issues. A company experiencing a severe decline in profits may hire a management consulting firm to develop a strategy for reversing the trend. Conversely, a company enjoying rapid growth and astoundingly high profitability may look to management consultants for a way to remain successful. Although the issues consultants examine are sometimes positive and sometimes negative, they all have significant implications for an organization's future. Management consultants are hired to predict these implications and to help a company seize control of its destiny.

In addition to working as business doctors, management consultants often fill a host of other roles: (1) officiating as experts in a given industry, operational function, or business situation; (2) serving as unbiased, external third parties to validate a concept or argument; (3) confirming a hypothesis or point of view through exhaustive analysis; (4) acting as conflict resolution mediators; (5) teaching organizations how to make decisions; (6) facilitating discussions to convert information into knowledge; and many more.

The list of roles is endless. New consulting firms offering unique specialties open every year, and continue to expand the competencies of the management consulting profession. Between 1995 and 2000, the demand for management consultants ballooned from $51 billion in total worldwide revenues to more than $114 billion, as is illustrated in Figure 1.1. And the industry is expected to continue growing at a similarly rapid pace, topping $200 billion by the year 2005.

Figure 1.1
The Global Consulting Marketplace, 1995–2005

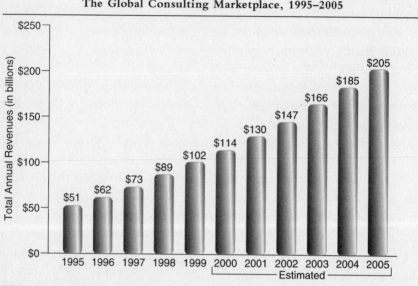

Source: The Global Consulting Marketplace: Key Data, Forecasts & Trends, 2001 Edition. Kennedy Information Research Group.

THE CONSULTING PRODUCT

What are consulting firms selling to generate such high revenues? The primary product is the intellectual capital of its consultants: quick and astute minds, proprietary business and organizational strategies, and an aptitude for managing relationships. Thus, the consulting product is actually a service that has an immensely valuable potential to bring about significant change. Because consultants are neither fortune-tellers nor magicians, they cannot guarantee a certain outcome from their work. They can only offer their best recommendation for success, stand prepared to respond to unexpected changes and roadblocks, and collaborate closely with their clients in developing a strategy to achieve a stated goal. Thus, the final outcome of a consultant's service is a goal rather than a certainty. Like teachers, who are compensated for helping others grow, consultants are paid for the objective of helping organizations improve. Therefore, the effectiveness of a consultant is only as good as the intellectual capital of the consulting team.

But when all firms claim to have the brightest and most astute consulting minds, how can a company know which to select? Consulting firms recognize this dilemma and attempt to attract companies by neatly packaging their intellectual capital under trademarked strategic frameworks, often derogatorily described as business buzzwords. A wide array of strategic frameworks have been promoted over the years; some of the most popular ones are presented in Table 1.1.

Table 1.1
Selected Consulting Concepts

Concept	Year	Consultant	Organization
Portfolio Analysis	1976	Henderson	The Boston Consulting Group
Five Forces	1980	Porter	Monitor Company/Harvard
Value Chain Analysis	1985	Porter	Monitor Company/Harvard
Core Competencies	1990	Hamel & Prahalad	Harvard/Michigan/Strategos
Customer Retention	1990	Reichheld	Bain & Company
Cycle Time Reduction	1990	Stalk	The Boston Consulting Group
Mass Customization	1992	Pine	Strategic Horizons/Diamond Technology Partners
Reengineering	1993	Hammer & Champy	CSC
Shareholder Value Analysis/Economic Value Added (EVA)	1993	Stewart	Stern Stewart
Value Migration	1996	Slywotsky	Mercer Management Consulting (Corporate Decisions, Inc.)
Value Net	1996	Brandenburger & Nalebuff	Harvard and Yale
Profit Zone	1998	Slywotsky & Morrison	Mercer Management Consulting

Source: The Global Management Consulting Marketplace: Key Data, Forecasts & Trends, 2001 Edition. Kennedy Information Research Group.

While some frameworks focus on growth and attempt to help organizations increase revenues and market share, others concentrate on cost-cutting initiatives to help organizations protect against losses. On the growth side, recent strategies include "The Profit Zone" by Mercer Management Consulting, and "Value Engineering" by Booz•Allen & Hamilton. And to evaluate the competitive dynamics of an industry to identify an attractive market niche, Monitor Company promoted Michael E. Porter's "Five Forces," and The Boston Consulting Group touted its "Growth-Share Matrix," now famous for its use as a portfolio strategy tool. On the cost-cutting side, CSC Index achieved astounding success by promoting "Reengineering," and was soon followed by a host of other firms offering similar products under different names.

THE RANGE OF CONSULTING FIRMS

Since consulting is generally considered a behind-the-scenes professional service, it rarely receives widespread press coverage—except, perhaps, from business publications. And since many consulting engagements involve unpleasant or not-so-glamorous issues (e.g., downsizing), companies undergoing such negative change do not want their consultants to discuss projects with the press. In fact, many companies keep the list of consulting firms they are working with a secret from the outside world. However, some organizations can gain from actively publicizing their consulting engagements, especially if the organization's stakeholders (investors, customers, employees) are likely to react positively to a serious investment in change (i.e., hiring management consultants).

Still, most consulting firms are not household names. The firms that have the widest name recognition tend to be the largest in the industry, and are often quoted in the business press. For example, you are probably familiar with most of the top 10 firms presented in Table 1.2, ranked by 1999 revenues. Accenture (formerly known as Andersen Consulting) is the largest consulting firm in the world, followed closely in size by PricewaterhouseCoopers. These firms are but a subset of the literally thousands of consulting firms that collectively comprise the industry. As you research the industry and begin to learn about individual firms, you

Table 1.2
Largest Management Consulting Firms by 1999 Revenues

Firm	1999 Revenues ($M)	Firm	1999 Revenues ($M)
Accenture	7,514	KPMG Consulting	3,500
PricewaterhouseCoopers	7,170	Cap Gemini	3,161
Deloitte Consulting	5,050	McKinsey & Company	2,900
Ernst & Young	4,050	Mercer Management Consulting	1,950
Computer Sciences Corporation (CSC)	3,640	Andersen	1,400

Note: Ernst & Young and Cap Gemini merged in 2000; Andersen was formerly Arthur Andersen.
Source: The Global Management Consulting Marketplace: Key Data, Forecasts & Trends, 2001 Edition. Kennedy Information Research Group.

should make a conscious effort to look beyond the largest and most widely recognized firms. A narrow view of the consulting landscape could cause you to overlook a potentially suitable firm. To help you avoid that trap, the following sections explain the many facets of the consulting industry. We introduce an approach for you to follow when thinking about which consulting segment is right for you.

SEGMENTING THE INDUSTRY

As illustrated by Figure 1.2, firms in the consulting industry can be segmented according to four broad dimensions: (1) the industries consulted, (2) the functional types of consulting performed, (3) the sectors from which clients are drawn (private, public, nonprofit), and (4) the firm's affiliation with its clients (external firms or internal corporate strategic planning units).

First, consulting firms can be segmented by the industries that the firms serve. Although some firms intentionally specialize in a particular industry, others work with a mix of industries, but focus on a smaller subset. For example, First Manhattan Consulting Group has traditionally positioned itself as a financial services consulting firm, focusing on banks, insurance companies, credit card issuers, mortgage lenders, brokerage houses, and so on. Other firms, such as McKinsey & Company and The Boston Consulting Group, consistently have

11

Figure 1.2
Segmenting the Consulting Industry

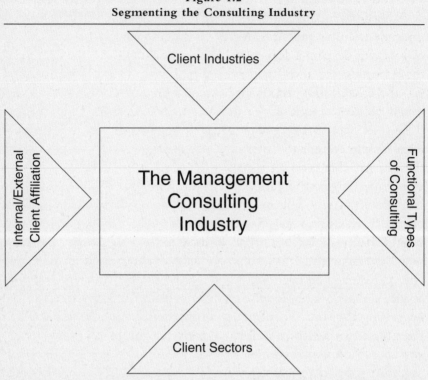

engagements with financial services clients, but are not limited to one industry—financial services is only one of their industry specialties. Single-industry firms tend to be smaller and less well known to the broader business and consulting community than firms that support multiple industry practices. In recent years, many of the best specialty firms have been acquired by larger firms, either to aggregate consulting market share in a particular industry or to accelerate entry into a new industry. IBM Consulting, for example, acquired the leading health-care consulting firm The Wilkerson Group (TWG) in 1995 as a means of quickly and credibly entering health-care consulting—TWG's clients became IBM's clients, and all of TWG's intellectual capital was available for the rest of IBM Consulting to learn from.

If you are interested in a particular industry area, you should consider both the smaller specialty firms and the larger firms that support multiple industry practices. Many consultants would argue that specialty firms develop a deeper, richer understanding of an industry since these firms spend all of their time thinking about the same industry. On the other hand, proponents of larger diversified firms would say this is nonsense, arguing that their approach provides superior consulting services by being able to draw insights and lessons from colleagues who consult to other industries. The decision as to which of these approaches is better is yours to make, but you should give both approaches fair consideration. Depending on your personal interests and learning styles, you may find certain firms more attractive than others. In addition, your prior professional experience may factor into your decision of what type of firm to select—if you were a senior manager at a commercial bank wanting to enter the consulting industry, for example, you may have an easier time securing a position at a firm that specializes in financial services. Alternatively, you may prefer to bring your expertise to a more diversified firm that has fewer industry experts so you can stand out from the crowd. Either way, you should do your homework on as many firms as possible before narrowing down your preferences. Be aware that not all consulting firms define their industry practices using the same terminology— one firm's "electronic commerce" industry practice, for example, may be another firm's "technology" practice.

The second method of segmenting consulting firms is to consider the functional practice, or type of work, being performed. Although different firms define functional practices in different ways, the most common include corporate strategy, product strategy, operations management, information technology (IT) strategy, and systems implementation. Firms with functional practices usually seek engagements that span all industries, since companies in entirely different industries face many of the same issues. The functional practice of corporate strategy, for example, is relevant to the management of just about every organization or entity.

One of the difficulties you will undoubtedly encounter with this segmentation strategy is with the definition of various functional practices. For example, one firm may offer "Information Technology (IT) Strategy" while another firm that offers the same type of consulting may call it "Systems Consulting." At face value, you might think these two practice areas were different, and only realize after digging deeper into the two consulting firms that they are actually quite similar. The lesson here is to do your homework and understand what lies behind the terms chosen by the firms (IT Strategy or Systems Consulting) to describe themselves. To help you begin segmenting firms according to functional practice areas, Table 1.3 categorizes some of the most recognized firms by four broad practice areas: Strategy, Information Technology, Operations Management, and Human Resources. These four categories are only a partial list of the wide variety of consulting practice areas, and each category could be further segmented if you desired a more granular approach (e.g., Information Technology could be segmented into Systems Integration, Website Development, Technology Outsourcing). The set of 10 firms that appears within each category is again only a partial list—these firms were chosen since they derive significant revenues from the category or categories they are listed under.

The third method for segmenting firms is by the sector in which their clients operate: private, public, and nonprofit. As you might expect, almost all large firms have a strong focus on the private sector and derive the bulk of their revenues from for-profit corporations. Yet what may be surprising is that many of these same large firms also have healthy nonprofit and public-sector practices, and increasingly seek clients in municipal, state, national, and international governments.

The firms that consult to nonprofit organizations are far fewer in number and generally smaller than firms operating in either of the other two sectors. Due to limited resources and earmarked contributions, nonprofits usually cannot afford to pay the high fees of private sector consulting firms. As a result, most of these firms can support only a few, experienced consultants, whose fees are generally less than those of their private sector peers. The small operating budgets of these firms limit their on-campus recruiting efforts, so it is up to graduating students to actively seek them out. Although some large private-sector firms do perform intermittent pro bono engagements for

Table 1.3
Leading Consulting Firms by Practice Area

Strategy	Information Technology	Operations Management	Human Resources
Accenture	Accenture	Accenture	Accenture
Arthur D. Little	American Management Systems	Andersen	Aon Consulting
AT Kearney	Cambridge Technology Partners (CTP)	AT Kearney	AT Kearney
Bain & Company	Cap Gemini Ernst & Young	Booz•Allen & Hamilton	Buck Consultants
Booz•Allen & Hamilton	Computer Sciences Corporation (CSC)	Cap Gemini Ernst & Young	The Hay Group
The Boston Consulting Group	Deloitte Consulting	Computer Sciences Corporation (CSC)	Hewitt Associates
McKinsey & Company	KPMG Consulting	Deloitte Consulting	Mercer Management Consulting
Mercer Management Consulting	Logica	KPMG Consulting	Pricewaterhouse-Coopers
Monitor Company	Pricewaterhouse-Coopers	McKinsey & Company	Towers Perrin
Roland Berger & Partners	Sema	Pricewaterhouse-Coopers	Watson Wyatt Worldwide

nonprofit organizations, their consultants obviously cannot work exclusively on no-fee projects. Therefore, candidates with a strong interest in nonprofit consulting may be better off finding a firm that explicitly consults to nonprofits for a fee, rather than working for a firm that consults primarily to the private sector and occasionally accepts pro bono engagements.

All three of these segmentations—by industry, by functional consulting practice, and by sector—are summarized in Table 1.4.

The final segmentation of the consulting industry is based on the affiliation of the consulting practice to the companies consulted: external or internal. Practices may be either independent of and external to the organizations they consult, or dependent on and internal to a specific company. Traditionally, management consultants have been thought of as independent, unaffiliated professionals who are retained temporarily by an organization for a project-based fee. However, this generalization excludes a growing circle of internal consultants who work for corporate strategic planning or business development groups. Figure 1.3 lists some of the major corporations that support internal consulting groups, and intend, through their investment in hiring consultants as full-time employees, to reduce expenditures on external management consultants and retain the knowledge gained from consulting projects in-house. Many of these groups operate in Fortune 500 companies, which also traditionally spend the most on external management consultants.

Typically, internal consultants are permanent employees of a company whose roles are identical to those of external management consultants. Their work has the same scale and scope as that of external consultants, and the stages of project engagements are usually the same. Internal management consultants now frequently displace external consultants and take on projects formerly handled only by external firms. Many internal consultants started their careers as external management consultants, but grew tired of adverse lifestyle requirements of external consultants such as extensive travel. As internal consulting groups have grown, so too have their on-campus and headhunter recruiting efforts. Large internal corporate strategic planning groups now compete

Table 1.4
Sample Segmentation Categories

Industry	Function	Sector
Communications	Corporate strategy	Nonprofit
Financial services	Human resources	Private
Health care	Information technology	Public
Insurance	Operations management	
Manufacturing	Reengineering	
Media and entertainment	e-business	
Oil and gas	Marketing strategy	
Retail	Mergers and acquisitions	
Transportation	Change management	

Figure 1.3
Selected Companies with Internal Consulting Groups

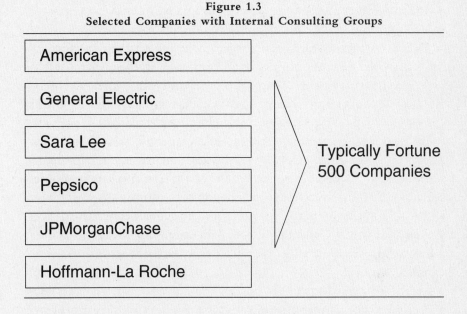

American Express

General Electric

Sara Lee

Pepsico

JPMorganChase

Hoffmann-La Roche

Typically Fortune 500 Companies

for the same student and professional candidates as external management consulting firms, and try to win the competitive recruiting game by promising a less demanding lifestyle, as well as the opportunity to interact daily with top management of Fortune 500 companies.

Each of these four segmentations should help you make sense of the somewhat chaotic diversity of firms. Confronted with literally thousands of firms performing widely varied tasks for many clients, you will need to use this tool to identify the types of consulting practices that appeal to you most.

THE EVOLUTION OF MANAGEMENT CONSULTING

Where did an industry with such rapid growth and huge candidate interest come from? How did the industry evolve into one of the hottest career paths available today? The answers lie in our earlier definition of a management consultant. Whether performing an economic analysis of a market, designing a new business, or justifying the release of

1,000 employees, management consultants perform a fundamental role: providing professional assistance to others, usually for a fee.

By this definition, consultants probably have been offering their services since the dawn of human civilization. Any person who used his or her competency or expertise to help someone else solve a problem could be thought of as an early consultant. In this sense, some American colonists could be considered consultants since they often extended their ideas and knowledge to others. Benjamin Franklin shared his knowledge of science, political philosophy, journalism, and diplomacy with others by forming the Philadelphia Library, the first public library in the United States that was established to bring "useful knowledge" to Americans across the colonies. And Thomas Jefferson, who was an architect, a gourmet cook, and an intellectual, used his skills as a statesman to help develop a system of government after the American Revolution.

Later, as a manufacturing economy took form during the industrial revolution, consultants with business and production acumen helped design and optimize assembly lines, build highway and transportation networks, standardize the size and shape of frequently used products to ensure universal compatibility, and so forth. Many specialists emerged, such as the engineer Frederick W. Taylor, who developed a system of production management and advanced the study of operations.

But the modern consulting firm did not exist until the mid-nineteenth century. Table 1.5 shows the founding dates of many recognized firms, going back to Foster Higgins in 1845, Sedgwick in 1858, and Arthur D. Little in 1886.

Many of these firms were founded by members of the engineering or accounting professions, who recognized the value of offering professional services on a project-fee basis. If we trace the history of some of these firms, we will see that many of them share a common heritage. In 1926, A.T. Kearney was founded by Andrew Thomas Kearney to provide accounting and budgetary controls to corporations. During that same year, James O. McKinsey left a public accounting firm to found McKinsey & Company, a consulting firm originally committed to providing management and financial advice to senior corporate officers. Later, consulting firms branched out beyond accounting

Table 1.5
Founding Dates of Selected Management Consulting Firms

Firm	Year Founded
Foster Higgins	1845
Sedgwick	1858
Arthur D. Little	1886
Arthur Andersen (now Andersen)	1913
Booz•Allen & Hamilton	1914
Buck Consultants	1916
A.T. Kearney (now owned by EDS)	1926
McKinsey & Company	1926
Towers Perrin	1934
Kurt Salmon Associates	1935
Hewitt Associates	1940
The Hay Group	1943
Watson Wyatt Worldwide	1946
Mercer Management Consulting	1959
The Boston Consulting Group (BCG)	1963
The Wilkerson Group (now IBM Consulting)	1967
Roland Berger	1967
Cap Gemini Sogeti	1968
Index Group (now CSC)	1969
American Management Systems (AMS)	1970
Bain & Company	1973
William M. Mercer	1975
Braxton Associates (now Deloitte & Touche)	1977
Marakon Associates	1978
First Consulting Group	1980
Monitor Company	1983
Corporate Decisions, Inc. (now Mercer Management Consulting)	1983
The LEK Partnership	1983
Computer Sciences Corporation (CSC)	1988
Cambridge Technology Partners (CTP)	1991
Sapient	1991
Answerthink	1997

Source: The Global Management Consulting Marketplace: Key Data, Forecasts & Trends, 1997 and 2001 Editions. Kennedy Information Research Group. Individual firm information.

and engineering and started to sell industry management expertise. McKinsey & Company attracted professionals from a variety of industries who could provide expert advice based on their experience. Then when a lawyer named Marvin Bower joined McKinsey & Company in 1933, the firm began to recognize the untapped value of taking the raw intellectual talent of freshly graduated college and graduate students and professionally training them to use the consulting tool set. McKinsey & Company reputedly became the first to hire consultants directly out of graduate business schools, cementing the connection between management consulting and rapid career advancement.

The turn of the century saw rapid growth in the demand for consulting services. As in any free market where demand outpaces supply, the consulting industry afforded firms liberal opportunity for growth. And as corporations with broad geographic operations approached firms like Arthur D. Little, McKinsey & Company, and A.T. Kearney, the need for widespread regional offices encouraged the consulting firms to expand nationwide.

Soon thereafter, the number of firms proliferated rapidly as partners from established practices acted on their entrepreneurial interests and founded their own firms. In 1963, Arthur D. Little saw Bruce Henderson leave the practice to work for the trust department of a Boston bank, where he created an internal consulting unit that later became The Boston Consulting Group (BCG). Ten years later, Bill Bain and a number of colleagues left BCG to found Bain & Company. Then, in the 1980s, several Bain professionals left to found their own practices, including Corporate Decisions, Inc. (CDI)[2] which, in the 1990s, saw one of its founding partners leave to form Vertex Partners. Since then, Corporate Decisions, Inc. was acquired by Mercer Management Consulting, and Vertex Partners was acquired by Braun Consulting. As a result, the industry has developed an extended and interrelated lineage, which continues to branch out to this day.

The recognized accounting firms—Andersen, Pricewaterhouse-Coopers, Deloitte & Touche, Ernst & Young, and KPMG—fueled significant growth in the industry by opening their own consulting practices. Having deep and long-standing relationships with the entire Fortune 1000, the accounting firms were in an ideal position to cross-sell consulting services to their existing clients by touting "solutions" consulting. Because the accounting firms had direct access to their clients' financial information, they were in the best position (or so they claimed) to understand and develop a strategy to meet the needs of those companies.

The sales pitch worked, catapulting the accounting firms into the world of consulting. In terms of revenue, Accenture is now the world's largest management consulting practice, reporting worldwide 1999 revenue figures of $8.94 billion and a staff of over 65,000 people.[3] In fact, the consulting groups of the big five accounting firms are all on the list of top 10 management consulting firms by revenue, and collectively account for nearly 45 percent of the revenues generated by the top 50 consulting firms.[4] Today, the consulting practices launched by the big five accounting firms continue to grow at some of the most rapid rates in the industry. The firms have vastly diversified their service offerings, running the gamut from high-level strategic consulting to more operational systems implementation. With a larger portfolio of consulting offerings, the firms have been able to attract broader and more diverse client bases, and rely less on the relationships of their accounting practices to generate consulting business. These firms have become aggressive marketers (a practice that was traditionally considered taboo) in the consulting industry to attract clients from all walks of life, purchasing primetime television and radio advertisement slots as well as entire sections of newspapers and magazines. It even seems that these firms have purchased every illuminated poster or billboard space in airports, plastering their names all over walls and kiosks to target business travelers who may one day hire a consultant.

But the success of these consulting firms has received criticism. The relationship of these firms with their sister accounting practices has raised questions of conflicting interests. In other words, the potential exists for an accounting firm to willingly ignore or hide financial figures of a given client when the sister consulting practice is busily earning millions in engagement fees from the same client. In 2000, concern with such a scenario led Arthur Levitt, chairman of the Securities and Exchange Commission, to propose limiting the relationships these firms could have with any given client to either consulting or accounting—but not both. Of course, any firm that willingly distorted a financial statement simply to protect a consulting relationship would compromise the integrity of both the consulting and accounting practice groups, each of which depends on its credibility to secure work. If revealed, such practices would cause significantly more damage than any single consulting engagement could be worth, which in theory protects the clients of these firms. Recently, some firms have addressed this concern by voluntarily separating consulting and accounting practices. The accounting practice Arthur Andersen and the consulting practice Andersen Consulting, for example, were split in 1989 into two stand-alone business units providing separate services. Although both business units reported to the same parent company, each operated independently from the other. But the two units squabbled over fee distribution and asset ownership until August of 1999, when Andersen Consulting decided to formally split from this arrangement and become an independent company. On January 1, 2001, Andersen Consulting was renamed Accenture to avoid any name association or confusion with Arthur Andersen.

With the rapid globalization of business and the proliferation of companies that manufactured and then sold products in countries outside of their own, consulting firms had to support international engagements. To meet the needs of multinational companies, management consulting firms have themselves become multinational with offices on other continents. And as businesses in emerging economies grow following deregulation and privatization, the demand for Western—and in particular American—consulting firms increases as well. Whether by acquiring a local consulting practice or sending a team of experienced consultants to open a new office, firms understand that they need scale to effectively compete for some of the most lucrative engagements. Not all management consulting firms have global aspirations, but all the large firms believe that global reach is a prerequisite to success.

Since 1990, overall revenues in management consulting have grown by more than 10 percent per year, and some firms have even reached 20 to 30 percent growth rate.[5] Although private sector engagements account for most of this growth, some consulting firms have made a substantial investment in servicing public and nonprofit organizations. In 1995, for example, KPMG, Andersen Consulting (now Accenture), and Coopers & Lybrand (now PricewaterhouseCoopers) collectively billed over $600 million to public sector clients.[6]

CONTINUED GROWTH OF THE PROFESSION

Although the management consulting profession attracts new recruits seeking professional stature and stratospheric salaries, three other key drivers underlie the continued expansion of the industry. First, management consultants are in demand during all economic cycles. During times of recession or economic instability, consultants are needed for their reengineering, cost-cutting, and defensive strategy competencies. Conversely, during times of positive economic expansion, consultants help organizations retain or even accelerate their growth, capture additional market share from weaker competitors, and predict and prepare for emerging economic trends. Unlike almost all other industries, management consulting is relatively well protected from economic cycles.

Second, the profession has low barriers to entry since intellectual capital is the primary input into the product. The main material expenses of starting a small practice are office space, the cost of accessing information, and the costs of communicating—computers and networks, telephone systems, video conferencing, and so on. All other expenses, such as travel, hotels, meals, shipping, and third-party subcontractors, tend to be billed back to clients as reimbursables. Although firms seeking high brand-name recognition must invest in sales and marketing, many consulting practices rely on the reputation of performing satisfactory work to capture clients.

Third, management consultants have attractive opportunities to exit the industry. Consultants are in high demand by organizations that are recruiting executive talent. Corporations that have hired consulting firms may seek to continue a relationship with members of the consulting team by extending full-time job offers to high-performing individuals. And most consultants are in frequent contact with head-hunters, who routinely harvest top candidates for industry positions from consulting. Like most firms, McKinsey & Company is proud of its alumni placement record and promotes consulting as a career accelerator when recruiting candidates. McKinsey & Company alumni can be found in most, if not all, of the Fortune 500 companies, linking corporate America in an extended web. Many of the most respected CEOs and chairmen in the world were trained by McKinsey & Company including CEO Harvey Golub of American Express, CEO Louis Gerstner Jr. of IBM, CEO Michael Jordan of Westinghouse Electric, CEO Gary DiCamillo of Polaroid, CEO John Sawhill of The Nature Conservancy, CEO Leo Mullin of Delta Airlines, and CEO Joachim Vogt of Hugo Boss AG, to name but a few. With proven and attractive exit options, consulting has become—and is predicted to continue to be—a natural stepping-stone for young professionals seeking rapid career advancement.

EMERGING TRENDS IN MANAGEMENT CONSULTING

Identifying general trends in an industry as diverse as consulting is extremely difficult. Simple characterizations are hard to apply to the industry as a whole, since firms have different industry focuses, methodologies, and lifestyles, for example. Still, consulting firms appear to have identified and are heeding two drivers of change in the industry, one on the supply side, and one on the demand side. On the supply side, the desire to capture additional market share is leading to the development of a full range of consulting services, from high-level strategy to detailed systems, e-business and technology implementation work. On the demand side, customers are holding firms increasingly accountable for the quality of their work.

Diversification of Consulting Services

Consulting firms are aware that a key to sustained success is diversification. By varying the industries served, services offered, and geographic areas reached, firms are better able to serve the needs of their clients. Diversification also builds additional intellectual capital and helps a firm capture a larger portion of the consulting pie. This quest for diversification, which has changed the face of consulting, is the driver behind three trends: (1) a substantial increase in firms acquiring or merging with other firms in a search for new competencies, (2) greater internationalization of firms seeking broader geographic reach to satisfy the needs of multinational corporations, and (3) the integration of information technology and strategy practices into individual firms. Let's look at these three trends in some more detail.

First, firms seeking to diversify their services have dramatically increased merger and acquisition activity among consulting practices. As Table 1.6 shows, M&A activity since 1987 has involved firms of many sizes, functional practice areas, and industry focuses. But acquisition does not guarantee success. In 1989, for example, McKinsey & Company acquired Information Consulting from Saatchi & Saatchi, in an effort to develop information technology capabilities. The result was a textbook case of culture clash, and the expected benefits were never realized. When acquisitions succeed, however, the result can be a tremendous gain to both parties. CSC's 1995 purchase of DiBianca-Berkman successfully brought new skills in change management to the strong information technology firm. Perhaps one of the most aggressive acquirers of consulting practices was the e-business consulting firm marchFIRST. The product of a merger between Whitman-Hart and USWeb/CKS, marchFIRST rapidly diversified its practice areas and acquired market share by purchasing client relationships and consultants. USWeb/CKS itself was a product of nearly 50 acquisitions, including Mitchell Madison Group (MMG) in the fall of 1999 and CKS at the end of 1998. And prior to merging with USWeb/CKS, Whitman-Hart also acquired a number of smaller consulting practices to boost its service offerings. Ultimately, the firm's inability to blend the many different cultures, offices, practice groups, and consulting approaches of its acquired firms, coupled with a simultaneous drop in demand for e-consulting services, resulted in the collapse of marchFIRST.

Table 1.6
Selected Consulting Firm Acquisitions since 1987

Buyer	Acquired Firm	Year	Size of Buyer ($M)	Size of Acquiree ($M)	Acquired Firm Specialty
Braun Consulting	Vertex Partners	2000	NA	NA	Customer-Oriented Growth Strategy
Cap Gemini	Ernst & Young	2000	NA	11,000	Systems Consulting
USWeb/CKS	Mitchell Madison Group (MMG)	1999	NA	NA	Strategy Consulting
USWeb	CKS	1998	NA	NA	Marketing Technology
Mercer Management Consulting	Corporate Decisions, Inc. (CDI)	1997	NA	NA	Customer-Driven Growth Strategy
CSC	APM	1996	4,242	85	Healthcare
IBM Consulting	The Wilkerson Group (TWG)	1995	600	NA	Pharmaceutical & Medical Strategy
EDS	A.T. Kearney	1995	8,600	346	General Management Strategy in Manufacturing
The Boston Consulting Group	Canada Consulting Group	1993	340	7	Strategy & Organization
LEK Consulting	Alcar Group	1993	85	NA	Valuation
Cap Gemini Sogeti	MAC Group	1991	1,700	74	Strategy
Staff Purchase	Hay Group	1990	Same	188	NA
Marsh & McClennan	Strategic Planning Associates (SPA)	1990	2,723	43	General Management
McKinsey & Company	Information Consulting	1989	635	20	Information Technology
CSC	Index Group	1988	1,150	25	General Management & Reengineering
Staff Purchase	Arthur D. Little	1988	Same	201	NA
Marsh & McClennan	Temple Barker & Sloane (TBS)	1987	2,147	52	General Strategy Consulting

Source: Management Consulting Marketplace: Mergers & Acquisitions, 1997 and 2001 Editions. Kennedy Information Research Group. Company press releases.

Second, the need for diversification encourages firms to build an international presence. It has almost become a requirement for large consulting firms to have global offices to remain competitive in attracting companies that are either already multinational, or are seeking to penetrate emerging markets. Accenture has offices in six continents, and many other firms have offices in five: McKinsey & Company,

Booz•Allen & Hamilton, Arthur D. Little, and Watson Wyatt World-wide, to name but a few. And firms that once concentrated on the United States, Western Europe, and Asia are now expanding into regions that have fewer consulting firms to choose from (e.g., Central Europe, the Middle East, and Africa).

Third, the quest for diversification is motivating consulting firms to integrate information technology services with business strategy. Most corporations are unable to fully capture the added value offered by rapidly developing technology and, as a result, increasingly seek the help of IT consultants. Furthermore, when strategy projects end, the next steps often involve significant information systems work requiring the continued assistance of these consultants.

In 2000, worldwide information technology and systems-related consulting totaled nearly $58 billion, and is expected to top $112 billion by 2005.[7] With the fastest growth rate in the consulting industry (14.3% per year through the year 2005), information technology is obviously an attractive practice area that strategy consultants want to tap.[8] Many strategy firms that did not have the competency have actively sought to add information technology and systems practices, primarily through acquisition (e.g., McKinsey & Company, Booz•Allen & Hamilton, and Monitor Group). The enormous success of Accenture's IT practice has opened the eyes of many firms to the impact of information technology and has encouraged IT manufacturers (e.g., IBM), systems integrators (e.g., CSC), and telecommunications companies (e.g., AT&T) to introduce IT consulting practices of their own.

Increased Firm Accountability

The second fundamental trend in the industry is the increased accountability of consulting firms for their services. This trend is driven largely by client dissatisfaction with the level of service and analysis received as well as by clients publicly voicing their complaints. In 1997, a client of Towers Perrin sued the firm on a charge that generic work was being peddled as unique analysis. And that same year, the former president of Club Med sued Bain & Company for alleged unsatisfactory work. These stories not only cast a dark shadow over the industry but also highlighted the growing doubt among many clients about the true value of hiring consultants. Other firms have also experienced the client backlash: The Boston Consulting Group was among a set of firms sued by the Cleveland-based conglomerate Figgie International for alleged overbilling and other errors, and Andersen Consulting was ordered by the British government to pay an $18 million penalty for not delivering a social security computer system on time.[9] The publication of books profiling client dissatisfaction, such as James O'Shea and Charles Madigan's *Dangerous Company: The Consulting Powerhouses and the Businesses They Save and Ruin* (New York: Random House, 1997), and Adrian Wooldridge and John Micklethwait's *The Witch Doctors: Making Sense of the Management Gurus* (New York: Random House, 1998), further reveals the growing determination of companies to hold consultants accountable for their work.

Partly in response to these client concerns, consulting firms have become more active in monitoring their own activities. They are placing greater emphasis on effective management of client relationships and on controlling client expectations. Some firms, have been known to not accept a fee unless a client is completely satisfied. And after completing projects, most firms routinely follow up with clients to monitor their satisfaction and offer additional guidance without charge.

As pointed out earlier, these trends serve as predictions but are by no means prescriptions of events to come. In fact, they are at best only a limited set of predictions since each day brings a new perspective on the future of the industry. We chose to not highlight some popular predictions, including the rise of public sector consulting, and the increasing emphasis on capturing institutional knowledge within the firm through formalized processes and electronic libraries. Because the future is uncertain, we prefer to focus on the key drivers of change that have fundamentally influenced—and will continue to influence— the evolution of consulting: extended service diversification and increased consultant accountability.

CHAPTER 2

THE CONSULTANT'S WORK
AND LIFESTYLE

Consulting is a highly stimulating profession, allowing intelligent, confident professionals the chance to work with similarly bright specialists on cutting-edge ideas and technology.
Maura Rurak and Perri Capell
National Business Employment Weekly

In this chapter, we will profile the consultant's work and lifestyle and describe what it is like to be a management consultant, in terms of the professional development opportunities and the day-to-day balancing of work and private life. We begin by describing the typical organizational structure and individual roles within a consulting firm, and the keys to achieving success in this environment. Then, we provide an overview of the consultant's work style: how consultants interact with clients and each other. Next, we will walk you through the steps of a typical consulting engagement, from its initial definition to the final presentation of recommendations. Finally, we conclude with two examples of the consulting lifestyle to compare with your own expectations.

THE MANAGEMENT CONSULTING FIRM

Although highly variable in size, number of offices, and work performed, management consulting firms tend to follow a similar operating model. Most large firms have an organizational structure similar to the one outlined in Figure 2.1: (1) Support staff in the library, recruiting, and production departments; (2) Research analysts or associates, who hold undergraduate degrees; (3) Consultants who most often have graduate business degrees as well as prior work experience; (4) Senior consultants, who have from two to three years of post-MBA consulting experience; (5) Managers or cast team leaders, who usually have started with the firm as consultants prior to promotion; and (6) Partners, directors, or vice presidents who are also likely to have started with the firm at a lower rank and worked their way up. Depending on the size of the firm, the complexity of the organizational structure will vary by the number of levels, specific roles, and titles.

Since consulting firms prefer to promote from within, they base the recognition and reward of their top performers on merit. Formal performance reviews, which usually occur twice a year, have a direct impact on a consultant's career progression and compensation. A firm

Figure 2.1
Typical Consulting Firm Organizational Structure

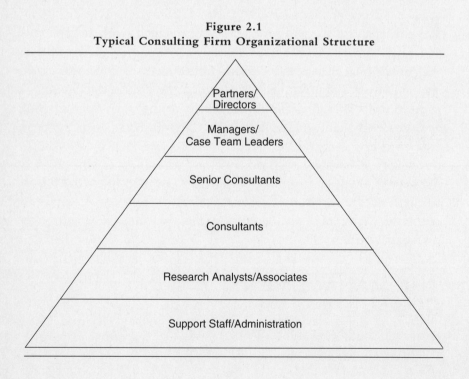

typically evaluates all its professionals using the same set of skill development criteria, such as analytics, teamwork, commitment and drive, presentation skills, time management, and people management. The list varies from firm to firm, but in all cases is designed to evaluate the key skills consultants need to lead people and manage work.

Different competencies are expected from consultants during different stages of their career. Figure 2.2 illustrates the progression of skills by consulting position. Research analysts are expected to focus on their analytical and client communication skills. Once they master the basic consulting skill set, they learn how to assume the greater responsibilities of consultant and senior consultant: managing projects and developing knowledge of industries and management functions. At the next professional level, managers take even greater responsibility and are expected to show aptitude for managing client relationships. At the highest professional level, partners generate new business and contribute to the growth and recognition of the firm through public speaking engagements, articles, and professional networking. Individual firms may diverge from this model. At smaller firms in particular,

Figure 2.2
Typical Skill Progression of Consultants

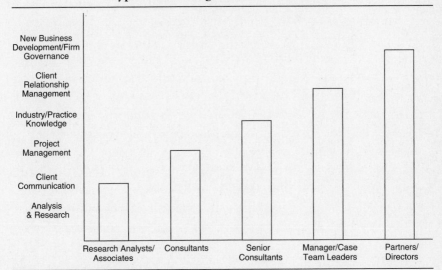

professional staff at each level may have greater responsibilities. Experienced senior consultants, for example, will probably participate in developing client relationships and selling new business.

Although the responsibility sets are usually clearly defined, the performance reviews based on them are, unfortunately, neither entirely objective nor scientifically performed. A subjective human element always creeps into such evaluations. Perception is reality, and individuals have to work diligently to manage the perceptions of their evaluators. The hard reality is that high-performing individuals can be perceived as poor performers if they never receive proper credit for their work. If taken too far, a meritocracy can produce a highly competitive atmosphere in which consultants vie for recognition or try to curry favor with the evaluators and senior members of the firm. In such a scenario, motivation comes from fear of failure, rather than from the prospect of reward. Our intent is not to undermine a system that works well for many firms and their employees, but rather to give you a complete picture of the structure you may encounter.

Most consulting firms prefer to hire consultants at junior levels and promote them through the ranks. Research analysts are commonly promoted to MBA-level consultant positions, and those who continue to be high performers may advance all the way up to the most senior partner levels. Instead of recruiting only established professionals who are recognized experts in specific fields, consulting firms have made a conscious decision to hire individuals who bring a fresh, can-do perspective. As a result, most firms rely on on-campus recruiting to fill their ranks, and invest significant time and resources to recruit top talent. In fact, some firms try to hold on to their top talent by paying for high-performing research analysts to attend business school, with the understanding that they will return to the firm after graduation.

Research analysts are usually hired during their senior year of college, while still working toward their bachelor's degrees. Consulting firms are generally attracted to students who have strong quantitative, analytical, and communication skills. Often students can demonstrate these skills through the courses they have taken and the extracurricular activities that they have been involved in. Research analysts generally have limited prior full-time work experience, but are likely to have held summer internships in business-related fields. They are recognized leaders in their schools, with strong records of academic achievement.

Consultant-level professionals are also hired through on-campus recruiting, primarily at graduate business schools. Since consultants at most firms are expected to supervise research analysts and manage projects, firms prefer candidates with academic and professional preparation that has taught them people and project management skills. And some firms actively seek candidates from the nation's top law and graduate programs, believing that these programs also develop high-caliber management competencies.

THE CONSULTING WORK STYLE

Teamwork is critical to the work of management consultants. Whether performing client work or working on internal office projects, consultants prefer to apply the collective minds of a group to a problem. Even though team members are drawn from various ranks in the firm, the work style is collaborative and tends to downplay hierarchical relationships. Teams can range from 2 to 15 people, depending on the scale and scope of a project. For example, a team comprised of 6 to 8 people would include a partner, a manager, 2 or 3 consultants, and 2 or 3 research analysts. Roles can vary dramatically depending on the size of the firm, and responsibilities can cross the lines of professional titles. But a common model in many recognized firms compartmentalizes roles by professional title in the following way: most data collection is performed by research analysts, who work closely with consultants and senior consultants to generate learnings; these three levels present their work to managers, who are primarily responsible for synthesizing team analyses into key lessons and next-step recommendations, and for leading presentations to the client. Partners are the primary liaison with clients, although all team members are likely to have client contact over the duration of a project.

At the same time, the client is likely to have created its own team to work closely with the consulting team throughout the project, with anywhere from 2 to more than 20 individuals pulled from various levels of the organization. Depending on the complexity, size, and duration of the engagement, client team members may either be fully or partially dedicated resources. Client teams commonly serve four purposes: (1) to provide information to the consultants as needed; (2) to serve as collaborative problem solvers with the consultants; (3) to absorb and retain knowledge from the project; and (4) to supervise the consultants in a way that ensures timely and effective delivery of the promised goal. Companies recognize that an effective consulting engagement is not one in which a large report is delivered after a number of months of behind-the-scenes work. Rather, it is one in which consultants and the client work closely together in a continuous learning arrangement. The degree of collaboration that is desirable or even possible is clearly dependent on the exact nature of the work that is being done, as well as the particular phase that the engagement is in.

Although most consulting firms use the same team structure, these teams interface with the client in two essentially different ways: either on-site at the client's offices for the entire duration of a project, or off-site at the consultant's offices with periodic visits to the client. Each of these models has positive and negative features, depending on the project. Consulting firms disagree on which model is better, as do companies hiring consultants. However, individual firms have migrated over time to one or the other model and have developed strong cultural attributes supporting their on-site or off-site practices.

On-Site Consulting

On-site firms are likely to argue that working in proximity to the client, surrounded by the people who the project directly influences, holds great value. On-site consultants can walk though manufacturing plants, view product testing and research facilities, speak with employees of all ranks, tap directly into corporate information systems, and observe day-to-day management and operation practices. On-site arrangements are more common for systems and information technology projects, as well as for implementation stages of work, each of which requires frequent and close contact with the company. Many companies prefer the on-site model since they can observe the daily work of the consultants and monitor their productivity. Furthermore, company employees are more likely to respect visibly hardworking consultants who interact with them every day. This respect helps to build the client's overall relationship with the consultants. This relationship is critical as the consultants convince the client to implement their recommendations and award new engagements to the firm. Consulting firms that are established with a particular client can use their strong relationship as a powerful barrier to other firms approaching that client. In contrast, consultants who work in their own offices and appear at the client site once a month may not develop these close working relationships and thus may not be as effective.

Still, the on-site model has several potential drawbacks. Consultants are inconveniently distanced from essential library resources located in their home offices. They are separated from the presentation production assistants and have to rely on phone, fax, mail, and e-mail channels to communicate with the department when producing a presentation. Support services may be difficult to use from a remote location, and consultants may have to work in very cramped quarters. Apart from the logistical challenges, many consultants find it difficult to think creatively and out-of-the-box when under constant surveillance by the client. Thus, on-site consultants may become risk-averse and fail to explore ideas simply because the client sees little value in them or wants to avoid them. In the long run, certain groups within the client organization may come to view the consultants as being politically aligned with other groups and thus may question the consultant's objectivity. The consultants themselves may truly begin to lose their objectivity if they are assigned to one client for long periods of time. Finally, professional growth for an individual consultant may be stunted if he is required to remain with a single client and not work with different organizations in different industries.

Off-Site Consulting

The second model, working off-site at the consultant's home office, avoids most of the disadvantages of the first model: library, production, and support resources are within easy reach, and the client is usually not smothering the consulting team. Working away from the client site may facilitate creative thinking and even enable consultants to share ideas with and receive feedback from colleagues who are working on other projects. Companies that hire off-site consultants may also prefer the model, especially for sensitive projects that involve mergers and acquisitions, layoffs, or reengineering. Because privacy can be an advantage in these cases, it makes sense to use off-site consultants. Company employees then have minimal contact with the projects, and little or no reason to become uneasy.

But, like the on-site model, the off-site model also has disadvantages. Clients may have difficulty following analyses if they cannot observe and participate in each step of the work. As a result, clients may question the value of their consultants and hesitate to implement their recommendations. To avoid these pitfalls, off-site consultants need to have frequent contact with clients to keep them abreast of progress and may have to hold more frequent interim presentations than their on-site counterparts do. Ultimately, it is vital for all consultants to develop working relationships with their clients that are based on trust and confidence. Off-site consultants need to be particularly sensitive to this because of the physical distance between them and the client.

STEPS IN A CONSULTING ENGAGEMENT

As you may have noted, the term *engagement* is used to refer to the multistep process of helping a client achieve certain objectives. Although the particular process used depends on the help a client needs, a prototypical consulting engagement can be segmented into four broad workflow steps: (1) problem definition and project planning, (2) analysis, (3) synthesis, and (4) presentation. This process, however, is not universally applicable to all projects. A consulting team may repeat steps before moving on to the next one, or even cycle through the entire four-step process multiple times before concluding an engagement. Still, this model makes two important points: Each step is critical to the overall success of the engagement, and a consultant needs a variety of skills to be successful. Figure 2.3 outlines a typical work plan for an engagement.

Step 1. Problem Definition and Project Planning

The first step involves clarifying the business issues the client faces, outlining the engagement's specific objectives and work steps, determining the deliverables to be turned in at the end of the engagement, and scheduling the time line for completion. It is important to note that prior to this first step, many of these items will have been considered, outlined, and presented to the client in the original statement of work. This first step will take these items to the next level of detail. Here, consultants need to differentiate between what clients are asking for and what they truly need, since clients who are stuck with their old habits may not be able to look at a situation objectively. Sometimes, clients are so involved in daily activities that they lack the perspective to identify the central issues behind their business problem. For example, is the client's problem a misalignment of its information

Figure 2.3
Typical Consulting Work Plan for an Engagement

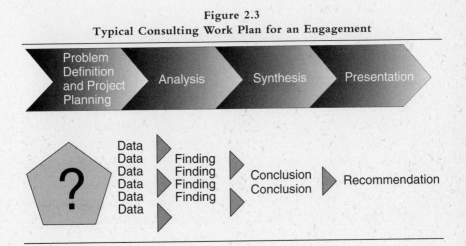

technology with its business strategies or, more simply, the lack of a business strategy in the first place? Consultants must bring a certain degree of skepticism to an engagement to question the client's perception of the problem and not simply accept an obvious answer. A consultant's ability to listen well, to consider the whole picture, and to draw on industry and business experience are critical to the success of this step.

Step 2. Analysis

The second step involves the gathering of primary and secondary data, building models and conceptual frameworks, soliciting feedback to ideas from experts and others with relevant perspectives, and analyzing the results of this research. Information may be gathered from surveys, telephone interviews, on-line searches, focus groups, and published materials. Models are workable abstractions of reality, ranging from highly quantitative financial models to qualitative assessments of public opinion. The challenge in building effective models and conceptual frameworks is balancing the need for abstraction with the need for complexity: they must be abstract enough to be useful, yet complex enough to be meaningful. And the analysis resulting from the synthesis of all the collected information should yield a set of alternative options based on a set of assumption-based scenarios. The consultant's ability to think in the abstract is crucial to success.

Step 3. Synthesis

As the name suggests, synthesis involves combining the individual conclusions into a single set of findings, from which recommendations are then formulated. Developing a cohesive set of findings may be more difficult than it sounds if some of the information collected over the course of the engagement is contradictory, or if the models and conceptual frameworks do not adequately capture the complexity of the issues. In this phase, a consultant must remain objective and level-headed to understand the underlying issues and construct appropriate and actionable recommendations.

Step 4. Presentation

The engagement usually concludes with a presentation of the findings and recommendations to the client. All the work done previously is useless unless the consultant can communicate the message effectively, enabling the client to learn from the process. If the consultant does not provide the client with an understanding of the critical issues and the appropriate next steps, then the project will have no impact, regardless of how much work went into the first three steps. But when the consultant makes the key lessons and recommendations clear, the client should retain enough of the analysis to facilitate the decision-making process. The presentation itself is generally made using some kind of presentation software (often Microsoft PowerPoint) and referred to as a *deck*. Depending on the particular style of the firm, decks are generally considered to be stand alone documents that can be left behind and understood by individuals not associated with the project. As such, consultants need to have a clear and concise writing style, and to be able to articulate a story that persuades the deck reader to take constructive action.

Although a typical engagement runs through these four steps, the final presentation does not necessarily mark the end of the project. Consultants may be retained for a second phase of work, which may involve additional analysis or even implementation of the recommended solution. Most consulting firms work diligently to extend projects, usually beginning to talk with the client about additional work as early as the second or third step of an engagement.

Through this four-step process, the client hopes to learn enough to make decisions that will bring the ultimate goal to fruition. And, admittedly, the consulting firm hopes to develop a deep and wide-reaching relationship with the client that creates a long-lasting revenue stream.

THE CONSULTING LIFESTYLE

So, how do the different operating models—on-site and off-site—affect the lives of the consultants who must work under them? To answer this question, we will first describe a typical week in the life of an on-site consultant. After spending the weekend at home, the consultant flies back to the client site on either Sunday night or Monday morning, depending on the distance traveled. She lives in either a hotel room or a fully furnished executive apartment for the next four days. Then, on Thursday night or Friday morning, she returns home, since on-site consulting firms usually try to bring their professionals back to the office one day a week.

From Monday through Thursday, the consultant works in her temporary office at the client site, adjacent to the offices of full-time employees. She probably has her own portable laptop computer from which she can dial in to her consulting firm's e-mail and intranet system. She also remains connected to her firm through her home office voice mail system, and her temporary phone line at the client site. Most of her consulting team, as well as the designated client team, are located in offices near hers. Her days are generally busy, and frequently long, since she spends only four weekdays on-site. She has been provided with a rental car to drive between the airport, her hotel or apartment, and her office, and typically has a daily expense budget, which should cover all meal, taxi, and telephone expenses. And her firm may reimburse other expenses, such as dry cleaning and team dinners. Her weeks on the project proceed in this fashion for the duration of the project.

Many on-site consultants enjoy this lifestyle. With constant client contact, they can continuously receive feedback and recognition. And the "high life" of business travel and on-site work can be exciting. On-site consultants may also benefit financially since meals are usually paid for, and the combined mileage of the flights, rental cars, and hotels can quickly add up to free vacations. But separation from family and friends for extended periods may prove difficult for some people, not to mention the physical toll of frequent travel and life out of a suitcase.

Now we will look at a typical week in the life of an off-site consultant. Unlike the on-site consultant, who has a routine travel schedule, our off-site consultant makes fewer trips for a shorter duration. On average, he travels one or two days a week, often returning late at night on the same day he flies out. He has a permanent desk in his firm's office, with a single phone and voice mail number. He spends most of his time in his firm's office, using the library and production resources, conducting interviews over the phone, or meeting with members of the client team who have traveled to visit the firm. His primary means of contact with the client is the telephone, with occasional face-to-face contact at the client site during meetings and presentations.

Off-site consultants would rarely trade their lifestyle for that of on-site consultants. They return to their own homes each night and spend more time with family and friends, especially on weeknights. These consultants may collect fewer frequent flyer miles than their on-site peers, but the reward of free trips, they argue, is not worth the cost of being away from home and family. Still, there are some negatives to off-site work. These consultants may complain about a lack of client contact and feedback, and as a result, feel less reward from their hard work than their on-site peers. Long work hours may go unrecognized by the client, perhaps leaving consultants feeling underappreciated.

Whether off-site or on-site, all consultants share several lifestyle similarities. In addition to their professional responsibilities, consultants are expected to participate in internal firm development activities, such as recruiting, interviewing, staff training and development, and preparation of annual off-site events. Work weeks average between 50 and 80 hours, not including travel time, with peaks occurring prior to presentations and due dates, and valleys for a short time thereafter. Consultants have typically lived by the motto, "work hard, play hard," although firms are now downplaying this theme in favor of promoting a "balanced lifestyle." The industry as a whole suffers from a high turnover rate among junior staff, but it is better at retaining senior management.

Firms that do a good job of rewarding their consultants and providing flexible work arrangements have tenures that exceed the industry average. Other firms, however, are notorious for employee burnout, and struggle to retain some consultants for more than a year. Still others are rumored to have an "up-or-out" policy, whereby consultants who are underperforming their peers must either improve within a specific time, or leave the firm.

But, regardless of a firm's working model or attitude toward long hours, certain people are just not built for the work and lifestyle of a consultant. Only those who can thrive under the pressure of hard work, can perform multiple tasks simultaneously, can cope with ambiguity and uncertainty, and can remain calm and collected when stressed or tired will be able to maintain a positive perspective on consulting and stick with it.

CONSULTING AS A CAREER ACCELERATOR

As this chapter outlined, the professional life of a consultant is not a simple one. Consultants are often asked to tackle difficult problems under stressful circumstances. They are asked to work long hours and sacrifice a certain amount of their personal life. However, in the process of doing their work, consultants develop a core set of transferable skills, gain a broad perspective of a variety of managerial and organizational issues, and fundamentally understand how to achieve results. These skills are highly sought after by companies outside of consulting, in a broad spectrum of industries. To attract former consultants, companies typically extend job offers that are at a higher level of responsibility than those offered to nonconsultants who worked an equivalent number of years within that industry. In this regard, consulting can accelerate an individual's career.

One consulting firm in particular, Stax Research, has taken advantage of this demand for former consultants and created an entire business using their talent: For temporary periods of time, companies (and incidentally, consulting firms as well) can hire former consultants to fill key job roles, perform critical work assignments, and serve as interim management. Stax represents and places hundreds of former consultants who used to work at the top firms. Many of these professionals decided to leave consulting to attend school, start a family, or simply pursue other interests, and are able to earn an income by working part time with Stax. Fortunately, for these individuals as well as for other former consultants, many companies believe the consulting experience develops a stronger and more diverse skill set than a traditional corporate environment. Former consultants are therefore brought in to be the "athletes" or senior managers of a company, and when hired full time they are often groomed to become the next generation of executive management. Such demand can significantly increase the market value of former consultants, and for many individuals, the long-term benefit is enough to outweigh the long hours and personal sacrifices of working in consulting.

CHAPTER 3

THE EMERGENCE OF
e-CONSULTING

The rapid development of Internet technologies and a growing awareness of the importance of the Internet as a business tool has led to an explosion of interest and activity in this emerging arena. Realizing the opportunities offered by the Web, entrepreneurs developed new business models and quickly launched ventures that ultimately changed the way we all communicate, shop, and conduct our daily lives. As these start-ups proliferated, they challenged not only the relevance of the old business models, but also the profits of the companies that adhered to them. The second half of the 1990s was a period of time when many young entrepreneurial companies, often led by inexperienced management teams, dominated the business landscape. The enormous amount of business activity pushed the U.S. economy, and arguably the world's economy, to new heights.

In this dynamic, high-growth environment, the need for consulting services quickly became apparent. The Internet pure-plays (companies whose business model is predominately dependent on the Internet) needed professional assistance in developing their business strategies and building on them. Traditional companies also needed these services as they scrambled to understand the emerging business models, their new competitors, and how they could create lasting competitive advantages.

Most consulting firms either introduced new e-business practices or broadened the definition of their existing technology and systems integration practices to include Internet-related activities. Simultaneously, a large number of new specialty e-business consulting firms were founded, including Viant, Scient, Sapient, and Razorfish. Many of these firms successfully attracted clients away from the larger brand-name management consulting firms, by offering end-to-end solutions and positioning themselves as innovative thought leaders.

Overnight, brand new firms as well as established consulting practices claimed to be experts in digital business building, when in reality they, like their clients, were just learning the basics about a nascent industry. This chapter provides an overview of the e-consulting industry by taking an in-depth look at the two fundamental e-business service offerings: e-consulting services and e-business incubation services.

E-CONSULTING SERVICES

What is e-consulting and how is it different from typical management consulting? Essentially, e-consulting though similar to management consulting, is fundamentally different in its focus and approach. Like management consultants, e-consultants work on a variety of business problems for their clients, approach these problems in a highly structured manner, work in teams at the client site or from within the home office, and live a consultant's dynamic, fast-paced lifestyle. However, e-consulting differs in two important ways: (1) e-consultants are required to have specialized knowledge of the Internet, and (2) the work requires a multidisciplinary approach. Let's look at these two differentiating characteristics in more detail.

A Specialized Knowledge of the Internet

The work of e-consultants involves the Internet. As such, e-consultants are required to have specialized knowledge regarding the Internet, particularly along three important dimensions. First, e-consultants need to have a broad understanding of the strategic use of the Internet. Why should a Fortune 500 company expand its retails sales into the Internet?

How will offline activities mesh with online activities to give the consumer a seamless experience with the company? Can the supply chain be made more efficient using the Internet? What impact will an online marketing strategy have on my offline brand? These are just some of the questions that e-consultants must be able to answer.

Second, e-consultants also need to have insight into the challenges of the man/machine interface. As the Internet grew, it became clear that a consumer's interaction with a company's site was critical to the site's success. A well laid out strategic plan could not compensate for a poor consumer experience. This experience directly shaped the consumer's view of the company. E-consultants must have an understanding of the consumer experience, since it is affected by a variety of factors including the functionality contained in the site, the number of clicks that a consumer is required to make to complete a business function, the time required to download a file or image, the use of graphics, and even the use of a color scheme. Although this seems far removed from the business courses that you may have taken, an understanding of consumer experience issues is critical for a successful e-consultant.

Third, a successful e-consultant must have a broad understanding of the technologies employed by the Internet. Although it is not always necessary to have the technical knowledge required to write code, e-consultants must have an understanding of the impact that technical limitations and advancements can have on the strategic options available to a client.

At this point you may be reconsidering any desire you had to become an e-consultant. The task of being knowledgeable in so many areas may seem daunting. But remember, as an individual e-consultant, you are required to build in-depth knowledge in one of the three areas, and maintain a broad knowledge in the others. The multidisciplinary approach of most e-consulting firms or groups will help you to quickly gain the depth of knowledge that you need.

A Multidisciplinary Approach

The second fundamental difference between e-consulting and management consulting is the multidisciplinary approach to the work. As a whole, an e-consulting firm must have resident experts who have a deep knowledge of the three critical areas mentioned above: Internet strategy, consumer experience, and technology. It is impossible to find a single individual who has deep expertise in all areas. As such, e-consulting firms typically employ a multidisciplinary approach to their work. An e-consulting team is commonly comprised of four disciplines: strategy, functional design, creative design, and technology. Table 3.1 illustrates some of the roles typically found in an e-consulting firm.

The unique nature of each project requires e-consulting firms to build teams that are composed of the appropriate number of strategists, technologists, creative designers, and so on. But generally, teams will have representation of each of these core functionalities. Individuals representing each of these roles will work together to collaboratively fulfill the requirements of a client engagement. An end-to-end engagement may be divided into three basic phases: (1) strategic planning, (2) consumer experience development, and (3) technology build-out. Table 3.2 illustrates these phases and the specific steps involved in each.

Most pure-play e-consulting firms offer a full line of services that would take a client from the strategic development to the technology build-out. Although many firms would like to work with their clients throughout the entire lifecycle of engagements, clients may or may not want a single firm to assist it throughout the entire process. For example, a single client may ask McKinsey to perform the strategic planning, then commission Razorfish to build the consumer experience, and finally have Sapient actually build the site based on the work of Razorfish and McKinsey. A rationale for such a division of labor would simply be that a single firm might not have the best resources or capabilities to handle each stage.

The actual composition of an e-consulting team will vary depending on the work stage of an engagement. As illustrated in Figure 3.1, strategists often dominate the team in the early phase. Functional and creative designers dominate during the second phase, and technologists dominate the final phase.

This multidisciplinary approach has several potential benefits along with a number of challenges. It is clearly a source of strength, since

Table 3.1
Typical Roles within e-Consulting Firms

Role	Description
Strategists	Strategists typically have a strong business background. They often work on a variety of activities including: conducting market research, developing overall strategic vision and direction, building supporting financial and operating models, developing the marketing strategy, conducting interviews and focus groups, and so on.
Technologists	Technologists often work a variety of tasks related to the planning, development, and actual technology build-out of the site. Specific tasks include: defining the physical architecture, researching and selecting the hosting provider, scoping the prototype, designing and constructing the development and testing environments, finalizing hardware requirements, and so on. Technologists generally have a solid understanding of Java, C++, Active Server Pages, and so on.
Content Architects	Content architects are generally brought in to identify functionality gaps, opportunities, determine site features, and so on. Specific tasks include: research competitive offerings and identify gaps, identifying opportunities for differentiation, identify and prioritize proposed customer functionality.
Functional Analysts	Functional analysts are experts in translating high-level business requirements into functional specifications that can be developed by other system programmers. Functional analysts will lead efforts in the functional use case analysis.
Information Architects	Information architects are responsible for the design of the information architecture, event flow, navigation scheme, and the user-interfaces of all interactive elements of a site. Information architects work closely with the functional analysts to develop a deep understanding of the user's requirements and the client's overall objectives. They are also generally responsible for leading the usability testing efforts.
Creative Developers	Creative developers often work very closely with graphic designers to turn design direction into actual code. Creative developers are generally proficient in using development technologies such as HTML and DHTML.
Graphic Designers	Graphic designers leverage their expertise to support specific business objectives. Their role is not merely to make the site look attractive. They are responsible for balancing the need to make the site visually engaging with the need to make the site functionally usable for a specified target audience. They typically have a solid understanding of graphic design software such as Photoshop, Dreamweaver, Director, and Flash.
Project Managers	Project managers are responsible for leading multidisciplinary teams from project inception to delivery. Project managers are responsible for the overall quality of the project work, developing the project plan, and managing the day-to-day efforts of the team.
Client Partners	Client partners are responsible for business development, bringing high-level expertise to the engagement, and have ultimate responsibility for client satisfaction.

Table 3.2
The Phases of an e-Consulting Engagement

Phase	*Example Work Steps*
Strategy Development	• Competitive analysis • Customer analysis • Market survey • Strategic plan development • Technology assessment: define capability map, component sourcing, and so on. • Operating model definition
Consumer Experience	• Marketing launch plan • Functional analysis • Information architecture • Creative/user interface design • Prototype development and technology infrastructure • Mock-up creation
Technology Build-Out	• Technical infrastructure set-up • Implementation • Testing • Production rollout and support • Operational planning and execution • Configuration management • Knowledge transfer

Figure 3.1
Approximate Work Allocation by Phase

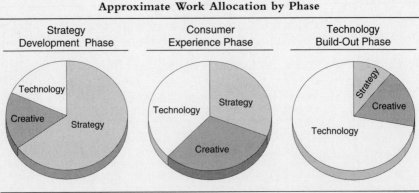

problems are viewed from a variety of angles, and solutions are investigated collectively and developed in a manner that is consistent across disciplines. A consulting firm that separates its disciplines could run into problems, where, for example, strategists are developing a strategic vision that is not realistic due to technology constraints, or creatives are developing a design that is not consistent with a central marketing message formulated by the strategists, or technologists are making changes during the build-out that fundamentally changes the strategic direction. By working together, solutions are created that make sense from the perspective of all disciplines.

However, this approach can also create significant problems in the way people communicate and work on a daily basis. The daily work environment can be significantly different from a traditional consulting firm. Differences could include a less formal dress code, a more hip office environment, and a more dynamic communication pattern among the disciplines. Interdisciplinary communication can become a serious challenge to completing project work. Misunderstandings could easily happen if the consultants are not sensitive to the communication style of their colleagues. The bottom line is that a multidisciplinary approach creates a more dynamic work environment. Applicants to firms that employ this approach would be well advised to carefully consider this and their personal ability to work and communicate with people from a wide variety of diverse backgrounds.

E-BUSINESS INCUBATION SERVICES

The second major type of service that e-consultants offer is incubation services. As the Internet boom continued and scores of companies began completing successful initial public offerings (IPOs) through the 1990s and into the 2000s, some of the most recognized consulting firms sought to maximize the value they could capture from this boom by establishing business incubators, or accelerators, that would develop new companies. Although incubators can take many forms, most provide start-ups with temporary office space, furniture and equipment, assistance with professional functions such as recruiting and legal affairs, and even dedicate full-time staff members to the start-up companies to temporarily fill empty roles. In return, incubators may receive cash payments and/or equity, and if an investment is made in a start-up, incubators usually take a very large chunk of the company's equity (sometimes in excess of 50%) priced at a very low valuation given the early development stage of start-ups. By some estimates, more than a thousand U.S. incubators were in operation as of 2001, led by recognized leaders CMGI, Hotbank, Idealab!, and Internet Capital Group (ICG). Many consulting firms believed they could enhance this formula by contributing their "expert" knowledge to the services offered by an incubator, and therefore build superior start-up companies in superior incubator facilities. Firms that launched incubators allowed their consultants, on a highly selective basis, to rotate through incubator engagements as a way of fulfilling personal entrepreneurial interests. But many firms only considered seasoned consultants for such engagements, and rarely if ever hired consultants directly into their incubator divisions. These incubators were supposed to showcase the best of the best consultants, since they were tasked with the high-risk job of building revolutionary new businesses.

Bain & Company, for example, has for years invested in companies through Bain Capital. But in the late 1990s, Bain introduced its new incubator under the name bainlab with the objective, as their Web site promotes, of ". . . helping Internet businesses succeed. We use our expertise to find the best Internet ideas and to help Web entrepreneurs, corporate entrepreneurs, and pre-IPO companies transform those ideas into commercial success."[1] bainlab invests capital in selected early stage companies, including seed-round capital, and provides strategic advice and guidance, as well as technical and management expertise.

On an even grander scale than bainlab, Accenture announced in February 2000 the introduction of their first Dotcom Launch Center, which by the end of 2000 grew to a network of over 25 locations around the world. The mission: to quickly propel the development of "New Economy" companies into scalable and viable businesses. But unlike many incubators that tend to work with start-up companies in their first six months of operation, Accenture's Launch Centers reportedly work with e-businesses that already have some financial support, a core management team, and some development activity underway. Like bainlab, the Launch Centers provide technical and management expertise, capital investments, and other tools and resources in return for significant equity stakes in the incubated companies.

Even McKinsey & Company entered the incubator game by launching The Accelerator @ McKinsey, which like the others invests capital in start-up companies, provides e-business strategy and development expertise, and accepts equity as a form of payment for services rendered. But in an attempt to differentiate itself, McKinsey distinguishes its accelerator from the pack of incubators: "The main difference between the Accelerator concept and conventional 'incubator' programs is that the latter typically provide small start-ups with seed funding, temporary office space, and limited advisory services," McKinsey explains, "The Accelerator @ McKinsey, on the contrary, focuses on incumbents and on start-ups in a later phase, providing clients, after initial funding, with objective expertise and deep industry skills to help management teams expand their reach dramatically."[2] Sounds a bit like Accenture's Launch Center concept, or arguably like bainlab since they will work with "pre-IPO companies," which are probably similar to McKinsey's "start-ups in later phase." Whether or not each of these examples can truly be differentiated from one another, one point is common to them all: The consulting parents of these incubators—or accelerators—share the belief that their e-business expertise enables them to build superior start-up companies.

By the end of 2000, incubators—or accelerators, launch centers, hatcheries, and so on—had fallen into ill repute due to the poor performance of many incubated companies and the accompanying fall in stock prices of the largest and most recognized incubators: CMGI, Hotbank, Idealab!, and ICG. Although the consulting firms that launched incubators continue to operate and promote their services, they have become much more conservative and have changed their screening criteria from seeking the hottest new ideas to seeking start-ups that will quickly become profitable and self-sustainable. As a result, incubators are accepting fewer new companies, and instead are focusing their resources on developing currently incubated companies into viable, self-supporting businesses. Consulting firms are likely to continue accepting equity as a viable payment currency for both consulting and incubation services, but their willingness to forego cash altogether is uncertain. The risk of accepting equity increased significantly at the tail end of 2000 and into 2001, as droves of dot-com and technology firms either closed their doors or missed expected performance targets, causing the bull market of the 1990s to look bearish. Only time will tell if the incubators founded and operated by consulting firms will themselves remain a viable service extension of consulting.

DETERMINING YOUR FIT WITH E-CONSULTING

Although e-consulting clearly offers a unique opportunity to become part of the Internet revolution without having to join any single dot-com or Internet technology company, there still are significant risks associated with joining a digital consulting firm. On the positive side, the e-consulting industry offers a unique environment in which to work: fast-track learning about the Internet, collaboration of strategists with technologists and creatives, launching new e-companies that promise to revolutionize the way businesses operate, and so on. The multidisciplinary approach, the focus on using technology as a transforming tool, and the opportunities to build from the ground up make e-consulting a potentially rewarding opportunity for many people.

However, on the down side, the sudden collapse at the end of 2000 and the beginning of 2001 of the market caps of many leading e-business consulting firms, such as Viant, Scient, Sapient, and Razorfish, reveals many of the risks associated with an e-business consulting job: high sensitivity to the general health of the U.S. economy and the technology sector, and the unproven sustainability of pure-play e-consulting firms (versus the more diversified offerings of traditional consulting firms like McKinsey and Pricewaterhouse-Coopers). As of this writing, many of the pure-play e-consulting firms are not even expected to survive, and consolidation in the sector is almost universally expected. With share prices in the single dollars, a number of the public e-consulting firms risk de-listing unless a dramatic change occurs in the perceived outlook of such pure-play consulting firms.

As you reflect on the e-consulting sector for yourself, you should recognize both the risks and rewards of joining a pure-play firm. The essay in Chapter 4 written by Glenn Cornett of Razorfish presents an insider's perspective on working in a pure-play e-consulting firm. Mr. Cornett shares his own thoughts on the evolution and turbulent nature of pure-play firms—like his own, Razorfish—and gives you tips on how to select an e-consulting firm for yourself. As you look into pure-play e-consultancies, you should also consider the alternative practice groups of larger, more diversified firms. Another essay in Chapter 4 by Joseph B. Fuller of Monitor Company is written from the perspective of a diversified strategic consulting firm that maintains a practice in e-commerce. Mr. Fuller presents some of Monitor's perspectives on how the Internet has changed and continues to change the rules of business, as well as the way consultants provide advice. Finally, you can read the essay on information technology (IT) consulting written by Rudy Puryear of Accenture to get a sense of how large systems consulting firms are helping companies adapt to the "New Economy."

These authors should help you understand three different approaches to e-consulting: (1) pure-play e-consulting firms, (2) diversified consulting firms with e-consulting practices, and (3) traditional large IT consultancies, and ultimately help you determine which approach is best suited to your own risk tolerance, learning objectives, and preferred working environment. Recognize that the landscape of e-consulting is shifting all the time. If you decide you want to pursue a career in e-consulting, be sure to collect as much firsthand information about the alternative firms as you can to build upon the advice and ideas our contributors present in Chapter 4.

CHAPTER 4

PERSPECTIVES ON CONSULTING

Now that you have a better understanding of the consulting industry and a sense of the work and lifestyle, you should meet some of the industry's leading consultants and strategic thinkers to gain firsthand knowledge of their own experiences. In this chapter, we have collected a set of personal essays that provide a rare insider's glimpse into the consulting profession. These original essays were written by individual consultants with your interests in mind, to answer some of the questions that you may presently have—and our contributing consultants once had—such as:

- Can consulting be a career?
- Should I go to a small or large firm?
- What is "internal consulting"?
- Should I be a generalist or specialist consultant?
- What is nonprofit consulting? Public sector consulting?
- Is there a relationship between consulting and venture capital?
- What do consultants do after consulting?

The essays are filled with personal stories and useful advice, and offer individualized perspectives on the profession. As you read through the essays, note the reasons why our contributors chose the profession of consulting, and what they consider to be the risks and rewards of their work. It may be useful to envision yourself in their shoes, to help you consider different industry and practice areas of consulting for yourself. Do you agree that generalists are more effective consultants than specialists, or do you favor the opposite point of view? Would you prefer to contribute to the growth of for-profit corporations, or work to refine the missions of nonprofit organizations? After reading these essays, you should have a better understanding of your own interests, and be able to focus your consulting job search on the types of firms and practice areas that you find most attractive.

The essays are grouped into six categories to help you select the essays that target your most pressing questions and interests:

1. *The Consulting Profession*

   The Work of Consulting, Gary Neilson, Booz•Allen & Hamilton

   Can Consulting Be a Career?, Bill Matassoni, McKinsey & Company

2. *Strategic Thinking and Innovation in Consulting*

   Business Strategy and Consulting: A Theorist's View of Practice and a Practical View of Theory, Barry Nalebuff, Yale School of Management

   Innovation in Consulting, George Stalk Jr., The Boston Consulting Group

   Customer-Driven Growth Strategy, Charles P. Hoban, Mercer Management Consulting

3. *Alternative Approaches to Consulting*

   The Generalist Approach to Consulting: The Strategic Value of Breaking Industry Barriers, Paul Smith, Bain & Company

   Selecting a Small versus a Large Firm, Ellen McGeeney, Braun Consulting

As a collection, these essays offer you a rare glimpse into the careers and perspectives of some of the industry's leading consultants and strategic thinkers. Although the essays cover a wide variety of topics, you will notice that a number of similar themes run through the collection, revealing many of the prevalent benefits—as well as the challenges—of consulting. We now invite you to enter the individual worlds of our contributing authors and share their thoughts and experiences.

The Work of Consulting

GARY NEILSON
BOOZ·ALLEN & HAMILTON

Gary Neilson is a senior vice president of Booz·Allen & Hamilton and leader of the Transformation and Organization practice. During his two decades with Booz·Allen, he has focused on organization and business process design, productivity improvement, and change management. Mr. Neilson has led the development of Booz·Allen's organization products—"Enterprise Value Engineering," "Creating High Performance Organizations . . . Making Strategy Work through Organization Capability," and "Theory P . . . Building Organization Capability through People and Business Processes." Prior to joining Booz·Allen, Mr. Neilson served on the financial staff of the IBM Corporation. He also served three years as a certified public accountant (CPA) with Arthur Young & Company. Mr. Neilson received a BS in Accounting from King's College and an MBA in finance from Columbia University's Graduate School of Business. At King's and Columbia, he graduated first in his class.

While I was earning my MBA at Columbia, I was attracted to consulting because it sounded like a continuation of business school—the chance to work on an assortment of the hardest, most critical business and organizational problems. But there would be a fundamental difference: as a consultant, I would be working "live" with real companies. The stakes and the pressure would be higher—these cases would involve real people and real capital—but so would the intellectual and financial rewards. Eighteen years later, my essential attraction to the profession has not dimmed.

This is a period of dramatic change. Call it the age of globalization, the age of information, or the age of knowledge, the business world cannot sit back and let history define it for us. Too much hangs in the balance. Someone has to find ways of translating these overwhelming forces into coherent ways of thinking and practical courses of action. That line between theory and action is where the consultant's work begins.

CONSULTANTS ARE PROBLEM SOLVERS

Companies do not bring in consultants for mundane problems. Although the consultant is an anonymous practitioner, there is glory in seeing your work in the second column of *The Wall Street Journal*, which is devoted to companies that are undertaking major initiatives. The visibility of your clients only adds to the stimulation.

We are outsiders. We are expensive, and we do not provide value if we are doing things that corporate staff members could do themselves, or if we are there to rubber-stamp management preconceptions. We have to know what we are talking about, we need the conviction to speak our minds, and we must be able to bring our experience to bear on client problems quickly and effectively. Our frameworks and platforms give us a ready-made set of standards to apply to each new situation and assess it expeditiously. We have established ways of proceeding and a conception of best practices.

This is not the much maligned cookie-cutter approach. We customize our work. However, while every situation is unique in its particulars, in broad terms it may have much in common with many other cases. Yet, the model is dynamic. Each engagement teaches us more. We are constantly refining our capabilities, improving our tools, and enhancing our practice.

Clients hire consultants who have seen problems before and understand the frameworks for solving them in as short a time as they responsibly can. The days are past when a company can afford to be smug about its own culture or its way of doing things. The competition is too intense.

When you are trying to merge one airline's routes, for example, into those of another airline by an announced date just a few months later, you do not want to reinvent the airplane—you want to get the job done. An engagement like this requires a vision that is both strategic and eminently practical. It needs to be done in a way that works. This involves tactical logistical thinking, such as ticketing, and making sure that the planes are available when the people are ready to depart. But it also requires ensuring organizational capabilities, such as scheduling, marketing, staffing, operations, and maintenance. Clients have all these capabilities in abundance, but extending them seamlessly across a much larger organization requires specialists who have seen it all before and know how it is done. That is what consultants can provide.

THE CHANGING ROLE OF CONSULTANTS

The center of gravity in my work has shifted as I have matured professionally. Early in my career, I was engaged primarily in analysis and the requisite fact gathering. The product of my work was typically a rigorous formal presentation of data and analysis, at the end of which was a recommendation about what management should do. These meetings were often contentious and intellectually stimulating. The more vociferous the argument, the more successful the presentation was, in my view, because it meant we were really disturbing the universe.

Of course, implementation was another matter. If your recommendations entail justifying major capital investments or a radical change in management style and methodology, the client must marshal the capital and will to effect the change. The disconnection between what to do and how to do it may account for the failures of so many efforts at corporate restructuring.

Today, fact gathering and analysis are still critical to consulting. But the work involves much more collaboration with the client throughout the engagement. We work with company teams specially chosen by senior management to arrive not only at a plan of action and a rationale, but a plan for implementation. The ultimate product is not our presentation; it is their presentation. The program is backed not only by our opinions as "outside experts," but by the mandate of insiders as well.

The best consultants, in my mind, help clients do things. They guide, they brainstorm, but above all, they coach them to think about their business and solve problems for themselves. Consultants believe that you should teach a man to fish rather than give the man a fish to eat.

THE CHANGING STRUCTURE OF COMPANIES

This mode of consulting ideally matches the needs of the emerging corporation, with a thin staff that bears scant resemblance to the corporations we knew years ago. In the new corporation, senior management must justify its existence by adding value every bit as much as the lines of business. Management is more likely to look outside to meet its needs—through outsourcing, strategic alliances, or vendor partnerships—than it is to create a new corporate department. Management consultants fit comfortably within that vision.

Keeping pace with this business takes a great deal of flexibility. You have to be temperamentally inclined toward a job-shop view of work—solid theoretical and methodological grounding, combined with an open mind. Alarms go off in my head when I interview a student who says he or she wants to be a partner. I ask myself, "How do they know? How can they be so sure?" I did not have that clear a vision of my future when I began. I wanted to learn as much as I could and have the chance to revisit my options. It turned out that I did become a partner, but only because this is a field where the challenges and opportunities constantly renew themselves. The field has changed, and I like to think I have grown.

CONCLUSION

I would like to end on a personal note. When I started out, I worked 15 hours a day, six or seven days a week. Then I met the woman whom I later married. I had the choice of continuing to work that hard or reengineering my own schedule so that I could have a life of my own. You would be surprised how efficient your own work processes can become when the incentives change. It is not that you do not occasionally work that hard or spend a great deal of time traveling. But weekends are much more clearly delineated on my calendar than they once were, and 6 P.M. on Friday is a more meaningful time.

Let me also mention that in the early days, before I began to limit my own hours, I much preferred working for people who had lives outside consulting than for those who worked as hard as I did. Lifestyle balance is not just a question of personal preference; it is a business necessity. If you work too hard, creativity and productivity begin to wane; and what is true for the individual is true for the firm. You cannot build teams or intellectual depth if you burn out each successive class of associates or partners. Any firm whose business is helping clients learn and change has to have the ability to learn about itself.

This is not an age for conventional thinking and closed minds. It is a time for learning, imagination, and perseverance. Our client companies and the people who depend on them deserve no less. Business history, like any other aspect of history, looks neat or inevitable only in hindsight. When we do our best, we help shape it for the better. That is the consultant's job.

———— ● ● ● ————

Can Consulting Be a Career?

BILL MATASSONI
MCKINSEY & COMPANY

Bill Matassoni is McKinsey's director of communications. His responsibilities include both external and internal communications, including several of McKinsey's key systems for sharing knowledge among its consultants. He joined McKinsey in 1980 and was elected partner in 1982. He received a BA from Harvard College in 1968 and an MBA from Harvard Business School in 1975.

Management consulting can be an ideal starting point for young professionals, but the reality is that most people who join consulting firms leave in a few years and take jobs outside consulting. Only a few stay long enough to receive more than one promotion, and even fewer are asked to become owners of their firms. Consulting gives professionals experience—lots of it, fast—and flexibility. It is an ideal professional development opportunity, but it is hardly a career.

A PROFESSIONAL TRAINING GROUND

If management consulting is a professional development opportunity rather than a career, then ask yourself this question: As you think about consulting in general and about individual consulting firms in particular, what kind of development would be good for you, and where are you likely to get it? To find your answers, consider the three elements that enable firms to help their clients: knowledge, skills, and people.

For some consulting firms, knowledge is their dominant source of value added. They may have a comprehensive database that is key to helping clients with purchasing problems, or they may know the software industry backward and forward—or at least the current key success factors. Knowledge can also be a combination of theory and methodology, such as with EVA (economic value analysis) that helps managers think more rigorously about actions that will increase their companies' market capitalization.

Skills can vary as much as knowledge. Skills may be simply relevant to a particular problem-solving approach. After running clients through a reengineering process 20 times, you get fairly skilled at it. But consultants need other skills, too: communications skills, project management skills, people development skills, and, at the higher levels, skills for interacting with senior management and keeping them involved in projects.

People, the last ingredient in this formula for a consultant's value added, is the hardest to pin down. People can be a synonym for leadership, values, commitment, professionalism, and trustworthiness. These are nice concepts, and all of us probably aspire to possess these attributes, but they may not always be required to have an impact on your client. A well-wrought combination of skills and knowledge, alone, may be enough to have an impact with your client. You are the expert, the gunslinger who comes in to solve the problem, and then moves on.

But most consultants who aspire to work on a client's key problems—whether organizational, strategic, or operational—understand that consulting is a very personal profession. You have to care about your clients, institutionally and individually, and they have to care about and trust you. There are many of us who believe that, even though our value to clients is delivered through a combination of people, skills, and knowledge, the quality of our people is, in the end, what really matters. The mission statements of most consulting firms emphasize not only their aspiration to have impact, but also to attract the best people and really help them grow. That is the case at McKinsey & Company, for example, where we have a saying, "At first you are known for what you do, then for what you know, and finally for who you are."

The implications for someone considering consulting are straightforward. If you are interested in developing a knowledge spike, look for consulting firms that have track records in practice development and research. Check out how often they publish and who gets to publish. If you want to develop analytical or people skills, consider their approach to training and how they do their day-to-day work. Is the emphasis on process or problem solving? How extensively are teams used, and are clients on them? What kinds of formal development systems do they have? To get a really good picture of which skills really matter, ask to see the complete list of new partners from the previous year (not just the "poster" partners in the recruiting literature), and see what kinds of background they bring and experiences they have had.

As for the people dimension, assess whether or not there will be real leadership opportunities for you early on. What kinds of roles do you get to play with clients? What kinds of clients are served, and what criteria are applied when considering the personal characteristics of prospective clients? Put more simply, will you get to work with real leaders? And have newcomers been involved in starting new practices and offices? These can be great opportunities for personal development because of their entrepreneurial nature. Or maybe the litmus test for assessing how well a firm develops its people is what its consultants do when they leave their firms. Do they go on to top positions in business, government, or academia?

AN AGENT OF CHANGE

Many consulting firms deliver on one or more of these dimensions of development, and that is what makes consulting so attractive. In fact, there has been a backlash in recent years because so many people find it attractive. Some critics have worried that with so much talent from business and other graduate schools going into consulting, American business and society are not being well served. That's not a fair argument. Indeed, consulting prepares many people to be successful, high-impact leaders. But some observers disagree, arguing that consultants do not implement anything, that they study things, give theoretical answers, and then leave. So, they argue, consulting does not prepare them for the real world. But what do these observers mean by implement?

- Do they mean developing a detailed plan regarding structure, systems, staff, and other key organizational changes, as well as a timetable for getting them done? Consultants do that.
- Do they mean giving top management real insight and conviction about what will create value in the future? Consultants do that.
- Do they mean experimenting on the front line with new approaches or prototyping new business models? Consultants do that.
- Do they mean marching people through a change process regardless of the situation? Some consultants do that, but it may not be right to do that.
- Do they mean running a client's business for them or usurping management's responsibilities? Consultants do not, or should not, do that.

The bottom line is that consultants do implement in many ways, and the best consultants, like their clients, cannot afford to just step back and study the situation. Russell Ackoff, a great thinker on strategy, once wrote:

Managers are not confronted with problems that are independent of each other, but with dynamic situations that consist of complex systems of changing problems that interact with each other. I call such situations messes. Problems are abstractions extracted from messes by analysis; they are to messes as atoms are to tables and charts. Managers do not solve problems; they manage messes.[1]

Management consultants confront messes, too. And in the ambiguity and turmoil of these messes are the real opportunities to help your clients and develop yourself. This is not to say that consultants have not, at times, been guilty of favoring elegant and theoretical solutions rather than practical answers. Writing about operations research, Ackoff lamented that it had become identified with techniques, mathematical models, and algorithms, rather than with "the ability to formulate management problems, solve them, and implement and maintain their solutions in turbulent environments."[2] Consulting in the 1980s could have been similarly criticized, but think about the challenges managers face today. Situations are fluid and problems are interconnected, and it is hard to determine cause and effect with certainty over time. What is needed under these conditions is what Schön and Ackoff described as the "active synthetic skill" of "designing a desirable future and inventing ways of bringing it about."[3]

A PERSONAL COMMITMENT

Helping clients design and invent—that is what consulting, at its best, is. It is not good enough to be right—your goal is to win. Your determination to help your client succeed goes beyond a professional obligation and becomes a personal commitment. As such, consulting can have a noble and admirable purpose, whatever the specific assignment and goal. It can mean helping a client develop and sell a terrific new product worldwide. It can mean helping a company in Kansas or Irkutsk stay independent and competitive. It can mean helping Glasgow renew its economy. It can mean helping a country's politicians understand how to create jobs.

Whatever the challenge, if you feel this sense of purpose when you consult, then the leadership, trust, skills, and knowledge that you aim to develop will all naturally result. And each year, when you ask yourself, "Should I keep doing this?" you will say, "Yes." But if that sense of purpose is absent, you have probably learned enough after a few years, and your answer should be, "No." It is time to move on.

—— • • • ——

Business Strategy and Consulting: A Theorist's View of Practice and a Practical View of Theory

BARRY NALEBUFF
YALE SCHOOL OF MANAGEMENT

Barry Nalebuff is the Milton Steinbach Professor at Yale School of Management. He graduated Phi Beta Kappa from the Massachusetts Institute of Technology in 1980, with degrees in Economics and Mathematics. A Rhodes Scholar, he received a doctorate in Economics from Oxford University two years later, and was awarded the George Webb Medley thesis prize. Before coming to Yale, he was a Junior Fellow at the Harvard Society of Fellows, and an Assistant Professor at Princeton University. Dr. Nalebuff is the author, with Princeton University Professor Avinash Dixit, of *Thinking Strategically: The Competitive Edge in Business, Politics, and Everyday Life,* and with Harvard Business School Professor Adam Brandenburger of *Co-opetition.* Dr. Nalebuff has co-founded two companies with his former students, Honest Tea and SplitTheDifference.com.

I believe that a theory of business will prove useful, perhaps even invaluable, to you. As a professor, what matters more than anything else is discovering truth. But that is not the way it works in the "real world." As a consultant, it is not enough to discover the right answer—the answer also has to get implemented. I am a game theorist and I apply

69

game theory to business strategy. But right now, I am writing about your future as a consultant and therefore better take heed of my own words. I recognize that my ideas, even if correct, do not count if you do not implement them. So now I must convince you.

A THEORY OF BUSINESS

Harvard Business School Professor Adam Brandenburger likes to say, "There's nothing so practical as a good theory." A good theory confirms the conventional wisdom that less is more: less because it does not tell people what to do; but at the same time more, because it helps people organize what they know and uncover what they do not know. And there is no better way to get someone to implement your ideas than for you to help them discover these ideas by themselves, so they think they came up with the ideas on their own.

Co-opetition (New York: Doubleday, 1996), the book I coauthored with Adam Brandenburger, develops a theory of business. It is a way to think about creating and capturing value. There is a fundamental duality here; whereas creating value is an inherently cooperative process, capturing value is inherently competitive. To create value, people cannot act in isolation. They have to recognize their interdependence. To create value, a business needs to align itself with customers, suppliers, employees, and many others. That is the way to develop new markets and expand existing ones.

But along with expanding the size of a pie, there is the issue of dividing it up. This is competition. Just as businesses compete with one another for market share, customers and suppliers are also looking out for their slice of the pie. Creating value that you can capture is the essence of business. To understand this duality, we use one of the key concepts of game theory, the idea of added value.

$$\text{Added value} = \frac{\text{Total value created}}{\text{with you in the game}} - \frac{\text{Total value created}}{\text{without you in the game}}$$

Game theory says that if competition is unfettered, no player will get more than his or her added value in a game. Thus, added value allows us to characterize who has power and who does not. It allows us to understand how a pie is created and how it is divided up. If truth be told, this one equation seems simple, perhaps even too simple. But its simplicity is deceptive.

The first thing to note is that added value is an allocentric concept ("Allo" means others and is the reverse of "ego" or self). Instead of asking what you can get on your own, it requires you to ask what others will lose if you go away. It forces you to imagine a world without you—not a pleasant task—and understand just what you bring to others.[4]

What is your added value? Where does it come from? And how can you make it bigger, much bigger? Doing something better or cheaper than others is an important source of added value, but it is not the only one.

Take Microsoft. Whether or not it does things better or cheaper than others is somewhat beside the point. A key reason for Microsoft's enormous added value is the existence of Intel and the complementarity between their products. The existence of complements will be a key determinant of whether the network computer, electric cars, DVD players, digital cameras, and a host of other new technology products succeed or fail.

COMPLEMENTORS

A complement to one product is any other product that makes the first one more, rather than less, attractive. Computer hardware and software are complements. So are hot dogs and mustard, cars and car loans, cable television and *TV Guide,* the Internet and high-capacity digital phone lines, catalogs and overnight delivery services—even red wine and dry cleaners, or Siskel and Ebert.

Traditionally, business strategy has largely focused on competition—Coke versus Pepsi—and in the process has underplayed complements. There has not even been a word to describe providers of complementary products. So we created one: "complementor," the natural counterpart to "competitor."

In new markets, paying attention to complements is a necessity. Without key complements, the market may never take off. In established markets, attending to complements has less dramatic but still valuable results. Here, complements most likely exist, but you can make your product more attractive by making the complements better, more plentiful, and less expensive.

Although your clients will probably know all about their competitors, chances are they will have thought less about their complementors. More to the point, which complementors are missing? Even a great product can sit on a shelf until key complements are developed. One cannot assume that the essential complements to a business are going to be there. And if the complements are missing, you cannot assume that the market will solve the problem. The company will have to work with others to create the complements, or create them itself.

Companies involved in today's information revolution are prime candidates for this focus on complements. A new system of creating and sharing information is evolving, and it has many complementary parts. It is not enough to invent one part of the new system; one has to pay attention to all the parts at once.

Intel understands this idea, and provides a lesson for every business. The company's engineers have done a brilliant job of developing increasingly powerful computer chips. But the chip is only part of a larger system, and most of us already have more processing power than we need to run our favorite applications. Thus, outpacing competing chip makers is not enough—Intel must also engineer demand for its next-generation chips. So Intel is on the lookout for complementors: video games on PCs, desktop video-conferencing, and more. As I write this in 1998, look for voice recognition as the next technology that soaks up processing cycles and bet that Intel will take an active role in bringing that technology to the market.

Added value can also be tied to some of the best-known concepts in business strategy. Consider, for example. Michael Porter's concept of "competitive advantage." This is typically understood to mean some activity or set of activities that one organization can do better or cheaper than others. If you can do some things better or cheaper than others, then without you in the game, the total pie would indeed shrink.

Added value also fits nicely with Hamel and Prahalad's concept of "core competence." You can think of a core competence as a source of added value. Would value be lost if you, along with that competency, were out of the game? How well can others fill in? How much value would be lost?

Added value offers a different way of looking at the world. Conventional economics takes the structure of markets as fixed. People are thought of as simple stimulus-response machines. Sellers and buyers assume that products and prices are fixed, and they optimize production and consumption accordingly. Conventional economics has its place in describing the operation of established, mature markets, but it does not capture people's creativity in finding new ways of interacting with one another.

CONCLUSION

In game theory, nothing is fixed. The economy is dynamic and evolving. The players create new markets and take on multiple roles. They innovate. No one takes products or prices as given. If this sounds like the free-form and rapidly transforming marketplace, that is why added value and game theory may be the kernel of a new economics for the new economy. You can say I told you so.

———•••———

Innovation in Consulting

GEORGE STALK JR.
THE BOSTON CONSULTING GROUP

George Stalk Jr. is a senior vice president at The Boston Consulting Group. He is worldwide chair of The Boston Consulting Group's innovation, marketing, and communications group and co-leader of the firm's global e-commerce business. Now based in Toronto, Mr. Stalk has also worked in BCG's Boston, Chicago, and Tokyo offices. His professional practice focuses on international and time-based competition.

The co-author of the critically acclaimed book on time-based competition, *Competing Against Time,* and of, *Kaisha: The Japanese Corporation,* Mr. Stalk has also been published in numerous business publications, including *Harvard Business Review.* He recently co-edited *Breaking Compromises and Perspectives on Strategy,* both anthologies of BCG writings. Mr. Stalk speaks regularly before prestigious business and industry associations and was identified by *Business Week* as one among a new generation of leading management gurus and by *Consulting* magazine as one of the world's 10 most influential management consultants.

Mr. Stalk holds a BS in engineering mechanics from the University of Michigan, an MS in aeronautics and astronautics from Massachusetts Institute of Technology, and an MBA from Harvard Business School. He held previous positions with Applicon, Inc., and Exxon Research and Engineering.

I was originally attracted to The Boston Consulting Group (BCG) because of its reputation for innovation. BCG's history is one of continuous innovation, including classics such as experience-based strategies, portfolio, stalemate, and average costing, and new wave strategies such as time-based competition, capabilities-based competition, and breaking compromises. And today, we pursue strategies based on the new economics of information. We are constantly searching for ways to compete that are not generally accepted, or that are overlooked, dismissed, or misunderstood.

THE COMPANY AS A LABORATORY

We have enormous opportunity to innovate in the consulting business because our clients represent an almost limitless laboratory. In helping our clients find solutions to the challenges they face—be they growth, turnaround, or repositioning—patterns emerge. These patterns enable us to understand cause and effect. Once cause and effect are clear, we are just a step away from identifying a strategy innovation. And once we identify the innovation, we can transplant it from one industry to another.

For example, almost all factories can be made flexible for faster throughput by just-in-time processes. But factories are just a collection of machines operated by a human organization. Should not all human organizations be amenable to being made flexible? The answer is yes. Just-in-time works in insurance companies and in the back office processes of a securities firm. In another example, the strategies for strengthening brands in consumer goods companies are very often just as effective for strengthening brands in financial service and industrial companies.

AN INNOVATION: TIME-BASED COMPETITION

Our work in making factories and other organizations flexible led us to time-based competition. The concept is simple: companies that meet the needs of their customers more rapidly than competitors do grow faster and are more profitable than others in their industries. We observed a pattern of faster throughput across a wide variety of factories that were made flexible. We incorporated speed into our strategy because we believe that time is the decade's most powerful competitive weapon and management tool.

And our beliefs were proven true. Companies of all sorts and sizes became or are becoming time-based competitors. By inspecting their processes and organizations through the lens of time, these companies found and are finding new ways to operate, satisfy their customers, compete, grow, improve quality, and invigorate themselves.

Time-based competition was directly lifted and applied to the management of hospitals. Karolinska Hospital, a leading research hospital in Stockholm, Sweden, used time-based competition to respond to reductions in government subsidies at a time when demand was growing. If people could get through the hospital faster, capacity could be freed up and costs reduced. At Karolinska, doctors were, at first, skeptical of the concept. How could they save time without risking quality, thereby imperiling patient care? In fact, they found that poor coordination and scheduling problems were not only reducing efficiency and inflating costs, but also causing patients unnecessary delay, inconvenience, anxiety, and, sometimes, health complications.

By redesigning operating procedures and staffing patterns, Karolinska cut the time required for preoperative testing from months to days. By compressing the operating room cycle from admission through operation, to intensive care, and out, the hospital was able to close 2 of 15 operating rooms and still increase the number of operations per day by 30 percent. Doctors could schedule operations in weeks rather than months. The result: better service for patients with no loss of quality (indeed, faster care is better care), less overhead, and more growth.

THE EXCITEMENT OF CONSULTING

The excitement of consulting is knowing that the patterns are out there to be observed, discovered, interpreted, and then transplanted. This excitement keeps many of us in consulting much longer than we anticipated when we first joined the profession.

Now, as a senior officer of BCG, I am extremely gratified to watch the progress of the bright, young people who enter consulting each year. As they develop tenure, their ability to innovate strengthens. First, experience brings stronger skills for faster pattern recognition and interpretation. Second, working with a client and an industry for a considerable period results in enhanced innovation. Clients do not keep consultants around to help with the same challenges over and over again. The bar keeps rising, and consultants must continually strive to hurdle it.

For example, I have been working as a consultant for an automotive OEM (original equipment manufacturer) since 1982. I have worked in component manufacturing, vehicle assembly, product development, and parts and services, and am now deeply involved in the distribution and retail end of the business. As I reflect on my years as a consultant, I realize that my tasks have become progressively more challenging.

This is frustrating and exciting at the same time. The frustration is that the job is not getting easier. The excitement is that the next request is always a more interesting and demanding challenge that will require innovation. Indeed, today we are questioning the fundamental structure of the automotive industry and how it will be affected by the forces of change, including the opening of markets, the restructuring of the supply base, electronic commerce, advances in technologies, changes in consumer behaviors, and changes in distribution and retail.

BUILDING LONG-TERM CLIENT RELATIONSHIPS

I know it is through innovation that we will be able to deliver the assistance and the value our clients seek. I also know that value will accrue to BCG since innovation in the client environment strengthens our firm. Indeed, many things we have done along the value chain of the automotive industry were precursors to changes in other industries, such as consumer goods, insurance, and banking. For example, the notion that growth opportunities are hidden in compromises that companies impose on consumers arose from trying to make dealers "customer friendly." Now, the notion of breaking compromises to release value and to grow is spreading through many industries.

When we review our largest, and longest, client relationships, we are always struck by how these relationships began with the client adopting an innovation and then seeking additional help, either in dealing with the ramifications of that innovation or in seeking other innovations. Innovation is important for getting impact because, in many companies, it is hard to achieve significant change by simply improving existing strategies. Another result of innovation is that we gain our clients' trust, which, in turn, allows us to help with their more difficult problems. This is a virtuous cycle that strengthens the consultant-client relationship and provides us with the laboratory we need to stay ahead in the game of innovation.

Customer-Driven Growth Strategy

CHARLES P. HOBAN
MERCER MANAGEMENT CONSULTING

Charles P. Hoban is a vice president at Mercer Management Consulting and head of the firm's Boston office. He specializes in the development of value-driven business designs for Mercer clients and is a leader of the firm's business design innovation practice in North America.

Mr. Hoban was a significant contributor to the development of the best-selling book *Value Migration,* leading the research team, managing the development of the manuscript, and articulating many of the book's basic frameworks. His ongoing work in understanding and quantifying the determinants of shareholder value creation has been integral to the continued development of Mercer's practice and the development of the follow-up best-sellers, *The Profit Zone* and *Profit Patterns.* In his 10 years of strategy consulting, Mr. Hoban has led several major consulting projects employing value-driven business design principles in the development of corporate strategy for major corporations. In particular, most of his recent work has been focused in technology industries.

Mr. Hoban has spoken at and led numerous management workshops on the topics of value migration and the profit zone at organizations including Microsoft, IBM, Mellon Bank, Hoechst Celanese, ABB, Motorola, and the Advertising Research Foundation's Leaders Forum.

Prior to joining Mercer, Mr. Hoban was a partner of Corporate Decisions, Inc., a strategy-based consulting firm that merged with Mercer. He was a founding member of CDI's European operation. Prior to joining CDI, he was an international copper and crude oil merchant for Cargill, Inc. Mr. Hoban holds a BA from Dartmouth College and a master's from Northwestern's Kellogg Graduate School of Management, where he graduated with distinction.

Management consulting is not a homogeneous industry. The issues addressed, the analytical processes employed, and the day-to-day activities of the project team can vary widely from one type of consulting to another. As you face the challenge of choosing your career path within the consulting industry, you have to dig beneath the surface of the recruiting pitches and ask yourself: What kind of consulting do I want to do?

CUSTOMER-DRIVEN GROWTH STRATEGY

If you were the CEO of a company in the 1970s, the rules were pretty simple. The number of things that you had to concern yourself with were relatively limited. It was a hard job because competition was fierce, but you knew how you were competing. You knew your competitors. You could count on certain economic rules applying. You wanted to gain high market share because that allowed you to advance down the experience curve. You wanted to get down the curve because that gave you a cost (and, therefore, profit) advantage. With that profit advantage, you could invest in the activities that allowed you to gain share. Your job as CEO was to lay out a plan to win at that game.

The consulting industry that grew up in the 1970s supported that task. Consulting was about experience curves, about relative cost positions, about pushing an organization to be more effective at that game. Even the 1980s' "paradigms"—total quality management, time-based competition, process reengineering—were all about making companies more competitive. In this world, "strategy" was sort of an academic exercise. Most companies knew where they were trying to go; they just needed help getting there.

Business has changed. Today, the number of strategic challenges facing a CEO is exploding. The amount of information available as input to decisions now seems infinite. The set of competitors is constantly changing. The traditional economic rules of the game do not seem to apply. Companies that got very good at competing in the old game may or may not be equipped to succeed as the game has changed. Too many companies have spent the past 20 years "getting competitive," only to find themselves looking up from that task to ask, "What am I competing for?" "Where am I trying to go?"

A client in a technology industry had long been successful by having the best products. They had invested in a product development capability that was world-class. They continued an unparalleled record of new product introductions, layering on new features at a startling pace. They were the market leader. In a matter of months, however, things began to shift. After years of impressive growth, three quarters in a row were disappointing. They were not getting the same kind of sales lift out of each new product. Something had changed, and they were just not sure what it was.

The client hired Mercer to help them develop a Customer-Driven Growth Strategy. While there were lots of theories within the management team about what was wrong, no one could prove any of their hunches. The internal processes all seemed to be working fine—quality was up, customer satisfaction was high, product development was hitting every milestone. But sales were slipping. The stock market was beginning to notice. The growth stock suddenly had stopped growing.

Setting strategic direction in this new environment requires a fundamentally different approach. You need to have a much more thorough and dynamic understanding of the external environment, and work "outside-in." While most of your effort has been focused on benchmarking competitors, now your focus must shift to the edges of the radar screen, to new and nontraditional competitors who may have more effective business designs than any of the incumbents. Similarly, customer understanding used to be the task of market research—gauging satisfaction, testing new products. Today, customer understanding is a complex task of analyzing the customer's decision-making process and environment. It involves a detailed understanding of decision economics, of trade-offs among factors, and of the effect of changing conditions on future behavior.

The scope of options and strategic implications of this dynamic environment has also exploded. Businesses are considering an increasingly diverse range of strategic moves. New business models—new ways of competing—are sprouting up every day. Our clients face bigger decisions, with bigger stakes, than ever before.

Mercer's case team initially focused on understanding how the external environment had changed. A particularly useful approach was identifying a set of new, very different companies that were growing rapidly. While they looked nothing like our client (they were not on the client's list of competitors), they were succeeding by offering a subset of the product bundle in a dramatically simpler way. These companies were changing the rules. They used different channels and had very different cost structures. And they were winning customers.

The case team then focused on identifying the business models that would be successful in the future. The new competitors were successful today, and they gave us early clues, but to respond to them directly would only put our client further behind the changing market. To anticipate the best moves to make, we worked to understand how customers were using the products. Our analysis focused on detailing the systems economics of the customer.

This changing environment has created a new kind of need for consultants. It has opened a new era of strategy. Strategy, no longer merely an academic question for a company's planning department, has moved to the top of the corporate agenda. Strategy now requires new approaches and new frameworks that allow a senior management team to sort through the flood of information to find the optimal value growth opportunities. The task is complex. That makes this an exciting time to be in the strategy consulting business.

Our analysis identified a series of business design moves for our client to consider. Ranging from adjustments to resource allocation and channel structure in the existing business, to entirely new businesses that anticipated the next wave of market changes, the client had to reinvent the way they did business. The old rules, the foundation of success, were no longer valid. Together with management, we designed an implementation program to begin the process of reinvention.

The change program is ongoing. The rules continue to change. Reinvention is now part of the management process.

It is an incredibly challenging time to be in the strategy consulting business. If all the old rules are no longer valid, consultants can no longer depend on traditional benchmarks and frameworks. We can no longer safely extrapolate the future from the past. Success depends on developing new and innovative ways of looking at dynamic markets and identifying new opportunities to create value. At the same time, the pace of change is accelerating. At Mercer, we have focused on developing and applying innovative frameworks that help our clients interpret the chaos surrounding them.

WHAT KIND OF CONSULTING DO YOU WANT TO DO?

My experience in the strategy consulting business has been extremely rewarding. I am as excited and challenged by the work today as I was when I started with Corporate Decisions, Inc. in 1990 (we merged with Mercer in 1997). Along with the many other attractions of consulting— rapid pace, smart people, learning about a variety of industries and issues—the content of the work has kept me motivated.

As a potential consultant, it is important to recognize the type of work that you like to do, that you are good at, and that will get you out of bed in the morning. Consulting of all types is demanding—clients expect excellence, energy, and a "pull out all the stops" approach. For that reason, you need to get a charge out of what you do. While many factors will determine the firm you want to join, the most important is the type of work they do.

The Customer-Driven Growth Strategy work that I have described is not for everyone. Understanding the external environment is, by definition, a boundless task. You never have "all" the information. Clients often ask you to deal with chaos and to put a structure on that chaos. You have to develop hypotheses and test them with the available information. Your research techniques must be creative. And you have to be willing to adjust your perspectives as you learn more about a situation.

By contrast, internally oriented consulting deals with more self-contained problems. The finiteness of the data leads to a different approach, and the process uses a different type of creativity for trying to find the right answer.

Take the time to understand the content of the work at the companies you are considering. Match that with the way you think, the way you learn. The right match can be incredibly exciting.

• • •

The Generalist Approach to Consulting: The Strategic Value of Breaking Industry Barriers

PAUL SMITH

BAIN & COMPANY

Paul Smith is a director and vice president in the Boston office of Bain & Company. He joined the firm in 1984 and was promoted to vice president in 1990. He specializes in the areas of high technology and telecommunications. In over 12 years of consulting, Mr. Smith has successfully led assignments in several industries, including telecommunications, information processing, high tech, healthcare, and technology. He has assisted clients in developing product technology, customer retention, reengineering, and turnaround strategies. Prior to joining the consulting staff at Bain & Company, Mr. Smith was employed at Burroughs Corporation, where he was primary designer of a new-generation series of mainframe computer hardware and operating systems. He earned an MBA from Harvard Business School with highest honors. Mr. Smith is a graduate of the University of California, where he received a BS in Mathematics and Computer Science with honors. In addition to his consulting activities, Mr. Smith has been actively engaged in the operations of Bain & Company's Boston office, heading the case assignment, evaluation, and compensation processes for Boston's consulting professionals for three years.

When I joined Bain & Company out of Harvard Business School in 1984, I planned to do consulting for a couple years, then get a job at Microsoft or Intel, three or four rungs up the product manager ladder from where I had left the high-tech industry. Born in Australia and raised in South Africa, I earned a degree in mathematics and computer science from UCLA. I moved first to Raytheon and then on to Burroughs to design computers. When Burroughs and Sperry merged to create Unisys, I took that opportunity to go to business school. As an R&D guy, I had very little exposure to the strategic aspect of the business. But I was intrigued by the consulting presentations I saw on campus. I saw that as a fairly junior consultant I could participate in many functional areas across multiple industries and have a lot of input into the most critical issues facing a company. The whole *results* pitch to develop practical strategic solutions that are implementable—which at the time no one else made—sold me on Bain & Company.

Within the context of Bain's generalist approach to consulting in a range of industries and functional areas, my high-tech experience and diverse geographic background have proved to be unexpected resources. I came expecting technology to be useless. But the true value of a well-run generalist firm is the ability to leverage knowledge. So, I find myself applying technology paradigms to nontech industries, and nontech modes of thought to our high-tech clients.

One significant—and unexpectedly positive—contrast with my background was doing something different every three to six months. The computer I designed at Burroughs took three years of my life and still did not come to market until three years after I left. In contrast, during the past 14 years I have worked on probably 100+ engagements: from pricing strategy and redeployment in the banking industry to product line profitability and sales force management in healthcare distribution; from business unit strategy and mergers and acquisitions for a software firm to divestment analysis for the airlines; from purchasing strategy for a conglomerate to turnaround on a major computer manufacturer; and even corporate strategy in women's undergarments.

A GENERALIST APPROACH TO FUNDAMENTAL STRATEGIC ISSUES

The generalist approach to strategy consulting is unusual in an industry of heavy specialization. Strategy consultants focus on issues that are of fundamental strategic importance to a business, unlike functional or systems consultants, who focus on operational, rather than strategic, issues. For example, if a business has run out of warehouse space and needs assistance in optimizing new warehouse locations or distribution points, a consultant specializing in logistics would be an appropriate choice. Systems or IT consultants would be required if the business has outgrown its current inventory tracking systems and needs a better solution. But if the real issue at stake is how the business should configure its distribution to attain maximum competitive advantage, whether to use direct or indirect distribution, or whether to use a single-tier or a double-tier system, then a strategy consultant is called for. At Bain, we define strategy as the science of allocating scarce resources, and strategy consulting as the art of helping our clients make the right decisions to capture and create value from those resources.

Our greatest "grand slams" in strategic decision making have usually been situations in which we have brought experience across an industry boundary. For example, our teams have taken loyalty work in financial services and applied it to the airlines. Using insights from completely different industries, we showed a major American automobile manufacturer how to think about product configuration and complexity. We constantly break traditional thought processes and work outside the barriers of industry paradigms. Because generalists are always learning, they ask questions that "industry experts" would never ask.

CHALLENGING ORTHODOXIES

Individuals are not expected to spend their careers in any single industry. While this approach may seem harder, our clients benefit immensely from the fresh perspective, and we learn a lot in the process. This insistence on challenging orthodoxies and searching out strategic innovations requires that, as a firm, we leverage knowledge across the board. The real value generalists bring to a company is the experience of making change happen, of working through each case from the very beginning, without relying on preconceived notions about industry norms that would prohibit the genesis of breakthrough ideas.

Off-the-shelf solutions simply do not allow clients to distinguish themselves from their competitors. As generalists, we benefit from being able to start from a strong base of industry knowledge but go beyond the cookie-cutter answers. Instead, we value superior analytic thinking that treats each client as the unique organization that it is. We work from the perspective of the CEO, and unlike industry gurus, we think the way a new general manager thrown into the client's firm would think.

STRATEGIC INSIGHT

The results of drawing on multiindustry experience are impressive. The following case study began with the question: "Why do we want to be in this business?"

The CEO of a $9 billion company came to us and said, "I have a division that is number 5 in this business worldwide, and I'm not even breaking even. I know number 5 businesses never survive. So why shouldn't I sell this thing tomorrow?" The division, at a little over $1 billion, was supposed to be a growth business, but wasn't making money. This CEO, a believer in the Jack Welch philosophy that "if a business is not number 1 or number 2, get out of it," asked us to validate that this business was a dead end and figure out how to exit it.

But our answer surprised the CEO: "Not only do you want to be in this business, but you should also invest in it!" Our work defied conventional wisdom and helped turn the division around to become a star performer in the company's portfolio.

We helped management understand how to target and capture the highest value customers in their market, how to take hundreds of millions of dollars out of the cost structure, gain market share to drive this multibillion dollar industrial products business from number 5 to number 3, and improve returns from −2 percent to 8 percent. The market cap of the parent has gone through the roof, and analysts and the press attribute much of this to the turnaround of the division.

So, what was the strategic insight? For the answer, we drew on our work in other industries, such as high-technology computer and software firms, in which the size and loyalty of the customer base drives the economics. What matters in an installed-base industry is how many people are using a particular product, not how many are sold every year—repeat purchase rates are the critical success factor. Historically, the company had been doing a strong business in North America and Europe, with developing markets in Eastern Europe, South America, and Asia. We decided we needed to understand how customer decisions were made in each of those markets, how pricing was done in each, and what it cost to serve customers across these markets.

By analyzing the customer base, we came up with an insight we often see in our work with clients in the financial services industry. The company would be more profitable if it focused on serving existing customers instead of engaging in dogfights over new customers in emerging markets. Our client was losing its shirt by offering huge discounts to new customers in Kazakhstan and Mexico rather than profitably capturing the next order from existing customers in Europe. It was a straightforward issue of customer retention. As in the insurance and credit card businesses, where customers are only profitable after many years, it was important for our client to understand how to run the business differently in areas where customers were already committed to them. The opportunity we identified for the client was to focus on servicing, follow-on sales, and adding the next set of features to a product, not just chasing new customers. We moved the best salespeople from new to existing accounts, helped change the sales and pricing incentives, and focused the business on where the profits lay.

Crossing not only industry boundaries, but also geographic lines, multioffice Bain teams throughout Asia-Pacific, Russia, Europe, and the Americas worked to customize strategies across the different markets for this client, as we rolled out the new strategy globally with management. For this particular client, the implementation of this strategy was a case in itself.

Within 12 months after our recommendation to stay in the business, the division had achieved 80 percent of its goal of a 10 percent return on sales, while continuing to accelerate its growth and removing hundreds of millions of dollars from the cost structure. Our work drew on our dealings with analogous situations of installed-base management in high-technology companies, retention in financial services clients, global competition in a consumer products client, and, of course, cost reduction in other industrial companies. And the end result was *results*.

REALIZING BUSINESS OBJECTIVES

This is precisely what clients care about: *results*. Success, in our clients' eyes, requires the achievement of tangible results according to specific business criteria that we determine together at the onset of a case. To achieve the goals developed by both the client and our consulting team, we have to maintain a clear and consistent interaction with the client organization at all levels, not just the ear of the CEO or senior management. "Perfect solutions" that cannot be implemented throughout the organization have no value—the end product is simply a hefty report, not true results. If nothing changes, nothing was accomplished.

I was drawn to generalist consulting because I wanted to learn more and get involved in creating new solutions. What I found is that it is all about results—it is the only yardstick at the end of the day that matters. And 14 years later (rather than the two years I expected to stay at Bain), this focus on results still has me captivated.

● ● ●

Selecting a Small versus a Large Firm

ELLEN MCGEENEY
BRAUN CONSULTING

Ellen McGeeney is vice president and co-founder of the eSolutions practice at Braun Consulting, where she co-founded the Communications and Technology practice. She draws on her experience in a variety of industries, including telecommunications, pharmaceuticals, consumer products, apparel, publishing, environmental services, and specialty chemicals. She has addressed problems such as aligning business objectives and strategy amid market turbulence, designing new market entry strategies, designing and managing revenue turnaround, and improving the effectiveness of large sales forces. Ms. McGeeney has also co-authored "Looking Ahead, Looking Out," an article confronting the challenges facing CEOs in the midst of turbulent markets and technology. Prior to joining Braun, Ms. McGeeney worked for Booz·Allen & Hamilton's consumer products practice. Before attending business school, she worked with the states of New York and Connecticut to implement a private-public partnership focused on reducing the welfare rolls. She received her BA with honors from Brown University, and her MBA from the Yale School of Management.

When choosing among myriad opportunities, many prospective consultants look to firm size as a metric to narrow the field. After all, large firms provide a stable opportunity, brand recognition, formal training, and access to a worldwide organization, whereas small firms offer collegial atmosphere, good growth opportunities, and less politics and bureaucracy. Right?

Well, not exactly. Although firm size can impact the work experience, not all important differences among firms are predictably correlated with size. In fact, the size of the firm is a relatively good indicator of only two attributes: brand recognition and your ability to have an impact on the firm. Small firms typically cannot offer the same blue-chip aura as the largest firms, but the brand-conscious should beware of the "brand value trap." Brand name alone will not do much beyond opening the front door, and the richness of your consulting experiences will count for more than the name on your resume.

If leaving your imprint is important to you, you should know that, while your impact is likely to be greater at a small firm, there is no guarantee. Entrepreneurial pockets can exist within large firms seeking fresh ideas and leaders to steer future direction. And, although small firms typically move more quickly and seek out those with entrepreneurial energy, they can lack the leadership or processes to channel that energy effectively.

Beyond brand recognition and your impact within the firm, size does interact with other characteristics to create the firm of your dreams or nightmares. When evaluating which firm to choose, you should explore four essential topics: the firm's growth trajectory, the project work, the people, and the culture.

GROWTH: GROWTH IS GOOD

Whether the firm you are considering is small or large, you must understand its growth trajectory to assess the opportunity. Senior consultants should be able to consistently and clearly articulate a compelling strategy for growth, and cite evidence to support the firm's progress toward achieving its growth goals. The firm's growth rate affects the risk profile of the opportunity, your career trajectory, and the balance between an exciting versus a stressful challenge.

People often look to firm size as a way to minimize risk and maximize reward, assuming that the stable option exists within the large firm. Just like any other high growth, competitive, and innovation-driven industry, however, consulting can be turbulent. Both large and small firms face layoff-generating hiccups in the revenue stream, and growth projections can be tough to meet at any firm, regardless of size. Adding to this risk, large firms can be plagued by greater political intrigues, leading to uncertainty for those whose careers are tied to specific partners. In comparison, a small firm with a strong growth strategy may provide greater upside potential for financial and personal reward.

The bottom line is slow growth can be a rate-limiting factor for your career. No matter how good you are, if the firm is not growing, your promotion track will be slow. This will frustrate you while you are at the firm and will not look good if you seek a job elsewhere. In contrast, too much unmanaged growth can wreak havoc on the worker bees (that means you). High turnover amidst growth is a sure sign of trouble and can quickly shift a challenging career into stressful overdrive.

PROJECTS: A PASSION FOR THE WORK INEVITABLY BREEDS SUCCESS

Ask most consultants who have remained in the field why they are still there. We love the work. We need to—after all, other careers offer comparable return for less stress and fewer hours. To see whether you will be able to sustain a passion for consulting, you must answer four questions about the work: (1) What mix of industries and client problems is the firm's practice based on? (2) At what level in the organization does the firm typically work? (3) At which stage in the problem-solving process does the firm do its work? (4) How are consultants assigned to projects?

Most candidates emphasize the firm's industry focus (e.g., healthcare, financial services) over the mix of client problems addressed (e.g., merger and acquisition strategy, reengineering, sales-force design and strategy). Industry focus should drive your decision if consulting is a transition to specializing in a particular industry. Otherwise, being exposed to a variety of client problems is far more interesting and valuable than ensuring that each case is in a new industry. Be wary of being pegged as operations-focused, for example, if you want to do strategy work.

The second factor to investigate is the level in the organization at which the firm typically works. Engagements that operate below the level of CEO or senior VPs who head major functional areas tend to attract minimal client interest, receive inadequate client commitment, and, as a result, can have limited impact. Problems that are frankly of minor importance to the client are far less interesting to work on, and may challenge and teach you less than you expect.

The third question, the stage of problem solving the firm focuses on, often determines several important aspects of the work: how much client interaction you have, how much number crunching you do, how much impact you are able to see, and the intellectual challenge you face. Most firms focus either on the strategy development or on the implementation phase of problem solving. And most prospective consultants I have spoken to are initially enamored with strategy work. However, CEOs increasingly value strategies that *work* over the big idea that they know will require a struggle for their organization to implement. In addition, it can be frustrating to repeatedly work hard on strategies that end up as reports, collecting dust on the CEO's bookshelf. What is more, pure strategy cases often involve lots of lonely analysis, with only the most senior members of the team having significant client interaction. Unless you enjoy computers more than people, you may want to ensure that your work will combine some measure of implementation with the strategy.

The final question you should investigate is how project staffing decisions are made. In theory, small firm size limits the variety of projects available to you, but in many firms, large and small, you quickly become tied to specific partners, and your project options are limited to the work they sell. Thus, the process of assigning projects is more important than firm size: find out whether the firm uses the "free market" or the "central clearinghouse" system. The free market system requires you to be proactive to ensure that you are in the running for the project you want. How effectively you market your skills can make or break your career. In contrast, the central clearinghouse system usually employs a full-time staffing coordinator whose job is to make sure that individuals' needs and interests are balanced with client and firm requirements in the staffing process. Most firms use a combination of the two approaches, but it is useful to understand which method dominates and which best suits your professional demeanor.

PEOPLE: THEY HAD BETTER PASS THE "AIRPORT TEST"

You will want to like and respect the people with whom you will be spending the majority of your time. Meet as many consultants as possible and give them the "airport test": if you got stuck in an airport with this person for five hours (it happens!), would you enjoy his or her company? Try to get a feel for whether or not your potential coworkers are happy with and challenged by their work.

In addition, look around for possible role models and ask people at different levels about the degree of interaction they have with partners or other senior mentors. Smaller firms may offer a more intimate and informal environment for building mentor relationships with senior partners, but larger firms can offer a bigger pool of mentors. In particular, if you are a woman or a minority member, check into how many others have made it to the top. If there are only a few, you may want to consider how great your desire is for blazing new trails. No matter who you are, make special note of those who have been successful. If you relate better to the people at the bottom than to those at the top, this may not bode well for your long-term prospects at the firm.

CULTURE: IT IS THE SUM OF ALL THE LITTLE THINGS

Here lies a frequently neglected aspect of candidates' decisions. People do not know how to evaluate culture, so they avoid the topic. But, as you will soon learn in your new consulting job, all things *can* be measured. Look for evidence of the culture you are seeking. It matters.

For example, if being in a learning organization is important to you, find out about both formal and informal training. Again, size is not a great indicator of the learning organization. Investigate how the firm manages and shares knowledge. How much publishing and speaking do people do? Are promotions and bonuses influenced by contributions to the firm's intellectual capital? How strong is the mentoring program? Which partners are most admired—the smart ones or the rainmakers?

If you are concerned at all about lifestyle, try to garner insight into whether face time or efficiency is more highly valued. At Vertex, we track hours closely, talk to individuals who are working too many hours to understand why, and pressure case managers to stick to time budgets. Another good lifestyle indicator is the firm's philosophy toward the professionals' time. Does the firm see consultants as a fixed cost investment with 24 hours of capacity that should be used however necessary to get the job done? Or, are consultants viewed as having a variable cost component that shows up in increased turnover and reduced quality? A firm's culture is the sum of many small things that add up to an environment that can foster your strengths or produce endless frustration. You ignore it at your peril.

CONCLUSION

Size matters far less than other characteristics of the firm. Although size can affect your work experience, you should not rely too heavily on it as the metric for the qualities you seek. You need to scratch beneath the surface to understand the opportunity the firm is offering. You have invested a tremendous amount of time and money into your education, so be equally thoughtful about your career decision.

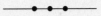

The Internal Consulting Practice of Strategic Planning

CATHERINE ARNOLD
SANFORD C. BERNSTEIN

Catherine Arnold is a senior research analyst and vice president of Sanford C. Bernstein, a unit of Alliance Capital Management LP. She provides institutional investors with equity research regarding the large cap European Pharmaceuticals Sector. Prior to joining Sanford C. Bernstein, Ms. Arnold spent four years at Hoffmann-La Roche Inc., a multinational pharmaceutical company, primarily in the Business Development and Strategic Planning Group. Preceding this, she was a management consultant for six years working for Booz·Allen & Hamilton and Ernst & Young. Ms. Arnold also worked as a registered nurse and holds a Master of Business Administration, Master of Health Administration, and Bachelor of Science, all from the University of Pittsburgh.

You may be surprised to learn that careers in consulting and strategic planning do not differ that much, particularly in terms of work content. Instead, the differences lie with the culture, lifestyle, variability, and predictability of the job issues. In fact, strategic planning can be thought of as a segment within the consulting profession.

CORPORATE STRATEGIC PLANNERS VERSUS EXTERNAL CONSULTANTS

Corporate strategic planners are a department or group of company employees responsible for ensuring that an organization's strategy is established, and that a plan to implement the strategy is executed. The strategy is usually developed through the interactions of strategic planners with the management team—the "client." Once the strategy is defined, strategic planners must see that it is effectively communicated throughout the organization. This communication is essential for promoting the client's use of the strategy in making decisions. If the client consistently considers the defined strategy when making short-, medium-, and long-term decisions, the strategy is more likely to be achieved.

Strategic planners know the organizational strategy intimately because of their role in developing it and supporting its execution. For this reason, they may also have responsibilities that require its intensive consideration, including corporate, business, or new business development.

Strategic planners are often viewed as internal company consultants because (like external consultants, but unlike most management personnel) they make recommendations, but typically do not have responsibility for implementing the tactics driven by those recommendations. The work of strategic planners is project-driven, and uses processes similar to those used by external consultants.

Recommendations made by both strategic planners and external consultants are typically a result of analyzing internal and external data. Given confidentiality concerns, strategic planners may have greater access to internal data than external consultants do; however, external consultants may access larger amounts of external industry data—partly to compensate for their lack of internal data. And finally, strategic planners tend to incorporate more of an organization's cultural and organizational context into an analysis than external consultants do.

THE PURPOSE OF STRATEGIC PLANNING GROUPS

Organizations—or parts of organizations—can conduct project work by "hiring" internal strategic planners, external consultants, or a combination of internal and external resources. Since all three options are viable, a company must decide which approach is most valuable. Most companies maintain an internal group, whose size and skills are determined by objectives defined by senior management. The organizational objectives for these internal groups are driven by:

- The dynamics and complexity of the business in which the company competes.

- The cultural preference for using internal versus external resources.

- The scope of responsibility of senior managers and other employees.

- The staffing philosophy regarding fixed and variable resources.

Regardless of the industry, business demands produce needs that can most easily be met by strategic planners. If management requires analysis and recommendations on specific business issues, their strategic planners can provide this analysis. Using internal resources over external consultants provides access to resources without going through a proposal process. Additionally, recommendations for highly confidential matters can be kept within the organization by using strategic planners.

The name "strategic planners" suggests that a primary objective of the group is to establish direction or strategies for the organization. The time period for these strategies may be short, medium, or long, depending on the company's needs. The company's organizational culture usually determines whether the process for developing strategies involves all levels of the organization or only top management.

Because strategies may involve new ideas or imperatives, these groups often have the responsibility for motivating change or paradigm shifts throughout the company. This may also be required in developing the strategy. Strategic planners are expected to motivate other employees to think "outside the box" to develop creative strategies, including "stretch goals" that enable the organization to seek a higher level of performance. Stretch goals will need to be adopted in the areas of an organization that will be held accountable for those goals. Strategic planners may find themselves operating as champions of these goals or other strategic ideas and directives to ensure their success.

Strategic planners are often given projects that require either a solution or a set of possible solutions. These solutions require "think tank" processes, whereby recommendations are supported by sound business data and cutting edge analysis. Intellectual capital tools may be developed to support this and other responsibilities of strategic planners, such as the analysis of relevant strategic business information. Table 4.1 shows typical organizational objectives for a strategic planning group.

Table 4.1
Typical Organizational Objectives for Creating
an Internal Strategic Planning Group

Strategic Planning Objectives	Descriptions
Make recommendations	Advise senior management of recommended next steps resulting from detailed analyses.
Establish direction	Facilitate the development of long-, medium-, and/or short-term strategies through the collection and synthesis of organizational ideas based on a competitive assessment. This is accomplished using one of three interactive approaches: top-down, bottom-up, hybrid.
Motivate change and/or paradigm shifts	Stimulate and/or propose provocative and possibly controversial business ideas or analyses that encourage managers to think of nonconventional strategies and/or tactics. Motivate others to implement organizational change through education and presentation of business concepts and strategy.
Analyze relevant strategic business information	Evaluate business situations and data for use by senior management.
"Champion" Ideas and/or "spread the word"	Encourage or convince relevant groups within the organization to adopt and integrate strategic direction and/or business ideas into their area of responsibility.
Provide intellectual capital for confidential and other business decisions	Create and maintain data sources and analyses to support senior management's knowledge and decision making, typically for a restricted pool of managers and for the most sensitive business decisions (e.g., mergers and acquisitions, etc.)
Serve as a "think tank"	Develop cutting-edge analyses and positions to resolve business issues and to support longer-term strategic planning.

97

PROFESSIONAL AND PERSONAL CHALLENGES

The challenges faced by strategic planning groups are similar across different organizations, since these groups usually report to senior management, who, regardless of the industry, make comparable types of decisions (see Table 4.2). Individuals seeking employment in this environment will be expected to maintain a broad or "big picture" perspective, and a current understanding of organizational and business issues. Although strategic planners are expected to be more objective in developing organizational recommendations because they are hired by top management and line functions, they are expected to customize their work product to consider the culture and characteristics of the company.

Strategic planning groups must adopt a credible work style to gain clients' confidence. As would be expected of an external consultant, strategic planners should consistently display creativity and superior analytical skills in their project work. Many of these projects may also demand the support of various levels of the organization. Strategic planners should define situations that require the input and buy-in of other employees and secure it.

To obtain support, strategic planners must deliver analyses and recommendations in a concise and meaningful manner. They must effectively communicate their conclusions or recommendations, especially when their ideas are to be delivered throughout a large part of the organization. Strategic planners may have to determine which processes best meet the needs of the specific situation, particularly when they are held accountable for the execution of their plans.

While strategic planners and external consultants have similar professional challenges, the personal challenges they face tend to differ, most importantly with respect to lifestyle, variability in the client, project work, and career pathways. As for lifestyle, strategic planners tend to travel less frequently and more predictably than do external consultants. This may be an important consideration if personal commitments demand less travel and more advance notice. Because strategic planners remain in one organization rather than changing clients, they

Table 4.2
Professional Challenges of Strategic Planners

Challenges	Description
Maintain a broad perspective	Consider the organizational impact in all recommendations even if the specific project if fairly compartmentalized.
Remain current	Keep in touch with organizational and business issues and incorporate this knowledge into the output of the group.
Customize work product	Develop recommendations and analyses that consider the culture the characteristics of the organization.
Maintain objectivity	Assess the strengths, weaknesses, opportunities, and threats of the company within the competitive environment without bias.
Demonstrate creativity	Consider and offer novel ideas in all deliverables.
Display analytical competence	Ensure the use of cutting-edge analytical (financial, strategic, and marketing) approaches and industry knowledge.
Rally support	Determine the need for input and buy-in from various levels within the organization, the secure it.
	Define, then satisfy, the organizational expectations for problem-solving and decision-making processes, including the required supporting data and analysis.
Present findings in a concise and meaningful manner	Develop communication vehicles (e.g., presentations, reports, and talking points) that relay only points of interest and relevancy, and maximize the audience's understanding.
Ensure plans are executed	Assure recommendations are implemented through the appropriate assignment of responsibility and the use of optimal processes.
Establish an effective means to communicate to the organization	Define and utilize processes to ensure the communication of strategy and other findings/recommendations developed by the group and approved by senior management.
Earn credibility	Exhibit a work style and provide deliverables that result in an organizational confidence enabling the group to meet its defined objectives.

tend to identify organizational issues and develop a foundation of knowledge about the company's product line (strengths and weaknesses) that they can continually use in project work. External consultants must climb the learning curve for each of these dimensions for each new client.

Depending on the strategic planning group's scope of responsibility, the projects they work on may be fairly consistent with regard to the issues they address. Lastly, corporate culture may allow for more flexibility in defining future job paths than would be available in a consulting firm. A strategic planner may choose between climbing the corporate ladder or remaining on a technical track. Planners can also move to another function within the corporation. In contrast, many consulting firms have an "up or out culture," meaning that you must continue to be promoted within the firm or be counseled out.

REQUIRED SKILLS

People interested in working as strategic planners must have certain skills for meeting both the challenges described in Table 4.2 and the project demands. Strong project management and interpersonal skills are a must. Because these projects are directed by top management, work plans must be completed on time and to specifications. Strategic Planning Managers must be able to collect and provide information throughout all levels of the organization using verbal and nonverbal communication techniques. To assure the most effective outcome, they must also feel comfortable challenging conventional thinking up through the highest level of management.

In addition to project management and interpersonal skills, well-rounded functional skills are needed. Almost all the business disciplines are used to some degree—finance, marketing, and strategy most frequently. The ability to exercise leadership supports the motivation of others toward project goals. Management experience lends an appreciation for the complexities involved in selecting and defending a recommendation among many alternatives. Finally, experience within the industry in which the organization competes is likely to increase an individual's opportunity to contribute quickly to the goals of a strategic planning group.

The rewards and challenges of a career as a strategic planner and an external consultant are similar, yet the intricacies of the job can differ significantly. You should contemplate these similarities and differences as you consider a job as a strategic planner, or as a management consultant.

● ● ●

Change Management Consulting

ARUN MAIRA
ARTHUR D. LITTLE

Arun Maira joined Arthur D. Little in 1989. He is leader of the Global Organization Practice and Managing Director of Innovation Associates Inc., an Arthur D. Little, Inc., subsidiary. Innovation Associates, co-founded by Dr. Peter Senge, author of *The Fifth Discipline: The Art and Practice of the Learning Organization* (New York: Doubleday, 1990), is the premier consulting company in the field of organizational learning. For over 30 years, Mr. Maira's work has focused on organization design and acceleration of change in large companies. He has worked as an executive at the board level of companies, and as a consultant to companies in many parts of the world and in many industries. This varied experience has given him practical insights into how to make change happen in large organizations. He is coauthor of a book, *The Accelerating Organization: Embracing the Human Face of Change*, (New York: McGraw-Hill, 1997). He has also written frequently for management journals and spoken at seminars for senior executives all over the world. Arun Maira who was born in India in 1943 holds an MS degree in physics.

Change management is one of the most important, and one of the least understood, services provided by management consultancies. Almost everything that a consultant does for a client, whether creating a new strategy or reengineering a process, requires the client's organization to make some kind of change. I will illustrate what change management encompasses with two case studies.

REACTIVE CHANGE

"Why does change have to take so long?" This question came from a chief executive of a successful company in North America that was faced with new, low-cost competition from international companies. He had sought help in improving his organization's production and distribution capabilities, and he had heard presentations by eight consulting companies. The consultants all agreed that trying to introduce new ways of working would inevitably meet with resistance to change. They said the culture of the company would have to be changed—a complex, time-consuming process.

They had all exhorted him, as chief executive, to take responsibility for bringing about this culture change and to be patient with the process. He responded to this suggestion:

> I am willing to give the process whatever time it takes, but I am afraid the world may not give my company the time you say the process needs. I want sustainable change—so that we do not have to keep turning to consultants to help solve our operating problems. And we need the change to happen fast. What is it about the approach to the process of transformational change that makes it take so long? Why can't we think about it as a process and improve it? After all, by thinking about our product creation activities as a process, we have been able to reduce the time required from several years to a few months. So, what are the essential activities in a transformation process, and in what order and combinations should they be done? Where is the real leverage in the process?

A multifunctional team from Arthur D. Little helped this chief executive and his organization answer these questions. We worked with our client on the business challenge of improving operating performance and changing the culture. At the same time, we examined the change models of all the leading academics and consultants and delved into the experience of our own firm with clients all over the world. Together with our client, we developed new thinking, and we customized approaches for their organization. They achieved what they needed: faster change than they had imagined and sustainable change. They have used their new knowledge about creating faster change to improve the performance of several companies they have acquired around the world. And they are taking the battle back to the home grounds of their competitors and are becoming a successful global company.

ANTICIPATORY CHANGE

On the other side of the world, the chief executive of a high-performing Asian company sensed that the world around his company and his country was changing in fundamental ways. These changes required rethinking his company's business model and competencies. The company needed to be much more innovative—in its strategies and in its product and service offerings. At the same time, it had to maintain, and perhaps even improve, its operational efficiencies. There was no immediate threat, but the company wanted to be able to change quickly to avoid being blindsided or caught flat-footed as the environment around it changed.

So how could the company be more innovative and more efficient at the same time? And how could it be even more responsive to local customer needs while being more global in its perspectives? This chief executive asked:

> What are the organizational competencies we need to manage these paradoxes of innovation-and-efficiency, local-and-global, change-and-stability? And how will we develop these competencies quickly and cost-effectively?

He had already heard from several consultancies and concluded:

> The advice of all consultancies, after all the arm-waving, always seems to boil down to choosing one thing or the other, rather than having both. Their industry experts have their views about where the

industry is heading. And their process of strategy-making is about choosing a particular path, for which the organization is then designed. But what if the environment changes and we have to change our path? What we need is a new model of organizing which gives us more flexibility while improving our current performance.

A multifunctional team of consultants from Arthur D. Little, as well as from Innovation Associates (the "Learning Organization" consultancy, which is now part of Arthur D. Little), worked with the client's organization on this issue. We looked for new principles for organizing businesses that would be more flexible and innovative and better tuned to their environment. We turned to the fields of complexity and biological evolution. And we examined business organizations around the world that have displayed, at some time in their histories, the qualities we were looking for. The client organization learned in action. They acquired the ideas, customized them, implemented them, observed results, and amended the solutions as required. They are becoming the innovative-cum-efficient, faster-learning organization they set out to be. Their multiple stakeholders have responded positively to the changes in the organization. Business analysts have talked up the stock price of the company. Market share is increasing. Employees at all levels are participating in the management of the paradoxes.

NEED FOR CONTINUING INNOVATION

These two cases illustrate the two principal, interrelated thrusts of Arthur D. Little's Global Organization Practice: change management and organizational transformation. Our practice has been greatly enriched by the merger with Innovation Associates, which brought us valuable knowledge and consulting skills around issues of leadership development, systemic thinking, and team learning. These competencies are, invariably, key leverage points for change management and organizational transformation.

These three competencies, as well as the broader capabilities for change management and organizational transformation in our

Organization Practice, are often combined with other functional strengths of Arthur D. Little. Thus, we can help clients effectively manage more focused business needs. For example, with our Strategy Practice, we can help clients to develop "ambition driven" strategies and to manage mergers and alliances. With the resources of our Technology Management and Information Management Practices, we can help clients improve their innovation and knowledge management processes. Our Practices are centers of excellence, which combine their competencies to address our clients' important business issues.

Our collective mission is to increase our clients' capabilities to produce results they have not produced before. To do this, we must continuously innovate, combining the world of ideas and the world of action. Our clients expect us to have our heads in the clouds and our feet on the ground. It is a challenge: sometimes we may appear too theoretical to the client, and sometimes we may seem like just an extra (and expensive) pair of hands. But when we get it right (which we generally do—or so our clients say) not only do we add great value to our clients, but we also learn and acquire new capabilities.

CONCLUSION

I came to consulting with Arthur D. Little after a satisfying career as an executive with a large operating company, where I had successfully solved many strategy, organization, and operations problems. To paraphrase Robert Frost, a few years ago, I came to a fork in the road, and took the road "less traveled by." As a consultant, I now work with clients in many industries and in many parts of the world, helping them create the new knowledge and competencies they need and want. Not only do I get to take action with my clients, but I also have the satisfaction of seeing the results emerge. As a consultant, I am at the intersection between the world of ideas and the world of action, the space in which real innovation takes place. It is a place for great challenge and great satisfaction.

———•••———

Information Technology Consulting

RUDY PURYEAR
ACCENTURE

Rudy Puryear is the global managing partner for electronic commerce and information technology strategy at Accenture. Based in Chicago, Mr. Puryear joined Accenture as a partner in 1991. He has over 25 years of experience in information technology, and has spent more than 20 years consulting to major organizations regarding IT strategy and planning. He routinely leads consulting assignments for large, complex multinational organizations addressing strategic technology issues. He frequently advises senior executives on critical IT issues and their relationship to business strategy. He is one of the firm's leading experts on electronic commerce and the implications of operating in the evolving electronic economy. His clients come from a broad cross-section of industries worldwide, and he regularly speaks before business audiences around the world. Prior to joining Accenture, Mr. Puryear was the managing director for Nolan, Norton & Co., an IT Strategy consulting firm. He did his graduate and undergraduate work in computer science at North Carolina State University.

As a strategy consultant who has surveyed the business landscape for a number of years, I have seen the power of information technology (IT) increase exponentially, and the role of IT in setting business strategy change dramatically. As a result, strategic IT consulting is now playing a critical role in helping organizations maximize their performance and stake a claim in the emerging electronic economy, or e-economy.

THE CHANGING ROLE OF INFORMATION TECHNOLOGY

Information technology has become a critical business enabler that is at the heart of every form of business consulting today. But to fully understand and appreciate the importance of IT today, we need to look back at its evolution.

Over the past 30 years, as the global marketplace has shifted from an industrial economy to an e-economy, IT has evolved through three fairly distinct periods: data processing, information systems, and knowledge management. Throughout each period, the role that IT has played in helping organizations develop and execute business strategy has changed, too.

In the 1970s, data processing automated business tasks, streamlined operations, and made things more efficient. Mainframe computing provided useful data for transactions, but the technology and the IT consultants of that day generally sat in the back room. Their role was primarily to track and report on the business, and provide business managers with the information they needed to execute against an existing strategy. Their job was not to identify strategy, and therefore IT was not a critical element in business strategy in the 1970s.

In the 1980s, sophisticated information systems provided user-friendly software applications, and hardware advancements gave the business environment efficient facsimile machines, desktop computers, modems, cell phones, broadband cable, fiber optics, satellite communication channels, and wide and local area networks. All this enhanced our homes and workplaces because it gave us the power to do things faster and with more geographic reach. In the workplace, technology evolved from simply reporting on business to actively conducting business. As a result, business began to rely more heavily on IT, and became more mindful of it.

The primary goal of the IT consultant at this time was to transform data into useful market information that could be strategically capitalized on. This information and the IT that supported it still did not drive strategy, but it became a critical tool for implementing strategy, and as a result IT became more respected for its overall contribution to the business.

During the 1980s, the challenges associated with using new and unproven technologies, platforms, and communications protocols created barriers that often impeded rapid strategy implementation and restricted strategic options. I remember one telecommunications client in particular that was trying to launch a new service. They needed the service and the associated billing systems to be ready at the same time, but because their product development cycle was 90 days long and their systems development cycle was two years, they had to hold back. That kind of scenario was fairly common in those days, and it placed a strain on the relationship between technology and strategy. Consequentially, the business strategists of the 1980s respected the potential of IT, but they were frustrated by the time and effort required for solution implementation.

In the 1990s, the focus shifted from business information to market knowledge. Laptops, high-speed modems, and desktop processors can now manage data and information at speeds unimagined by the mainframe programmers of the 1970s. In just 30 years, we have seen over a 50-millionfold increase in the price-performance of technology. Had the same productivity been applied to the automotive industry, you would have been able to purchase a Rolls Royce for under 10 cents today.

With the performance and implementation challenges of the 1970s and 1980s behind us, businesses are now able to turn IT loose on the challenges of complex, rapidly changing global markets. In these markets, knowledge is power. Specifically, managing the intellectual assets of the organization to turn market information (today's trends) into market knowledge (knowing your customers and suppliers so well you can drive tomorrow's trends) has become a key strategic weapon.

A CRITICAL DRIVER OF STRATEGY

Today, as we prepare to enter the twenty-first century, IT finally has the capability to create business strategy, not just support it. For example, a major auto manufacturer recently asked our consulting practice to study the effectiveness of their IT. Years ago, this request would likely have resulted in a detailed functional review that would have uncovered processing inefficiencies and cost overruns. But once executive management recognized that IT was a key business enabler and not just a tool to support their operations, the project quickly became an opportunity to envision how IT could help reshape their business. The results were exciting. We helped the client totally redefine their customer relationships and make the transition from being a mass-marketing organization to becoming a relationship-marketing organization. We did this by helping them focus on their customers as individuals. We used technology—such as new data mining techniques, and technologies that allow business to be conducted independent of time and location—to make it easy for the customer to do business with the company instead of the other way around. The impacts were dramatic.

Bottom line, it is no longer enough for companies to use IT simply to support business strategy. More and more, they must embrace IT as the means to create business change throughout all levels of their organizations. Today's successful enterprises use IT to enlighten their strategy process and determine their tactics. They rely on IT strategy to drive and enable successful business strategy and its implementation. They also realize that IT must be considered during, rather than after, the strategy formulation process.

CHANGING THE PRACTICE OF CONSULTING

IT strategy consultants are on the cutting edge. Now that IT has become so tightly interwoven with business strategy, individuals who truly respect and understand the power and potential of technology have become extremely valuable business strategists. Today, my colleagues in IT practices around the world work at the boardroom level with the most exciting and aggressive companies, assisting them in their quest to become market leaders in the new e-economy. We are defining and implementing meaningful and distinctive Internet strategies; we are designing revolutionary technology-enabled delivery models that allow business to be conducted independent of time and location; and we are helping clients discover new methods of differentiation through creative deployment of technology. These are exciting times.

Working every day at the crossroads of information technology and strategy, IT strategists possess the essential knowledge and skills to lead the changes demanded by today's complex marketplace. From our vantage point, we anticipate and monitor technology innovations that shape market trends and redefine entire industries. We understand the vital role IT has in setting business trends. And, most importantly, we help our clients anticipate and manage for these trends.

IT strategy consulting is a rewarding path to long-term success and satisfaction in a volatile business world. If you can bring to bear a strategic perspective on IT as a business enabler, you will have the opportunity to create real change and value. Moreover, if you became a consultant because you wanted to make things happen, you should most definitely consider a career in IT strategy consulting.

● ● ●

The Evolving Role of Health Benefits Consulting

BRUCE KELLEY
WATSON WYATT WORLDWIDE

Bruce Kelley is a senior consultant with Watson Wyatt Worldwide. He has more than 20 years of experience in the areas of health promotion, disease prevention, self-care, information-based benefits decision support, and managed healthcare. He has presented at many conferences, published extensively, and is frequently quoted in the professional and popular press. Previously, Dr. Kelley was a Principal and National Practice Leader for Health Management in William M. Mercer, Director of Client Services for the Central Region with the MEDSTAT Group in Ann Arbor, MI and Vice President of Analytical Services with Health Risk Management (HRM) in Minneapolis, MN. Dr. Kelley's undergraduate degree was a BS with a major in Economics and a minor in Human Resources Planning. He earned MS and PhD degrees in Preventive Medicine from the College of Medicine at Ohio State University.

The benefits industry has changed rapidly over the past few decades and, as a result, so has benefits consulting. New regulations, more complex plans, and increased technological capabilities are just a few of the factors affecting the way employee benefits are administered today. But, even though the emphasis and the means of performing tasks have changed, employers must still help their employees face the same contingencies—retirement, savings, medical expenses, and death and disability. And now, more than ever, to help attract and retain employees, companies must provide competitive but affordable benefits. The benefits consulting industry has evolved to help companies meet these basic objectives and prepare for the future.

A BRIEF HISTORY OF BENEFITS CONSULTING

When the first major benefits consulting firms were founded in the 1930s and 1940s, all were rooted in the insurance industry, either through actuarial work or the sale of insurance products. Without the numerous laws and regulations that burden the industry today, life in the benefits consulting business in the post-World War II era was much simpler and proved to be a time of slow, steady growth. Benefit and contribution calculations required the work of actuaries and administrators, and the consulting profession was more than happy to help supply the expertise.

The state of the industry became more complex with the passage of the Employee Retirement Income Security Act (ERISA) in 1974, which ushered in an era of legislative activity in benefits. Over a dozen major pieces of legislation were issued during this time, including the Tax Equity and Fiscal Responsibility Act, the Deficit Reduction Act and the Retirement Equity Act. Because employers needed help in complying with these new regulations, consulting firms were hard-pressed just keeping up with the increased demand. By the late 1970s, more than half of all business conducted by the major consulting firms related to defined benefit plans. The rest of the consulting business comprised thrift plan and profit-sharing work, executive compensation, health and welfare plan design, and some human resources functions.

HEALTH BENEFITS CONSULTING

Health benefits consulting has been driven—and is even more driven today—by employers' need to recruit and retain employees and to motivate them to higher levels of performance. At any point in time, the primary focus of health benefits consulting is influenced by the national economy and the economics of employers and health plans. When the economy is strong and the labor market is tight, plan sponsors tend to enhance health benefits. Periods of health benefits enhancement are followed by excessive escalation of the cost of health benefits. The focus of health benefits consulting then shifts to benefit cost management. These periodic shifts in the focus of health benefits tend to follow shifts in the business cycle, normally a six- to eight-year cycle, and the underwriting cycle, which, until 1990, was a six-year cycle.

The current health benefits consulting cycle began about 1990 with the beginning of the business cycle that continues today. At that time, businesses began to trim inventories, seek favorable financing of debt, shed obsolete assets, and lay off nonproductive workers. By 1992, healthcare benefit costs had flattened for most plan sponsors. This was attributable mainly to the growing penetration of managed healthcare, which began with the prior cycle's focus on cost management. And it may also have been attributable to the fact that management did not offer—and workers did not demand—many health benefits enhancements during a time characterized by labor force reductions.

Wages have been rising since 1993. Unemployment has declined to levels below what economists define as full employment. Yet, inflation in the general economy has remained low; corporate revenue continues to increase; and profits remain strong. It has become obvious that increases in productivity are the engine driving the current stage of the business cycle. These factors drive the current health benefits consulting cycle, which will probably continue for at least several years.

Many health plan administrators and provider organizations are beginning to increase premiums and prices again. However, this may not immediately provoke employers and other plan sponsors to focus vigorously on cost management. Senior and operations managers appear to be pressuring human resource managers to focus more on contributing to the business goals of their firms. Thus, it appears that human resources and, therefore, health benefits consulting will attempt to influence both the cost and the contribution of labor, which will translate to improved productivity of labor.

COST OF LABOR

The cost of health benefits plays a role in the cost of labor. However, in most industries, health benefit costs comprise less than 20 percent of the cost of labor. Other factors have a much more direct and significant impact. There are early signs that management of these factors will become more central to human resource management and, therefore, to health benefits consulting.

In a tight labor market, the costs of recruiting and of not retaining productive employees are substantial. Employers will likely examine how health benefits can contribute to recruitment and retention. They may respond sympathetically to the concerns of employees—and of providers and legislators—about managed healthcare. Thus, employers may ask consultants to help them remove some of the limitations on access and significant contribution or out-of-pocket expense differentials associated with managed care. As a result, employers may accept greater increases in health benefit expenses to achieve reductions in the cost of recruiting and retaining employees.

To offset employees' negative perception of managed care portions of the health benefits package, employers may also seek (relatively) low-cost benefit enhancements that employees perceive to have high value. These enhancements may take the form of nurse advice line services, health promotion programs, disease management services, coverage of alternative medicine, and so on. Employers may ask consultants to identify and develop a business case for such services.

CONTRIBUTION OF LABOR

Continuing to increase the contribution of labor may become even more important to employers. By raising morale or creating a sense of greater security, health benefits may have an indirect effect on employees' productivity. However, health benefits can affect whether employees are present at work. Health benefits consultants may be called on to help workers maintain their health and slow the progression of disease. They may also help workers avoid taking time off from work for unnecessary visits—their own or their dependents'—to medical professionals. In these areas, consultants can either help clients directly or work with their health plans to: cover preventive medical procedures cost-effectively; take a risk management (instead of an entitlement) approach to health promotion programs; provide self-care/nurse advice line services; implement disease management programs; and put in place integrated disability management programs.

CONCLUSION

As the benefits industry changes, so do the needs of employer and the role of benefits consultants. Health benefits consulting now encompasses much more than matchmaking between clients and vendors and supporting clients in plan administration. It also includes helping clients manage benefits while keeping an eye on the bottom line. Health benefits consulting is part of a broader approach to human resource consulting.

Health benefits consulting is changing because human resource management is changing. More and more, senior and operations managers are directing corporate benefits managers to make benefits contribute directly to productivity, profitability, and other fundamental business goals of firms.

In the future, employers may hire benefits consultants primarily to learn how to use benefits as tools that encourage employees to perform at higher levels. Employers will more likely want to focus on how benefits can fulfill employees' fundamental needs for security and quality of life, which will motivate them to achieve higher levels of productivity.

● ● ●

Consulting to the Nonprofit Sector

LAURA FREEBAIRN-SMITH
GOOD WORK ASSOCIATES

Laura Freebairn-Smith is a partner at Good Work Associates, a consulting firm that specializes in the three areas of strategic planning, team development, and diversity development. Its primary mission is to help people understand and overcome obstacles to group effectiveness. After receiving her BA in Philosophy and Political Science from the University of California at Berkeley, Ms. Freebairn-Smith moved to Asia. She spent four years on the Thai-Cambodian border serving as the Education Coordinator for the International Rescue Committee in Khao-I-Dang. This work sparked her interest in how organizations operate and how people within an organization work together. Ms. Freebairn-Smith earned her Master's in Public and Private Management (MPPM) from Yale School of Management in 1986. During the past 12 years, she was Chief Operating Officer for Jobs for the Future and Managing Director of the Gesell Institute of Human Development. She is an instructor at Yale University, and has taught at Central Connecticut State University and the University of New Haven. She also speaks at numerous workshops and seminars.

To effectively help nonprofit organizations, we, as consultants, must have a strong understanding of the nonprofit sector and its typical organizational structures. We need to convince our nonprofit clients that we have strong functional and industry expertise. And we also have to prove that we understand the organizational behaviors arising out of the three economic sectors: private, pubic, and nonprofit. Since organizations tend to experience similar issues regardless of sector, the solution to a nonprofit's problem may be similar to those for the private or public sectors. As a result, we can ask the same question of any of the three sectors: How does being a nonprofit—or a for-profit, or a public—organization either affect or create the issues our client faces? Although this question applies to all three sectors, the context within which we ask it leads to very different answers.

THE THREE SECTORS OF THE U.S. ECONOMY

Each sector has its own distinct relationship among owners, customers, decision makers, and other constituents. The nonprofit sector fills a critical market niche by providing services and products for subsets of the population—services and products that are not provided by the other two sectors. Nonprofits fill the gap between market-driven and publicly provided goods, as Figure 4.1 shows.

As a culture, we are willing to pay taxes for certain goods—protection, clean air, education—products that we believe all people

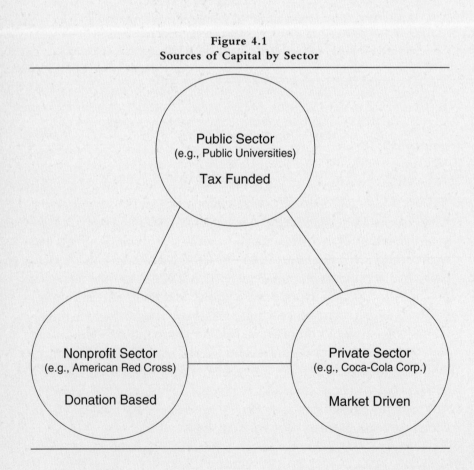

Figure 4.1
Sources of Capital by Sector

should have and from which no one should profit. These are publicly provided goods. The private sector, on the other hand, provides goods that we all believe are profit-driven. Coca-Cola, for example, is not essential to a functional society (although the students in my early morning classes might disagree).

The nonprofit sector provides goods and services of two primary types. First are those that we, as a society, believe no individual organization should profit from, and only a subset of the population believes are important to society's well-being. It would be considered morally inappropriate, for instance, to profit from providing housing for the homeless or food for the hungry.

Second, the nonprofit sector provides goods and services that we feel the public sector is often not suited to provide. The bureaucracy of the public sector can inhibit its ability to respond to crises, except through public organizations specifically designed for that purpose, such as the military, police and fire departments, and emergency medical teams. For example, the Red Cross manages the national blood supply. We do not feel that the public sector is capable of managing this type of operation since the technical knowledge required to run a blood bank is not the same as the knowledge required to be a good soldier or fire fighter. We look to the nonprofit sector to provide specialized skills or services to fill just such gaps between the public and private sectors. Table 4.3 summarizes the key differentiating characteristics of each sector.

THE NONDISTRIBUTION CONSTRAINT OF THE NONPROFIT SECTOR

The nonprofit sector involves three parties: the donor, the organization, and the recipient of the service or goods. That is, this sector is funded by donors, who pay for an organization to deliver a product to needy recipients.

Unlike the private sector customers, the customer of a nonprofit may never have a financial transaction with the organization; the donor provides the funds that are transformed by the organization into

Table 4.3
Key Characteristics of the Three Economic Sectors

Sector	Goods and/or Services	Owners	Customers	Source of Funds	Customer's Recourse	Key Decision Makers	Managers
Private	Market-driven goods (e.g., Coca-Cola houses)	Shareholders	Purchaser of good or service	Customer purchase; borrowing; equity of-ferings	Stop purchasing item	Board and top managers	Hired managers
Public	Public wel-fare goods (e.g., clean air, public education policing)	Unclear (Taxpayers? Voters? Citizens?)	Unclear (All citizens? Voters? Taxpayers? Users of the service?)	Taxes, fees, bonds	Withhold votes; lobby; run for office	Legislators	Government employees
Nonprofit	Gray mar-ket goods (e.g., some cancer re-search)	None; quasi-"owners" are members of the board of directors	User of good or service	Donations, grants, borrowing, fees (not commonly paid by users)	Limited; stop using good or service	Board of directors and execu-tive director	Hired man-agers and executive director

goods or services for the "customer," without accruing a profit for the effort. Thus, nonprofits are subject to the "nondistribution constraint."

The nondistribution constraint provides the psychological trust donors need when giving money. The blood bank, the soup kitchen, and the homeless shelter are all examples of organizations that must not accrue a profit or, more accurately, must not distribute profit to any one individual or group. For example, the donor believes that when she gives her $1,000 to CARE (a worldwide agency working to eliminate hunger), most of the money will be used for the "consumer" or client, with some portion of the donation going to operating or fund-raising expenses. She believes that no single person or group will reap personal wealth from her donation. Without this psychological contract, which is encoded in law, the nonprofit sector could not exist.

The nondistribution constraint, and the donors' trust it generates, is the primary differentiator of how nonprofits operate. Still, some 80 percent of the organizational issues occurring in nonprofit organizations are the same as in the private sector: teams still start, stop, succeed, and fail for many of the same reasons. And strategies are conceived and carried out for many of the same reasons.

The remaining 20 percent of the organizational issues are unique to the nonprofit sector because the nondistribution constraint drives nonprofits to pursue a mission—not a bottom line, as in the private sector. Nonprofits do not pursue missions such as "the best customer service in the world," or, "the largest bank in the universe." Rather, nonprofits must strive for missions that serve either the nonmonetary purposes of a group of people or the higher good of humankind.

A CAREER IN CONSULTING TO NONPROFITS

What does this mean for a career in consulting to nonprofits? Primarily this: A "nonprofit" consulting focus works only to a certain extent—one also needs to acquire both industry (e.g., healthcare, transportation, education) and functional (e.g., human resources, marketing, finance) expertise. All too often, nonprofits are lumped together, and consultants assume they can provide services to any nonprofit. This may work for certain functional issues, but a consulting practice focused on nonprofits must be enhanced by elements other than a generic "nonprofit expertise." For example, a few areas of expertise are particular to consulting to nonprofits: developing a board of directors, managing endowments, and fund-raising. The following discussion is an example of one we frequently have with applicants:

> A young, recent MBA graduate is sitting across from me at my desk. He eagerly asserts, "I want to be a consultant."
>
> I look at him with curiosity, "Why?"
>
> After a very brief pause, he responds, "I like to work on a variety of projects and I do not mind working long hours," having practiced his response in many interviews.
>
> "Well, that tells me *how* you like to do your work, but it still does not answer why consulting? And why Good Work Associates?" I ask.
>
> Earnestly, he replies, "I really care about the nonprofit sector—I want to help make the world a better place."

When we encounter such unbridled and idealistic enthusiasm, we are certainly pleased by the candidate's good intentions. But we are also concerned that the candidate has not seriously thought through his consulting interests. All candidates, before interviewing, should recognize three characteristics that are essential to success as a consultant, and determine the degree to which they possess each:

1. Consultants do not simply "want to be consultants." Consulting is the means to an end, a path to achieving some larger vision.

2. Good consultants not only have a passion for a topic or field, but they also have a strong liberal arts curiosity. Are you broadly trained? Are you fascinated by Plato, sundials, and the Aztecs? Do you write well? Are you reading *Harvard Business Review* as well as E. Annie Proulx's latest novel? Successful consultants can distill and integrate ideas from the past and from around the world and use those ideas for creative problem solving.

3. Consultants should have a sense of their path of personal development; they should seek to improve both themselves and the working world. And we believe consultants should aspire to balance the "three legs of life"—work, family, community—throughout the three concurrent phases of life—learning, earning, and returning.

Many of our young applicants see consulting as a way to make a lot of money or to build their resume. We believe that both goals are ultimately disappointing to everyone involved—the firm, the employee, and more importantly, our clients. We hope that our staff will see consulting as a means to several ends—an improved society, a meaningful career, and better workplaces for our clients.

───● ● ●───

Consulting to Government and Nonprofit Organizations

BRIAN MURROW

PRICEWATERHOUSECOOPERS

Brian Murrow leads the PricewaterhouseCoopers e-philanthropy practice. This practice works with nonprofits, dot-coms, and large multi-national organizations to develop and implement Internet strategies, create customized Web-based applications, and encourage and foster inter- and intra-sector collaboration of Web-based tools and standards. For its clients, PwC's e-philanthropy practice has created online volunteer listing and management systems, Internet donation and corporate intranet pledge systems, and online auction and commerce applications. A sample of Brian's e-philanthropy clients include America's Promise, The Alliance for Youth, CreateHope.org, an online giving portal for organizations' employees, MissionFish.com, an online auction that benefits nonprofits, and SERVEnet.org, a volunteer listing and management Web site.

In addition to the area of e-philanthropy, Brian has experience in the design and implementation of large-scale Web sites, Web-based applications, financial management systems, customer relationship management systems, and large-scale statistical, econometric forecasting, and marketing models. Brian's clients have included large multinational corporations, housing finance agencies, federal and state government agencies, and start-up businesses. In addition to consulting to clients, Brian managed a $150 million private investment portfolio. He regularly speaks at industry conferences on e-business and e-philanthropy, regularly publishes and is quoted on e-business, and appears on business-oriented television programming. Brian serves on various boards of foundations and nonprofits.

A career with PricewaterhouseCoopers (PwC) has given me the opportunity to work with a wide-range of organizations through a rich variety of consulting engagements. These experiences have included designing and implementing large-scale decision support systems for a secondary mortgage market lender, building and operating performance measurement systems for a large worldwide logistics organization, building corporate Internet and intranet Web sites, and building custom financial systems. In more recent projects over the past few years, I have transferred the knowledge and lessons learned from these experiences to the nonprofit and government sectors, by helping clients reach strategic goals more efficiently and effectively using advanced, Web-based technologies. When consulting to government and nonprofit sector clients, I often draw from my private sector consulting experience.

Similar to the broad-based skills required for private sector consulting, management consultants working for the nonprofit and government sectors need to bring an equally diverse skill set. Government and nonprofit organizations increasingly expect their consultants to transfer private sector skills and knowledge to their organizations, especially in today's fast-paced technology environment. The private sector continues to advance its strategic goals at a blinding pace. By applying this knowledge to nonprofit and government communities, through best practices and lessons learned, consultants will be able to help nonprofit and government organizations meet their strategic goals in the most effective and efficient ways possible.

To give you a flavor of the consulting work I perform, I will highlight two of the many challenges that are fundamental to public and nonprofit sector consulting, and draw illustrations from my prior client engagements.

CHALLENGE 1: BALANCING GOVERNMENT POLICY OBJECTIVES WITH FINANCIAL RESPONSIBILITIES

In the private sector, success is typically measured in profits. Activities that lead to increasing current or estimated future profits are considered prudent investments. However, in the public or government sector, there is an additional—and significant—element that must be considered in the decision-making process: public sector organizations must balance financial responsibilities with overall policy objectives. A public sector organization must ensure that the execution of its program meets specified policy objectives, in addition to being fiscally prudent. Even routine administrative functions, such as personnel employment or supply procurement, are often performed in a manner that supports policy objectives.

For example, when I was consulting with a large federal government agency in the telecommunications industry, I worked on a project team that was engaged to reengineer an acquisition process. Since our client was a public sector organization, we had to adopt a decision-making process that was different from that used for private sector clients. In the private sector, the decision-making process aims to minimize the total cost of acquisition to result in the "best value" for the products and services acquired. "Best value" refers to the minimization of the price of the product or service to achieve the desired quality. However, in the public sector, the decision-making process must take into account the overall policy objectives of the agency, in addition to the objective of realizing the "best value."

My client wanted to reengineer its procurement process to assist small and disadvantaged businesses. Our objective as consultants was to design a procurement process that allowed the government agency to achieve its policy objectives, while also ensuring that the government continued to procure "best value" goods. This added a considerable amount of complexity to our task, especially since the economies of scale in the telecommunications industry often resulted in the lowest prices coming from the larger vendors. But what appeared to be an insurmountable economic hurdle ended up holding the key to our recommended solution: large and small vendors would be required to work together to provide competitive pricing, and a significant portion of business would be directed to small and disadvantaged organizations as subcontractors to the larger businesses.

In other engagements, I worked with state and federal mortgage insurance organizations. Again, I found that balancing policy objectives with financial responsibilities was a vital aspect of the decision-making process. Mortgage insurance, as you may already know, insures the borrower's mortgage payment to the lender. The presence of mortgage insurance results in lower interest rates, thereby lowering the monthly payment to the borrower. Mortgage insurance is typically required on low down payment loans, including both single-family home loans and the loans for owners of multifamily apartment buildings. There are many federal and state programs that subsidize these insurance programs to keep mortgage insurance premiums low, and to make housing more affordable for low- and moderate-income families.

Government-sponsored insurance programs need to continually balance responsible financial decision making with the interests of the citizens they serve. For example, government-sponsored insurance programs may want to lower mortgage insurance premiums to reduce the financial burden on homeowners and help achieve the policy objective of making housing more affordable. But such a move would reduce the reserve funds that are held to cover payments to lenders in the event that borrowers default on mortgage payments. Facing a similar problem, my team at PwC and I created financial simulation models for a mortgage insurance client that maximized the policy objective of increasing home ownership while minimizing the financial risk to the government in the event of an economic downturn. The client utilized our recommendations in restructuring a large federal housing insurance program, and our recommendations have remained virtually intact for over 10 years. As you can see, one of the perks in government sector consulting—where public policy is balanced with principles of good management—is the knowledge that your recommendations have helped put more Americans in homes, or supported the welfare of small disadvantaged business owners.

CHALLENGE 2: USING WEB-BASED TECHNOLOGY TO FURTHER A NONPROFIT ORGANIZATION'S CAUSE

An emerging area in consulting to the nonprofit sector, and the area in which I have recently devoted significant time, is called e-philanthropy. I broadly define e-philanthropy as, "Internet-based activities and tools that help to intermediate the market more efficiently between the resources nonprofits *need* and the resources individuals and businesses *have* to fulfill this need." There are a number of effective e-philanthropy tools that supply the nonprofit industry with the resources they need to achieve their missions more effectively. I have worked with clients over the past few years to design and build these tools, which include: online volunteer listing and management tools, corporate employee-giving intranet tools, cause-related portals, on-line charity malls and affiliate programs, online charity auctions, and online fund-raising tools.

In one engagement, a national nonprofit organization needed a so-lution to make its volunteer recruitment and management processes more efficient. Nonprofits generally need volunteers to help imple-ment their charitable programs, such as building houses, mentoring at-risk youth, or staffing soup kitchens. But the time it takes for volunteers to sign up or prepare for an activity can reduce productivity and be extremely costly to nonprofit organizations. Web-based technology can significantly reduce administrative time through process au-tomation and simplification.

To illustrate, let's suppose a large multinational manufacturing or-ganization, employing over 400,000 people, allows each employee to take 16 hours of paid time off to volunteer for community service. A Web-based volunteer search and coordination tool could shave at least five minutes off of the time it took for each volunteer to find and prepare for every two-hour volunteer activity. This type of Web-based solution would result in over 260,000 additional hours per year to ded-icate to community service, benefiting both the sponsoring multina-tional manufacturing organization and the community.

For a national nonprofit client seeking a means of reducing re-cruiting expenses, we designed and developed a Web-based tool to in-crease the efficiency of signing-up, training, and deploying volunteers. We created a system that was easy to find and simple to navigate, thereby empowering volunteers to self-select and self-register for al-ternative volunteer opportunities over the Internet. Detailed informa-tion on each opportunity was available to help volunteers prepare for their selected activities. To help the nonprofit better manage its vol-unteers, we built tools that tracked the activities each volunteer per-formed over time. And to help businesses that were interested in supporting employee volunteer programs, we made sure the solution contained tools that enabled employers to track employee volunteer activities.

Another client engaged PwC to build a workplace donation application that would enable businesses to run paperless fund-raising campaigns through corporate intranets. Workplace pledging, which enables an employee to make a donation to the nonprofit of his or her choice through payroll deduction, has traditionally been a manual process. To help nonprofits and businesses improve the efficiency of their workplace pledge campaigns, we designed and developed a Web-based solution that not only automated the process, but also offered resources to educate donors about participating nonprofit organizations.

CONCLUSION

As a consultant at PwC, I apply private-sector experiences and tools to my work in the government and nonprofit sectors. Over the past decade, the federal government and national nonprofit organizations have made significant progress in increasing their operational efficiency and in achieving their policy objectives. Being involved in this progress as a consultant is an extremely satisfying experience, especially when you can watch your own recommendations further policy and organizational objectives. Over the next 10 years, the government and nonprofit sectors will continue to advance their deployment of Web-based technologies and further increase their effectiveness. Such Web-based technologies include e-learning, e-procurement, and delivering services through online interfaces. As the government and nonprofit sectors continue to adopt this technology, the demand for public sector consultants will continue to increase, and the opportunity to have a positive impact on the public sector will likewise grow.

● ● ●

Consulting in the World of Electronic Commerce

JOSEPH B. FULLER
MONITOR COMPANY

Joseph B. Fuller is a founder and CEO of Monitor Company. He joined Monitor at its inception and currently oversees its consulting operations globally. During his tenure at Monitor, Mr. Fuller has worked with clients in a wide variety of industries. His particular interest is in industries undergoing structural transition. This has led him to work in a wide variety of industries over the past 20 years, including life sciences and a number of high-technology industries. He is an internationally recognized expert on telecommunications and has advised some of that industry's leading companies.

Mr. Fuller has contributed extensively to Monitor's conceptual work. In recent years, he has focused his attention on the interaction of market forces and companies' decision-making processes, helping to create Monitor's Organizational Strategy practice. His interest in research began during his collaboration with Professor Michael Porter of Harvard Business School on the development of the concepts presented in Porter's book, *Competitive Advantage*. He has also authored articles for the *Harvard Business Review, CEO,* and *Across the Board* magazines.

Mr. Fuller is a *magna cum laude* graduate of Harvard College, where he was a Charles Warren Fellow. He is a graduate of the Harvard Business School, where he was an honors student. He currently serves as a director of the Phillips-Van Heusen Corporation, Merrimac Industries, and eMergent Information Technologies.

Strategy consulting offers the best career option I know for pioneers and explorers, for people who like to operate on the frontier, for people who want an early look over the horizon at the big new issues facing global industry. A perfect case in point is the growing surge of interest in Electronic Commerce (e-commerce)—that emerging arena of economic activity defined by the convergence of telecom, computer, communications, software, hardware, and other information-related businesses. By any relevant standard, this process of convergence is a major development in the business world, confronting managers with seminal choices about where, how, and over what to compete.

For consultants on such a frontier, the challenge, of course, is to learn how to get quickly beyond the hype to a robust understanding of the real choices managers face. Make no mistake, there is plenty of hype to get beyond. You probably recognize the rhetoric:

> Something important—something major—is happening. From whatever angle you look, it represents a paradigm shift in the world of business. And given the magnitude of this shift, the whole apparatus of established ideas, analytical frameworks, and consulting approaches is suddenly obsolete. Sweep it all into the trash. Here—and here only— is the one true road to competitive success in so brave a new world.

This is, of course, nonsense. The old rules and the old logic may no longer blindly apply to businesses engaged in e-commerce, but that does not mean they do not apply at all. The task is to determine on a case-by-case basis how far to push the rules and where they are most likely to need amendment or qualification.

MIGRATION TO AN ELECTRONIC ENVIRONMENT

For some companies migrating to e-commerce, the process of transition is pretty much a question of using the Internet to reshape and reconfigure assets and processes that already exist for an electronic environment. If a PC manufacturer originally sold directly to end users through catalogs, advertisements, and a toll-free telephone number, for example, how should it supplement those efforts with, or migrate them to, a Web-based system for online sales? Or how might a pharmaceutical firm allow a potential customer to research—in private—basic information about drugs for a socially embarrassing condition such as incontinence, before talking about it with his or her doctor?

For other companies, the main question has to do with selecting features and prices for products designed to support electronic commerce: software for ordering over the Web, for example, or databases for recording Web-based purchases or prestructured information about potential customers to better target marketing initiatives.

For still others, the new technology enables a more thorough redefinition of key parts of the underlying business model. Consumers who used to purchase books and recordings only if they happened to be immediately available at a local bookstore or music store can now access a much wider inventory of titles through Web sites like Amazon.com, and CDNow. What are the likely economic effects of such changes? Do they provide a plausible foundation for building competitive advantage? Or for building a sustainable advantage?

All these examples are linked by a common theme: moving into the world of e-commerce forces companies to make strategic choices about their primary mode of participation. Should they be a provider of content, or of the interface between Web and consumer, or of the means for product distribution? Or, finally, a provider of some combination of distribution, interface, and content? True, the specific business content of these choices, as well as the context in which they sit, may be novel, but the need to make such choices is a familiar part of what managers do when addressing basic issues of strategy.

EROSION OF INDUSTRY BOUNDARIES

At the same time, however, our work on questions related to e-commerce regularly leads us onto new theoretical ground. As the boundaries between previously distinct industries become ever more permeable, the range of expertise needed to frame effective choices, let alone implement them, expands geometrically. And as the intensity and complexity of competition heighten, it becomes increasingly difficult to act as if a one-dimensional relationship exists between our clients and other companies operating in the same general industry space—or to act as if the classical laws of economics have remained unchanged.

Because a single company might simultaneously be a competitor, a complementor, a partner, an informal collaborator, a supplier, a distributor, a licensee, a licensor, and/or a customer of our client, we have to bring to our industry analyses an understanding of the mechanics of what my friends professors Barry Nalebuff and Adam Brandenburger call, "co-opetition." Moreover, because such multidimensional, fluid industry settings are best thought of as interdependent ecosystems— and not as traditional competitive environments populated by independent entities—we must be sensitive to the ways in which the various participants in an industry co-evolve. Further, because the ecosystem of e-commerce is being shaped by the convergence of leading-edge technologies, we cannot assume that, other things being equal, a participant's economic returns will tend toward equilibrium. We must be alert to the possibility of what Professor Brian Arthur calls "lock-in" effects: an economics of increasing, not decreasing, returns, where early movers can lock in sources of advantage—new technical standards, for example—that become more valuable as well as more defensible over time.

ENRICHMENT OF STRATEGIC ANALYSIS

Equally important, the new ground associated with work in the e-commerce domain also extends and enriches the practical, hands-on analyses associated with strategy consulting. Of the many possible examples, I will briefly mention five. First, given both the speed with which e-commerce-related markets develop and the degree of uncertainty associated with those developments, we have found it extremely important to help managers carefully frame the questions they ask. Quite often, they express concern about selecting the best set of features for a new product or service when they really should be asking—at that stage of the market's evolution—whether they should be in it at all. And if they should not be in it at the moment, the next question is how they might best reserve the option to participate later.

Second, given the capabilities inherent in e-commerce-related technologies, it is now reasonable for companies to review the pockets of "trapped value" in their industries. The purpose is to see if those capabilities might provide a cost-effective means for unlocking the traps and capturing the hidden value. As a rule, value gets trapped when extant modes of communication and coordination lock clusters of economic activity into inefficient structures and processes. Think, for example, of the huge amounts of money spent on business travel or document delivery services or the processing of paper-based transactions that could be freed up through better application of network and information technologies. Or of the proliferation of safety stock in a multitiered distribution system.

Third, as the economics of e-commerce businesses become more transparent and as comparative information about their products and services becomes more widely available, consumers will expect access to the best prices and deals. They will also begin to demand control of, as well as economic value in return for, information about themselves generated as part of Net-based transactions. The availability of information is starting to outrun traditional efforts to segment markets, to calculate the cost to serve each segment, and to decide both how and among whom the value generated by economic activity gets divided. How, then, should segmentation be approached in an information-rich environment? And which segments should a company aspire to serve?

Fourth, given how quickly things are moving—a doubling of Web pages every nine months, for example, or the coming explosion in transmission capacity through wave division multiplexing in long-haul transmission and broadband wireless for local connectivity—the state of the Net-based art changes faster than the adoption and decision cycles of most companies. How, then, should they choose in their business planning whether to aim at the current state of the art or out ahead of the target—and, if the latter, out ahead by how much?

And fifth, because the Net-related choices that companies make can significantly affect their relative competitive position over the long term, on what basis should they decide whether to make a large, upfront bet about the future (like Dell, say, in computers, or Fruit of the Loom with its new online ordering system), or buy "insurance" against the destabilizing effects of new technology (like Compaq making on-the-Web ordering available in response to Dell's success), or wait for things to become clearer?

CONCLUSION

Our work in these areas leads us to wrestle with a host of other recurring problems, including the innovation of performance metrics for companies engaged in e-commerce, the selection of infrastructure optimally suited to support them, and the design of policies and procedures to promote the development of effective leadership. We have found absolutely no merit in the common assertion that patterns of industry evolution and technological change in the rest of the economy have no light to shed on the world of e-commerce. Our challenge, then, is to understand what lessons do apply, how they need to be amended or qualified, and what new lessons need to be added.

———— • • • ————

Digital Consulting

GLENN CORNETT
RAZORFISH

Glenn Cornett has had an illustrious career in consulting, working with some of the top firms in the world. Most recently Dr. Cornett served as vice president, Strategy, Europe for Razorfish. He had responsibility for strategy work in North America and Asia, and contributes to general-strategy work in Europe as well.

Prior to joining Razorfish, Dr. Cornett worked as a strategic consultant at McKinsey & Company and in strategy, business development, marketing and sales positions at Eli Lilly. He has worked as a policy analyst and scientific consultant at Los Alamos National Laboratory. He was also president and founder of Metastrat, a company that helped explore, structure, and negotiate Internet-related strategic deals.

Dr. Cornett holds an MD with Distinction in Research from the University of Michigan and a PhD in neuroscience from the Brain Research Institute at UCLA. He has a BA with University Honors in chemistry from Brigham Young University. He also did a brief postdoctoral fellowship in artificial intelligence and health at a joint Harvard/MIT laboratory.

Digital consulting companies are known by many different terms: digital consultants, Web consultants, e-business consultants, digital-solutions providers, and so forth. The proliferation of these terms is perhaps itself an indicator of the evolving and turbulent nature of this segment. The services each company provides is a function both of reputation and capability, but tends to involve a mixture of strategy, design and creative services, technology, and project and delivery management. I focus on the strategic services provided by firms in this segment.

By late February 2001, the past 12 months had not been easy for a number of digital consulting companies: Scient, Viant, Sapient, Razorfish, Proxicom, marchFirst, and their same-space competitors. Currently, the clients that are typical to these firms (Fortune 2000 companies and their international equivalents) no longer have a sense of urgency about fending off new "Internet pure-play" entrants such as Amazon.com. The economy has slowed down, resulting in tighter consulting budgets. As a result, business development, once largely a function of deciding which telephone calls to return so that contracts could be negotiated quickly, now frequently involves lengthy discussions in highly competitive bid situations. The sales cycle has lengthened, and cash flow issues are now critical at some of the digital consultancies. Most of these companies (if they have made it through IPO) have seen their market capitalization fall roughly 80 percent to 95 percent; several have laid off roughly 30 percent of their employees. The economy in general—and this segment in particular—is widely expected to get worse before it gets better. Indeed, the digital-consulting sector may have seen significant consolidation by the time you read this.

WHY CONSIDER DIGITAL CONSULTING NOW?

With all of the current challenges in this segment, what rational basis would anyone have for joining a Web consultancy at this time? There are actually several reasons to enter this sector, particularly for those looking at strategy roles:

1. *Relevance, scarcity, and value.* Despite the arrogance, hyperbole, and naivete that have characterized the excesses of the digital boom, the economic basis for digital business remains strong. With all of the displacement from the dot-com shake-out, and the parallel disappointments with digital initiatives at more established companies, clear strategic thinking is becoming more, not less, relevant in the digital realm. In particular, the following abilities will continue to be both scarce and valuable:

   - Scan rigorously yet efficiently across a broad array of digital opportunities.
   - Focus on the most-promising opportunities.
   - Produce robust, quantitative arguments for selecting and pursuing opportunities.
   - Work with clients to provide actionable, effective implementation plans.

   Clients increasingly need "hard" numbers to back up their proposals to pursue digital initiatives. Those able to drive rigorously and credibly to such numbers, and develop action plans to achieve them, should be able to gain the trust, appreciation, and repeat business of clients.

2. *Growth opportunities.* Arguably, many digital consulting firms have swung from being overvalued to being undervalued. For talented people with high-risk tolerance, joining a digital consultancy offers the possibility of significant growth (both personal and corporate), accompanied by an attractive financial upside.

3. *Preparation for a better business climate.* Severe tightening of venture capital and other private funding has hampered much of the start-up environment. Public funding for new digital companies is also tenuous at this time. An increasing number of talented, entrepreneurial people are finding the digital consulting arena an attractive venue for:

- Riding out the current economic storm.

- Bolstering their digital/business experience so that they are well prepared for senior or founding roles at start-ups when the economic climate improves.

This is already happening at senior levels; many of the better senior strategists at digital consulting firms have experience at top-tier strategy consulting firms (e.g., BCG, McKinsey), followed by technology start-up experience.

4. *Preparation for senior roles.* Just as the traditional strategy consulting firms have provided excellent preparation for senior roles at traditional business firms (e.g., the Fortune 500), the digital consulting firms should provide excellent preparation for senior roles at digitally oriented companies.

5. *Alternative to traditional strategy consultancies.* The tightening economy can be expected to result in at least a flattening if not a decrease in hiring activity at the traditional consulting firms, thereby making positions more competitive at the top firms. Decreased access to venture capital and a more-difficult stock market in general has reduced the number of people entering start-ups, creating significantly more competition for positions at the most-desirable strategy consulting firms. The digital consulting firms are therefore likely to be an attractive alternative to those who have difficulty entering a traditional strategy consulting firm. Additionally, the lifestyle at most digital consulting firms tends to be less demanding ("brutal" is frequently the preferred term) than that of traditional strategy consultancies.

CHOOSING A DIGITAL CONSULTING FIRM

At the risk of stating the obvious: Company soundness, cultural fit, and your intended personal career path should all factor into your process of selecting a digital consultancy. A higher level decision could be between joining a digital consultancy, or one of the older consultancies such as the IT firms (e.g., the former "Big 5," EDS), or a traditional strategy firm (e.g., BCG, McKinsey). Those tolerant of, or more pointedly driven toward, the iconoclastic, counterconformist, risk-tolerant cultures of some of the digital consultancies might not have a positive experience in some of the older consulting firms. On the other hand, there are significant cultural differences among the older consultancies. Many of the older consultancies might have smaller groups or "islands" in which "digital nonconformists" are quite comfortable and successful.

Let's look at each of these factors in making a choice:

1. *Company soundness.* There are many who expect that several digital consultancies will either merge or go out of business altogether over the next year or so. I will avoid the temptation to predict winners and losers here, but will be happy to point at some relevant indicators. While the rational-markets hypothesis has proven amusing (if not downright laughable) to some over the past two years, use of market valuation as an indicator of future viability does have merits. Doing yourself what equity analysts do (e.g., assess company financial statements, leadership, business pipelines, reputation, quality of employees, other drivers of success) could be a useful exercise. Perhaps most importantly, getting a reliable source inside or close to the companies under consideration should provide critical information such as morale, momentum, and talent pool. For instance, I recently advised a highly talented friend to avoid a particular digital consultancy neither on the basis of its pipeline nor its recent financial performance, but rather because much of its critical talent pool had been trickling away for several months.

2. *Cultural fit.* There are distinct cultural variations among the different digital consultancies. Culture should be examined both in terms of organizational personality and individual personalities. These two are not necessarily the same, particularly in rapidly evolving companies and industries. Tensions between

the two can be healthy, and even drive the development of a company; on the other hand, they can also be disastrous.

- *Organizational personality.* Some companies have earned a reputation for being quite similar to the former "Big 5" in their predictable (some would therefore say "less innovative, less fun," while others would say "more reliable, more-consistently valuable") approach to planning and executing work. At the other end of the spectrum, some are known for being so fun and innovative that they might not survive 2001 as a stand-alone, ongoing concern. Assessing trade-offs between thirst for innovation and tolerance of risk is important here.

- *Individual personalities.* Superimposed on organizational personality (and not necessarily mapping with a high correlation against it) are the personalities of the individual employees—some open and friendly, some arrogant, some stodgy. Arguably, some of the major problems experienced by digital consultancies have been the result of being innovative, open-minded organizations with dour, arrogant, and/or stodgy personalities.

3. *Personal career path.* Allow me to share a personal experience: I interviewed with a half-dozen digital consulting firms before taking this position. I found the organizational personality (stated philosophy; objectives of senior people) of one of the firms to be consistent with my risk-tolerance profile and career goals. It also helped that the salary range discussed was highly attractive. After a few discussions with search consultants (i.e., headhunters) and three or so interviews with senior people at the firm, I was told that I could have an official offer in about 10 minutes if I wanted one. I was thrilled, but asked if I might meet a couple more of their people before accepting an offer. They agreed, and flew me to a couple other cities, where I met slightly less senior people at various airports. By the end of the circuit, it was evident to me (and I think to some of them) that I would find a better fit elsewhere. Following through on that impression has proven fortunate.

SECURING A POSITION AT A DIGITAL CONSULTANCY

The flip side of choosing a company is getting them to choose you. In general, consulting firms look for (1) problem-solving skills, (2) influencing and interpersonal capability, and (3) cultural fit. Other sections of this book should help you with those issues. Please note that many firms (digital and otherwise) consider their culture to be their most valuable asset. In particular, some digital consultancies pride themselves on their nonconformist tradition; if you do not find a particular company's stance attractive in this regard, there are probably other digital firms where you will have a better experience. Prior to your interviews, try to get pointers on a company's culture (and determine how you would interact with it) from informal contacts (e.g., via your school's alumni network). Of course, you can use the same opportunity to get pointers on influencing styles, and on successful case question/problem-solving responses. By tapping into your network of contacts, and drawing on available resources like this book, you should have the tools you will need to evaluate firms, practice your interviewing skills, and influence your choice firms to select you as a new hire.

● ● ●

Consulting and Venture Capital

ANDREW L. BUSSER
JEFFREY S. EDELMAN
WILKERSON PARTNERS LLC

Andrew L. Busser is a principal at Wilkerson Partners. He has spent his entire career in the healthcare industry, most recently as a consultant at IBM Healthcare Consulting/The Wilkerson Group (TWG), a leading global healthcare consulting firm. At TWG Mr. Busser worked with major biotechnology and e-health companies, and specialized in developing new business models to take advantage of emerging technologies in the healthcare industry.

Prior to TWG, Mr. Busser was with IBM's Healthcare Industry Solutions Unit, leading a global business development strategy with technology partners focused on the pharmaceutical industry. Before joining IBM, Mr. Busser spent nearly five years at the DuPont Merck Pharmaceutical Co. in sales and marketing management, where he focused on the cardiovascular and neurology markets. Additionally at DuPont, Mr. Busser was a business leader for several information technology efforts directed toward increasing sales force effectiveness and sales force automation. He received a BA in History in 1991 from Colgate University, where he currently serves on the Alumni Board of Directors.

Jeffrey S. Edelman is a principal at Wilkerson Partners. He joined the firm in February 2001 bringing a unique background of healthcare experience as an operating executive, management consultant, and investment banker. Most recently, he was director of corporate strategy at SelfCare where he refined the long-term growth strategy for the company, worked with the senior management team to raise $105 million of venture capital funding, and negotiated more than $100 million of strategic alliances with leading online and offline companies. SelfCare was acquired by Gaiam (Nasdaq: GAIA) in January 2001.

Prior to joining SelfCare, Mr. Edelman was a senior consultant with L.E.K. Consulting, where he served as a core member of both the Healthcare and Internet practice groups. Among other assignments, he evaluated the healthcare investment portfolio of a leading commercial bank, prioritized the strategic partnering plan and clinical development program for a gene therapy company, and served as a ghostwriter of equity analyst research for a boutique investment bank. Prior to joining L.E.K., Mr. Edelman was a consultant with McKinsey & Company, and an investment banker in the healthcare group at Alex, Brown & Sons. Mr. Edelman is also a founder of and advisor to an Atlanta-based distributor of biological materials.

Mr. Edelman received a BA in Economics with high honors from Dartmouth College in 1992, where he was awarded the Lewis H. Haney Prize for his honors thesis on reverse LBOs. In 1996 he received an MBA in Healthcare and Strategic Management from The Wharton School of the University of Pennsylvania, where he was awarded a Kaiser Foundation Scholarship.

There is an established relationship between the consulting and venture capital industries, typically with venture capital firms being clients of the consultants. Venture capital firms rely on consulting

firms and independent consultants to help them make better decisions, understand their challenges and opportunities, and ultimately
to make more money. In this section of the book, we discuss relationships between consultants and venture capitalists, the value consultants bring to venture capital, and how and why some people make a
career progression from consulting to venture capital.

CONSULTING AND VENTURE CAPITAL: A BRIEF OVERVIEW

We examine the relationship between consultants and venture capitalists from the perspective of a consultant. Thus, we examine venture
capitalists as clients, and the first thing we want to know about any
client is: What do they do, and how do they make money?

Venture capitalists are in business to invest in and help build emerging growth companies. They make money only when their investments
in these companies become liquid, typically through sale of common
stock in the public markets (through an IPO) or through sale to another company. To provide a framework for understanding different
types of venture capitalists, we begin by breaking the industry into
four stages of investor:

1. *Angels.* These are typically high net worth individuals who invest small amounts of money in very early stage companies. Typically, these companies are at the idea stage and have no
   product, service, revenue, or employees. Angels will invest at this
   stage because they believe in the idea or management. A standard investment at this stage is likely $10,000 to $500,000.

2. *Early or seed stage.* These are the first institutional investors in a
   company, typically investing when the company has just a few
   employees, little or no revenue, and is still developing its technology, service, business model, and operations. A typical investment at this stage is $250,000 to $5,000,000, depending on
   how far along the company is in its development, and what its
   capital needs are.

3. *Second round investors.* These are the investors who really accelerate growth of a company that has begun to prove itself, either through successful development of technology, or initial success in the marketplace. A typical investment here is $2 to $20 million, again depending on development and needs.

4. *Mezzanine private equity.* These investors are focused on companies that have significant revenues, but need additional growth capital to get to an IPO (initial public offering), or to get to profitability. A typical investment here is $5 to $50 million.

Venture capitalists and venture funds typically choose to invest where they think they can make the best return and add the most value to the company. Unlike most investors in the public markets who have little control over the growth or operations of the companies in which they invest, investors in private companies, such as venture capitalists generally take a very active role in building their companies. This is often where consultants can play a role by leveraging their knowledge of a market, operational expertise, strategic relationships, and other key skills that will help build a company.

In addition to understanding the stages of venture capital investment, it is important to understand the types of risk that venture capitalists take when they consider investments. In many cases, it is the need to understand, evaluate, and mitigate these risks that drives venture capitalists to work with consultants:

- *Technology risk:* Will the technology work?
- *Market risk:* Is there a market for the product, and will customers pay enough for it to build a sustainable business?
- *Management risk:* Can the management team build this business, or do they need more help?

In the course of making an investment, considering follow-on investment, or determining how best to help a portfolio company move its business to the next level of success, venture capitalists will work with consultants.

141

CONSULTING TO VENTURE CAPITAL: EXAMPLES FROM OUR EXPERIENCE

We started Wilkerson Partners for the purpose of advising a select group of venture capital and private equity clients that invest in healthcare. Indeed, our firm was "incubated" within the offices of Galen Partners, a large successful healthcare-focused private equity firm that remains our anchor client, and with whom our principals have had long-standing relationships. As Wilkerson Partners has continued to grow and evolve, we continue to focus significant energies on Galen and mid-to-late stage private companies. Our job is to bring value to venture investors and portfolio companies by providing objective insight through multiple channels including:

- Objective primary and secondary research.
- Structured analysis.
- Industry and market expertise.
- Strategic relationships.

Our clients rely on us to bring healthcare industry expertise. This is not to say they don't have it themselves—they definitely do. But we bring added breadth, depth, focus, and experience in specific segments of the healthcare industry. Essentially, we provide added leverage to the market.

Let's explore how these values can be applied to venture capital clients. The first and most basic application in our experience is in the due diligence process. Due diligence describes the process through which potential investments are evaluated. A venture investor will work with us to examine key issues about a company's product or service, its management, technology, customers, legal and patent position, and many other issues. Often during this process we can leverage our significant relationships, previous operating and consulting experience, and methodical research approach to provide significant insight into a company's operations, market opportunity, competitive landscape, and other issues that will affect its potential as an investment candidate.

In addition, we often work with venture investors to determine strategic options for a company in the portfolio. Examples of this include looking for M&A opportunities, strategic partnership opportunities, or helping them find new markets for a product. Again in all cases, we are leveraging expertise, relationship, and a methodical research approach that achieves insight.

As another example, we often work with operating companies directly after an investment is made to help the company continue to grow. It is likely that after receiving an infusion of invested capital, a company will be in a fast-growth phase in an effort to hit key milestones and maximize value creation for shareholders. This requires tremendous operational focus by the management team, but the company must continue to plan strategically for the medium and long term as well. In this latter regard, we often play a role as an "outsourced strategic planning" department within the company. We bring value through objective research and analysis that helps management and venture investors see important issues on the horizon, while allowing management to focus its energies and execute its business objectives in the current environment. While this need is common among larger companies as well, there is a special need among growing venture-backed companies who simply can't afford to build and manage in-house strategic planning resources with the breadth and depth that an external consulting firm can bring.

A final example of a consulting role in venture capital is being an "outsourced venture partner." By this we mean bringing deals to our client and helping them through the investment process. This is a great benefit to both the consultants and the venture capitalists. We as consultants benefit by creating an opportunity for upside gains in equity issued to us during the investment process, and the venture capitalists gain by bringing in a prescreened investment they may not have found otherwise. If the investment is a success, everyone wins. It may also create a consulting opportunity for us to work with the company on an ongoing basis in this capacity.

CAREERS: MOVING FROM CONSULTING TO VENTURE CAPITAL

Given the frenzy of activity in private equity markets in recent years, many consultants have been intrigued to move from consulting into venture capital. Their premise is that they feel they can leverage their expertise into greater upside as investors than as consultants. There are a very limited number of consultants who actually make this move successfully, but for those who do, there are several key skills they bring to venture capital. These key skills include:

- *Industry expertise.* This includes knowing how an industry works, who the key players are, what the key drivers of business success are, and where the profits are. Typically, this is a source of enormous competitive advantage because it enables the venture capitalist to separate companies that seem like a very good idea from companies that will be viable businesses in a marketplace.

- *Strong analytical skills.* Being smart is good, but the real value is being able to apply intellectual horsepower to determine differences in business models, customer needs, and viable strategies. As in consulting, this requires asking tough questions, finding unique sources of information, exploring all sides of an issue, and coming up with a rational conclusion.

- *Financial analysis skills.* This is often where many consultants are weakest due to lack of experience. The later in the investing cycle that a venture capitalist invests, the more important this skill becomes, as terms become more complex and valuations become more difficult to determine. Consultants who can develop financial analysis skills, including development of negotiating skills and deal terms will have a much better chance of moving into successful venture capital roles.

- *Relationships.* A key to developing a successful consulting practice is developing high-level relationships with clients. This is true in venture capital as well. The more senior level relationships a person can develop in consulting, the better chance that person can bring those relationships to bear in venture capital when looking for potential co-investors, strategic partners for a portfolio company, or conducting due diligence on a potential investment.

Overall, it is the consultant who is creative, entrepreneurial, inquisitive, disciplined, and focused that will be most likely to make a successful move into a career in venture capital.

● ● ●

Life after Consulting

EILEEN M. SERRA
MCKINSEY & COMPANY (EMERITUS)

Eileen M. Serra is the chief operating officer of FrontLine Capital Group, a holding company that develops and manages businesses that provide outsourcing and infrastructure solutions to small and mid-sized enterprises and mobile workforces of larger companies. Ms. Serra oversees both the strategy development and operations at FrontLine Capital Group and provides strategic guidance to FrontLine's partner companies. Ms. Serra joined FrontLine from the American Express Company where she was the senior vice president and general manager of Financial Services for the Small Business Services Division. She was responsible for achieving significant and rapid growth of the financial services business and leading the new business strategy and initiatives for the small business market. Prior to this role, Ms. Serra was senior vice president of Strategy and Business Development for American Express where she worked with the office of the CEO and Business Unit presidents on major new growth initiatives. Before joining American Express, Ms. Serra spent more than 11 years at McKinsey & Company, where she was a partner in the New York and Los Angeles offices. At McKinsey she advised leading consumer products and services companies on strategy and organization issues. She earned an MBA from the University of Chicago and a BS in Food Chemistry from the University of California.

145

I joined McKinsey & Company with the typical new associate attitude: Stay for two years to become an engagement manager, learn something about solving problems, build my resume, and then get a real job. It was more than 11 years later, before I decided to leave McKinsey to join the American Express Company. During my time at McKinsey I learned many valuable lessons. I'd like to share some of these with you: First, consulting can be a "real job"; second, the opportunities for personal and professional growth are almost limitless; and third, consulting is a wonderful steppingstone to other careers. I hope you will come to appreciate the value of a career in consulting, however long that career may be, by reading about some of my thoughts on my own experience. Consulting can offer you a rewarding and sustainable career in itself, while also preparing you for a series of accelerated post-consulting careers.

MY CAREER WITH MCKINSEY

I knew little about consulting before I joined McKinsey & Company. There were few resources available that described a consulting career. My interest in consulting was generated by a friend who joined McKinsey a short time earlier. He spoke enthusiastically about the fast pace of consulting, the project-based nature of the work, and the opportunity to work with very senior executives on critical issues. Consulting sounded like it would be a great experience. As I went through the interview process with McKinsey, I connected extremely well with the people I met, and formed a chemistry that ultimately persuaded me to join the firm.

My first six years with McKinsey were based out of the New York office. I had a strong interest in consumer-focused industries, like packaged goods and retailing, and spent virtually all of my time serving clients in this arena. As I developed a strong industry focus, I also worked across a wide range of issues and functional areas (e.g., strategy, operations, distribution, sales force management, and marketing). Such diversity provided me with an opportunity to build a broad set of functional skills, while also gaining in-depth expertise about an industry. By

146

maintaining a balance between industry and functional expertise, I was able to take a broad perspective in solving client problems.

Shortly after I was elected a partner, my husband and I decided to relocate to Southern California and I transferred to the Los Angeles office. I continued my focus on consumer goods but added media and entertainment companies to the mix. McKinsey was in the process of building its West Coast consumer practice, which provided an opportunity for me to work with colleagues across California. I also assumed the coleadership role of the North American packaged goods practice. Such firm-level leadership roles were very rewarding, and provided me with new development opportunities.

Throughout my consulting career, I was very active with people-related initiatives in the areas of recruiting, professional development, and performance management. In consulting, the ability to develop and lead people is critical to your success—both to have an impact on a client engagement and to ensure that the consulting firm continues to attract, develop, and retain exceptional people. It was tremendously satisfying to recruit highly talented people to McKinsey, and to help them develop and grow into outstanding professionals. As you can see, my McKinsey career was multifaceted. In addition to performing consulting activities, I was also deeply involved in knowledge development and people leadership within the firm.

CONSULTING AS A STEPPING STONE

A career in consulting can be challenging and rewarding, and it can also be a great way to quickly prepare for a wide range of alternate careers. The project-based nature of consulting engagements, the broad diversity of experiences, and the high caliber of the people you interact with all work to create a unique learning environment with an incredibly steep learning curve. While at McKinsey, I watched consultants learn the basic skills that I believe are critical for success in any career, and then move on to become leaders in fields outside of consulting. Let's look at some of these fundamental skill areas in more detail.

Learning How to Think

No matter where you work—a large company or a small, a service business or an industrial manufacturer, a for-profit company or a non-profit organization—your success will be dependent on your ability to think, to solve problems, and to create opportunities. As a consultant, you will first learn to solve problems. This is the most fundamental building block in your skill development process. Consulting will help you develop critical thinking skills to disaggregate problems, develop hypotheses, structure analyses, and synthesize information into insights or conclusions. You will learn to rely on your judgment and intuition to make decisions. Not everything can be (or should be) analyzed to death. The ability to recognize patterns can be instrumental in developing the insight and the confidence one needs to make quick decisions, and then act on breakthrough opportunities. The project-based nature of consulting provides the opportunity to observe many different types of problems, within different industries and different functional contexts. This exposure is invaluable and occurs much more frequently and at a more sophisticated level in consulting than in a typical corporate environment—especially during the early stages of your career.

As you become more experienced in solving business problems, you will find that some problems are so complex or so poorly understood that your clients themselves have difficulty coping with them. Your clients will look to you for help, and expect you to cut through the confusion to structure a clean and logical approach to solving the problems. Being able to deal with ambiguity is critical to your success in any business environment. If you don't develop a basic comfort level with ambiguity, you can become paralyzed. Some individuals don't know where or how to get started on a difficult problem; they need someone to structure the work for them. Consulting is a wonderful environment to learn to deal with ambiguity, since every engagement begins with a clean sheet of paper, and often the first task of a consultant is to help a client understand and articulate the problem.

Learning How to Communicate

Consultants quickly learn that their problem-solving skills are only as good as their communication skills (e.g., the ability to structure a logical argument, to articulate ideas clearly and concisely, to persuade others to see alternate viewpoints or new insights). If a consultant cannot express her ideas in both oral and written form, her analysis will have little impact. Successful consultants are able to capture the imagination of their clients through persuasive communication and encourage them to take action by describing new possibilities for success.

Given the diversity of the individuals you will work with as a consultant, you will have many opportunities to practice alternative communication styles and to see what works and what does not work in different situations. You will learn to tailor your communication style to the way individuals hear and process information, and to proactively manage the way you interact with people to achieve your desired objectives. Since the skills are valuable in any work environment, your consulting experience will be transferable to a wide array of professions outside of consulting.

Learning How to Lead

The third skill learned by a consultant is the ability to lead others. Over the course of your career, both in consulting and afterwards, you will see a wide variety of leadership styles and develop your own perspective of effective leadership. While there are some common elements to great leaders—such as the ability to influence others and gain their support for your ideas, the ability to have conviction in your own ideas and the courage to uphold them, the ability to anticipate the need for and bring about change—the development of a leadership style is highly personal.

Consulting provides a rich environment for you to formulate and experiment with your own leadership style. As a consultant, you will have exposure to very senior people across many client organizations. You can observe leaders and form your own opinions about what works and does not work when it comes to leading others. Since consultants work as members of engagement teams that change from project to project, you will have a variety of opportunities to try-on different leadership styles and see what works best for you.

LIFE AFTER MCKINSEY

Although I thrived in the consulting environment, I was ready to move on to my next career after 11 years with McKinsey. I realized that my professional aspirations could not be achieved solely through a consulting career. I wanted to be accountable for the financial success of a business. I wanted to see my ideas and my vision for a business implemented in the marketplace. I was ready for a new set of challenges.

I left McKinsey in 1996 to join American Express as the senior vice president of Strategy and New Business Development. It was a terrific opportunity to transition from a consulting environment to a corporate environment, and to bring my consulting skills to an internal strategy group. After about a year, I moved into a line position in the Small Business Services Division of American Express to become the senior vice president and general manager of Financial Services. I was responsible for building the lending business as well as managing the new business development arena. This was a great position, since small businesses comprised a very large and high-growth market, and American Express had a strong competitive position within this segment.

After focusing my energies on creating American Express products and services for entrepreneurs, I got the entrepreneurial bug myself, and decided that my next position would be within a small company environment. At the end of 2000, I became the chief operating officer of FrontLine Capital Group, a publicly traded holding company with a portfolio of infrastructure and technology companies that support the operating needs of small- to medium-sized businesses.

In each of these positions at American Express and FrontLine Capital, the skills I developed as a consultant at McKinsey were invaluable.

They helped me pinpoint the critical issues and opportunities for the organization, ensure organizational alignment behind key priorities, recognize the need for change and providing structure and support during change processes, quickly build relationships with other people, and lead an organization. Consulting does not provide all of the skills required to lead a successful post-consulting career. There are clearly new things to learn and new dimensions to experience in a line position, three of which in particular stand out:

1. *The value of focus.* In a consulting environment, when you get a bunch of smart people in a room, you always come up with three new ideas. Typically, the best ideas come up at the eleventh hour. However, in a line organization, the creation of new ideas needs to stop at some point, and the organization needs to execute if it is to achieve its goals—which brings me to my second point.

2. *The importance of execution.* Ultimately, it is not the smartest idea that wins in the marketplace, but the idea that is best executed. Line executives need to ensure that the solutions or ideas that are generated are not beyond the capacity of the organization to implement. Only those ideas that can be executed—and executed well—by the organization will produce the optimal results.

3. *The impact of accountability.* When mapping out a strategy or a plan of action to achieve a desired goal, line managers know they will be held accountable for the success or failure of their efforts. Although line managers may hire consultants to help them develop this plan of action, consultants are not accountable for achieving the goal—line managers are. As a line manager, I am accountable for delivering tangible results, and I am measured by how well I meet or exceed my financial targets. Every day, line managers need to make decisions that balance short-term financial performance with long-term growth commitments. In many cases, these decisions impact both customers and employees so there are significant, and at times irreversible, consequences to these decisions. The stakes feel much higher as a line manager than they do as a consultant.

REFLECTIONS ON MY CAREER

I am currently in the third phase of my career. My first was in consulting, my second at a Fortune 500 financial services company, and my third at an entrepreneurial venture capital firm. I don't know where my career will lead next, but I do know that McKinsey was the best place for me to have started. My skill set increased exponentially as a consultant; the exposure I had to people and problems in my 11 years at McKinsey were equivalent to double or triple that of a more traditional corporate job. The intensity of the consulting work environment also fostered the development of extremely close working relationships. As a result, I have an incredible network of friends and colleagues who have provided support and counsel to me well past my McKinsey days. It opened up many doors of opportunity.

Consulting can help you get a "real" job, but the experience is so much more valuable than simply being a career stepping stone. My decisions to join McKinsey and then stay there for 11 years were the right decisions for me, both from a personal and a professional perspective. My subsequent opportunities and career choices have been greatly influenced by this experience. Consulting provided me with the foundation I needed as my career continued to evolve.

CHAPTER 5

PLANNING YOUR CONSULTING CAREER

Prestige may be the most important factor when it comes to recruiting. . . . Many students are heavily indebted upon graduation, and may migrate to prestigious firms in search of high compensation.
Kennedy Information Research Group

Prestige and compensation are powerful incentives for applying to consulting firms. In fact, many candidates base their entire job search on these two objectives. But such a shortsighted decision can lead to a mismatch between the individual and the firm. Choosing a firm is a much more complex decision than many applicants realize. Since more than half of your waking hours will be spent in the office, the right firm will offer not only adequate compensation and prestige, but also interesting work, an enjoyable office culture, and opportunity for career advancement. When consultants are professionally satisfied, they and their firms—as well as their clients—are likely to have a more productive and enjoyable relationship.

As stressed in Chapter 1, the complexity of the industry can make identifying and selecting the right firms a difficult task. And when it comes to applying, many candidates are so discouraged by the required preparation that they decide to avoid the profession altogether. Oddly enough, the application process itself is often one of the highest barriers to entering the profession.

This chapter will help you hurdle this barrier by providing a step-by-step way to pin down your own personal and professional interests, identify and select consulting firms that promise to meet these interests, and develop practical strategies for researching, contacting, and securing interviews at these firms. By the time you finish reading this chapter, you will have the tools you need to sell yourself on paper and get your foot in the door.

FINDING YOUR NICHE IN CONSULTING

Before applying to a single firm, you should first reflect on your professional goals and personal interests, and then identify the types of consulting that best suit these interests. These initial steps are often overlooked or ignored by eager candidates who use simplistic criteria when pulling together their list of targeted firms. Rationales such as "I like strategy consulting," or, "I'm going to apply to all the big consulting firms," reveal a candidate's limited understanding of the need for serious research. These are the candidates who apply to as many firms as they can using a mail-merge, even though they know little to nothing about any individual firm. Casting a wide net over so many firms in the hope of catching the interest of a few is time and resource consuming, and it could possibly place you in an unsuitable position.

To find your niche, you need to invest time into the iterative process of continuous learning, as illustrated in Figure 5.1.

Whether applying for full-time or summer internship positions, you should choose a firm that suits all your needs, rather than a firm that would only strengthen your resume. Only if you understand your personal and professional objectives can you evaluate the opportunities afforded by different firms and their multitude of consulting practice areas. Then, as you learn more about the work and lifestyle of consulting, you will be able to clarify your objectives and, ultimately, distill your list of firms into the most attractive set.

Start your introspective learning by asking yourself forward-looking questions: Do you want a consulting job because you think it will help you get into graduate business school or, perhaps, into a law or doctoral program? Or, are you about to receive your MBA and believe

Figure 5.1
Finding Your Niche in Consulting

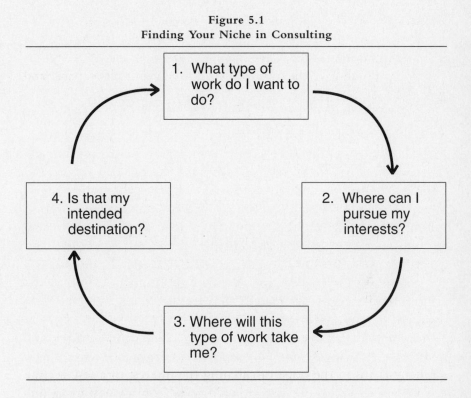

that a consulting position will most rapidly accelerate your career? And how long do you envision yourself staying in consulting—only two or three years, or alternatively until you become a partner? These are the critical questions you must answer before you can identify firms that might be right for you. Ask yourself, "Where do I want to be in five years?" With this vision in mind, set some interim goals, and identify the consulting experience that will help you achieve them.

Once you have gained a basic understanding of your personal and professional goals, you are ready to begin researching the industry. Learn as much as you can about the different areas of consulting and its many firms, and try to envision yourself working at each. As you understand the industry better, you are likely to need to revise your initial self-assessment—after all, you are in a better position to know what you want to get out of consulting once you know more about the industry. So go back and reconsider your goals, and repeat the itera-tive process of comparing the industry's opportunities to your own personal aspirations until you find your proper niche.

RESEARCHING THE INDUSTRY

With thousands of firms in the industry, it is impossible to research all of them. But in Chapter 1, you learned how to efficiently sort through them and focus on those that have the most to offer you. There, we introduced a technique for segmenting firms according to four di-mensions: (1) the industries consulted, (2) the functional types of con-sulting performed, (3) the sectors from which clients are drawn (private, public, nonprofit), and (4) the firm's affiliation with its clients (external firms or internal corporate strategic planning units). By screening firms this way, you should be able to focus your research efforts and concentrate on only those firms that best match your per-sonal and professional goals.

Are you attracted to a particular industry? Then you probably want to use the first segmentation dimension to eliminate firms that do not service companies in that industry. Or perhaps you have a background in engineering and want to leverage that experience by performing reengineering projects? Then rely on the second dimension to screen out firms that do not have reengineering practices. What if you want to develop growth strategies for a single company operating in the private sector? Then you should use a multidimensional screen to find strategic planning groups that belong to for-profit organizations.

You may understand the framework, but how do you locate the in-formation you need? Although we live in the age of information, find-ing the right data to answer specific questions can be difficult. As the saying goes, you may be drowning in data, but starved of knowledge. Start your research by reading materials written by people who know the industry best: practicing consultants and leading strategy thinkers. By reading the personal essays in Chapter 4, you have already begun to learn about some of the latest thinking on the industry, and should have a sense of the kind of consulting you find attractive. Next, you can quickly find information on specific firms by visiting their Web sites, many of which have "career" sections that describe the available positions. Other useful resources include the recruiting and promotional brochures distributed by the firms, consultants' speeches from forums sponsored by organizations like The Conference Board, and consultants' articles published in periodicals such as *Harvard Business Review, McKinsey Quarterly,* and *Strategy & Business.*

If you are an undergraduate or graduate student with access to a career planning office, finding primary research may be easier. You are likely to find a tremendous amount of information at on-campus events, delivered right to you by the consultants themselves. Firms that formally recruit new graduates will hold presentations so that you can meet them—and so they can meet you. These events give you a unique opportunity to ask targeted questions and to have short, one-on-one conversations with consultants in a relatively non-threatening setting. Just be aware that not all firms can afford the time and money required to visit campuses. If you limit your primary research to on-campus events, your picture of the industry will be incomplete, and you may overlook a potentially attractive position at a smaller firm that relies on recruiting channels other than on-campus visits.

Those of you who are particularly interested in strategic planning may find that few, if any, corporations recruit on campus for their internal consulting positions. Because strategic planning groups tend to be smaller, they often expect candidates to approach them. Your primary research strategy will, therefore, have to be proactive. A proven, though time-consuming, method of finding strategic planning groups is to simply compile a list of companies you might want to work for, and then call their corporate switchboards to ask if they have strategic planning or business development groups. When organizations do not actively seek you out, you need to be creative. Also note that some strategic planning or internal consulting groups only hire seasoned consultants, and may not offer entry level positions. But don't be discouraged—there are plenty of groups that do.

If you are in graduate business school, many of your classmates may have worked at the very firms and companies you are researching. Ask them for their perspectives on their former employers, and collect contact names of consultants at those firms to talk to later. On rare occasions, having an insider contact can actually swing a candidacy from a "ding" to an "accept." And if you are a first-year MBA student looking for a summer position, speak to your second-year classmates who just completed internships at consulting or strategic planning groups for even more contact information.

You can also research available consulting positions by using some of the popular online job sites, such as monster.com, hotjobs.com, headhunter.net, or cruelworld.com. The Web sites will allow you to search available positions by defined criteria (i.e., geography, professional level, salary range), and apply for positions online without a charge. On occasion, consulting firms as well as internal corporate strategic planning groups post listings for consultants on these sites—particularly during the times of year when consulting firms are traditionally not in active on-campus recruiting mode, such as the middle of summer. Although this approach is a useful way to supplement your other research, it is inadvisable to rely solely on Web listings. Not all consulting firms use these sites, and in many cases the listed positions are for senior-level consultants (which may be useful if you have extensive work experience and can convince a firm that you are suitable for a more senior position). Nevertheless, the sites are worth a visit since the listings change daily.

Widely used secondary sources are also available to further your research. You could start with Appendix III of this book, which provides a directory of 100 consulting firms. Table 5.1 provides a partial list of additional directories, industry guides, periodicals, and electronic sources that may help your research. Although this is only a partial list, it should get you well on your way to developing a more complete understanding of the industry and its firms.

NARROWING YOUR LIST OF FIRMS

As you learn more about the industry and begin to prioritize your interests, you may find your list of attractive firms becoming unreasonably lengthy. To narrow your list, select other dimensions for screening firms such as firm culture, firm prestige, anticipated

Table 5.1
Sample Research Sources

Directories and Industry Guides	Organization
Ace Your Case! Consulting Interviews	Wet Feet Press
Career Guide to the Top Consulting Firms	Kennedy Information Research Group
Consultants and Consulting Organizations Directory	Julie A. Mitchell, Editor
2000 Consultants Directory	Canon Communications
Directory of Management Consultants	Kennedy Information Research Group
Harvard Business School Guide to Careers in Management Consulting	Harvard Business School Press
Killer Consulting Resumes	Wet Feet Press
The Vault Career Guide to Consulting	Vault Reports
The Wharton MBA Case Interview Study Guide	Wharton MBA Consulting Club

Periodicals	Organization
Consultants News	Kennedy Information Research Group
Harvard Business Review	Harvard Business Review
The McKinsey Quarterly	McKinsey & Company
Strategy & Business	Booz•Allen & Hamilton

Electronic Sources	Organization
FindConsultancy.com (www.findconsultancy.com)	FindConsultancy.com
Information Central for Management Consulting Worldwide (www.mcninet.com)	Management Consulting Network International
Vault Reports (www.thevault.com)	Vault Reports
Wet Feet Press (www.wetfeet.com)	Wet Feet Press
Yahoo! Management Consulting Directory (www.yahoo.com)	Yahoo!
About Management Consulting (www.about.com)	About.com

Strategy Books	Author	Publisher
Co-opetition	A. Brandenberger & B. Nalebuff	Doubleday, 1996
Competing in the Information Age	J.M. Luftman	Oxford University Press, 1996
Competing for the Future	G. Hamel & C. K. Prahalad	HBS Press, 1994
Competitive Strategy	M. Porter	Free Press, 1980

(continued)

Table 5.1   (Continued)

How Digital Is Your Business?	A. Slywotsky & D. Morrison	Crown, 2000
Leading the Revolution	G. Hamel	HBS Press, 2000
The Loyalty Effect	F. Reichheld	HBS Press, 1996
The Mind of the Strategist	K. Ohmae	McGraw-Hill, 1991
Modern Competitive Analysis	S. Oster	Oxford University Press, 1994
People, Performance & Pay	T. Flannery	Free Press, 1995
The Profit Zone	A. Slywotsky & D. Morrison	Times Books, 1998
The Strategy-Focused Organization	R. Kaplan & D. Norton	HBS Press, 2000
Strategic Management of Non-Profit Organizations	S. Oster	Oxford University Press, 1995
Taking Charge of Change	D. Smith	Addison-Wesley, 1995
Thinking Strategically	A. Dixit & B. Nalebuff	Norton, 1991
Value Migration	A. Slywotsky	HBS Press, 1996

lifestyle, number and locations of offices, and estimated starting salaries and signing bonuses. As you select the dimensions you find most important, rank them by degree of significance.

For example, if you dislike the rigors of extensive travel, but would love to join the Rolls Royce of consulting firms, then you will have to decide which of the two attributes—balanced lifestyle or prestige—you value more. Every firm offers a different mix of benefits and requires different sacrifices. Without some ranking of these preferences, your shortened list may not be very meaningful.

Attributes like firm culture, firm prestige, and balanced lifestyle are subjective and consequently difficult to research. Two consultants from the same firm may have completely different subjective opinions of their firm's culture. As you research subjective attributes of different firms, speak with as many current and former consultants as you can to get a wide variety of perspectives. There are plenty of primary and secondary sources of information that will help you narrow your list of firms and focus on the subset that is the best fit for you.

PRIORITIZING SHORT-TERM VERSUS LONG-TERM INTERESTS

As you select your screening criteria, decide explicitly whether you are more interested in satisfying short-term or long-term interests. Short-term considerations, such as starting salaries and signing bonuses, start dates, and initial office or client assignments, often dominate because they provide immediate gratification. A gigantic signing bonus, after all, can be very gratifying to one's financial health and may even eliminate a student loan in one fell swoop.

Consulting firms clearly recognize the importance of short-term considerations when persuading an applicant to join the firm. In 2000, average starting salaries for undergraduate recruits were $40,000 to $50,000, with signing bonuses from $5,000 to $10,000; for top MBAs, the average base salary reached $100,000, with signing bonuses as high as $40,000. These big numbers can overshadow all other considerations, to the detriment of both the firm and applicant. Once you experience the day-to-day realities of being a consultant, the money may no longer seem so attractive if, for example, you discover that you really place greater importance on a more balanced lifestyle, with a 9 A.M. to 6 P.M. job.

Explicitly considering your long-term objectives will help you make a more rational—rather than emotional—decision. Company A may be offering a starting salary of $92,000, with a $35,000 signing bonus, but how will an experience with Company A position you for future professional endeavors? What skills will you add to your resume? Conversely, Company B, with an $80,000 starting salary and a signing bonus of $10,000, may have a less attractive package, but it may also offer far superior opportunities for professional growth. And some firms with lower starting packages may offer more frequent and higher raises than others, which, in the long run, may result in significantly higher compensation. As all these considerations suggest, when you are comparing firms and potential offers, it pays to think ahead and weigh the relative importance of future rewards against immediate rewards.

GETTING YOUR FOOT IN THE DOOR OF A FIRM

Once you have selected a group of firms to contact, how do you get them to recognize you? As shown in Figure 5.2, getting your foot in the door involves a four-step process: (1) perform targeted research on an individual firm; (2) adjust your resume to suit the firm; (3) speak to individuals with direct exposure to the firm; and (4) write a cover letter that will capture the firm's interest. Although this may seem overly methodical, you should consider each step as a unique piece of the job-search puzzle, since a mistake at any one step can eliminate your candidacy altogether.

Step 1. Performing Targeted Research

Although you will have invested hours in your initial research on the industry and its firms, you will probably need to perform additional research on the firms you are targeting. You need very specific information to complete the next few steps: the exact title of the position you are applying for; the office location you prefer; the exact name of the practice group you seek to join; an accurate name and address of the recruiting coordinator; and other details that will give your application the polish it needs to impress. A small mistake, such as incorrectly referring to the position of "Associate" as "Research Analyst" in a cover letter, has in the past been responsible for an immediate decline or "ding" decision.

You should review all the firm's promotional materials, watch videotapes of on-campus presentations you might have missed, and perform targeted literature searches using search engines such as Dow Jones or Lexis/Nexis to find the most current information available on a firm. If you are applying to an organization that does not participate in formal on-campus recruiting, you might even want to ask for an informational interview in the company's office. In addition to giving you direct access to a potential employer and enabling you to ask targeted questions, informational interviews give you a chance to impress, and to establish a positive reputation with the firm even before submitting your application. Remember, targeted research can also have the proactive effect of promoting your candidacy.

Figure 5.2
Getting Your Foot in the Door

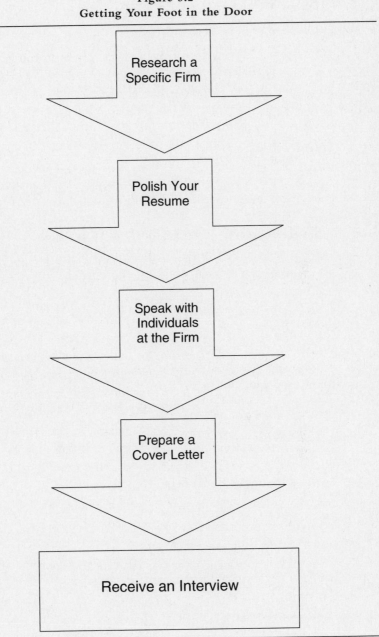

Step 2. Refining Your Resume

In the second step, you need to tailor your resume to the specific firm or company you are targeting. Your resume may be the most critical element of your application, since it usually carries more weight than your cover letter or your (rarely requested) recommendations. As you may have guessed, a poorly written resume can ruin your chances of getting an interview. But what you may not realize is that a winning resume for a consulting application is slightly different from a resume written for other jobs. When consultants review applications, they look for specific attributes that they consider to be critical to a successful consulting career. Some of the most sought-after attributes are presented in Table 5.2.

A resume designed for a consulting firm must highlight a candidate's competencies. Each bullet point should begin with an action verb that emphasizes a critical skill area. Your goal is to prove to the reader that you have already developed, through your academic, professional, and extracurricular experiences, the minimum required skill set to become a consultant.

Each statement on a resume should also be results-oriented. For example, a candidate who analyzed the cost structure of a surgical procedure with the objective of reducing reimbursement claims for an insurance company could explain her experience in two different ways:

Example: Cost Analysis for an Insurance Company

Option 1: Built an excel model to profile the cost distribution of stereotactic radiosurgery.

Table 5.2
Key Competencies of Qualified Candidates

•Academic achievement	• Extracurricular involvement
•Analytical skills	• Leadership
•Communication skills	• Quantitative skills
•Creativity	• Results orientation
•Drive and commitment	• Team orientation

Option 2: Led analysis to determine the cost distribution of stereotactic radiosurgery, resulting in an estimated savings of over $10,000 per patient treated.

The second option is better because it goes beyond a simple description of the task and acknowledges the longer term impact. But be careful: as you phrase your achievements and experiences according to the terminology consultants look for, do not stretch the truth. If you falsify any information on your resume—even unintentionally—and are later discovered, you will likely lose your job and jeopardize the applications of all future candidates from your school.

A consulting resume is not carved in stone. Different firms may stress different competencies, and therefore should receive customized versions of your resume. You can expect to spend hours reviewing and revising your resume for each application. Consulting resumes need not be entirely formal—include some information about your personal interests at the end to show that you are a person who has a life too. A consultant reviewing your resume will want to know if you are someone who would be pleasant to work and travel with for long hours. Make sure you convey that you are an interesting, as well as bright, person.

The format of your resume should meet certain minimum standards. No resume for an entry-level consulting position should exceed a single page. If you need two pages, you need to be more selective with your bullet points and less verbose in your descriptions. Noting that you won your state's spelling bee, for example, is just not necessary once you have an MBA. The one-page limit forces you to judiciously choose the experiences you want to highlight, and the words you want to use. Avoid colored paper in favor of standard white and off-white stock. Likewise, avoid unusual fonts, and certainly never put graphic images on your resume—not even your photo. Always maintain a high degree of professionalism and let the content of your resume speak for itself. An extremely unconventional approach will draw attention to you for all the wrong reasons.

Finally, have others critique your resume before sending it off. Academic institutions often have dedicated resources to help students with their resumes, and your peers who are also going through the job search can offer additional perspectives. But the best proofreader may, in fact, be a consultant. If you have family, friends, or even willing alumni from your school who are consultants, ask them to read your resume as if you were applying to their firm. They will be able to provide current, relevant, and personal commentary on your resume. But never ask consultants at the firms to which you are applying to proofread your resume; they are likely to question your judgment—and with good reason!

Step 3. Speak to Knowledgeable Individuals

Once you have the basic information about a firm and your resume is almost ready, you may want to compare notes with people who have had direct exposure to the firm. Family, friends, professors, and even "safe" consultants (e.g., individuals who have recently graduated from your school and are willing to speak with students in confidence) are all sources you might want to use. If you decide to contact "safe" consultants, select those who are close to the professional level that you plan to enter. For example, if you are about to graduate from college, speak to a research analyst at your targeted firm.

A more formal approach is to arrange an informational interview with a consultant at the targeted firm. As a proactive strategy, this may expose you to greater risk, but it may also let you leapfrog ahead of your competition if you make a good impression. In contacting these people, your objectives are to gain further insight into the firm and to demonstrate that you are serious about consulting and about that firm in particular. Ask questions that seek their opinions, rather than statistics that you could have looked up elsewhere. After all, that is why you wanted to speak with them instead of simply reading about the firm. Appropriate questions would be: What are the rewards of working for Mercer, and what are the sacrifices? What experience did they have before joining the firm? Which academic courses best helped them to prepare for consulting? But inappropriate questions would be, How big a firm is Mercer? Does the firm have a business strategy practice? How about an office in London? These are questions that reveal your lack of preparation, and could have been looked up prior to the interview

To arrange an informational interview, fax or mail your resume and a short letter to either a consultant or the recruiting coordinator, and then follow up with a call shortly thereafter. In the letter, explain how you got the person's name, who you are, and what your objective is for the interview. Close the letter with an action statement letting the addressee know that you will make a follow-up call on a specific date. Before you make that call, prepare your questions, since the individual may decide to use that moment to conduct a quick phone interview instead of arranging a later meeting. You may get only a few minutes of the person's time and should be respectful of his or her busy schedule. So do your research, prepare a list of questions in advance, and be ready to explain why you are interested in the firm—and even why they should hire you.

After the informational interview, close the loop by writing a thank-you letter. It should be short, but personal enough to remind the reader who you are and what you discussed. And since this was only an informational interview, do not conclude with a statement such as "I look forward to your response."

Step 4. Write a Cover Letter

Here is where your research efforts really pay off. When writing your cover letter to formally apply for a position, you should address three essential topics in a single page. First, in the opening paragraph, state who you are and why you are writing: "I am a first-year graduate student at The Wharton School seeking a summer position at Hewitt Associates," or "I am a vice president of Marketing at Procter & Gamble interested in transitioning to management consulting." Refer to the title of the position you are applying for, and identify the office location you prefer. This will demonstrate that you have done your homework. If you have spoken with anyone at the firm, mention that person as a point of contact who confirmed your interest in the firm.

Second, in the next paragraph or two, bring your resume to life by highlighting your skills. Explicitly connect your competencies to consulting, and convince the reader that you possess the necessary skills for the profession. If there are weaknesses on your resume, explain them here, and preferably describe a weakness in a way that makes it appear to be a strength. For example, if you worked at three companies in three years, explain how your apparent lack of commitment actually gave you a broader skill set by exposing you to a range of industries and responsibilities. Tell the reader why you would be a valuable addition to the firm, as well as a close personal fit with the firm's culture. Although this is a lot of information to convey in a single page, the keys to an effective cover letter are directness and conciseness.

Third, end your letter with an action statement. Like the letter you wrote requesting an informational interview, your cover letter should include a request for an interview and state when you will call to follow up. Recruiters at large firms review hundreds of resumes and cover letters a day. Part of your objective, therefore, is to convince them to select yours from the pack and to agree to meet with you.

The rules governing the format of your cover letters are the same as for your resume. Do not use paper of an unusual color, and make sure the cover letter paper exactly matches your resume paper. Avoid small or unusual fonts, and never use graphics. These comments should come as no surprise, but we mention them because we have seen far too many letters that violate these simple guidelines.

Be extremely careful to address the letter to the right recruiting coordinator, and at the right office address. Large consulting firms typically have multiple people in charge of different types of recruiting, such as an undergraduate recruiter, an MBA recruiter, an international office recruiter, and a professional hire recruiter who works with headhunters. Some firms may allocate their coordinators to specific schools, and in many cases, offices located in other countries have separate coordinators. Firms expect you to do your homework and find the right recruiter. If you make a mistake, your entire application could be sent to the wrong address and land in the trash.

Once you have completed all of these steps, you are ready to submit your application. Firms recruiting on campus often ask career planning offices to collect applications and mail them in all at once, rather than have students mail their applications directly to the firm. Pay close attention to submission deadlines: Almost all firms stop accepting applications after a certain date, no matter who you are or what you say.

The competition for consulting positions is fierce, and little things can sway the end result. If you end up getting turned down, do not take it personally. You have to be thick-skinned during this process. "Ding" or "bullet" letters are so plentiful that many students wall paper their dorm rooms with them. Once you get over the initial frustration of rejection, take a close look at the resume and cover letter you sent, and try to identify ways to improve them. With proper preparation next time, you can dramatically enhance your chances of securing an interview.

When your application is accepted and it is time to meet with the firm, the game changes entirely and presents a completely new set of challenges. In Chapter 6, we describe the process of case interviewing, and show you how to convert face-to-face meetings into a job offer.

CHAPTER 6

MASTERING THE CASE INTERVIEW

You have been warned. The gentle job interview is dead. These days companies ask applicants to solve brainteasers and riddles, . . . act as managers of make-believe companies and solve complex business problems.

Nina Munk and Suzanne Oliver
Forbes

You have worked hard to secure an interview. You have diligently researched the firm's background, spoken with their consultants, polished your resume, and written a winning cover letter. Now, the only obstacles standing between you and the offer are the infamous rounds of case interviews. This chapter will help you hone your skills through practice and prepare you to succeed at case interviews. But your preparation cannot wait until the last minute. You should begin to practice immediately, and continue to do so throughout the entire application process.

Most candidates who fail the case interview do so because of inadequate preparation. They simply read through a list of sample case questions and think about how they would answer them. But when they are faced with the pressure of an actual face-to-face case interview, these candidates suddenly realize how inadequately prepared they are. Passive preparation is not enough; preparing for case interviews requires an active investment of time into practice.

This chapter begins by reviewing exactly what a case interview is, and then teaches you practical techniques for mastering each of the interview's component parts.

THE PARTS OF A CASE INTERVIEW

A traditional interview includes three parts: an initial greeting, a discussion of the candidate's resume, and a final question-and-answer session. What, then, is a case interview? It is an expanded version of the traditional interview, which is uniquely characterized by its inclusion of a fourth part: a case question. These questions can ask you to discuss almost anything, from estimating the number of gas stations in the United States, to measuring the impact of online travel booking sites on traditional bricks-and-mortar travel agents. The case question is intended to test a candidate's ability to think and act like a consultant in an intense face-to-face situation. By simulating a client-consultant interaction, interviewers are able to observe firsthand how a candidate would manage a discussion with a client. Case questions are intentionally abstract, usually obscure and puzzling, and often technical. They are designed to test your ability to think creatively, make sense out of ambiguity, handle abstraction, and systematically derive an answer when an answer seems next to impossible.

But remember that the case question is only one part—albeit the most important part—of the overall case interview. The case question will usually require 50 percent to 80 percent of the time allocated to a case interview, with the remainder of time allotted to the other three parts of the interview. Most case interviews follow this basic format, as presented in Figure 6.1.

Although the length of case interviews may vary between 30 and 45 minutes, they will typically proceed through each of the four parts. Rarely will an interviewer skip a step. Each part is deliberately designed to test for a different set of attributes. Therefore, an interviewer who overlooks a part may have to base a decision on relatively incomplete information.

The following sections cover the four parts of a case interview. As we describe each part, try to internalize the process by envisioning yourself proceeding through it. Although no two interviews will be identical, the process outlined here will provide you with the tools to navigate through any case interview.

Figure 6.1
The Four Parts of the Consulting Case Interview

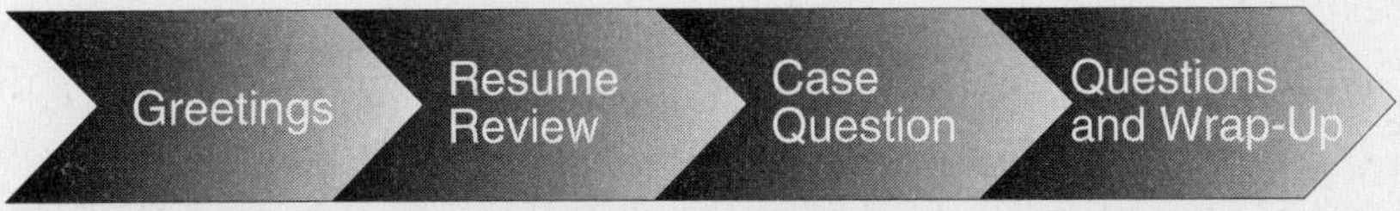

| Greetings | Resume Review | Case Question | Questions and Wrap-Up |

Timing (minutes)			
45-minute version 1	10	30	4
30-minute version 2	5	20	3

PART I. GREETINGS

From the moment the interviewer extends her hand, she has begun to evaluate you—she is judging a book by its cover. Whether consciously or not, she notices the way you dress, the way you sit, and many other superficial elements of your appearance. If this first impression is positive, the interviewer is more likely to begin the interview with a favorable attitude toward you. Conversely, if the interviewer finds something odd or unexpected in your appearance, this negative perception of you may lead her to look for other reasons to not accept you. People have a tendency to be selectively rational—we register only those pieces of evidence that support our initial hypotheses. Perception, after all, largely forms our understanding of reality.

So to take control of the interviewer's first impression by paying close attention to the initial greetings. This is the time to put both yourself and the interviewer at ease, and to control her perception of you by building a positive rapport. This is also your chance to pass what is euphemistically known as the "airport test": If the interviewer were stranded with you at a snowed-in airport, would she enjoy your company? Practically all consulting firms emphasize this test. Since consultants tend to spend long hours together, and actually do get stranded in airports from time to time, it is best if they enjoy spending time together. You may be an outstanding candidate in all other respects, but unless you pass the airport test and make a social connection with your interviewer, your chances of being hired are slim.

Experience has shown that interviewers typically prefer well-groomed candidates who give firm handshakes, look them directly in the eye, have a clear and confident voice, and show no signs of nervousness. Dress professionally and conservatively, regardless of the firm or company you are interviewing with. Women should wear either pant or skirt suits, preferably of a muted pastel or dark color, with limited jewelry and perfume. Men should likewise wear muted or dark suits, a tie, and polished shoes. Arrive early enough to prevent appearing harassed, and to have enough time to acclimate yourself to your surroundings.

What should you bring to an interview? The short answer is: as little as possible. You are likely to need a pad and pen to work through case questions, and you may want to carry them in a small portfolio. To refresh your memory just prior to the interview, bring a few notes on the firm or company and a list of questions you would like to ask. But do not carry books or volumes of information on the company or firm; instead, memorize anything you think you may need to know. Business cards, if you have them, are useful but not necessary, and a poorly prepared interviewer may ask for copies of your resume. Do not, under any circumstances, bring a calculator to an interview. In fact, you are likely to be tested for your ability to manipulate numbers in your head. Finally, do not chew gum or eat candy or other food during an interview; but if you are offered a drink, it is usually alright to accept.

How should you use the things you bring to an interview? Sparingly. Present your resume only if the interviewer asks for it or has not seen it before. Use your pad and pen only to jot down some simple notes during the case question. Too many candidates become dependent on their pads and write continuously during an interview. Before they know it, they are speaking into the pad, and forgetting to look up and make eye contact with the interviewer. Reference your notes on the firm and look at your list of questions before, not during, an interview. Memorize everything you may need to know.

After the interviewer leads you into a private meeting room, select a high-sitting chair, if possible, rather than a soft couch; your physical stature will undoubtedly have a direct impact on your level of confidence. Although case interviews can be stressful, try to remain relaxed. Smile, be enthusiastic, and do not be afraid to laugh, even if the interviewer seems stern. The best and easiest advice to follow is to be yourself. Remember: if the interviewer does not like who you are when you are yourself, chances are you would not want to work with that person, either. These simple, commonsense tips will give you a polished presence and increase the interviewer's confidence in your candidacy.

PART II. THE RESUME REVIEW

After greeting you, the interviewer will typically launch into a 5- to 10-minute discussion of topics drawn from your resume. Work experience, academics, extracurricular pursuits and interests, and even hobbies are all fair game for this discussion. Interviewers use this opportunity to delve into your past and understand how you have grown from prior experiences. They hope to learn about your strengths and weaknesses, and to evaluate your professional and personal "fit" with their firm. Interviewers may even use this time to test your "business sense" (e.g., can you explain the business objectives of a former employer?) and to see if you keep up to date with your former employers (e.g., do you know what their current stock price is?).

Sounds simple enough, but you need to learn how to interpret their questions. When asking a question, interviewers tend to have a predetermined idea of a "good" answer, which rarely includes obvious responses. There is a difference between what the interviewer asks and what the interviewer means. For example, if an interviewer asks, "What did you do as an intern at IBM?" he is not looking for a list of tasks. Rather, he wants to see if you can take a broader perspective and articulate the competencies you developed and the impact that your work had on the company. His question should, therefore, be read as, "How did your position at IBM improve your professional skills?" Or better yet, "How did your position at IBM prepare you to join us?"

Similarly, if an interviewer asks, "How do you like Yale?" his true meaning is likely to be "Are you doing well at Yale?" or even "Are you a top performer at Yale?" Questions relating to hobbies or interests can be more difficult to interpret. For example, a question of "So, you like to ski?" is soliciting more than a confirmation from you. The interviewer wants to see if you can articulate the reasons why you like to ski and even convince him to try the sport himself.

To put it simply, you should use the Resume Review to sell yourself (but without being too boastful). Simple questions are actually invitations for you to provide a richer, more impressive description of your skills and abilities—and interviewers hope that you will use their questions to do just that. Although you can interpret a question in many ways, you should routinely try to step back from a simple answer, and instead offer a broader explanation of your skills to prove that you are an impressively competent candidate.

To prepare for the Resume Review, evaluate yourself introspectively, and identify the key skills you want to highlight. You actually began this process when you wrote your resume—a topic we covered in Chapter 5. By using action verbs such as "managed" and "supervised" to begin each bullet point on your resume, and by taking a results-oriented approach to describing the tasks you performed (e.g., ". . . resulting in an estimated savings of over $10,000 per patient treated"), you highlighted the evidence that proves you have certain skills. Then, when you wrote your cover letters—also covered in Chapter 5—you bundled the evidence into a smaller set of key skills and demonstrated that you have what it takes to be a management consultant.

Essentially the same process is required in the Resume Review: When an interviewer invites you to discuss a specific event on your resume, you have to demonstrate how that event taught you an essential skill for management consulting. And for each Resume Review question that an interviewer asks, you have the opportunity to highlight a different skill. You should thus be able to explain how any and all of the bullet points on your resume endowed you with a valuable competency.

So how should you characterize your competencies? If you recall, Table 5.2 provided a list of key competencies that interviewers want to see, and taught you to highlight as many of these skills as possible in your resume. This "core skill set" is what we call your "commercial": the summary of who you are and what you bring to the table. Although we would all like to think that we possess every skill listed in Table 5.2, in reality, we have different selling points, and hence, different commercials. Your commercial makes you unique, and tells the interviewer why he should hire you. Before an interview is over, you will want to talk about each and every one of your core skills. Practice answering Resume Review questions with these skills in mind, and, as explicitly as possible, link them to your academic, professional, and extracurricular experiences. When you can adeptly convert almost any set of Resume Review questions into a discussion of your entire commercial, you will be ready to conquer the Resume Review.

Successful candidates report that the best way to remember a commercial is to create a mnemonic. For example, a candidate who has Communication, Analytic, and Teamwork skills could think of herself as a "CAT." Add in Organizational skills, and she could then become a "TACO." Although you should not get carried away with this idea (we would hate to turn the consulting applicant pool into a zoo or restaurant), in the stressful atmosphere of an interview, it is much easier to think of your commercial as a single word than as a series of three to five words. Experiment with the skills of your commercial, and have some fun characterizing yourself.

Finally, prepare to answer open-ended questions, such as "Who are you?" or, "Why should I hire you?" A partial list of such questions is provided in Table 6.1.

By asking these questions, the interviewer is testing your reaction to an unexpected question. Your best bet is to fall back on your commercial, and use the open-ended question to sell yourself. For example, if your interviewer asks, "Who are you?" you have a perfect invitation to recite your commercial: your key skills, and the experiences that

Table 6.1
Common Open-Ended Interview Questions

What are your greatest strengths? Weaknesses?

Why should I hire you?

Tell me about yourself.

Who are you?

How do you like your school?

What is your favorite book and why?

What are your three greatest achievements?

What are your three greatest failures?

What three things must you do in your life?

What are your dreams?

Where do you see yourself in five years? Ten years?

What kind of people do you like? Dislike?

What would you like me to know that is not already in your resume?

How do you spend your free time?

Why are you here?

How would you describe your ideal job?

Which other companies are you interviewing with? Why?

What do you know about our firm?

How will an experience with us help your career?

Why did you choose to go to school A? Why not school B?

Why did you leave your last job?

Which courses have you liked the most? The least?

Do you like to travel?

What do you think of the stock market's performance?

What have you done with your life over the last few years?

developed and demonstrate these skills. Or, if your interviewer asks, "What is your greatest weakness?" you should think of a weakness that could also be considered a strength, such as paying meticulous attention to detail. Naturally, you can not anticipate and practice all the open-ended questions that you may get. But with some practice, you can avoid becoming flustered, and learn to deal with the tough questions by falling back on your commercial.

PART III. THE CASE QUESTION

We finally come to the case question. You have had your chance to develop a rapport with the interviewer in the first few minutes, and explain why you possess the skills required to be a consultant in the subsequent 5 to 10 minutes. Over the next 20 to 30 minutes, you will have to prove that you can think "on-the-fly" and actually behave like the consultant you promise to be.

As mentioned, case questions are intentionally abstract, usually obscure and puzzling, and often technical. Their primary purpose is to test a candidate's ability to think and act like a consultant in a live simulation, and to verify whether a candidate truly has the skills claimed in the resume and cover letter. Case questions challenge you to discuss hypothetical situations using either information the interviewer provides, or assumptions you must make based on other, commonly known information. Even if you have no background to help you with the case, you will still be expected to address the question thoughtfully under pressure. Do not be surprised if the interviewer unexpectedly becomes impatient or irritable when discussing the case question. This may just be part of his strategy to test your ability to handle ambiguity in a pressured face-to-face interaction.

Case questions are infinitely variable. They can be based on any industry, company, or organization, and may be either reality based or entirely fictional. Although most deal with business situations, some cases may have to do with everyday life activities (e.g., "Why do the hands on a clock turn clockwise?"). Although cases vary greatly from requiring intense quantitative analysis to demanding purely abstract thinking, most case questions can be grouped into 10 broad types. Table 6.2 illustrates these types with a sample case question for each.

You will find a set of 100 case questions in Appendix II, along with 10 sample answers (one answer for each broad type of case question). Remember that the type of case question is more important than the actual question itself. The set we have provided in Appendix II is merely illustrative and by no means encompasses even the smallest portion of all the possible cases you may get. But if you learn how to recognize each of the types of cases, then you should be able to handle any variety of questions within that type.

Cases are not always clearly stated; interviewers occasionally turn a Resume Review question into a case without telling you. An interviewer may ask, "I see you worked at a bank last summer. Could you

Table 6.2
Ten Types of Case Questions

Type	Example
1. Brain teaser	Why are manhole covers round?
2. Business strategy	Should an airline offer fee services, like travel insurance?
3. Human resource management	What should banks do with their tellers as ATM networks expand?
4. Market entry	How should a gourmet coffee chain locate its stores?
5. Market sizing	How many people surf the Web in a single weekday?
6. Mergers and acquisitions	Should a gin distillery buy a beer company, or chip-dip company?
7. New product introduction	Should a food canning company offer olives with pits, or without?
8. Opportunity assessment	Should a soda bottler backward integrate into the manufacturing of syrup?
9. Pricing	How does the U.S. Post Office price a first-class stamp?
10. Profitability loss	A pharmaceutical company is losing money. What should it do?

tell me about something that didn't work well at the bank and how you would have improved it?" This question may actually be a "business strategy" case rather than simple interviewer curiosity. Although most interviewers stick to more traditional case questions and make a clear transition from the Resume Review to the Case, you should pay close attention to questions that raise hypothetical situations, and be ready to treat scenarios arising from your own experience as case questions.

Even though cases come in many shapes and sizes, they are all designed with the same objective: to test your ability to rationally, methodically, and persuasively discuss the relevant issues of a question, and, ultimately, work your way toward a possible conclusion. Always remember: Interviewers primarily want to see how you think—not whether you can get the right answer. In fact, many interviewers have no idea what the "right" answer is! Instead, most interviewers will grade your performance along the predetermined dimensions of an interview evaluation form, a version of which is presented in Figure 6.2. You will notice that getting the right answer is not one of the dimensions.

Now that you have an idea of what interviewers are looking for, how will you navigate your way through a case? Figure 6.3 outlines a proven five-step process to help you structure your thinking, and methodically work through a case from start to finish. Each step is reviewed in detail in the pages that follow.

Case Step 1. Listen to the Question and Repeat

The first step in answering a case question involves careful, active listening. Too many candidates fall into the trap of misinterpreting the question and then talking on and on for 20 minutes about an entirely different subject. These candidates are doomed from the start, no matter how well they performed on the Resume Review. Interviewers

Figure 6.2
Sample Interview Evaluation Form

Candidate Name	Interviewer Name
School/Company	Title
Job Position	Resume Topics
Round	Case Topic
Date	Location of Interview

	1 Low Performance 5 High Performance 10
Communication Skills	1 ←———5———→ 10
Leadership	1 ←———5———→ 10
Team Orientation	1 ←———5———→ 10
Analytic Skills	1 ←———5———→ 10
Quantitative Skills	1 ←———5———→ 10
Interest in Firm/Consulting	1 ←———5———→ 10
Interpersonal Fit	1 ←———5———→ 10
Presence/Maturity	1 ←———5———→ 10

Areas to probe further _____   Recommendation: ◯ Bring back ◯ Reject

Figure 6.3
The Five Steps of Answering a Case Question

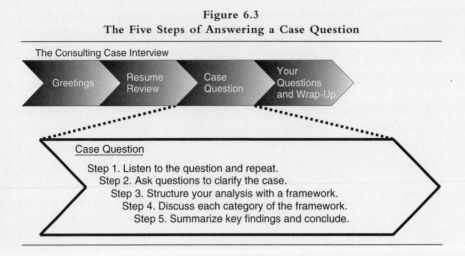

The Consulting Case Interview

Greetings | Resume Review | Case Question | Your Questions and Wrap-Up

Case Question

Step 1. Listen to the question and repeat.
Step 2. Ask questions to clarify the case.
Step 3. Structure your analysis with a framework.
Step 4. Discuss each category of the framework.
Step 5. Summarize key findings and conclude.

may or may not be considerate enough to guide them back on track, and some interviewers are actually entertained by watching candidates crash and burn.

While the interviewer is explaining the question and providing some background information, you may want to take a few notes on your pad. Jot down the question at the top of the page and circle it for easier future reference. Record any numbers or figures you are given, including the units (i.e., dollars, thousands, pounds), and be sure to label what you have written so you won't forget. On occasion, your interviewer will present you with a visual: a chart, graph, set of data points, and so on. Jot down any observations made by the interviewer when presenting the visuals, since these are the "so-what's" that the interviewer evidently finds most important. But remember: Your pad is only a tool to help you recall crucial information; do not take too many notes, and be sure to look up and make eye contact with your interviewer. Once the interviewer has finished, you should mentally review the question and then repeat it to the interviewer for validation—we call this the "question check." Only after the interviewer agrees with your version of the question should you then proceed to the next step. We do have one caveat, however: if the question is simple enough to understand at first blush (e.g., "Tell me how many gas stations are in the United States."), then you probably should not embarrass yourself by mindlessly repeating the question.

Case Step 2. Ask Clarifying Questions

Many case questions are abstract and ill-defined. This is intentional. The interviewer wants to see if you can organize your thoughts and structure a logical discussion. In these situations, you will need to ask some clarifying questions of the interviewer to solicit additional information. For example, a case simulation commonly places you in the consultant's seat and the interviewer in the client's, and requires you to interview the client as if you were in a real consulting engagement. Your client has a great deal of information but does not know which information you need until you ask for it.

Ask questions that will provide you with additional context and background. Take, for example, the following case question: "My company is losing money. What should I do?" You will want to find out what industry the company is in, how long the company has been losing money, and what products or services the company provides. Each of these clarifying questions will help you add structure and lucidity to an ambiguous case. Try to limit the amount of time you spend asking clarifying questions. The purpose here is simply to collect enough information to clarify the question, and be able to move on to the next step: structuring your intended path of analysis by developing a discussion framework.

Case Step 3. Structure Your Analysis with a Framework

Before you jump into the discussion of a case, you should outline your intended path of analysis. Not only will this help you structure your thinking, it will also give your interviewer a road map for following the logic of your discussion. Consultants refer to this analytical outline as a "framework:" an intellectual tool that directs an analysis toward the critical issues of a case in a logical manner. Frameworks, such as Porter's Five Forces or BCG's Growth-Share Matrix, are frequently used in business strategy classes. Others, such as the 4-P's (Product, Price, Place, Promotion) and the 3-C's (Company, Competitors, Customers), are frequently used in marketing classes. These and many others are listed in Table 6.3 and described in more detail in Appendix I.

You should use a framework as a mental checklist of the topics you intend to discuss. Frameworks will help you identify the critical issues logically and systematically, help you reorient your train of thought if you become confused or lost, and recharge your analytic creativity if you begin to run out of ideas. In themselves, frameworks will not give you answers; but they will orient you in the right direction and provide a structure for your thinking.

When selecting a framework for a case, you may want to look beyond the preceding list and develop your own. Use your imagination to build a framework that suits the unique needs of a case. If, for example, you believe that a discussion should revolve around only three of the four P's, then go ahead and use a "3-P's" framework and forget about the fourth. Or, if you believe that a situation is best analyzed by looking at customer fads, weather patterns, and the fuel efficiency of car engines, then offer these three categories as your framework. Do not be afraid to sketch out framework ideas on paper as they come to

Table 6.3
15 Essential Frameworks

1. 3-C's (Company, Competitors, Customers)
2. 4-P's (Product, Price, Place, Promotion)
3. The Boston Consulting Group Growth-Share Matrix
4. Breakeven
5. Cost-benefit analysis
6. Internal-external
7. Life cycle
8. McKinsey 7-S's (Style, Staff, Systems, Strategy, Structure, Skills, Shared Values)
9. Porter's Five Forces
10. Profits
11. Ratio analysis
12. Supply and demand
13. SWOT (Strengths, Weaknesses, Opportunities, Threats)
14. Value chain
15. Value net

mind—a visual image may actually make your task of developing a framework easier.

Many interviewers prefer to see candidates display their creativity and initiative by generating new frameworks, rather than using traditional ones. Some interviewers may even deduct points if a standard framework is inappropriately used, and most will cringe if the popular framework of Porter's Five Forces is mindlessly applied to an analysis. Under no circumstances should you force a case into a framework; rather, always build your framework around the case.

Do not be afraid to take a minute to think in silence when developing a framework. Most interviewers will understand your prudence and appreciate your desire to offer an intelligent—and intelligible—discussion. Even though silence may make you feel uncomfortable, it is well worth the effort to carefully plan the framework that will drive your ensuing analysis. But be aware of the interviewer's response: if he is visibly impatient, or if you take more than a minute out of an already short interview, you should immediately begin introducing your framework. If you are quiet for too long, the interviewer may assume you are frozen by confusion and unable to manage the case question.

After you have outlined your intended path of analysis, ask the interviewer what he thinks: "Does this framework seem reasonable to you?" We call this question the "directional check": seeing whether the interviewer thinks your framework will lead you in the right direction to identify the relevant issues. If you receive agreement, then proceed with the next step. But if the interviewer attempts to direct you in a different direction—"You might want to consider the customers as well," for example—then be sensitive to her advice and adapt your framework accordingly.

Case Step 4. Discuss Each Category of the Framework

Once you have outlined your framework and received agreement from your interviewer, you are ready to tackle the case. Steps 1 through 3 should have taken you no more than 5 minutes, leaving you with a residual 20 to 25 minutes. Pay close attention to the time: If you have a four-part framework such as the 4-P's, then you should allocate approximately 5 minutes to each part, keeping in mind that you will need a few minutes at the end to summarize your thoughts. Consulting interviews are hard to come by; you would not want to be eliminated from the running simply because you ran out of time.

Your discussion of the case should closely follow your framework. Cover one part of the framework at a time, moving sequentially through each of the parts within the allotted time. Try to discuss all the issues relevant to one part of the framework before moving on to the next. Do not jump back and forth from one part to another—after all, the ability to organize your thoughts into a structured analysis is one of the key skills being evaluated.

Be careful to explain each step in your discussion and avoid making logic jumps. Assume that the interviewer has little to no knowledge of the topic and needs a full explanation of your assumptions and conclusions—unless, of course, the interviewer instructs you otherwise. A good indicator of your performance is the interviewer's body language and facial expression. Does he look confused? Perhaps you are making leaps in your logic that he cannot follow. Is he bored? This is probably a sign that you are either belaboring a point or failing to hit the most important points. Not all interviewers will stop you when you are heading in the wrong direction, but many may inadvertently reveal their thoughts through their demeanor.

As you work your way through your framework, be flexible enough to respond to the interviewer's comments. If you are redirected or instructed to look into a particular area in more detail, then do so. If you learn something new from the discussion and feel that an alternative framework would be more appropriate, then offer to adjust your approach, and have the interviewer approve your suggestion. Again, your primary objective is to prove to the interviewer that you are an active and structured thinker. By changing your mind and admitting a mistake, you are demonstrating your ability to self-improve.

When discussing highly quantitative cases, you want your numbers to be reasonably correct. To help you accurately approximate and calculate your numbers, Table 6.4 provides some useful statistics, many of which (but certainly not all) you may want to memorize.

Table 6.4
Useful Statistics

U.S. Statistic	Figure
Total population	281 million
Number of women	139 million
Number of men	133 million
Number of families	71.5 million
Number of households	104 million
People per household	2.6 people
Number of single-person households	27 million
Median household income	US$40,816
Median sale price of new single-family house	US$160,000
GDP	US$9.3 trillion
People below poverty level	32.3 million
Annual births	3.95 million
Annual deaths	2.36 million
Annual marriages	2.34 million
Annual divorces	1.15 million
Occupied housing units	105 million
Motor vehicle registrations	216 million
Airline revenue passengers	635 million
High school graduates	2.9 million
Higher education enrollment	15.07 million
Bachelor degrees awarded	1.15 million
Master degrees awarded	380,000
Doctorate degrees awarded	40,000
Number of metropolitan statistical areas (MSAs)	276
Population in metropolitan statistical areas (MSAs)	218.6 million
Total number of farms	1.9 million

Source: U.S. Census Bureau (all statistics are the latest available as of 2001).

Interviewers deliberately use quantitative cases to test your comfort with numbers and to see if your calculations are not only accurate, but also within a sensible range. You should get into the habit of subjecting your numbers to the "sanity test" by mentally checking them for reasonableness, and by comparing them with other numbers that you know.

For example, if you are calculating the number of gas stations in the United States and assume that a single station services 5,000 cars a day, you can subject the number to the sanity test by figuring out how many minutes per car this would equal. You probably know from your own experience that filling and paying for a tank of gas takes approximately five minutes. So, if your sanity test reveals that each of the 5,000 cars can be serviced by a station in five minutes, then the assumption is reasonable. Assume an average station has four pumps and is open from 6 A.M. to 9 P.M., or 15 hours a day: 4 pumps × 15 hours × 60 minutes = 3,600 pump-minutes. When 3,600 pump-minutes is divided by 5,000 cars, the answer tells us that each car is allotted less than a minute, which is ludicrously low. Thus, the assumption that a station can service 5,000 cars a day is over six times too high! A more reasonable assumption, therefore, would be about 700 cars per day instead of 5,000. By checking your numbers this way, you will end up with more accurate quantitative assessments, and you are even likely to earn points with your interviewer.

What should you do if your numbers are completely off? Or worse still, what if your entire analysis—both conceptual and quantitative—has gone awry in the middle of your discussion? First, do not panic. You may still be able to save your interview. Second, admit your mistakes rather than trying to hide them, and push on. Most interviewers have a strong familiarity with their cases and will not be easily distracted from noticing your mistakes. If you do not admit your error, your interviewer is likely to give you a low score for analytical thinking. On those occasions when you do have to admit a mistake, you should always identify where you made your error and how you would correct it—and then actually make the correction if you have time. This will show that in addition to having an analytical mind, you have the confidence to admit mistakes, and the drive to succeed.

Case Step 5. Summarize and Conclude

As you approach the last few minutes of the case question, you should summarize your thoughts. This is your opportunity to give your discussion closure, to make sure it is not left dangling. Because many interviewers evaluate candidates by their ability to achieve results, they may evaluate your summary as an indication of your aptitude. Your summary should always refer back to the original question—the one that you circled at the top of your pad when you began the case—to ensure that you have directly answered it. Pull together all the conclusions you derived while proceeding through your framework, and summarize what you have learned. Then, offer the appropriate conclusion: a recommendation (e.g., the company should acquire its competitor), a decision (e.g., do not launch the product), or a number (e.g., there are *n*-number of gas stations in the United States).

If you have identified all the critical issues and made a convincing argument, you will probably receive an "ah-ha" reaction from the interviewer. He will be supportive of your effort and perhaps even smile with satisfaction. In most cases, you will know you performed well if your reasoning was structured, logical, and rational. And in the best scenario, you will have learned something, and maybe even have enjoyed the case.

PART IV. QUESTIONS AND WRAP-UP

When you have completed the case, your interviewer will typically finish the interview by asking if you have any questions. Our advice here is simple: You should always come prepared with questions to ask. This is your last chance to show that you have a strong interest in the firm or company, and to prove that you are serious about joining. Last impressions count, and you should do your best to control how your interviewer perceives you. To the extent that your questions are insightful or unique, you may stand apart from the crowd. You can quickly generate a list of questions by reading through promotional materials, browsing Web sites, or reading annual reports, if available. The research you performed earlier when writing cover letters is useful here as well.

Examples of effective questions include: "A number of strategy firms are developing IT practices. Is yours planning to do the same?" or, "How will your firm respond to the unique needs of companies in emerging markets?" Conversely, any question that could have been answered by simply reading the firm's literature or browsing their Web site would be considered a "poor" question (e.g., "Do you have an office in Tokyo?" or "Do you have a financial services practice?").

These questions signal poor preparation and a possible lack of interest in the firm.

Make sure your questions are appropriate to the interviewer's position. You probably will not want to ask a partner or vice president, for example, about the local night life in Chicago. Avoid questions about your interview performance or chances of getting an offer, which could be interpreted as symptoms of poor self-esteem or confidence as well as poor judgment. And never, under any circumstances, ask questions relating to salary or compensation packages until you are extended an offer.

When the interview is over and your interviewer stands to leave, extend a firm handshake, thank him for his time, and mention that you are looking forward to hearing from the firm. Just as first impressions counted when you met your interviewer, here, too, last impressions count as well. A confident and mature "thank-you" puts the final polish on your performance.

PRACTICE MAKES PERFECT

Now that you understand the four parts of the typical case interview, you are ready to develop your case skills through practice. Get together with another person and alternate roles of interviewer and candidate. Or better yet, since it is admittedly difficult to think of interview questions while simultaneously evaluating a candidate's performance, grab a third person to play the role of an outside observer. You may want to photocopy the evaluation form in Figure 6.2, and fill one out for each practice interview.

Run through each of the steps of a case interview, including the greetings and good-byes—and try not to laugh! The closer your role-play replicates the intensity and pressure of an actual case interview, the more you will learn and the better prepared you will be. You should take time in advance to develop challenging "Resume Review" questions from the other person's resume to replicate the Resume Review, and draw case questions from those provided in Appendix II (you may want to start with the ones that have sample answers to get properly oriented). If the candidate is practicing for upcoming interviews at a particular firm, have the candidate bring questions to ask at the end of the interview that relate to that firm. If you know that an upcoming interview will last only 30 minutes, then practice within that time constraint, and cut the candidate off if he runs over. After a few rounds, you may want to change the members of your role-play group to get a diversity of opinions and see a variety of styles.

Do not underestimate the importance of role-playing; there is no better way to learn than through experience. Even if you feel confident after reading through this chapter, you may be caught off guard when it comes time to actually work through a case. Speaking about yourself is harder than you think, and dealing with ambiguous cases can be a nearly impossible task if the interviewer is particularly obnoxious. This process takes time, so you should set time aside to prepare in advance. It will pay off once your real interviews begin.

POST-INTERVIEW FOLLOW-UP

After every round of interviews, mail a thank-you letter to each of your interviewers within a few days, regardless of whether you get called back or receive an offer. It is a polite gesture that has become an accepted practice. Your letters should be typed, written professionally, and as short as possible without seeming like a generic template. Avoid sending handwritten notes, cute cards, or e-mails; faxes may give the impression that you are overeager. If you are writing to multiple people at the same firm, send each person a different letter, since the letters will likely be entered into your personal file and may be compared. Try to personalize your letters by highlighting at least one element of each interview discussion. Reiterate your interest in the firm or company, and tell them you are looking forward to meeting with them again—assuming that you are, of course.

RESPONDING TO REJECTION

What should you do if you are not invited back or are "dinged"? You have invested hours in researching, applying, preparing for case interviews, and meeting with firms—but to no avail, right? Wrong. Being rejected is a natural part of the process of getting hired. Not every firm will like you. And the people around you who are getting offers are also likely to have ding letters wallpapering their rooms. Instead of giving up, use this occasion to learn from your mistakes by proactively requesting feedback from your interviewers.

Call your interviewers and ask for specific reasons for having been rejected. Did you inadequately convince them of your leadership abilities? Was your case performance subpar? Did you use an inappropriate framework? You might also ask for a relative scale ranking of your performance compared with other candidates: Were you a top runner-up, or toward the middle of the pack, or honestly at the bottom? Do not be afraid to push them for concrete answers. It is their responsibility to provide them. Unless you know the reasons for your rejection, you will have no way to improve. But try not to use this information to compare your personality or credentials with those of the candidates who were called back. Since you were not present during their interviews, you cannot judge from their resume and character alone why they were selected over you.

Just remember: You are not deficient if you get rejected. After all, the firm wanted to interview you, and you beat out the competition to get your foot in the door. Your resume was impressive enough to warrant the interview. What you need to do now is take your paper credentials and bring them to life in a face-to-face situation. Go back and practice your case interviews some more, paying particular attention to the improvement areas identified by your interviewers. This is a continuous learning process—think of how far you have come to get to this point.

CHAPTER 7

NEGOTIATING YOUR OFFER

Congratulations! The many hours spent on researching your targeted firms, polishing your resume, and practicing cases have finally paid off with an offer. You have had your last interview, and all you have to do is sign on the dotted line. Right? Wrong. You are not done yet. An important phase of the interviewing process is still before you: negotiating the terms of your offer.

Although the importance of this phase may seem obvious, prospective consultants often find it intimidating and difficult to navigate. Dr. Keith Allred of the Kennedy School of Government at Harvard University has developed a framework for successfully negotiating the terms of an offer. This chapter presents his framework, which highlights the critical issues you will need to think through, and provides step-by-step guidance on how to succeed in the negotiation process.

Negotiating the Terms of an Offer

KEITH G. ALLRED

HARVARD UNIVERSITY

Keith G. Allred is an assistant professor at Harvard's Kennedy School of Government, where he teaches and conducts research on negotiations. He is also a member of the Negotiation Group and Negotiation Roundtable at Harvard Business School, and the Project on Negotiation at Harvard Law School. Before coming to Harvard, Dr. Allred was on the faculty at Columbia University. Dr. Allred has a PhD in Organizational Behavior from UCLA's Anderson Graduate School of Management. Together with Sarah Sandberg, Dr. Allred founded DynamicFeedback.com, a firm that provides online 360-feedback and training services to businesses, law firms, and government agencies.

Receiving an offer from a consulting firm can justifiably feel like the successful conclusion of the rather arduous interviewing process. But after taking much-deserved time to celebrate that success, you will want to think through the next brief, but important, step toward your management consulting career. If you are fortunate, this time will be complicated by the need to choose between multiple offers. In any event, it is time to negotiate the terms of the offer. One of the simplest, yet most important, points in this chapter is that the initial offer you receive from a firm is not necessarily final. Although this can vary widely, many firms expect some negotiation of the terms of the offer. In fact, many of the offers are carefully crafted to begin the negotiation process on terms favorable to the firm.

This chapter provides you with guidelines for succeeding in three critical dimensions of negotiation performance: claiming value, creating value, and maintaining relationships. First, it is important to note that you and the firm will inevitably share both compatible and incompatible interests. One compatible interest would be that the firm wants you to work for them, and you, presumably, also want to work for the firm. A competing interest might have to do with salary: you would rather earn a higher salary, but they would rather pay you a lower one. These are just two of the most obvious examples of many competing and compatible interests. The mix of interests you and the firm share gives rise to the first two dimensions of negotiating the terms of your employment: claiming and creating value.

The mutual interest shared by you and the firm creates a certain amount of mutual value. The firm can generate more revenue by hiring you, and you can generate income and valuable experience by working for them. Thus, the first dimension of negotiation relates to how well you can claim a portion of the value generated by joining the firm. This is the value-claiming, or distributive (i.e., how the available value is distributed), dimension of negotiation.

Beyond the mutual value you and the firm create by joining forces, however, there may be creative ways of integrating your interests with the firm's interests, thereby making your relationship even more mutually beneficial. The extent to which you and the firm realize such opportunities for further joint gain is the value-creating, or integrative, dimension of negotiation.

The third dimension of negotiation reflects that you are entering into an ongoing relationship with the consulting firm. If you are highly successful in obtaining favorable terms for yourself, but sour your relationship with the firm in the process, you will have been less successful than if you had managed the same deal for yourself while still maintaining a good relationship with the firm.

In this chapter, I offer strategies and tactics you can use to claim value, then to create value, and finally to maintain your relationship with the firm. Of course, it is not always easy to succeed in the three dimensions simultaneously.

NEGOTIATING A FAVORABLE DEAL FOR YOURSELF: THE ART OF SUCCESSFULLY CLAIMING VALUE

Throughout this chapter, the fictional example of Ann and Enterprise Consulting Partners (ECP) will illustrate effective negotiation strategies. Ann is about to complete her MBA. After three rounds of interviews,

ECP, a medium-size, rapidly growing management consulting firm offers her a position. ECP's package includes an annual base salary of $60,000, an offer Ann is thrilled to receive. She thinks ECP is an exciting and interesting firm, and the thought of $60,000 in annual salary is a relief as she contemplates her student loans that will soon be coming due. Yet she certainly would not mind earning more than this and actually has friends who have received higher base salaries at similar firms. She starts to consider how she might negotiate with ECP for a better salary.

A number of concepts are useful in thinking about how Ann might proceed. First and foremost, Ann needs to consider what her best option would be if she did not accept an offer from ECP. In *Getting to Yes*, Fisher, Ury, and Patton[1] refer to this point as one's "Best Alternative to a Negotiated Agreement" (BATNA). Second, Ann will want to estimate ECP's own BATNA, which is probably a function of the next most attractive candidate they have identified for hire. Assume that Ann's BATNA is defined by an offer she has from a different firm for $55,000. Aside from differences in salary, she finds this other firm similarly attractive. Assume further that Ann believes ECP has identified another graduating MBA who is as attractive as she is, and that ECP estimates this other candidate would agree to work for them for $75,000.

These two BATNAs—Ann's and ECP's—define what is called "the settlement range," as seen in Figure 7.1. At any offer below $55,000 from ECP, Ann would prefer to go work for the other firm. At any offer for Ann above $75,000, ECP would rather hire the other candidate. Within the settlement range from $55,000 to $75,000, both parties would prefer to conclude a deal with each other rather than go to their best alternative. This means that there is $20,000 ($75,000 − $55,000) worth of value to be claimed between Ann and ECP. The question is: How much of that $20,000 will each party get?

Because BATNAs define the settlement range, Ann's BATNA will be her primary source of leverage in the negotiation with ECP. If Ann had an offer from a similarly attractive consulting firm for $70,000, she would be able to negotiate a better deal for herself than with the offer for $55,000. This illustrates one of the most important points to be made. You should do everything you can to secure the best alternatives for

Figure 7.1
Ann and ECP's Settlement Range

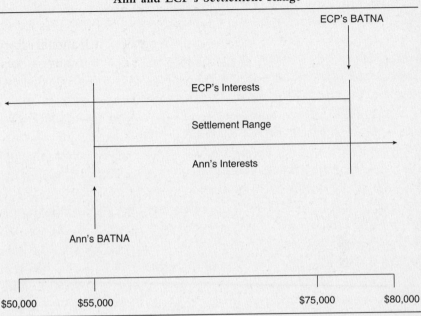

yourself. Even if you have your eye on a particular firm, you need to seek out possibilities elsewhere. Furthermore, once you receive an offer from your preferred firm, you should not necessarily turn down other offers right away. Continuing to get as many offers as you can that are as attractive as possible is one of the best strategies for successfully claiming more value for yourself.

There is a deeper point to be made here: Your BATNA will largely determine your negotiation leverage not only in your current negotiation, but also in negotiations throughout your career. The attractiveness of the alternatives available to you is a function of the skills, abilities, knowledge, experience, and contacts that you bring to your career. This suggests that jobs, particularly early in your career, that provide you with valuable opportunities to develop yourself are of great long-term value because they will allow you to generate future attractive alternatives. Although in the consulting industry there is likely to be a positive correlation between how developmentally beneficial a position is and the salary it offers, the correlation is far from perfect. If you have one offer that provides a lower salary but a better developmental opportunity, and another offer that provides a higher salary but a less interesting opportunity for development, there is much to be said for taking the greater developmental opportunity and accepting the lower salary. It is an investment you will be able to amortize over the entire length of your career.

Returning to the example of Ann, note that ECP's negotiation leverage is similarly a function of their best alternative to Ann. If they identify a candidate as attractive as Ann whom they could hire for $60,000, they should be able to negotiate a more favorable deal for themselves than if they could only hire a similarly attractive candidate for $75,000. Undergraduate and MBA students often feel that all the negotiation leverage is in the hands of the consulting firms. After all, the firms have jobs to offer or not offer. But the preceding analysis should help you realize that consulting firms do not necessarily have more leverage. Rather, their relative leverage is a function of how attractive their alternatives are (i.e., other candidates they can attract) relative to yours (i.e., other offers you can attract).

As the first chapter of this book indicated, management consulting has been growing at extraordinary rates. This means that the demand for management consultants has increased at a similarly extraordinary rate. While the supply of management consultants—people like yourself interested in going into management consulting—may have grown to a degree, it appears to have grown slower than demand over the past decade. This means that the BATNAs of candidates and, thus, their negotiation leverage, have improved relative to those of consulting firms in recent years. Take heart. You are not necessarily without alternatives!

It may be helpful to break down the negotiation process itself and see how the strength of one's BATNA plays out. In Ann's case, ECP offers her $60,000; she has an offer from a similarly attractive firm for $55,000; and she believes that ECP's best alternative is a candidate they could hire for $75,000. What should she do? If she is reasonably sure that she will not get additional offers, it would not be unreasonable, given that her next best alternative is a $55,000 offer, for her to accept the $60,000 offer from ECP. However, because she thinks ECP's best alternative is to hire someone else for $75,000, it would also be reasonable for her to seek a higher salary—up to the $75,000 limit.

When deciding how aggressively to pursue a higher salary, Ann faces a double-edged sword. The more aggressive she is, the greater potential she has to capture value. However, just as in financial investments, moves with higher potential gains also expose one to greater risk of loss. Specifically, research on the effects of the positions that negotiators take can be divided into opening positions or offers, intermediate positions or concessions, and final positions or final offers. The more extreme one's opening offers, the more stingy one's concession making. And the more aggressively one uses final offers, the more likely the negotiation will end in no agreement. But if an agreement is actually concluded, it will be all the more favorable.

Ann should take into account these potential benefits and risks when choosing her course of action. Two rules of thumb are helpful in thinking about an opening offer to make in response to the offer of $60,000. First, research suggests that negotiations typically settle at the mid-point between the two opening offers. So if she offers $70,000, chances are they will settle at $65,000. Second, Lax and Sebenius[2] suggest that Ann should make an opening offer that she is 90 percent to 95 percent certain is higher than the highest figure ECP is willing to pay.

Assume that Ann decides to ask for a salary of $75,000. Given that ECP has offered her $60,000, one or both sides will need to concede, or the negotiation will obviously end in no agreement since ECP could hire the other equally attractive recruit for $75,000. But if concessions are made, how large should they be? If it is likely that there will be a couple of rounds of counteroffers or concessions, it is generally wise to graduate the level of concessions. If Ann expects to make two more counteroffers before it is all concluded, she will want her second concession to be smaller than her first. Imagine that ECP counters her $75,000 with $65,000. She could now counter with $70,000, a concession of $5,000 over her prior offer. If ECP now counters with $67,000, she could counter that with $68,000, a concession of $2,000 over her last offer. By making a second concession that is substantially smaller than the first, Ann signals that she is approaching a point beyond which she will not go.

At some point in this process of concession and counterconcession, one of the parties may concede as far as it is willing and will then make a final offer. The implicit meaning of a final offer is that the party is willing to walk away from the deal rather than concede any further. In other words, the party is making a final commitment to that offer. As mentioned, however, Ann faces a double-edged sword here. The more ironclad she makes her commitment seem, the more likely it will be successful in inducing ECP to give her that salary amount. In the event that ECP is unwilling to settle at the point where Ann commits herself, however, this same appearance of commitment creates a situation from which it is difficult to extract herself. Either she must hold to the commitment and lose the job, or she must find a way to communicate that she was not committed to the offer after all, and is actually willing to concede. It is obviously more difficult for her to make a credible commitment after having a prior commitment unmasked as a bluff.

To summarize, when seeking to claim value, you must make a choice between more aggressive, higher risk, higher potential gain moves, and less aggressive, lower risk, lower gain moves. Two additional general points should be made about claiming value. First, firms vary widely in the extent to which they are willing to negotiate the terms of the offers they make. Some firms come in with their best offer up front and stick with it, refusing to negotiate with any recruit. Some firms make a policy decision that, because of the value they place on maintaining equity among members of the firm, or because of financial constraints, they will not offer different recruits different compensation packages. Of course, firms can also intimate that they have such policies as a negotiation ploy, when, in fact, they do negotiate.

It is difficult to get reliable information on how willing a firm is to negotiate, but you should learn what you can. Speak to consultants who have been recently hired by the firm. You will have to judge whether there are individuals with whom you feel comfortable discussing this topic. You might also try to identify friends or associates who have secondhand knowledge of your firm through acquaintances who have recently joined that firm. Or speak to pioneering classmates who have also received offers and have already attempted to negotiate. Not only do you want to find out whether the firm will negotiate the terms of the offer, but also the extent to which they will negotiate, and on which terms they are most willing to negotiate. In the Ann and ECP example, I have used base salary as the only issue under negotiation. This, in fact, is the one component that consulting firms are often least willing to negotiate. Frequently, firms are more flexible on issues such as the amount and timing of signing bonus, annual bonus, profit sharing, moving stipends, or tuition reimbursement.

When deciding whether to negotiate, it helps to know the typical range of consulting compensation packages. Although the figures are not the result of a scientific survey, I can provide a general sense of the range of recent compensation packages based on figures reported by Kennedy Research Group,[3] and by informal polling of recent recruits. The ranges can differ according to a number of factors, including prior experience, education, and the size of the consulting firm. In 1998, undergraduates taking entry-level consulting positions tended to earn an average annual salary of $40,000 to $45,000, with some firms offering a modest signing bonus of around $5,000. For MBAs from top schools, average starting salaries were approximately $92,500, with signing bonuses ranging from $30,000 to $40,000. At most firms, year-end bonuses ranged from 10 percent to 25 percent of salary.

In addition to annual salary, signing bonuses, and year-end bonuses, candidates often receive some financial support for their relocation. Sometimes this comes in the form of a cash amount, but more often it is provided as a reimbursement for moving costs actually accrued, up to a predetermined limit. The moving reimbursement or stipend may range from $0 to $20,000. And candidates are sometimes offered, or negotiate for themselves, reimbursement for costs incurred during a housing search (e.g., realtor fees, travel, and hotel charges).

ENLARGING THE PIE: THE ART OF CREATING VALUE

Now you know that negotiation is a win-lose proposition. A gain in salary for you represents an equal financial loss for the firm and vice versa. However, favorable changes in the terms must not necessarily come at the expense of the consulting firm. In other words, besides claiming a portion of the value pie for oneself, it is often possible to increase the overall size of the pie by dovetailing the two parties' interests in creative ways. The most common method of creating value can be illustrated by introducing the issue of a signing bonus into the negotiation between Ann and ECP.

Imagine that as Ann nears the end of business school, having had two years of very little income and high expenses, she is in a cash crunch. She is near her credit limits on her credit cards, and she knows that she will have considerable expenses over the next few months before starting her full-time job. Her old, unreliable car will no longer suffice, and she will have to trade it in for a new one. She needs a serious wardrobe upgrade to be ready for her new job. And, if at all possible, she would like to go to Europe with several business school friends after graduation. They will all be starting jobs with enormously demanding schedules, and this will be their last real opportunity for some recreation.

Imagine, also, that Ann spoke with another recent hire at ECP and discovered that ECP will negotiate salary, but only within a restricted range. The firm hesitates to bring in new recruits at different salaries due to equity concerns. Moreover, ECP would prefer to keep the monthly fixed cost of paying Ann's salary to a minimum. However, ECP is willing to negotiate the signing bonus since it is a one-time variable cost. This situation could be represented by the payoff schedules in Table 7.1. The numbers in parentheses indicate the relative value to each negotiator of concluding a particular issue at a particular level.

The point values in this case reflect Ann's preference for a higher salary and signing bonus (i.e., the greater the salary and the greater the signing bonus, the more points she gains) and ECP's preference to give her a lower annual salary and signing bonus (i.e., the lower the salary and the lower the signing bonus, the more points they gain). However, salary and signing bonus are not of equal importance to the two parties. Because of her current cash crunch, Ann is more interested in the signing bonus than in the salary amount within the range under consideration.

Table 7.1
Payoff Schedule

Ann's Payoff Schedule		ECP's Payoff Schedule	
Annual Salary	Signing Bonus	Annual Salary	Signing Bonus
$69,000 (100)	$13,000 (250)	$69,000 (50)	$13,000 (20)
68,000 (80)	11,000 (200)	68,000 (100)	11,000 (40)
67,000 (60)	9,000 (150)	67,000 (150)	9,000 (60)
66,000 (40)	7,000 (100)	66,000 (200)	7,000 (80)
65,000 (20)	5,000 (50)	65,000 (250)	5,000 (100)

This difference in relative weight is reflected in the greater points allocated to the signing bonus figures (i.e., an additional 50 points for each additional increment of signing bonus versus an additional 20 points for each additional increment of salary). In contrast, ECP's point allocation reflects the importance the firm places on salary level due to internal equity issues and a desire to limit fixed monthly costs relative to the less important one-time cost of a signing bonus (i.e., an additional 50 points for each lower increment of salary versus an additional 20 points for each lower increment of signing bonus).

Ann and ECP have offsetting priorities on these two issues. This creates integrative potential or the potential to increase the size of the pie that will be divided between them. Imagine that Ann responds to ECP's opening offer by saying, "I would prefer to receive a salary of $69,000 and a $13,000 signing bonus." ECP responds with a counteroffer of $66,000 and a $7,000 signing bonus. Through this typical dance of counteroffers, Ann and ECP haggle to the midpoint of the ranges for both issues, coming to an agreement in which Ann receives a salary of $67,000 and a signing bonus of $9,000. That agreement would be worth 210 "points" to each of them, for a total pie worth 420 points.

Now assume that Ann follows a different strategy. Drawing on the information from the recent hire at ECP, she responds to ECP's initial offer by saying, "I understand that you are particularly concerned with the salary amounts you offer because of fixed-cost and equity issues. Since I have some pressing financial needs at the present time, I'm willing to concede to a salary of $67,000, if you will give me a $13,000 signing bonus." Recognizing the opportunity for joint gain, ECP responds by saying, "We will come up to $13,000 on the signing bonus, if you'll agree to a salary of $65,000." Ann accepts, resulting in an agreement that is at the lowest end of the range on salary and at the highest end of the range for signing bonus. This agreement yields 270 points to each, for a total pie of 540—120 points more than the prior agreement in which they haggled to the middle on both issues.

This strategy, in which each party concedes on their issue of lesser importance to gain on their issue of greater importance, is known as "logrolling." You can use this strategy to create value anytime you and the firm attach offsetting values to different issues. The logrolling approach to creating value suggests a deeper point: It is critical to think through the relative importance of various issues in advance of your negotiation. Since it is unlikely you will be able to get everything you want, you need to focus on getting what is most important to you.

Once you clarify the relative importance of different issues for yourself, you face another dilemma in choosing how forthcoming and explicit to be in communicating those relative preferences to the firm. By telling ECP that she cares more about the signing bonus than about salary, Ann makes it more likely that she and ECP will discover a mutually beneficial trade-off. However, she also exposes herself to possible exploitation.

Imagine that ECP is actually willing, if necessary, to pay Ann both a $75,000 annual salary and a $13,000 signing bonus, and that their initial offer was just a way of trying to start the negotiation on terms favorable to the firm. Upon hearing that Ann has a preference for an increase in signing bonus over an increase in salary, the firm may respond opportunistically. They may disingenuously say, "Since the signing bonus represents an out-of-pocket expense long before you begin to really contribute to the firm's profitably, it is a particularly important issue to us as well. But we want to be responsive to your wishes, so we would be willing to give you a $10,000 signing bonus if you are willing to recognize the up-front cost we have to take and accept a salary of $62,000."

As you decide how forthcoming to be with information about the relative weights you attach to different issues, you will want to consider both the potential for discovering mutually beneficial trade-offs and the risk of exploitation. At a minimum, if you come to feel that you will have to make concessions to reach agreement, be sure to concede on issues of less importance to you before conceding on issues of greater importance.

MAKING ALLIES OUT OF YOUR NEW COLLEAGUES: THE ART OF MAINTAINING AND ENHANCING RELATIONSHIPS

As you negotiate the terms of your offer, remember that you may eventually work with these same people. On occasion, an aggressive recruit can take advantage of an excess demand for consultants in a limited supply market to negotiate an extraordinary deal for herself. While a firm may agree to an unusually generous package to win an attractive prospect away from competing firms, the firm can end up begrudging it after the fact, and resenting the recruit who extracted the generous offer. This can make working relationships difficult once the new employee starts. Besides being the object of resentment, the unusually well-compensated recruit may become subject to extremely high work load and performance demands from the firm. This much you can usually count on—your firm will make every effort to get the full dollar's worth out of you.

Research indicates that ill will related to job offer negotiations is only partly a result of the firm resenting the recruit's success in negotiating a favorable offer. The resentment can be even greater if the firm feels as though the negotiation *process,* rather than the outcome, was unfair or unsavory. If the members of the firm involved in the negotiation come to feel like victims of extreme gamesmanship, or if they believe that the recruit exhibited an arrogant or disrespectful attitude, then the candidate will later pay for the lucrative package through the ill will it generated.

The same principles apply to you. If both the process and outcome of the negotiation leave you feeling exploited, you may want to reconsider whether these are the people with whom you want to spend the lion's share of your waking hours. Generally, consulting firms try to put their warmest and friendliest face forward during the recruiting process. But in the negotiating process, you may find the firm less friendly—and you will rarely find it more friendly.

CONCLUSION

You would be well advised to do as much planning and preparation as you can prior to negotiating the terms of your offer. As mentioned, try to generate as attractive a set of alternatives as you can, and try to gather as much information as you can about how firms tend to negotiate with recruits. With that information in mind, plan your approach. Use the strategies in this chapter to achieve the goals of claiming value for yourself, creating value where possible, and maintaining a good working relationship with the firm. While planning is extremely helpful, you must also be ready to change your plan as new information comes to light during the negotiation.

Finally, remember that what you offer the firm is as valuable to them as what they offer is to you. The fact that they have made you an offer in the first place is evidence of this. Moreover, the current situation of demand for new recruits exceeding supply should give you a heightened sense of confidence as you enter your negotiations.

EPILOGUE

Now that you are armed with a powerful set of negotiating techniques, you have all the tools you need to jump into the consulting career search. The process is challenging, but you have already separated yourself from the pack by reading this book. You have overcome the first challenge of understanding the process. We have covered a great deal of material, detailing each of the steps you will have to go through to get a job in consulting. At this point, you should have a realistic understanding of what consultants do, how you can successfully gain entrance to the industry, and finally, how you might negotiate the best offer for yourself.

The second challenge in the job search is execution. Understanding the consulting industry helps, but it does not get you through rounds of interviews. You should now read through the following appendixes, which have been carefully designed to jump-start your research and to sharpen your case interviewing skills. If you use these appendixes properly, you should be able to hurdle the challenge of execution, and develop consistently dependable and impressive interviewing skills. Remember that the more you know about the industry and its entrance requirements, the more confident and relaxed you will be when working your way to an offer. And the more you practice case interviews, the better prepared you will be and the more enjoyable you will ultimately find them to be.

We are confident that you will learn a great deal about yourself through this process, and are even likely to surprise yourself with newfound analytical prowess. By practicing case questions, you will learn how to approach problems in an entirely new way, and to apply common sense and rational insight to questions where you might previously have had no idea where to begin.

Getting a job in consulting is challenging, but you have the tools to succeed. Now is the time to sharpen your tools, and to convince your interviewers that you are the candidate they want. We wish you the best as you work your way toward your new position.

APPENDIX I

FIFTEEN ESSENTIAL FRAMEWORKS

Before you begin to practice case questions, you should familiarize yourself with the most common business frameworks. This section will provide you with a basic understanding of the 15 frameworks most often used to answer case questions. Although many of them may seem familiar, you should use the frameworks as you practice answering case questions to truly become comfortable with them. The descriptions that follow the frameworks are simplifications and are intended either to refresh your memory if you have had prior framework experience or to provide an introduction to the fundamentals if you have not. If a framework is new or unfamiliar to you, we highly recommend reading additional texts to fully capture their nuances.

As you practice answering case questions, remember three things: First, well-prepared candidates will have learned to use frameworks as a mental checklist of topics to discuss. Some of the mnemonics used to name the frameworks (e.g., 3-C's, 4-P's, or 7-S's) may seem a bit foolish at first, but they are intentionally simplified to serve as memory hooks and to help you discipline your thinking as you answer case questions. In addition to helping you think through a case question, frameworks also help interviewers follow your analysis.

Second, the frameworks presented here are a mere subset of the limitless number you could generate. Feel free to use your creativity and generate your own. Recruiters appreciate intellectual creativity and may give you points for taking risks. Third, you should never try to squeeze a case into a framework; rather, the framework should be carefully selected or designed to suit the case. Only select or build a framework for a case once you have a clear understanding of the question and its relevant issues.

Please note that not all candidates will be expected to have the same level of understanding of frameworks. Business school students will be expected to have a thorough understanding of all the frameworks and how to properly apply them. Other graduate school students, career-changing professionals, and undergraduate students are advised to be familiar with all the frameworks, but mose likely will not be held to the same high standard of expertise as business school students.

3-C'S (COMPANY, COMPETITORS, CUSTOMERS)

The 3-C's is a classic marketing strategy framework. An effective marketing strategy leverages a company's relative competitive advantage (RCA) which is the term used to describe the degree to which a company possesses unique properties that enable it to outperform its competitors. The analytical model most commonly used to identify the sources and strength of a company's RCA is the "3-C's" framework depicted in Figure AI.1, which explores the interaction of a company with its competitors and customers.

Company

The strength of a company's RCA is partially determined by the unique advantages the company possesses over the competition. Sources of advantage include distinguishing core competencies, such as product innovation, production efficiencies, responsiveness to changing customer needs, and ability to optimize market-entry timing. Proprietary corporate resources such as patents, established supplier and

Figure AI.1
3-C's Framework

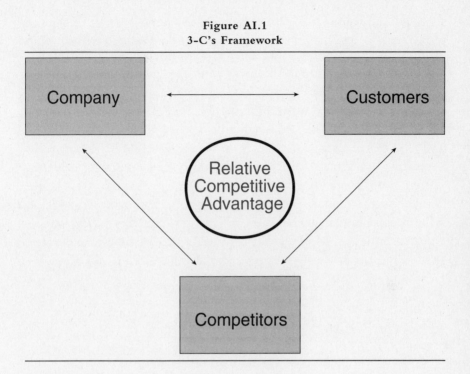

buyer networks, and exclusive technology capabilities may also provide competitive advantages to a company, as can structural arrangements such as joint ventures or strategic alliances.

Competitors

Similarly, the competition may possess unique core competencies that could weaken the company's RCA, such as superior production technologies or distribution networks, preferential sourcing relationships, or superior market positioning (i.e., the highest share of customer spending in a market). And the business strategies of the competition may impact the company's RCA over time: Predatory strategies are likely to pose serious threats, whereas collaborative or complementary strategies may actually benefit the company by increasing overall industry profitability.

Customers

As purchasers of products and services, customers are the final judges of a company's marketing strategy. Companies that understand the interests, needs, and behavior patterns of customers are able to produce superior goods, and thus strengthen their RCA. Persuasive marketing messages can be constructed around the behavior patterns of customers, and used to lure customers away from the competition. And companies can target emerging pockets of opportunity by monitoring changing customer needs and innovating their products or services accordingly.

An integrated analysis of the 3-C's enables a company to assess its relative competitive advantage in an industry, take the appropriate actions to either build or solidify its RCA, and ultimately generate a marketing strategy that captures optimal value from its RCA.

4-P'S (PRODUCT, PRICE, PLACE, PROMOTION)

The marketing strategy of a product must be sensitive to the interrelated forces operating within the market where the product will be sold. A 4-P's analysis will provide the necessary context, and will enable a company to generate a superior marketing strategy by evaluating the product, its pricing strategy, its place of sale, and its means of promotion, relative to the competition. A schematic of this framework is provided in Figure AI.2.

Product

The attractiveness of a product to a customer is in part determined by its characteristics and features. Products that appear to offer greater value to a customer relative to competitor products, either through superior functionality, style, durability, or cost-effectiveness, may have the advantage of differentiation. However, products in commodity markets are perceived by customers to be similar if not identical in value regardless of feature or characteristic, and are typically only differentiated by low price. Over time, a product tends to pass through a

4-P's (Product, Price, Place, Promotion)

Figure AI.2
4-P's Framework

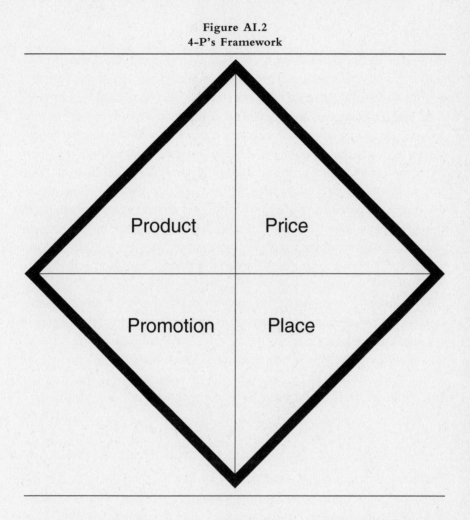

series of "attractiveness" stages, depicted by the product life cycle curve (described later in this appendix): New products are developed and introduced to the market; they then gain share and reach a natural maturity once sales plateau; thereafter, the product tends to decline in popularity due to either obsolescence or competitive substitution, and eventually production may be discontinued altogether. Understanding how customers perceive the value of a product with respect to substitutes is critical to the development of an effective marketing strategy.

Price

The price of the product must be sensitive to customer perceptions, as well as to the product's features and characteristics. Products that are perceived to offer superior value relative to the competition merit premium prices, whereas products that are not differentiated will rarely sell at a premium, and must instead be priced below the market reservation price for the product. In a perfectly competitive market, the price of a product will over time equal the marginal cost of production. But in a monopoly, the market price will exceed the perfectly competitive price, and the quantity supplied will be less than the amount supplied in a perfectly competitive market, allowing the company to earn excess profits. But price-setting can be more than reactive—it can also be an active driver of a company's product strategy: a product's price can be set below market average to drive higher sales volume (a "volume-play" strategy), or it can be set high to maximize the unit margin (a "margin-optimization" strategy). Or the company may try to maximize profits by price discriminating (charging different customer segments different prices), or by extending special pricing offers such as volume discounts, rebates, limited-time promotions, or bundled prices (i.e., reduced price when purchased together with another product).

Place

The place of sale, or sales channel, determines how a product will come in contact with customers. Alternative sales channels include retail, catalog, door-to-door, and e-commerce. Not all products are suited for all sales channels, and conversely not all sales channels can effectively sell all products. The choice of sales channel has a direct impact on sales volume and pricing: a broad retail network will likely drive high sales volume and a higher price to cover the costs of delivering the goods to market; conversely, a narrower direct sales channel such as mail-order catalogs or the web may limit sales volume due to more limited customer exposure, and perhaps offer lower prices due to the absence of middlemen (e.g., third-party wholesale distributors) who tend to charge for additional services (e.g., storage, delivery, financing, payment processing, and promotion).

Promotion

The promotion of a product is critical to raising customer awareness, and to inducing trial of the product through a purchase. Promotions can be broad-based, attempting to communicate a single message to multiple customer groups simultaneously, or it can be targeted, tailoring specific messages to different customer segments. A product's degree of differentiation will naturally make it more attractive to certain customer segments than others. Similarly, a product's price may attract only certain customer segments, and its primary sales channel may give it access to even fewer. Here, again, targeted promotions may be preferable.

The product, price, and place dimensions all have a direct impact on promotion, and collectively, the four dimensions characterize the environment within which a product strategy must operate.

THE BOSTON CONSULTING GROUP GROWTH-SHARE MATRIX

The growth-share matrix characterizes the relative attractiveness of a company within its industry according to two dimensions: relative market share, and rate of industry growth. All companies can be placed into one of the four quadrants displayed in Figure AI.3.

Companies that are considered to be worth starting, buying, or investing in lie within the upper right or "star" quadrant (high market share and high growth). These companies are expected to flourish because they are already the dominant players, and over time will become even more dominant in a high-growth market. Conversely, companies that should be sold, closed, or avoided as investments are situated in the lower left or "dog" quadrant (low market share and low growth). These companies are weak and relatively small, existing in stagnant markets. Lower right "cash cow" companies, due to their low growth

Figure AI.3
The Boston Consulting Group Growth-Share Matrix

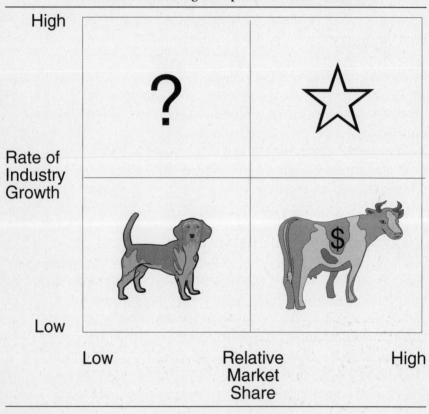

High

Rate of
Industry
Growth

Low

Low   Relative   High
Market
Share

and high market share, should be run with the primary purpose of capturing the maximum short-run value—or simply stated, milking the company for all its worth. These companies are worth a lot today, but may not continue to be so in the future. And lastly, companies in the upper left "question mark" quadrant have an uncertain future due to their low relative market share, and are not guaranteed to become attractive over time even though they operate in a high growth market. They may or may not be able to capture the value that is being generated by the market's growth, since their small size may make them vulnerable to the competition.

The growth–share matrix can also be used to discuss product differentiation: brand managers would be advised to focus marketing investments on products in either the star or cash cow quadrants (and arguably even the question mark quadrant), since their high relative market share is likely to secure a high return on marketing investment. New product developers would be wise to invest R&D dollars on products that are likely to lie in the "star" quadrant—high industry growth and high relative market share—since these promise to offer the longest-term profitability.

The matrix is versatile and can also be used to segment markets, or to discuss the evolution of a product over time from a question mark, to a star, to a cash cow, to eventually a dog (i.e., obsolescence).

BREAKEVEN

The attractiveness of a new business venture or product introduction can be evaluated using a breakeven analysis, which determines the minimum profitability required for an operation to pay for its startup and operating costs without losing or making money. Figure AI.4 details the required inputs into a breakeven equation, with fixed costs (e.g., start-up costs of purchasing equipment, technology, facilities, etc.) in the numerator and operating profits (e.g., the money left over

Figure AI.4
Breakeven Equation

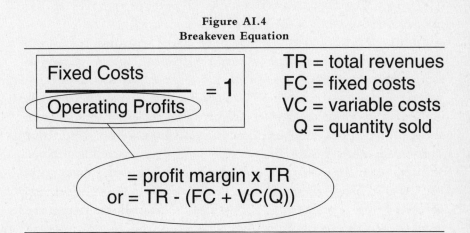

217

from sales after the variable costs of production are deducted) in the denominator, all set equal to zero.

If, for example, you know the fixed costs of a new business venture and are trying to decide whether to launch the business, you can use the breakeven equation to determine the minimum sales the business will require to make zero profits. If the resulting sales figure seems reasonably attainable, then the business venture may be attractive; but if the required sales are ludicrously high, then the venture has little hope of succeeding. This same type of analysis can be performed if you know the operating margin of a business, for example, and need to determine the minimum number of product units sold to cover the fixed costs. Or if you know the total profits of the venture over a given period of time (e.g., have a contract to supply a certain amount of product to a single buyer with a predetermined price markup), then you can calculate the maximum amount of money the business can spend on start-up costs without losing money. So long as you have data for either the numerator or denominator of the equation, you should be able to calculate the other variables, and make a decision.

COST-BENEFIT ANALYSIS

Cost-benefit analysis helps to determine whether the beneficial outcomes of a project are sufficient to justify the cost of undertaking the project. This approach is often used to assess capital expenditure projects. The strength of this framework is its simplicity and wide applicability. Simply stated, if the benefits of a project outweigh the associated costs, then the project is worth completing, as seen in Figure AI.5.

For example, assume that you are considering opening a lemonade stand. Assume that you can operate your lemonade business for only one day. Should you do it? Using a cost-benefit framework, you would first look at all the potential cost drivers for your new project: ingredients, plastic cups, materials to construct an advertising sign and stand, and so on. Then you would compare these costs against the expected benefits (i.e., the number of cups of lemonade you expect to sell during a single day). If the difference is positive, then you should

Figure AI.5
Cost–Benefit Analysis

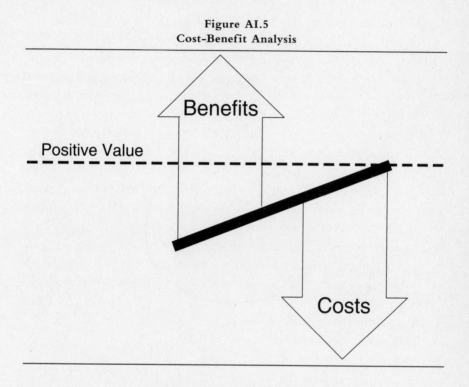

begin your business. In finance, net present value (NPV) analysis is a slightly more sophisticated version of this because it takes into consideration the impact of time, risk of failure and the cost of financing the project. Although a simple cost–benefit analysis alone will rarely get you through a complex case, it can help you structure your thinking in identifying all the drivers that need to be considered.

INTERNAL-EXTERNAL ISSUES

The internal-external framework simply divides the analysis of a case into two parts, as seen in Figure AI.6: internal issues (e.g., within a company, an industry, a country), and external issues (e.g., outside the same company, industry, country).

Because of its simplicity and generic applicability, this framework can be helpful in starting an analysis to a case question, especially when

Figure AI.6
Internal-External Issues

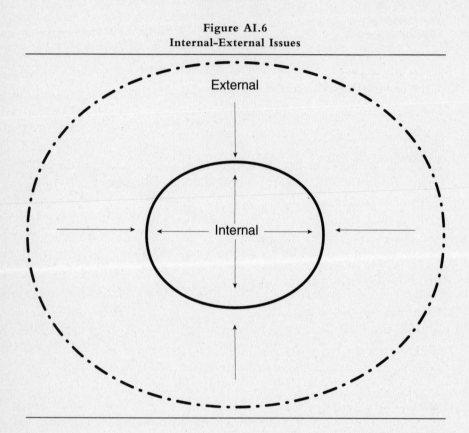

you are flustered. For example, if an interviewer wanted you to determine why profits at a company had been steadily decreasing for the last year, you would naturally want to use the profit equation (described later in this appendix). But what if you could not remember the profit equation? You could save yourself by using an internal-external framework to look for causes of declining profits first inside the company, and then outside the company.

Looking internally, you could discuss the elements of the balance sheet to determine whether the cause is hidden there. Perhaps a new factory was built recently that necessitated a rise in prices? This, in turn, might have negatively impacted sales because of a highly elastic consumer demand function, and therefore the decline in profits would likely be due to diminishing revenues. Notice that we took an internal diagnosis and moved our analysis to the external in this example. We started by evaluating the impact of a new fixed asset, and ended by linking the cause of the decline in profits to the elasticity of consumer demand.

LIFE CYCLE

Although life cycles have multiple applications, they all have the unique feature of discussing business issues over time. For example, a product life cycle is used to explain the evolution of product attractiveness over time, from the product's introduction, to growth, to maturity, to decline. As a product evolves through each of these stages, its sales will fluctuate, resulting in a slanted "S-shape" curve like the one displayed in Figure AI.7.

Similarly, a service life cycle can be used to describe the changing demand for a service over time, such as for travel agencies, which were once essential to the planning of almost all trips, but today are losing market share to direct-booking channels, such as Internet sites like

Figure AI.7
A Product Life Cycle

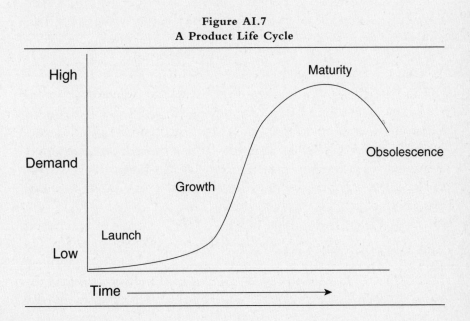

Expedia or Travelocity. Or a life cycle can be used to describe the spending patterns of an individual over the course of his life, from childhood, to having a family, to retiring.

In each of these cases, life cycles can be used to develop strategy. Brand managers, for example, will most likely want to introduce new products when their existing products approach the zero-growth stage, so that the sales growth of new products will compensate for the expected decline of existing products. Life cycles can also be used to describe seasonality (e.g., snowblowers sell more rapidly during winter months than summer), and as a result be schematically drawn as a series of cycles, or a wave.

MCKINSEY 7-S'S (STRATEGY, SKILLS, SHARED VALUES, STRUCTURE, STAFF, SYSTEMS, STYLE)

The McKinsey 7-S framework was developed to evaluate the effectiveness of an organization by explicitly considering seven critical elements of a firm: strategy, institutional skills, shared values (firm culture), structure, staff (people), systems, and style. As Figure AI.8 shows, the key elements of a company are interdependent, and thus, must work together to produce an effective organization.

Strategy

A strategy is a map or a plan of an integrated set of actions designed to achieve specific corporate objectives (e.g., operational efficiency, growth, shareholder value). The strategy is important because it gives direction and purpose to the company, sorts and identifies key organizational needs, and provides a benchmark for measuring the company's success.

Institutional Skills

Institutional skills refer to an organization's capabilities as well as the abilities of its managers and staff. Institutional skills drive organizational

Figure AI.8
7-S's Framework

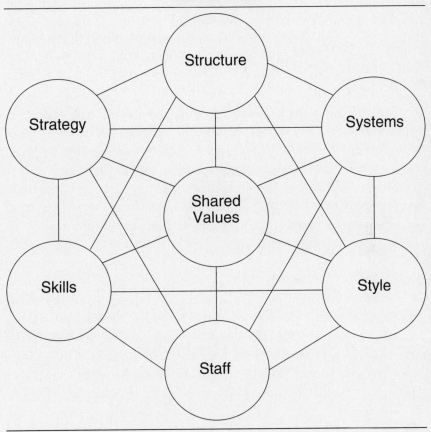

Source: T.J. Peters and R.H. Waterman, *In Search of Excellence* (New York: Warner Books, 1983).

design. That is, other organizational elements must be designed to either build needed skills or properly exploit existing skills. Strategy development is incomplete without explicit consideration of the institutional skills necessary to execute the strategy.

Shared Values

Shared values refers to the culture of the company. Although it is difficult to objectively evaluate company culture, shared value attributes include attitude toward work, competitive/cooperative nature among colleagues, and communication with corporate leadership. Although this is the most difficult "S-dimension" to influence, it may be shaped by frequent, and consistent communication from top management.

Structure

Structure refers to the organization of the company: who reports to whom, and how tasks are divided up and integrated. The structure of the organization should be designed to facilitate coordination and integration between the layers of management and staff and focus the organization's attention. The structure should be consistent with the company's culture and skills. The type of structure (e.g., degree of centralization) is one of the key considerations of this dimension.

Staff

This refers to the company's people in terms of their capabilities, experience, and potential. A company's staff ultimately determines whether the company is able to deliver superior products or service value. Staff composition and productivity are important determinants of present and future strategic success. Key issues include where to look for new hires, who to hire, how to train, and how to properly structure incentives.

Systems

Systems refers to the processes and procedures that facilitate daily activities. Some important systems include management information systems, incentive systems, and communication. When evaluating the systems of a company, it is important to consider formal or institutionalized systems, and informal or ad hoc systems.

Style

This refers to the style of leadership that guides a company or organization. At an individual level, a leader's style can be characterized by his or her prevailing approach to decision making and management (e.g., supportive or aggressive, analytical or emotional). An individual's style can be revealed by how that person speaks and conducts meetings, works with partners and negotiates agreements, what questions he or she asks, and what settings he or she appears in. At a higher organizational level, leadership style can refer to the corporate culture that influences the way decisions are made and employees interact with each other (e.g., cut-throat or collaborative, top-down or bottom-up). Leadership style, at either an individual or an organizational level, has the power to shape corporate values and reinforce strategic initiatives.

PORTER'S FIVE FORCES

Michael Porter's Five Forces model characterizes the dynamics of competitive rivalry within an industry. Figure AI.9 schematically illustrates

Figure AI.9
Porter's Five Forces Industry Analysis

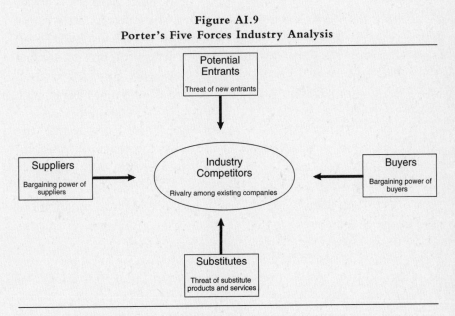

Source: Porter, M. *Competitive Strategy: Techniques for Analyzing Industries and Competitors* (Boston: Harvard Business School Press, 1980).

the set of players that collectively shape an industry, and depicts the competitive forces that determine an industry's overall profitability.

The five forces interact as follows: (1) Within an industry, *companies* compete for market share by attempting to win customers and capture business from rivals. An activity of one company is likely to be met with a competitive reaction from another company, which in turn is likely to generate other competitive activities from other companies. Industries that have a high number of competitors are likely to face more intense competitive rivalry, and as a result the overall profitability of the industry will tend to be lower.

Influencing this cycle of rivalry are other competitive forces: (2) *Suppliers* (entities that provide necessary inputs to the production of the industry good) may be large enough to wield bargaining power over a company, or may band together to generate greater collective bargaining power. Powerful suppliers can increase the costs of inputs, and as a result reduce the profits of the input user. (3) Similarly, *buyers* (customers that purchase the good produced by the industry) may individually or collectively purchase enough quantity of the good to wield bargaining power over a company, and be able to drive prices down. (4) Potential *new entrants* into an industry may threaten to steal market share from existing industry competitors by offering unique customer benefits, for example, or by benefiting from preferential agreements with buyers or suppliers. (5) The industry's product may be threatened with replacement by *substitutes* from other industries.

The collective activity of all five forces produces a competitive environment in which each rival company must respond to, and more importantly anticipate, each other's competitive actions, to protect their own interests.

PROFITS

The profit equation is a function of two drivers, as seen in Figure AI.10: revenue and cost. Two versions of the equation can be written to encompass different levels of detail.

The profit equation can be used as a guide to step through most profit-related case questions, such as companies losing money, or

Profits = Total Revenues – Total Costs
or
$$\pi = (P \times Q) - (FC + VC(Q))$$

π = Profits   P = Price

TR = Total Revenues   FC = Fixed Costs

VC = Variable Costs   Q = Quantity Sold

incurring significant costs, or encountering sudden sales declines. To use the equation, look at each of the two drivers separately, breaking each down into its component parts. As the second, more detailed version of the equation shows, there are essentially four inputs that affect profit: price, fixed costs, variable costs, and quantity sold. If price increases, profits should increase. Likewise, if quantity increases, so too should profits increase. However, if either fixed costs or variable costs increase, profits should then decrease. The profit equation gives you a structure for remembering not only what the elements are, but also whether the elements cause profits to increase or decrease. For example, an interviewer may ask you the following question:

Company A makes one variety of widgets. The widget market is currently booming. Company A is selling everything they can make. The huge demand for widgets has even caused the price to rise slightly. But despite all this good news, their profits have been falling. In fact, the more they sell, the worse their profits become. Why?

Using the profit equation, you can quickly highlight a potential cause of diminishing profits: variable cost. As quantity rises, so too might the variable costs of overtime wages, which ultimately may exceed the profit margin on a widget.

RATIO ANALYSIS[1]

Ratio analysis assesses a company's financial performance and health. This is achieved by evaluating the company's ability to execute the key drivers of profitability and growth: product market, and financial market strategies. As Figure AI.11 shows, these strategies are implemented through the four "levers" of operating management, investment management, financing policies, and dividend policy. Ratio analysis directly evaluates the general profitability of a firm, as well as management's ability to operate each of the four levers.

Ratio analysis can be used in three ways. First, the ratios of a company can be compared over time to determine relative performance improvement or decline. Second, ratios for one company may be compared against the aggregate ratios of other companies (which is a proxy for overall industry performance) to evaluate relative performance. Third,

Figure AI.11
The Components of Profitability and Growth

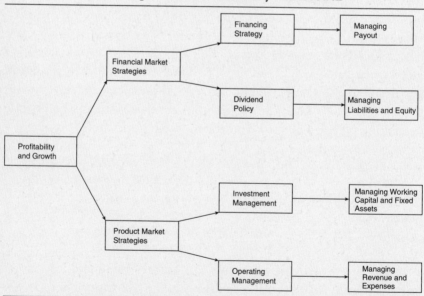

Source: K.G. Palepo, V.I. Bernard, & P.M Healy, *Business Analysis & Evaluation: Using Financial Statements* (Cincinnati: Southwestern Publishing, 1996).

ratios may be compared with a benchmark value to evaluate performance to some predetermined standard (e.g., a financial performance goal). Table AI.1 presents a list of useful ratios and their definitions, which some case interviewers may expect you to be familiar with.

Return on Equity (ROE) is a good indicator of a company's general profitability because it indicates how well the company is using the capital invested by its shareholders (equity) to generate returns. As Table AI.1 shows, there are many ways to measure ROE. Another method of calculating ROE is to use return on assets (ROA) and financial leverage. ROA indicates how much profit a company is able to generate for each dollar invested (assets), and financial leverage indicates how many dollars of assets the firm is able to deploy for each dollar invested.

Table AI.1
Ratio Analysis

Category	Ratio	Definition
General profitability	• Return on equity (ROE)	= NI/SE = (NI/assets) × (Assets/SE) = ROA × financial leverage
Operating management	• Net profit margin	= NI/Sales
Investment management	• Current asset turnover • Accounts receivable turnover • Days' receivable • PP&E turnover	= Sales/CA = Sales/(CA − CL) = AR/Average sales per day = Sales/PP&E
Financing strategy	• Current ratio • Quick ratio • Cash ratio • Operating cash flow ratio • Debt-to-equity ratio	= CA/CL = (Cash + Short-term investments + AR)/CL = (Cash + Short-term investments)/CL = Cash flow from operations/CL = Total debt/(Total debt + SE)
Dividend policies	• Dividend payout ratio	= Cash dividends paid/NI

Note: AR = Accounts receivable, CA = Current assets, CL = Current liabilities, NI = Net income, PP&E = Property, plant, and equipment, ROA = Return on assets, SE = Shareholder's equity.

Operating management involves the management of a company's revenues and expenses. Net profit margin (NPM) indicates the residual portion of revenues that the company can keep as profits for each sales dollar. Thus, NPM shows the profitability of a company's operating activities.

Investment management involves managing a company's working capital and fixed assets. There are several good measures of investment management. Current asset turnover, accounts receivable turnover, and days' receivables are all helpful in analyzing a company's working capital management. Current asset turnover indicates how many dollars of sales a company is able to generate for each dollar invested in current assets. Accounts receivable turnover measures how productively accounts receivable is being used. And finally, days' receivables indicates the number of days of operating activity that are supported by the level of investment in the company's receivables. In terms of fixed asset management, property, plant, and equipment (PP&E) is the most important long-term asset on a company's balance sheet. Thus, PP&E turnover provides a metric for measuring fixed asset management because it shows the amount of sales generated by a dollar's investment in PP&E.

Analyzing a company's *financing strategy* involves evaluating its policies as they relate to their liabilities and equity. Analysis in this area may be divided into two broad categories: short-term liquidity and long-term solvency. The following ratios are helpful in evaluating a company's ability to meet its short-term obligations: current ratio, quick ratio, cash ratio, and operating cash flow ratio. The first three focus on a company's short-term assets, which could be used to repay short-term liabilities. The fourth focuses on a company's ability to generate the resources to repay the short-term liabilities. In terms of long-term solvency, debt-to-equity ratio indicates how many dollars of debt financing a company is using for each dollar invested. This ratio, along with a few others, is helpful in evaluating how well a company is using debt.

Finally, a company's *dividend policy* can be measured by the dividend payout ratio, which has an inverse relationship with the company's sustainable growth rate. If the dividend payout ratio increases, the sustainable growth rate of the same company will decrease.

SUPPLY AND DEMAND

Supply and demand are the fundamental building blocks of economics, describing the market interaction between customers and producers. Although the framework is simple, it is a powerful tool that can help you perform three functions: (1) organize information, (2) gain insight into the effects of a change (e.g., increased government regulation, decrease in quantity supplied), and (3) develop strategies to achieve a given objective. The basic elements of this framework are a supply curve, a demand curve, an equilibrium price, an equilibrium quantity, consumer surplus, and producer surplus, all of which are related to each other in Figure AI.12.

Figure AI.12
Supply and Demand

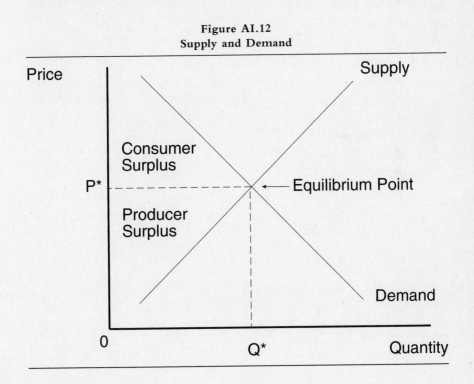

First, the supply-and-demand framework is useful for organizing information. For example, suppose an interviewer asks you to determine the quantity of a good that will be sold, in the long run, given an equilibrium price of P* in a perfectly competitive market. To answer this question, you could quickly sketch out the supply-and-demand chart presented in Figure AI.12 and indicate that supply equals demand at the price of P*, and therefore the quantity of the good that will be sold in the long run is Q*—the associated quantity equilibrium point. By using a graphic construct, you are able to convincingly argue your answer, as well as provide an analytical approach to your work.

Second, supply and demand can also be used to understand the effects of a change. For example, consider a technological breakthrough that enables an increase in the production of widgets. If we assume that all companies have this new technology, what would be the effect on the market? The new and more efficient production process would cause a shift in the supply curve outward, reflecting an increase in production. Holding all else constant, this outward shift would result in a decrease in price and an increase in quantity demanded. And the final effect on consumer and producer surplus will depend on the elasticity of the demand curve (i.e., the slope of the demand curve). Thus, by using the framework, you can provide a much more robust and analytical answer.

Third, supply and demand can also help you develop a strategy to achieve a given objective. For example, suppose a company set an objective for itself of increasing revenues. How would it do this? By using a supply-and-demand framework to map out the consumer surplus region, you can see that the company could increase revenues by capturing some of the consumer surplus value. This might be achieved by setting prices higher—but would this drive price-sensitive customers away from the product? Perhaps, so the best strategy would be to price discriminate—segment customers into different groups according to their sensitivity to price, and charge each group a different price. Hence, the supply-and-demand framework is a useful tool for strategy development.

SWOT (STRENGTHS, WEAKNESSES, OPPORTUNITIES, THREATS)

Unlike Porter's Five Forces, which structures the analysis of industries around five distinct and well-defined dimensions, the SWOT framework, illustrated in Figure AI.13, offers a less restrictive industry analysis framework by using four broad categories—strengths, weaknesses, opportunities, and threats—that have a great deal of definitional latitude.

Figure AI.13
SWOT Framework

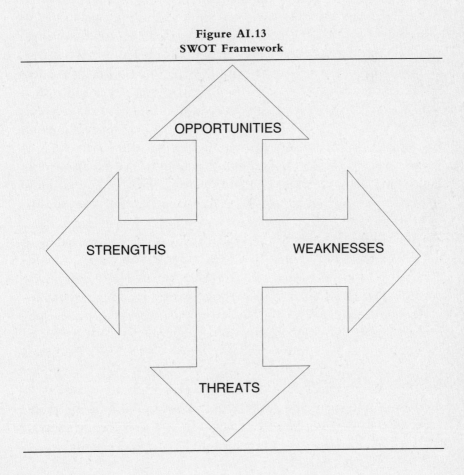

You may be attracted to the framework because its flexibility enables it to be applied to a broad range of case questions. But you should recognize that the framework's flexibility requires greater effort on your part to clarify the key issues of the case before dropping them into the four buckets. And be careful before you pass judgment on what a strength is versus a weakness, or what an opportunity is versus a threat.

A company's strengths and weaknesses can, at times, be hard to define. What may be a strength to one company may actually be a weakness to another. And similarly, a company's strength today may become a significant weakness tomorrow. For example, you might be told that a company enjoys dominant market share in an industry, and that the industry has high barriers to entry due to the high fixed cost of investing in production equipment. Here, you might immediately conclude that the company's dominant market position is a strength. But what if you were then told that the industry was actually doomed to become obsolete through technological innovation? Then, all of a sudden, today's apparent strength becomes an incredible weakness because the company's investment in the high fixed costs of production equipment now locks the company into a dying industry.

Likewise, a company's opportunities and threats may also be hard to define, since an opportunity may actually pose a threat, and a threat may conversely lead a company to discover a new opportunity. For example, the pursuit of an opportunity like a new product launch may actually threaten the core business of a company by diverting resources and funds toward a highly risky venture. And conversely, the threat posed by the entry of a new competitor into an industry may actually become an opportunity by scaring an established company into improving its product quality, production efficiencies, and so on—investments that in the long run may yield higher profitability for the company.

VALUE CHAIN

A value chain, also known as a business system, is a descriptive framework used to detail a sequence of operational or functional events. The example in Figure AI.14 uses a value chain to describe the production stages of a product.

Figure AI.14
Value Chain Example

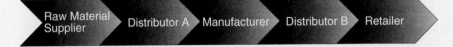

Value chains assume that the links are not in competition with each other but rather in collaboration, working toward the same collective end goal. Each link in a value chain represents an entity that adds value to the end product or service. Only when the final stage of the chain is reached will the product or service be considered complete. Value chains can also be used to describe other events, such as the process of bringing a finished product to market (e.g., from manufacturer, to shipper, to distributor, to another shipper, to retail store). And each link of a value chain most likely has its own underlying value chain (e.g., a raw material supplier must buy access to its product, perform extraction activities such as quarrying, and then process and refine the product for sale). Any individual link in a chain may seek to backward or forward integrate (i.e., assume responsibility for performing the tasks either ahead of or behind the initial link) to capture greater additional value. And if a single company performs the steps in all the links, it is said to be "fully integrated." Multiple value chains can be used to describe the same process, by breaking down the stages involved in bringing a product to market into discrete steps. As a result, two or more value chains can operate in parallel to achieve greater production efficiency.

VALUE NET

The Brandenburger and Nalebuff Value Net characterizes all relationships among players in the game of business. Traditionally, a company produces a good using inputs from suppliers, and then competes with other producers to win the favor of customers. With the Value Net, Brandenburger and Nalebuff introduce a new dimension into the game of business: complementors—"those who provide complementary rather than competing products and services."[2] Figure AI.15 schematically describes this dynamic.

The Value Net emphasizes the element of symmetry in relationships. For example, there are competitors and complementors with respect to both customers and suppliers. A company's customers have other suppliers. If those other suppliers make the company's products or services more valuable to the customer, then these companies are complementors. If they make the products or services less valuable, then they are competitors. Similarly, a company's supplier has other customers. These other customers are either competitors or complementors depending on whether they make it more expensive or cheaper for the supplier to produce its products (or services) for the original company. Everything about customers applies to suppliers and everything about competitors applies in reverse to complementors.

It is important to remember that customer, supplier, competitor, or complementor is a role that companies play and the same company will often have multiple roles. To develop an effective strategy, a company must understand the interests of all four roles each player might have.

While Michael Porter's Five Forces framework (described earlier in this appendix) is typically associated with discussions of competition between the five types of players in an industry, Brandenburger and

Figure AI.15
The Value Net

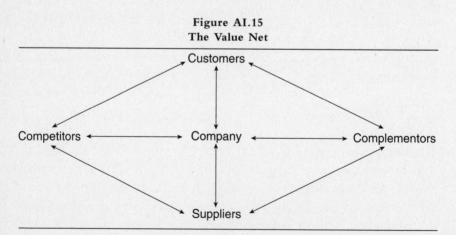

Source: A. Brandenburger and B. Nalebuff, Co-opetition (New York: Doubleday, 1996).

236

Nalebuff introduce a sixth force to the Porter model, namely comple-mentors. This sixth force is not more important than the others, but it is as important and often less well understood.

Another difference between the Value Net and Five Forces is that Porter focuses on the division of the pie, while the Value Net empha-sizes both the creation and division of value. Dividing the pie is a zero-sum game, and who does best is determined by the relative power of the players in the game. The Value Net emphasizes the dual aspect of com-petition and cooperation. Companies work with their customers, sup-pliers, and complementors to create value (win/win). At the same time, they are in a contest with their customers, suppliers, complementors, and competitors to capture portions of the pie (win/lose). This combi-nation of competition and cooperation is called co-opetition.

APPENDIX II

ONE HUNDRED CASE QUESTIONS AND TEN SAMPLE ANSWERS

Your key to successfully navigating the case interview is practice, practice, and more practice. We cannot overemphasize the value of role-playing when learning how to tackle ambiguous and almost certainly unfamiliar questions. Voluminous reading about cases cannot adequately prepare you for the intensity of an actual face-to-face interview.

As you will recall from Chapter 6, the questions asked by consulting firms can be grouped into 10 broad types, presented in Table AII.1. This appendix contains 10 questions from each category. Answers to the first question of each category are presented at the latter half of this appendix. As you begin your preparation for case interviewing, first, make sure that you practice every type of question. Avoiding questions that you find challenging will only hurt your overall preparation. By practicing a variety of question types, you will develop the confidence you need to succeed at any case interview.

Second, consider the relevance of the case questions to different business topics when formulating your answer to a case. If the question involves issues of organizational behavior, for example, it may not be appropriate to answer it using an economics framework (even though you may know economics very well).

Table AII.1
Ten Types of Case Questions

1. Brain teaser
2. Business strategy
3. Human resource management
4. Market entry
5. Market sizing
6. Mergers and acquisitions
7. New product introduction
8. Opportunity assessment
9. Pricing
10. Profitability loss

Third, when practicing case questions, follow the steps detailed in Chapter 6: (1) listen to the question and repeat it, (2) ask clarifying questions, (3) structure your analysis with a framework, (4) discuss each category of the framework, and (5) summarize and conclude. The more you use this step-by-step approach, the better you will become at answering cases in a methodical, rational, and compelling manner.

Fourth, the cases provided here can be answered in many different ways, using a variety of frameworks and approaches. The sample answers provided are merely illustrative. They are not definitive examples of the "best" possible answers. Read through the sample answers within each type of case question, paying careful attention to recognizing patterns of structure and approach among the group, and then practice applying these patterns to the remaining 90 questions. Remember that the answer to a case is less important than the approach you use to work through the problem. Simply getting an answer right is not enough—interviewers are looking for discussions that are rational, systematic, and persuasive, and only after these three tests are passed will the answer or conclusion be important.

Fifth, work through these cases in role-playing groups of two to three people. Two people can exchange roles as interviewer and interviewee, and critique each other's performance (while also learning what it is like to be in the interviewer's shoes!). With three people, you can add the role of "observer" into the same exercise, which is often more instructive than the role of interviewer. You should also be careful to work with different people over time, since everyone has a different interviewing style, and you may find yourself becoming too accustomed to one.

Be sure to set time aside each day for practice. In time, you should not only find yourself excelling at cases, but also actually enjoying them.

APPENDIX II

SAMPLE CASE QUESTIONS

TYPE 1 BRAIN TEASER

Case 1.1   **Weight of a Boeing 747**
Answer: p. 264 How much does a Boeing 747 jumbo jet weigh?

Case 1.2   **Manhole Covers**
Why are manhole covers round?

Case 1.3   **Microsoft Windows**
Why do you have to push the "start" button to shut down Microsoft Windows?

Case 1.4   **Bottle Tops**
Why do bottle tops unscrew counterclockwise?

Case 1.5   **Coffee Cans**
Why are coffee cans cylindrical in shape?

Case 1.6   **Concorde**
Why does the nose of a Concorde passenger jet move up and down?

Case 1.7   **House Construction**
In what ways does a house in New Hampshire differ in construction from a house in Florida?

Case 1.8   **The Sun**
How many ways can you tell if the sun is burning or glowing?

Case 1.9   **CEO Office**
Why is the CEO's office often on the top floor of a corporate tower? Are there reasons why it should not be?

Case 1.10   **Clocks**
Why do the hands on a clock turn clockwise?

TYPE 2 BUSINESS STRATEGY

Case 2.1   **Home Improvement Retailing**
Answer: p. 266 A nationwide retail chain sells both soft (e.g., clothes) and hard (e.g., hardware) goods in each of its mall-based stores. Consumers, however, find this

mix odd, and the CEO has determined that shoppers of soft goods are very different from shoppers of hard. As a result, he decides to take the hard goods departments out of the stores and build a new chain of stores selling only hard goods, but does not know what format or size would be optimal. Given the information presented in the accompanying chart (Figure AII.1), what would you recommend he do?

Case 2.2

Small Business School

A small business school in southern Illinois wants to be recognized as a "top 20" business school in the next 10 years. How should the school do it?

Figure AII.1
Home Improvement Retail Industry: Average Sales per Square Foot

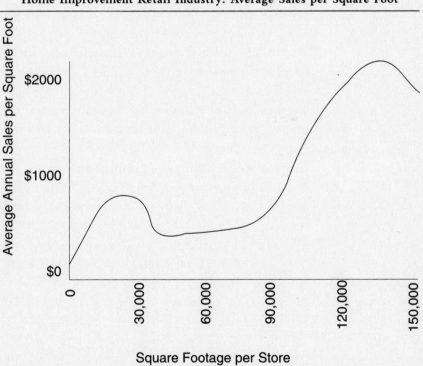

Case 2.3	**Hollywood Film Production**

A Hollywood production company knows that only 1 movie out of every 20 is a blockbuster. How should the company decide which films to produce, and what should its marketing strategy be?

Case 2.4	**Pharmaceutical Patents**

A pharmaceutical company has 20 patented prescription drug products that all face patent expiration in two years or less. A generic brand drug manufacturer has offered to purchase 10 of the patents at a price to be negotiated. If the sale is approved, the pharmaceutical company would have to cede all production rights over the 10 drugs to the generic company for the remaining life of the patents. Should the company sell? If so, then for how much?

Case 2.5	**Entertainment Conglomerate**

An entertainment conglomerate in southern California owns an entertainment complex that consists of multiplex movie theaters, concert halls, restaurants, and theme parks. The facilities all share one parking complex, which was recently expanded using every available piece of remaining land. But customers are still being turned away due to a lack of parking space. What should the conglomerate do?

Case 2.6	**Consumer Products Competition**

A consumer products industry has three manufacturers that collectively own 100 percent of the market. Company 1 has 50 percent market share, company 2 has 40 percent market share, and company 3, your client, has the remaining 10 percent. Consumer research has found that your company's product is far superior in quality to those of the other two, but customers simply do not recognize your brand. Furthermore, your small share means that your company has higher distribution costs, higher manufacturing costs, lower manufacturing capacity, and poor negotiating power with stores for shelf space. What should your company do to increase market share?

Case 2.7   **Resuscitation Device**

You are developing a new resuscitation device which has two components: (1) a piece of permanent equipment and (2) disposable attachments. You will be ready to sell the equipment next month, but the disposable attachments will not be ready for six months. Your competitor is developing the same device and will be prepared to release both the equipment and the disposable attachments six months from now. What should you do?

Case 2.8   **Starting a Firm**

You and several close friends are considering leaving your consulting firm to start your own. Is this a good idea, and if so, what kind of firm should you open?

Case 2.9   **Wonder Drug**

On a recent trip to South America, you discovered the Salito flower. Locals claim that the petals from the Salito flower can help people lose weight. How can you make the Salito flower the next Echinacea, without scientific proof and with a very small advertising budget?

Case 2.10   **Advertising Strategy**

Your marketing strategy group has developed clever albeit childish advertisements attacking the number one and number two companies in your industry by exaggerating their weaknesses. You are concerned with the reaction to the ads, both by customers and competitors. Should you approve the ads?

TYPE 3   HUMAN RESOURCE MANAGEMENT

Case 3.1   **Recruiting**

Answer: p. 271 You are the recruiting director of a major consulting firm. Your firm has traditionally been known for very bright and innovative consultants. But what candidates do not know is that the office atmosphere is "cutthroat." Informally, you have been told by several senior partners that the atmosphere needs to change, but they fear that a selection bias in the recruiting process is perpetuating the cutthroat atmosphere. How would you begin to investigate this hypothesis?

Case 3.2 **High Tech Start-Up**

The CEO of a leading high tech start-up company is concerned by a recent exodus of nearly 50 percent (or 35 people) of his software engineers. During exit interviews with some of those who resigned, he learned that his company's compensation package of base pay, annual bonus, benefits, and stock options, is anywhere from 20 percent to 200 percent lower than those offered by the competition. However, as a start-up, his company is cash constrained and is resistant to putting additional stress on cash flow. How should he evaluate the situation, and what should he do to stop the exodus and ultimately revitalize his engineering staff?

Case 3.3 **Downsizing**

You are the CEO of a company that has just reported its third consecutive annual operating loss of over 100 million dollars. A consulting firm you hired to reengineer the company has recommended that you reduce operating costs by 40 percent through forced retirement or release of 2,000 middle management employees. How will you identify your targets, implement the decision, and position the downsizing effort to the company and investor community?

Case 3.4 **Leadership**

You are the manager of a consulting team that has been helping a company develop a new electric automobile. Having successfully developed and tested a prototype, the company is ready to establish a new car division around the product and build 10,000 units for sale. But you have serious concerns about the leadership competencies of the individual nominated to head the division, even though she was working on the project since the beginning. On more than one occasion, you had to bail her out to avoid seriously embarrassing or disastrous consequences. What should you do?

Case 3.5 **Conflict Management**

A real estate developer has had to stop construction of a 50-story luxury apartment building after its general contractor unexpectedly filed for bankruptcy. As a result, all the stakeholders in the project have threatened to file lawsuits against the developer to get their money back: investors, individuals who purchased apartments in advance, and the subcontractors who performed work and have yet to be paid by the general contractor. The developer wants to hold the project together, and needs one month to find additional project financing and a new contractor. How should she manage the impending conflict between the vested parties, and buy herself some time?

Case 3.6 **Profit Sharing**

Cross Cultural Air (CCA) is an international airline with routes to various cities in the United States, Asia, Europe, and Africa. Five years ago, CCA was hailed as a cutting-edge airline when it instituted a generous profit sharing plan. The plan called for crews (pilots, flight attendants, etc.) to share profits based on the profitability of the route they serve. The idea was that crews who only flew short domestic flights should not get the same profits as those who served longer and more strenuous, international flights. In the five years since the plan was instituted, CCA noticed that morale has declined, and the recruiting and retention of new pilots has been more difficult. This is very surprising, considering that the plan was designed to specifically address these issues. What should CCA do?

Case 3.7
Scapegoat
You are the Senior Vice President at Brettenham Pharmaceuticals, the U.S. subsidiary of Brettenham Holding Group (BHG), a British holding company. Senior officials from BHG are planning a U.S. visit to inquire about the recent failure of Facor, a fat-reducing drug. You have been made aware of a plan to fire the product manager for Facor. You know BHG wants an explanation and action for the failure, but you feel that it is unfair to blame a single person. What should you do?

Case 3.8
New Technology
You are the new CEO of Winston Auto. Winston has a long tradition of building some of the finest automobiles in the world. Each model is hand-built requiring over two months and thousands of worker hours. Winston has two plants in the United States. Although Winston enjoys strong customer loyalty, growth has been stagnant for the past 10 years. It is your responsibility to increase either profits or revenues—or preferably both. You are considering automating a portion of the construction process, thereby reducing your costs and turning out more cars, but your employees are opposed to this. They have informed you of their intention to strike and begin a negative public relations campaign. Customer loyalty, as well as attracting new customers, is crucial for Winston's continued survival. What should you do?

Case 3.9   **Corporate Culture**
You are the president of a large advertising firm. Several months ago, your company purchased a small PR firm. You thought that the merger was going well. However, it has come to your attention that the employees of the new firm are unhappy with the small kitchen that was installed in their new office space. You thought they would be delighted to have a kitchen at all because no other floor in the building has one. And now your employees are grumbling that the employees from the acquired company are being given too much. You want the merger to work, but you do not want to upset your existing employees. What options do you have?

Case 3.10   **Consulting Engagement**
Your consulting team has been working diligently on a project for the past two months and is now nearing completion of the final presentation. But when you called one of the client team members this morning to verify some information, he unexpectedly told you that the vice president who hired your firm feels unacceptably distanced from your team's work, and is likely to reject all your firm's recommendations, believing that they are unfounded and inadequately researched. What should you do?

TYPE 4   MARKET ENTRY

Case 4.1   **Italian Pottery**
Answer: p. 273 A family-owned pottery manufacturer in Assisi, Italy, has decided to export its handcrafted wares to the United States, but needs your help to determine how. The manufacturer is considering three options: (1) sell directly to stores; (2) sell to distributors, who then sell to individual stores; and (3) open its own chain of proprietary stores. What should the manufacturer do?

Case 4.2   **Consulting Firm**
A Boston-based start-up consulting firm has grown from 3 consultants to 100 in two years. It is now prepared to expand overseas and work with global clients. How would you help the firm develop a strategy, and what would you recommend?

Case 4.3   **Sports League Expansion**
You are the Commissioner of the NFL, and have learned that the League's profitability has leveled over the past 10 years. You are considering expanding the league to include teams in foreign countries to increase profits. Which countries should you enter, how, and when?

Case 4.4   **Auto Franchises**
A Korean auto manufacturer wants to enter the French market and is looking for franchise distributors. The company will supply 50,000 luxury cars per year at a wholesale price of $20,000 each, and suggests a retail price of $30,000. How many individual franchise distributors should the company establish in the first year?

Case 4.5   **Baby Clothes**
Your company is the number one manufacturer of baby clothes. Recently, a leading designer of women's apparel, Marie Briscoe, has launched its own line of baby clothes. What should your response be?

Case 4.6   **Electric Car**
You have just developed an electric car that has a top speed of 90 miles per hour, and a total battery operating time of six hours. Your production costs per car total $9,000, which is less than half of the cost of the closest competitor. Where should you first sell this car, and what would be your long-term strategy?

Case 4.7   **Water Filter**
Water filtration products have traditionally not sold well in rural U.S. communities because of the purity of local reservoirs. However, your boss believes that rural markets are the next growth area for water filtration devices, and has asked you to devise a rural market entry plan. What would you recommend?

Case 4.8   **Donut Chain**
A Texas-based chain of donut shops, A-Donut-A-Day, is considering nationwide expansion. How should the chain determine where to locate the first 100 company-owned shops?

Case 4.9   **Web Site**
A nonprofit environmental action group is considering building a Web site, since most of its peers have already done so. Why would the organization want to have a Web presence? What should be the content of the Web site?

Case 4.10   **Airport Gates**
A Midwest regional airline is prepared to expand its routes to the West Coast, but finds that all the gates at the San Francisco airport are rented to other airlines for at least five years. What should the regional airline do?

TYPE 5   MARKET SIZING

Case 5.1   **Gourmet Coffee Shops**
Answer: p. 277 **Part I:** A large coffee processing company has seen sales of its well-known supermarket brand coffee drop 15 percent per year over the past five years. As a result, manufacturing costs per pound of coffee are increasing, since 25 percent of the machines are no longer being used, and monthly production has dropped by 50,000 pounds. Meanwhile, gourmet

coffee chains are growing rapidly across the United States. Should the company try to capture some of this growth by opening its own proprietary chain of gourmet coffee stores?

Part II: How many individual coffee stores could the company supply, if it has 50,000 pounds of excess monthly production capacity? Assume one pound of coffee yields 10 cups of brewed coffee.

Case 5.2 **Gas Stations**
How many gas stations are in the United States?

Case 5.3 **Ridership of New York City Subways**
How many people ride the New York City subway during the morning rush hour?

Case 5.4 **College Pizza Consumption**
How many square feet of pizza are consumed on a college campus in a year?

Case 5.5 **Airplanes in Flight**
At noon on a typical weekday, how many airplanes are flying over the United States?

Case 5.6 **Diaper Demand**
Determine the annual demand for diapers in the United States.

Case 5.7 **Windshield Wipers**
How many pairs of windshield wipers are manufactured in the United States each year?

Case 5.8 **Fortune 500 Market Value**
What is the cumulative market value of the Fortune 500?

Case 5.9 **Lightbulb Sales**
How many lightbulbs were sold in the United States last year?

Case 5.10 **Tea in China**
Determine the annual demand for tea in China.

TYPE 6 MERGERS AND ACQUISITIONS

Case 6.1   **HMO Acquisition**

Answer: p. 282 A New York based health maintenance organization (HMO) is considering expanding its operations. They currently have the funds to purchase another HMO. Their internal M&A group has identified two possible targets: Allied HMO in Miami, and Washington Health in Seattle. Which should they purchase?

Case 6.2   **Merger Discontinuance**

Your company has been engaging in merger discussions with another company for the past year, and as a result the stock prices of both companies have risen by 30 percent. However, the two companies have come to a mutual realization that their businesses are not as compatible as previously thought. How should the companies announce their decision to remain independent, while still protecting their stock prices from sudden collapse?

Case 6.3   **Auto Parts Chain Acquisition**

A publicly held supermarket chain seeks profit-generating opportunities to increase its stock price and offer higher earnings per share. An undervalued auto parts chain has been identified, and evidently needs a cash infusion to pay off its mounting debt. Should the supermarket acquire the auto parts chain?

Case 6.4   **Air Conditioner Company Acquisition**

Our client is a conglomerate. One of its subsidiaries is a manufacturer of air conditioning systems that also performs the service of installing the sold units. In the past, there was a fierce price war between this conglomerate and an independent, family-owned air conditioning business. Recently, the family has approached the conglomerate and offered its company for sale. Should the conglomerate buy the family business? If so, what would the contractual and pricing arrangements be?

Case 6.5   **Airline Synergies**

Two major U.S. airlines have discussed the advantages of forming one airline and are now considering two scenarios: (1) One airline could simply purchase the other; or (2) the two airlines could merge under one name, and fully integrate their reservation systems, flight routes, and rewards programs into one. Which of the two options would be optimal for both airlines?

Case 6.6   **Oil Exploration**

A major U.S. oil company has been approached by an oil exploration company with a proposal to merge. Should the oil company agree, or instead continue to contract out all of its exploration?

Case 6.7   **Cement Company**

A cement company has just acquired another cement company that owns a 1,000 acre forest located 200 miles north of San Francisco. Our client would like to know what to do with the forest?

Case 6.8   **Chemical Conglomerate**

A holding company that owns 10 small chemical manufacturing companies has recently purchased an 11th one. Should the conglomerate operate all 11 companies under one consolidated name, or continue to operate them independently under their original names?

Case 6.9   **Company Valuation**

You are considering buying a start-up company that is trying to develop a new polymer but as of yet does not have a product to sell. How would you determine the value of the company?

Case 6.10   **Gin Distillery Acquisition Options**
Should a gin distillery expand by acquiring a beer company, a fruit juice company, or a chip dip company?

TYPE 7   NEW PRODUCT INTRODUCTION

Case 7.1   **Cricket Ball Exports to the United States**
Answer: p. 285 A U.K.-based cricket ball manufacturer seeks sales expansion opportunities in the United States. Current production is at full capacity, but US$500 million has been allocated to build additional capacity. Should the company introduce the product in the United States?

Case 7.2   **Nylons-R-US**
Nylons-R-US (NRU is a subsidiary of Athena Conglomerate) has developed a new hosiery that is 300 percent more durable than regular brands. The lifespan of the product is twice that of the old. Athena requires that all new projects show $100 million in U.S. revenues by the fifth year after launch. NRU is considering setting the price at $1.00 per unit. Should NRU go ahead with this project?

Case 7.3   **Olive Canning**
A food product canning company has decided to introduce a new canned olives product. Should the company offer prepitted olives, or olives with pits?

Case 7.4   **Hayatem**
Zorost Pharmaceuticals has been developing Hayatem, a revolutionary new weight-loss drug, for the past seven years. Clinical trials have shown that Hayatem, along with proper exercise and diet, can safely help individuals lose weight. Zorost has been simultaneously developing an over-the-counter version of the drug and a prescription version. Unfortunately, Brein, the leading weight loss drug, was linked to breast cancer and was hastily pulled from

the market. The public seems to have a general distrust about weight loss drugs in general. Should Zorost introduce any of the drugs, and if so, how?

Case 7.5   **AME Biotech**
AME, a large, multinational biotech, is searching for new products to develop. You have a meeting with the CEO in a few hours. He wants three alternative methods for developing new products, and your recommendation of the one AME should pursue.

Case 7.6   **Cereal Manufacturer**
A major U.S. manufacturer of breakfast cereals currently produces 10 different brands, and collectively has a 30 percent market share. Five of the brands are positioned to attract children, while the other five tend to be purchased by health-conscious adults. Since the total U.S. cereal-eating population has remained relatively constant in size, the only way the company can increase market share is by taking sales away from the competition. To do so, the company seeks to develop five new cereals within the next year, and hopefully capture customers who previously did not buy the company's brands. What step-by-step strategy would you advise to help the company develop and introduce five new cereals?

Case 7.7   **Home Diagnostics**
Smith Labs, a diagnostics company, is seeking ways to expand its core competency: diagnostic services. It is currently completing the development of a multiuse home diagnostic kit, targeted to homebound elderly patients who need diagnostic services. The kit's final design will depend on the marketing strategy for introducing this product. What should the strategy be, in terms of price, promotional strategy, and distribution channels?

Case 7.8   **Small Business**
Heartland Consulting Group is a small management consulting firm based in Columbus, Ohio. They specialize in small business consulting and are about to launch an Internet-based consulting tool for small businesses. The program will be able to help small business owners with basic management questions. How should the product be designed to add value to the customer without taking business away from Heartland?

Case 7.9   **Personal Computers**
A major manufacturer of personal computers is going to design a desktop model to suit the needs of a specific customer segment: homemakers. What design process would you recommend to ensure a close "fit" between the features of the model, and customer needs?

Case 7.10   **Rewards Program**
An Internet-access provider is considering offering a points-based rewards program to its subscribers. One point would be credited for every dollar spent by a subscriber, in any of the following activities: (1) paying the monthly membership fee of $19.95, (2) purchasing items through the provider's on-line shopping service, and (3) signing up additional members. How should the company decide whether to offer this rewards program?

TYPE 8   OPPORTUNITY ASSESSMENT

Case 8.1   **On-line Bookstore**
Answer: p. 289 If a book distributor were thinking about launching an online bookstore, what would be its estimated annual sales?

Case 8.2   **Light SUVs**
A small automobile company in Japan is considering developing a new lightweight sport utility vehicle

(LSUV). The car is designed to attract women who want the size of an SUV, but also want a vehicle that drives like a car. The company has a $10 million R&D budget with a monthly burn rate of $200,000, and knows that development costs will be high. Venture capital funds are likely to be needed, but VC firms are only interested in projects that have a very high upside. The meeting with a potential VC investor is next week. What should the company tell the investor?

| Case 8.3 | **Profitability of Backward Integrating** |

Could a juice manufacturer significantly increase its profitability by backward integrating?

| Case 8.4 | **Express Mail** |

Could an overnight express mail company build a viable new business by introducing two- and three-day delivery service? If so, how would it differentiate itself from the competition, and by approximately how much would its revenues increase?

| Case 8.5 | **Microbrewery** |

A restaurant-based microbrewery in Montana produces three types of beer: a dark stout, a medium amber beer, and a light pale ale. All three have been very popular among customers, and are often sold out. As entrepreneurs, the owners of the brewery have naturally thought about expansion, and now have dreams of selling their beers nationwide. How would you help them evaluate the idea? If it seems to be a viable business opportunity, what strategy would you suggest?

| Case 8.6 | **Pastry Shop** |

A famous European pastry chef has for decades owned and operated a café in New York City. With a flair for the dramatic, the chef has become renowned for catering special occasions, such as weddings, New Year's parties, and black-tie dinners. He would now like to offer a new "breakfast in bed" service, where customers could arrange in advance for delivery of an elegant breakfast or brunch spread to their apartments, complete with flowers, chinaware, and fine linen. How many "breakfast in bed" customers would you expect the café to attract? With what pricing scheme? Could you improve on the business concept?

Case 8.7   **Device Manufacturer**

A venture capital firm is considering investing $5 million in a start-up device company that is developing a somewhat controversial method of storing blood products. The VC will be given a certain equity stake in the company for its investment. They have asked you to develop a model to determine how equity should be shared between the company and the VC firm.

Case 8.8   *Woman's Week*

Woman's Week, a newsstand magazine, is considering using the Internet to increase its readership. Would you recommend this strategy?

Case 8.9   **DLS Consulting Group**

DLS Consulting Group has a well established strategy-based consulting practice, and is considering offering information technology consulting services. The primary motivation of this interest is not to enter a new consulting field, but rather to increase the firm's profit margin. Is this a good way for the firm to improve its profitability?

Case 8.10   **Eye Care Center**

The Eye Care Center has developed a new technique for correcting nearsightedness. The technique involves using a microscalpel, and is considered a somewhat risky procedure. But if successful, the surgery permanently corrects the problem. What should their optimistic, pessimistic, and realistic market demand forecasts be?

TYPE 9 PRICING

Case 9.1
Answer: p. 292

Amtrak Rail Ticket
How does Amtrak price a rail ticket from Boston to Washington, D.C.?

Case 9.2

Pharmacies
You own a pharmacy that promises to meet or beat any competitor's prices. Your brother-in-law's pharmacy next door is exactly the same size, shares the same product mix as you, and advertises the same price guarantee. You both have the same volume of customers, but your brother-in-law's revenues are much higher. Why?

Case 9.3

U.S. Post Office Stamps
How does the U.S. Post Office price a first-class, 1-ounce letter stamp?

Case 9.4

Stock Exchange
How are the stock prices on the New York Stock Exchange determined?

Case 9.5

Flat Tax Rate
If the United States switched to a flat income tax, what percentage tax rate would enable the government to collect the same level of revenue as today?

Case 9.6

Sports Car Development
An Italian car company wants to develop and introduce a new sports car in the United States. What considerations should be taken into account when determining the style, features, target customers, and ultimately the price of the car?

Case 9.7

Airline Seat Pricing
Passengers on any given flight rarely pay the same price for seats in the same class. How do airlines determine the optimal mix of prices?

Case 9.8	**Red Wine**

Red Wine
How is the retail price of a bottle of red wine determined?

Case 9.9
Valentine's Day
On Valentine's Day, how should a florist price flowers other than roses?

Case 9.10
Newspaper Pricing
The price of a one-year subscription to a newspaper is higher for the online version than the paper version. Does this make sense?

Type 10   Profitability Loss

Case 10.1
Answer: p. 295
Pharmaceutical Drugs
The CEO of a major pharmaceutical company wants to know why the profits of one of its leading over-the-counter drugs declined by 25 percent over the past year.

Case 10.2
Blacksmith Shop
A blacksmith in Vermont owns and operates a custom wrought-iron shop, specializing in artistic gates and fencing. Over the past decade, the blacksmith has enjoyed steady business and has been able to develop a reputation of high quality and reliability. As a one-man shop, he has always had more work than he could handle, and could afford to be selective in the commissions he accepted. However, over the past two years, his annual income has dropped dramatically. Why?

Case 10.3
TLJ Hot Dogs
TLJ sells hots dogs from a small vending stand on the corner of 57th and Madison in New York City. TLJ actively price discriminates, by selling different hot dog combinations (i.e., toppings) for different prices at different times of day. Does this maximize his profits? Under what conditions

would this approach fail? In answering this question, consider the practical barriers to perfect price discrimination.

Case 10.4   **Lumber Company Profit Loss**
A medium–size lumber milling company in Oregon has recently been experiencing a dramatic loss in profits. It owns and operates two mills located 25 miles apart, and also owns and operates a large tree farm. Approximately 50 percent of its wood is supplied from the farm, while the remaining 50 percent comes from sources in Canada. Should the company close one of its mills and consolidate operations? If not, what should it do?

Case 10.5   **Price Maintenance**
In the competitive game of airline pricing, airlines are encouraged to undercut their competitors to win customers. However, if prices continue to fall as competitors promote lower and lower prices, eventually zero if not negative profits will be made by all competitors. How can an airline attempt to control the pricing market, and not get trapped in a zero-profit price war?

Case 10.6   **Takamiya**
Takamiya Computers builds and sells hardware to Fortune 500 companies. However, they have noticed that their profits have leveled off over the past three years. How can they boost their profit margins?

Case 10.7   **Custom Windows and Doors**
A leading manufacturer of custom–made wood windows and doors located in Maine has developed a reputation for high quality, on–time, and competitively priced work. Over the past two years, however, the manufacturer has earned zero profit despite a backlog of work. Evidently, the costs of labor and wood materials have risen dramatically.

What options does the company have, and what actions would you recommend to restore the company to profitability?

Case 10.8
Deseret Printing Shop
Deseret Printing Shop has been automating certain functions within their shops (six sites across Utah, Colorado, and California), but they have not yet realized their expected profit increases. Why?

Case 10.9
Outlet Malls
The largest outlet mall in the United States is being developed outside Chicago. For the development group to maximize profits, how should it organize the mall, and which retailers should be invited to open stores in the mall?

Case 10.10
Atlantic Daily
Atlantic Daily is a newspaper with a circulation of 250,000 subscribers. After two other "specialized" newspapers came into the market, Atlantic saw its profits dwindle. Since a recent survey showed that people are reading more newspapers as the number of papers increase, why are profits for Atlantic going down? How should Atlantic respond?

SOLUTIONS TO SELECTED CASE QUESTIONS

TYPE 1   BRAIN TEASER

Case 1.1   **Weight of a Boeing 747**

How much does a Boeing 747 jumbo jet weigh?

Elements of a Basic Answer

Framework: Divide a 747 into variable and fixed-weight components, and calculate the weight of each.

1. Variable weights:
   - Passengers: A 747 can hold approximately 400 people. At 150 lbs per person, the total weight of the passengers is 400×150 lbs = 60,000 lbs.
   - Baggage: If each person carries two suitcases, weighing approximately 50 lbs each, then the total baggage weight is 400×50 lbs $\times 28$ bags = 40,000 lbs.
   - Cargo: In addition to the baggage, a 747 can carry other cargo such as mail and overnight packages. To simplify the calculation, let's assume it is at least equal to the weight of the baggage: 40,000 lbs.
   - Supplies: Each of the passengers must be provided with meals, drinks, and other necessities. If we assume that each passenger accounts for 10 pounds of such supplies, we then have 400×10 lbs = 4,000 lbs.
   - Fuel: A 747 can travel as far as New York City to Tokyo. Since a New York City to Tokyo round trip will usually provide a passenger with a free domestic US ticket on a frequent flyer program, we can assume the round-trip mileage to be 25,000 miles (the average required mileage for a free domestic ticket), and the one-way trip to be 12,500 miles. A 747 has four engines, each of which consumes much more fuel than a car engine; therefore, we know that each 747 engine must get far fewer than 25 miles to the gallon. To be conservative, we can assume that each engine gets 1 mile to the gallon. Thus, the total fuel consumed on the longest one-way trip is 12,500 miles $\times 1$ mile/gal $\times 4$ engines = 50,000

gal. In terms of weight, we can assume 1 gallon equals 3 pounds, so 50,000 gallons equals 150,000 pounds.

2. Fixed weights:
   - The structure: We can estimate the weight of a 747's fuselage, wings, engines, and all other component parts by comparing the size of a 747 to the size of another unit of machinery that we are more familiar with, such as a car. If we assume the weight of an average car is two tons, or 4,000 pounds, we can estimate the weight of a 747 by approximating the number of cars that will fit into a 747. A simple approach would divide the number of passengers that can ride a 747 (400 people) by the number of passengers that can ride in a car (5 people), thus approximating the number of cars that would fit in a plane: $400/5 = 80$ cars. The weight of these 80 cars is $80 \times 4,000$ lbs $= 320,000$ lbs.

3. The total weight of a 747 is simply the sum of each of these component weights:
   - People   60,000 lbs
   - Luggage   40,000
   - Cargo   40,000
   - Supplies   4,000
   - Fuel   150,000
   - Structure   320,000
                          614,000 lbs

(Boeing reports that the maximum take off weight of a 747–100 is 735,000 lbs)[1]

Elements of an Outstanding Answer
An outstanding answer would refine the total weight figure through two additional steps:

1. Identify the weight components which could vary considerably according to the distance of the flight, such as fuel.
2. Dissect the fixed weights into their components (i.e., seats, overhead bins, toilets, steel body, and wings) to derive a more "accurate" calculation.

TYPE 2   BUSINESS STRATEGY

Case 2.1   Home Improvement Retailing

A nationwide retail chain sells both soft (e.g., clothes) and hard (e.g., hardware) goods in each of its mall-based stores. Consumers, however, find this mix odd, and the CEO has determined that shoppers of soft goods are very different from shoppers of hard. As a result, he decides to take the hard goods departments out of the stores and build a new chain of stores selling only hard goods, but does not know what format or size would be optimal. Given the information presented in the accompanying chart (Figure A.II.1), what would you recommend he do?

Elements of a Basic Answer

Framework: First interpret the chart to learn as much as possible about the retail environment, and then perform a 3-C's analysis: Company, Customers, and Competitors.

1. Chart interpretation:
- This chart displays the average sales per square foot of all retail home improvement stores in aggregate, including hardware stores, specialty home improvement stores (paint, carpet, etc.), and "big box" superstores.
- Evidently, sales per square foot increase dramatically as small stores increase in size, but then taper off again. Similarly, large stores also exhibit a rapid increase in sales per square foot as size increases, but then again show signs of diminishing returns as the square footage approaches 150,000. All the stores in between the two peaks appear to have nearly identical sales per square foot, regardless of size.
- Small stores are likely to be hardware stores, located within cities. Due to high city rents, hardware stores tend to be smaller than 5,000 square feet, and quite cramped. The merchandise offered will cater to the apartment dweller, who will usually only enter a hardware store to purchase items for a repair or small

project. Similarly, contractors are likely to make only "convenience" or "emergency" purchases at a hardware store, and prefer larger non-city stores for significant purchases. As a result, customers shopping at city hardware stores will typically purchase only one or two small items. To compensate for low sales volume and high rents, hardware stores charge much higher prices than other home improvement stores. Why do customers pay these higher prices? Simply for the convenience of only having to walk down the street. The chart supports this argument by showing that small stores typically have higher sales per square foot than medium-size stores.

- The medium-size stores are likely to be suburban specialty home improvement stores, such as paint stores, tile stores, or carpet stores. These stores sell only one (maybe two) home improvement categories, and serve as a destination for customers who have a specific project to perform. Although both consumers and contractors are likely to shop at a specialty store and purchase multiple items, these stores still display lower sales per square foot than either the small or large stores. Why? This is most likely due to a number of factors: a poor ability to encourage customers to purchase incidentals (e.g., batteries); an inability to benefit from customer cross-shopping (e.g., a customer who came to the store to buy paint also realizing that she needs plant food); and a weakened ability to serve as a one-stop shop for customers needing items in multiple product categories. As a result, the combination of larger stores and fewer customers is responsible for lower sales per square foot.

- Large stores capture the highest sales per square foot for two reasons: (1) they are one-stop shops, offering not only the greatest selection within a product category, but also the greatest number of categories; (2) a large percentage of sales come from contractors, who may purchase thousands if not millions of dollars of merchandise from a single superstore in one year. Customers who shop at superstores hardly ever "just drive by;" rather, they make a conscious decision to drive to the store and sacrifice time for the benefit of selection, lower prices, and ultimately the convenience of not having to make a second trip to another store.

Now that we have interpreted the chart and learned about the industry, we can return to the original question of what retail size and format our client should adopt.

2. Company:

- The size and format of the new store should be designed to maximize sales per square foot. But it would be hasty to immediately recommend a big box format due to its superior sales performance, since we do not know if the current home improvement section in the department store has enough product categories to fill a superstore.

Q What product categories do we currently sell?

A We sell hand and power tools, hardware, electrical, plumbing, appliances, and paint and wallpaper.

- With so few categories, we can see that a big box store would be hard to fill. We currently have no experience with lumber, roofing materials, building materials, and lawn and garden, to name a few. Suddenly, the superstore format seems less attractive. But should we alternatively recommend a medium-size specialty store, or a hardware store at this point? We first need to know more about the competitive advantages of the store's hard goods to decide.

Q What brands do we carry?

A Some of our categories carry all the major brands, such as power tools, but others only offer our own proprietary brands such as hand tools. In fact, our hand tools brand has been proven through customer research to have the strongest reputation of quality and reliability. In addition, we also have our own brands of paint, and appliances, but carry other brands as well.

- If we have a superior hand tool brand, perhaps we should open a specialty hand tool store. But then what should we do with the other categories? Eliminate them? We need to know more about our customers before we can make such a decision.

3. Customers:

Q Who are our primary customers?

A We currently attract both consumers and contractors. Hard goods consumers tend to shop for a collection of items, and never even enter the soft goods sections of the store. Most consumers come back again at a later date to do more shopping. Contractors, on the other hand, typically come in to buy our proprietary brand of hand tools, and occasionally buy from the other categories at the same time, but rarely frequent our stores.

- Based on this response, it appears that the store benefits from having multiple product categories. A hand-tools-only store might not offer a strong enough reason for a consumer to enter, and while it may be attractive to contractors, this format would not be able to cross-sell additional products to contractors.

Q Do our customers also shop at other home improvement stores?

A Yes. Consumer research shows that most of our customers also shop at hardware stores for convenience, and big box stores for variety. They shop with us when they either need one of our superior hand tools, or would like advice on an item or project from one of our respected associates, or want one of our brands of appliances or paint. In short, we represent reliability and trust to our customers—that's why they come back.

- We have now learned that the store offers other respected brands in addition to hand tools. A hand-tools-only store can now be rejected in addition to the big box format.

4. Competitors:

- With two of the three format options eliminated, we should now test the concept of a hardware store.

Q Since our customers shop at all three types of stores, I would assume that our competition includes all home improvement retailers. But to what extent do hardware stores steal our customers away from us?

A Hardware stores have only a small impact on our competitiveness, primarily because of their superior neighborhood convenience. Our customers are willing to drive the extra mile, however, just to purchase our brands and talk to our respected associates. Ironically, we lose more customers because we are located in malls, and because we also sell products like underwear and designer suits, than because of the home improvement competition.

- At this point, we have enough evidence to strongly support a "hybrid" store format, one that is large enough to offer each of our product categories, and is also located outside the high-rent cities (since our customers are evidently willing to drive to us). We could call this format a "large suburban hardware store," a format that is new to the industry. These stores would allow us to continue to offer our proprietary brands, which are critical to getting customers in the store, and at the same time satisfy their cross-shopping interests. We would not have to learn how to merchandise new product categories, and could operate stores similar in size to the current hard goods department. Finally, we would avoid direct competition with the city hardware stores, and offer an easier, more convenient shopping experience for consumers and contractors that do not have the time or energy to navigate voluminous superstores.

Elements of an Outstanding Answer
Although no numbers were provided, an improved answer would include a brief quantitative analysis to determine if the hybrid format could break even.

1. Store revenues
   - Approximate sales per square foot of a 5,000 square foot store (from chart): $200
   - Expected sales of entire store: $5,000 \times \$200 = \$1,000,000$
2. Fixed store expenses
   - Cost of constructing 5,000 square feet of converted warehouse space: assume $100 per square foot: $\$10 \times 5,000 = \$500,000$
   - Assume cost of leasing land is $25 per square foot per year: $\$25 \times 5,000 = \$125,000$

3. Variable store expenses
- Make a conservative assumption that the average store margin is only 10 percent, after all variable costs are recognized.

4. Store profitability
- Sales of $1,000,000 with a 10 percent margin produces annual profits of $100,000. At this rate, the store would require approximately 6 years to cover the fixed cost of the building.

Since our margin estimate of 10 percent is conservative and the store, under the experienced management of the company, will likely earn a higher annual margin, we can assume that the breakeven point will arrive in less than six years. We will therefore still recommend that the store adopt a hybrid format.

• • •

TYPE 3   HUMAN RESOURCE MANAGEMENT

Case 3.1   Recruiting

You are the recruiting director of a major consulting firm. Your firm has traditionally been known for having bright and innovative consultants, but what candidates do not know is that the office atmosphere is "cutthroat." Informally, you have been told by several senior partners that the atmosphere needs to change, but they fear that a selection bias in the recruiting process is perpetuating the cutthroat atmosphere. How would you begin to investigate this hypothesis?

Elements of a Basic Answer
Framework: Internal–External.
As mentioned earlier in this book, it is very important that you answer the question that is asked and not the one that is anticipated. This case is a good example of an unexpected question attached to the end of a normal case. The case is not asking you to find a way to make the office less competitive, or to find out all the reasons why the office is overly competitive. It is only asking you to investigate the possibility of selection bias.

The generic nature of the internal/external framework makes it very useful in this case. Selection bias may occur because of the internal process that the firm uses to determine the best candidates. Or it may occur externally by the type of individuals who are attracted to the traditional image of this firm.

1. Internal:
   - Internally, three key elements may drive selection bias: the firm's target schools, the interviewing process, and the interviewers themselves.
   - Students at some schools traditionally have been more competitively inclined than at others. Is there a procedural bias toward these schools? How does the firm decide which schools to target? Are these targeted schools known for their cooperative or competitive student body? Are target schools determined by size of the alumni base at the firm or some other method (e.g., geographic proximity, popular press rankings)?
   - The interviewing process may effectively be screening out those applicants who may potentially be more cooperative in their work. What criteria are used to screen candidates during the initial resume review? On what attributes are candidates judged during the interviewing process? Is this rigid or flexible? How involved are the partners in the interviewing process?
   - There is a great deal of subjectivity in the interviewing process. Consequently, the personalities of the interviewers may intentionally or unintentionally influence those candidates who are selected. What type of consultants are allowed to interview? Have they observed any difference in competitive behavior from consultants from different schools?

2. External:
   - Externally, self-selection bias may be driven primarily by perceptions of the firm. How is the firm perceived by the candidates, particularly, in terms of the office culture, and promotion policies? Is it considered a high-stress environment where only those individuals who are willing to work long, difficult hours

survive? Do candidates believe that the firm has an up-or-out policy?

- The firm may be projecting an image that it does not intend. How does the firm present itself to students?

Elements of an Outstanding Answer

- An outstanding answer would consider how indirect forces may be influencing selection bias. For example, the company's internal promotion policies may develop competitive attributes in its consultants, who in turn may unintentionally have a bias toward those candidates who are more competitive.

———— • • • ————

TYPE 4   MARKET ENTRY

Case 4.1   Italian Pottery

A family-owned pottery manufacturer in Assisi, Italy, has decided to export its handcrafted wares to the United States, but needs your help to determine how. The manufacturer is considering three options: (1) sell directly to stores; (2) sell to distributors, who then sell to individual stores; and (3) open its own chain of proprietary stores. What should the manufacturer do?

Elements of a Basic Answer

Framework: Review the 4-P's (Product, Place, Price, Promotion), and then evaluate the three options.

1. Product:

- Italian pottery is typically produced in relatively small batches, and is glazed with unique patterns that are hand-painted by artisans.
- Complete sets of pottery can be obtained with the same glazing: serving platters and bowls, dishes, pitchers, mugs, storage containers, and even soap dishes and matching mirrors.

- Colorful glazes are typically painted on white backgrounds, and are organic in nature (vines, birds, and abstractions of other natural forms).
- Italian pottery has many substitutes, including all other types of dishes and serving platters.
- Still, Italian pottery is differentiated by its handcrafted artistic origin, and by unique patterns that are difficult to replicate.

2. Place:
   - Handcrafted artisan pottery is currently sold through only a few channels in the United States: upscale department stores, specialty home stores, and mail-order catalogs.
   - Occasionally, museum stores and even some gourmet coffee chains sell selected pieces.
   - Very few if any stores that are entirely devoted to the sale of artisan pottery exist, other than individual stores located at pottery manufacturing sites.
   - Stores that sell pottery typically offer a wide variety, imported from many different countries and regions.

3. Price:
   - European artisan pottery tends to be sold at a premium in the United States, due to its upscale image, its uniqueness, its fragility, and the middle and upper-class incomes of its primary customers.
   - Prices must be set high enough to cover the aggregate costs of manufacturing, distribution, financing, and allowances for loss/breakage, while still offering acceptable profit margins for all the players involved in the venture. The price and margin captured by the Italian manufacturer depends on the distribution channel selected.
   - Pricing decisions for the Italian pottery should also consider the price levels of substitutes. Consider the pricing decision of an Italian dining plate: if the closest substitutes (e.g., artisan dining plates imported from other countries) are priced at $10 each, then to remain competitive, the Italian plate should also be priced at $10. Only if customers perceive the manufacturing or artistic value of the Italian plate to be higher than that of the primary substitutes can the price exceed $10, at say $12 or even $15.

Similarly, if either the manufacturing or artistic quality of the Italian plate is perceived to be subpar, then the price should be set below $10, say at $8.

- If Italian pottery has had little exposure in the United States, or has had trouble capturing market share of the artisan pottery niche, then an alternative pricing scheme could be adopted undercut the prices of substitutes to develop customer interest and to encourage a trial purchase of the product, which in the long run may lead to repeat sales.

- Finally, pricing schemes need to consider customer perceptions: lower prices may attribute lower quality and uniqueness to the pottery, while higher prices may be translated into higher quality. Similarly, bundling schemes that offer lower prices when multiple pieces are purchased together may also connote lower quality.

4. Promotion:
- Italian pottery is likely to be difficult to promote, given the unique nature of each piece sold and the relatively limited quantities manufactured.

- If the pottery is sold through upscale department stores or home stores, then most of the promotion will likely be performed by the stores themselves, rather than either the manufacturer or distributor.

- Customers typically purchase artisan pottery for the following reasons: to buy a unique item as a gift, to buy a set of serving and dining ware for special occasions, or simply to satisfy an impulse urge when browsing through a store. As a result, customers may or may not have a predetermined intention to purchase artisan pottery before entering a store.

Let us now evaluate our three options.

Option 1: Sell directly to stores:
- This strategy would allow the manufacturer to bypass all middlemen and as a result capture greater profit. The manufacturer would also be able to carefully select the stores, and reject those that either do not support the upscale image of the product, or

carry too many substitute products, or are not committed to promoting the product.

- However, it may be difficult for an Italian-based manufacturer to identify American stores that may be interested in carrying the product. To be selective in its choice of stores, the manufacturer must have enough alternative stores to sell to.

Option 2: Sell to distributors:

- Given the difficulty of identifying American stores from Italy, the manufacturer may benefit from selling to distributors who already have store relationships. By working with multiple distributors, the manufacturer could indirectly increase sales by encouraging distributors to compete with each other and increase their sales efforts to stores.
- However, the profit earned will have to be shared with the distributor. Moreover, the distributor may not be as discriminating as the manufacturer when selecting stores.

Option 3: Open a chain of proprietary stores:

- This option might allow the manufacturer to capture the greatest profit from the venture, since it would be fully vertically integrated. The manufacturer would have full control of the display and design of the store, and would make all retail pricing decisions.
- On the other hand, the expense of opening retail stores may substantially reduce if not consume all the profit earned. The manufacturer has no experience with retailing, and is likely to have little knowledge of markets in the United States. Finally, there is little evidence that stores selling only artisan pottery could even survive.

The lowest-risk option is clearly number 2: sell to distributors. Other than building relationships with distributors, the manufacturer would not have to develop additional competencies. The cost of establishing retail outlets would be avoided, as would the cost of selling to stores. Although the manufacturer might not capture as much profit from each unit sold, the costs associated with this option are also the lowest.

Elements of an Outstanding Answer

- This entire analysis was performed without even questioning the fundamental idea of selling Italian pottery in the United States. Perhaps alternative strategies would yield preferable results, such as selling pottery to stores in Italy or other parts of Europe, or teaming up with tour agencies to bring vacationers to the factory store.

- An outstanding answer might also propose additional U.S. distribution strategies, such as mail-order catalogs, or sales though the World Wide Web.

—————•••—————

Type 5   Market Sizing

Case 5.1   Gourmet Coffee Shops

Part I: A large coffee processing company has seen sales of its well-known supermarket brand coffee drop 15 percent per year over the past five years. As a result, manufacturing costs per pound of coffee are increasing, since 25 percent of the machines are no longer being used, and monthly production has dropped by 50,000 pounds. Meanwhile, gourmet coffee chains are growing rapidly across the United States. Should the company try to capture some of this growth by opening its own proprietary chain of gourmet coffee stores?

Part II: How many individual coffee stores could the company supply, if it has 50,000 pounds of excess monthly production capacity? Assume one pound of coffee yields 10 cups of brewed coffee.

Elements of a Basic Answer

Framework: **Part I:** 3-C's: Company, Customers, Competitors.

Part II: Bottom-up breakeven: estimate the number of customers who visit a gourmet coffee shop in a month, then translate visits into the number of pounds of coffee required to brew the cups consumed. Divide

50,000 pounds of excess monthly capacity by the total pounds of coffee consumed at a single shop in a month, to determine the total number of shops the company could supply.

Part I

1. Company:

- We should begin to answer the question by understanding whether the company needs to look outside its existing sales channels at all. Although sales have been declining, the company may be able to fix its current core business before exploring alternative ones.

Q Does the company sell its coffee only through supermarkets, or are additional channels used?

A All the coffee is sold in pressure-sealed cans through supermarkets and general food stores. No other channels are used.

Q Have supermarket and general store sales of coffee dropped overall, or only for this company's brand?

A Market research indicates that all the brands sold through these channels have experienced the same rate of sales decline.

- It appears that the channel is driving the company's declining performance. Although the company could attempt to capture greater market share through aggressive pricing schemes, the channel appears to be losing attractiveness overall. An alternative channel may indeed be an attractive way to solve the excess capacity problem.

- We should now assess the competencies of the company, to determine how well positioned it is to open coffee shops.

Q How well known is the brand? Does the company have more than one brand?

A The company sells all its coffee under a single brand, but the brand has universal recognition in the United States. It has been around for nearly a century as a household name, and is currently supported through an extensive television and print advertising campaign.

Q How many different products are offered under the brand, and which are the best sellers?

A The company produces regular, decaffeinated, gourmet, and instant. Their best selling coffee is regular, and very little of the gourmet is sold.

- The company is an established brand, with a complete array of products. But a weak gourmet product does not support the idea of opening a chain of gourmet coffee shops. The brand name may have strong equity, but it appears to be associated with more generic coffee products.

Q Does the company have any retail experience?

A No. Sales have always been through the same supermarket and general store channels.

- Not having a competency in retail management could threaten the success of a gourmet coffee shop venture. The company will either have to slow the rate of opening stores to learn from mistakes and build expertise, or buy managers from another company at great expense.

2. Customers:
- The strength of the brand lies in the loyalty of its customers. We might argue that a chain of gourmet coffee shops operating under the same brand name as the supermarket coffee will attract people who already select the brand.

Q How would you define the primary customers of the brand?

A Most customers are located in suburban or rural areas, and are of lower- to middle-income levels.

- Already, the argument looks weak. Most gourmet coffee shops are located in urban centers, but evidently the company's primary customers live elsewhere.

Q Is it fair to assume that most purchase this company's coffee to brew at home?

A Yes, or at the office.

Q How brand-loyal are people who purchase the canned coffee?

A Hardly. Price seems to be the primary driver of a purchasing decision, although some people stick with certain brands, believing that they taste better.

- If customers who already purchase the company's canned coffee are only weakly loyal, then they are unlikely to be any more attracted to a gourmet coffee shop under the same brand name than anyone else would be.

- In fact, the high recognition of the company's brand may actually be a handicap. It is undeniably ironic for a gourmet store to be named after a supermarket brand of generic household coffee.

3. Competitors:
- If the company were to open a chain of coffee stores, it would most likely be the third or fourth (or higher) entrant in any given market. The company would be fighting an uphill battle from the very start.
- Many competitor chains have national coverage, and operate hundreds of stores in most major cities. They already have the exposure to build a strong gourmet brand identity, and have spent years building customer loyalty.
- The competition has had years to test and refine their retail concept, and to work the operational kinks out of stores.
- Most of the prime real estate in many key gourmet coffee cities, like Boston, New York, and San Francisco, is already owned by the competition.

The evidence stacks up against the idea, and the company should not open a chain of gourmet coffee shops.

Part II   Treat this part of the case as a market sizing calculation.

1. Estimate the number of customers who visit a gourmet coffee shop in a day:
- Assumed number of cash registers in one shop: 2
- Estimated time to service one customer: 1 minute
- Number of customers serviced in one minute:
2 registers $\times$ 1 customer per minute = 2 customers per minute

- Hours of store operation
  (assume 6 A.M. to 12 midnight): 18 hours
- Number of daily hours that are "peak"
  (assume 7 A.M. to 10 A.M., 12 P.M. to 1 P.M.,
  and 8 P.M. to 10 P.M.): 6 hours
- Number of customers serviced during "peak" (assume lines are long and the flow of customers is constant):
  6 hours × 60 minutes × 2 customers per minute = 720 customers
- Number of customers serviced during "nonpeak" (assume traffic flow is half of peak levels):
  12 hours × 60 minutes × 1 customer per minute = 720 customers
- Total number of customers serviced during hours of operation:
  720 + 720 = 1,440 customers

2. Estimate the number of pounds of coffee required to service customers in one month
   - Number of customers visiting in one month:
     1,440 customers × 30 days = 43,200 customers
   - Number of cups of coffee consumed
     (assume 1 house coffee per customer): 43,200 cups
   - Equivalent number of pounds of coffee:
     43,200 cups/10 cups per pound = 4,320 pounds.

With 50,000 pounds of excess monthly production capacity, the company can service 50,000 pounds/4,320 pounds per shop = almost 12 shops. We now have yet another piece of evidence to argue against the gourmet coffee shop idea: to successfully compete against the established chains, the new chain needs a presence that is broader than 12 shops.

Elements of an Outstanding Answer
Rather then opening a proprietary chain of coffee shops, the company should become a supplier of coffee to existing shops. This strategy would build on the strengths of the company (coffee processing and distribution), would eliminate the need to develop new competencies (gourmet brand identity, retail experience, loyal customer base), and would allow the company to sell its excess production capacity to

exactly 12 shops. Since the primary objective of the company was to restore production to prior levels of efficiency, this solution will achieve the desired result without creating any new problems.

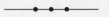

TYPE 6 MERGERS AND ACQUISITIONS

Case 6.1   **HMO Acquisition**

Question: A New York based health maintenance organization (HMO) is considering expanding its operations. They currently have the funds to purchase another HMO. Their internal M&A group has identified two possible targets: Allied HMO in Miami, and Washington Health in Seattle. Which should they purchase?

Elements of a Basic Answer

Framework: 3-C's: Company, Customers, Competitors

When considering M&A questions, it is very helpful to first identify the purpose of the merger or acquisition. Often, candidates assume that the intent of the merger is to have a positive impact on the company's balance sheet. However, the actual purpose could be to improve the strategic positioning of the company, send a signal to the market, or eliminate a competitor. A company could have many reasons for choosing to merge or acquire another company. Understanding the original intent will guide the rest of the answer. In this case, the intent is to improve the geographic coverage of the HMO.

1. Company:
- At a minimum, you will want to determine if there is a cultural fit between the two companies. Significant cultural fit issues have the potential to sour any M&A activity. Other issues to consider include a company's public image, and its relationship with its doctors. Questions may include the following:

Q What is the leadership style at the New York HMO (NY HMO)? And how does this differ with the other two companies?

A NY HMO's former CEO developed a strong hierarchy of leadership within the company. The President, CEO, and COO decide most management issues. By contrast, Washington Health gives its individual divisions a great deal of autonomy. They developed a Leadership Board composed of the vice presidents of all the divisions. This approach is mirrored at Allied HMO. Allied makes a conscious attempt to include a wide variety of people in its decision-making process, through its Leadership Board, employee suggestion box, and a strong open-door policy.

Q Does the new CEO adhere to the old hierarchical approach? How open is this person to change? How open is the company to change?

A NY HMO's new CEO was recruited from a manufacturing firm. Consequently, she has not been indoctrinated into the traditional approach. As the COO of the manufacturing firm, she instituted policies that essentially decentralized the manufacturing process. Because of high wages and generous benefits, turnover at NY HMO is very low.

• Although there may be a cultural fit problem with acquisition targets, the new CEO may be able to resolve them.

• We should determine whether the corporate reputation of NY HMO among patients and physicians fits with those of its acquisition targets. A mixed reputation could potentially have a severe impact on the ability for an HMO to function well.

Q How is NY HMO viewed by the public? Is it viewed as an HMO with cutting-edge technology and methodologies? Does it have the best doctors? How does this image differ with those of the two acquisition targets? What is the relationship between doctors and NY HMO? Is this relationship similar to the other two acquisition targets?

A NY HMO is seen as the premier HMO in the New York and northern New Jersey areas. It is not a staff model (i.e., the doctors who serve NY HMO patients are not employees of the company). They recruit only the best doctors, keep close track of their performance with frequent customer satisfaction surveys, and generously compensate them for their work. Despite some late reimbursements, doctors are generally very pleased with their relationship with the company. Washington Health follows a traditional staff model. The doctors are well paid for their geographic region. Their reputation is strong in the area they serve. Allied is not a staff model and is considered average. Allied generally promises to help any company reduce its healthcare costs within two years. Because of this approach, they keep very close track of their doctors, but some physicians resent this level of scrutiny.

- Based on reputation, there seems to be a better fit with Washington Health.

2. Customers:

- If the intent of the merger is to expand geographic coverage, then the purpose of the merger is to better serve the customers. So first you need to understand their customer base.

Q What type of customers does NY HMO serve?

A The majority (75%) of NY HMO's customers are older patients, who are either on Medicare, or can pay for healthcare themselves.

Q What is the customer composition at the other two HMOs?

A Washington Health and Allied have a standard mix of customers.

Q Are there any other important demographic characteristics by which we could segment each HMO's customer base?

A Yes—money. NY HMO's customers are generally fairly well off.

- Customer composition is critical. In this case, it suggests that there may be behavioral aspects that should be considered.

Q If NY HMO's customers are relatively well off, do they travel frequently?

A Yes. They frequently travel to Florida for the winter.

- Since the intent is to expand geographic coverage, NY HMO should consider Allied despite the potential problems, given the travel patterns of its largest customer segment.

3. Competitors:

Q If NY HMO were to acquire Allied, what kind of competitive response could there be in the New York-New Jersey market and in the Florida market?

A The competitive response would be weak. Most HMOs are actively recruiting Medicare patients and are generally limited to a single state.

- In this case, competition is not a significant factor.

The evidence supports the acquisition objective, so NY HMO should acquire Allied.

Elements of an Outstanding Answer
A more in-depth analysis would include an abbreviated cost-benefit analysis. The acquisition of Allied may be strategically sound, but how much would it cost? Is the acquisition a positive NPV project?

Is NY HMO a public company? How would an acquisition impact their leverage ratios (ratios that indicate the long-run solvency of a company)? What kind of information would be needed? How would stockholders respond? Would stockholder objectives be different from that of management?

———— • • • ————

TYPE 7 NEW PRODUCT INTRODUCTION

Case 7.1   **Cricket Ball Exports to the United States**

A U.K.-based cricket ball manufacturer seeks sales expansion opportunities in the United States. Current production is at full capacity, but US$500 million has been allocated to build additional capacity. Should the company introduce the product in the United States?

Elements of a Basic Answer
Framework: Consider three topics: (1) the size of the current U.S. cricket ball market, (2) initiatives the company might take to promote the sale of cricket balls in the United

States, and (3) whether US$500 million is an adequate investment in production capacity to meet U.S. demand.

1. Size of the United States cricket ball market:
   - Approximate population of the United States: 250 million
   - Age bracket of people who may play cricket: 16 to 45
   - Percentage of population represented by this bracket using the following assumption:

Ages		
0–15	20% of population	
16–30	20	
31–45	20	= 40%
46–60	20	
61–80	20	
	100%	

   - Number of people of age to play cricket:
     250 million × 40% = 100 million
   - Assumption: only those people who have heard of cricket may play. Estimate 1 in 5 people have heard of the game:
     100 million × 20% = 20 million
   - Of the people who may play, only a few will actually play. Base this assumption on personal experience, by assuming that 1 in 20 people who have heard of baseball, for example, actually play:
     20 million × 5% = 1 million
   - But baseball is a much more widely played game than cricket, so we should scale this number down, say by 50% = 500,000 people
   - How many cricket balls will these people purchase? For baseball, only one ball is required for 15 to 30 people to play. So assume a similar ratio for cricket of 1 ball for 20 people:
     500,000 × 5% = 25,000 people
   - Would it be worth the manufacturer's effort to sell 25,000 balls per year in the United States? If each ball were priced at US$10.00, then the total revenue (assuming 100% market share) would be US$250,000. This could be worthwhile if the cost structure were low enough, but we do not have enough information to make a judgment.

2. The company could try to increase the market for cricket balls through a number of promotional initiatives:
   - Sponsor broadcasts of live cricket games over United States television to improve public familiarity of the game and even generate sustainable interest. However, this would be very expensive, and only a few viewers would purchase a cricket ball in response to the shows.
   - Sponsor cricket camps for children to encourage interest in the game at an early age. This would be less expensive, but the strategy has a number of problems: children do not purchase cricket balls, their parents do; and cricket camps can only attract children (and parents) who already have an interest or curiosity in the game.
   - Give away free cricket balls at other sporting events. This would introduce the game to a population that already has sporting interests; however, this could be extremely costly (especially when only 25,000 balls are expected to be sold in year one), and although people may appreciate the gesture, few of the balls would actually be used to play a game of cricket.
   - Promotional efforts are likely to face a number of hurdles: high cost of promotions, low public awareness, and a high degree of organization required to play game.

3. Assess the adequacy of US$500 million to cover the cost of adding additional manufacturing capacity.
   - To determine the marginal cost of adding a unit of production capacity, we need to understand the fixed costs associated with the existing facility. However, no information was provided. Instead, we can assume that the company would have to build additional production space, and possibly add a new warehouse. We can be generous and allocate US$10 million toward property enhancements. As for additional machinery, we now know that 25,000 balls must be manufactured each year, which when divided by 250 working days yields 100 balls per day, or 12.5 balls per hour of an 8-hour day. Need the company buy more than one machine to meet this demand? Probably not. In short,

US$500 million is an extremely large amount, and will certainly cover the cost of adding the requisite capacity.

4. So should the company introduce cricket balls into the United States? At this point, everything we have learned would support an answer of no: The market is too small, it is far too costly and difficult to promote the game, and with a cash reserve of US$500 million the company could easily explore other ideas.

Elements of an Outstanding Answer

Three other strategic options could be considered: (1) alternative markets, (2) alternative ball products, and (3) acquisition.

1. Now that we have rejected the U.S. market as too small, perhaps we could consider other markets, especially those in which cricket is already played. Australia, India, Pakistan, Hong Kong, South Africa, Ireland, and Scotland are but a few of the markets the company could consider. However, we do not know whether the company already sells to these markets.

2. Another option could be to manufacture other ball products, such as baseballs, soccer balls, and tennis balls. If the company adopted this strategy, then entry into the U.S. market could once again become a possibility. However, to be able to compete in the United States, the company's products have to be lower in cost, or superior in quality, or in some other way unique. Thus the market for these alternative products may be larger, but the company would have to learn the business dynamics of unfamiliar products.

3. If the learning curve of manufacturing new products is too steep, then the company could consider purchasing an established ball manufacturer, either within or without the United States. This way, the company could immediately acquire the sales volume of the other company, and expand without having to build a competency or production capability from scratch. Still, alternative investments of the US$500 million exist, and may offer a higher return at a lower risk (e.g., bonds).

Ultimately, the selection of a strategy depends on more than a simple interest in expanding sales. It is directly related to the interests of the company's constituents (e.g., shareholders), and the competencies and vision of management.

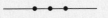

TYPE 8   OPPORTUNITY ASSESSMENT

Case 8.1   On-line Bookstore

Question: If a book distributor were thinking about launching an on-line bookstore, what would be its estimated annual sales?

Elements of a Basic Answer

Framework: Estimate the annual sales of a Web-based bookstore using a top-down approach.

1. Number of Americans with Internet access:

- Number of people in the United States: 250 million
- Age bracket of primary Internet users: 16 to 45
- Percentage of population represented by this bracket using the following assumption: 40%

Ages	0–15	20% of population
	16–30	20
	31–45	20
	46–60	20
	61–80	20
		100%

$\left. \begin{array}{c} \\ \\ \\ \end{array} \right\} = 40\%$

- Number of people within primary bracket:
250 million × 40% = 100 million
- Percentage of people within bracket who own computers with modems using the following assumptions:
  Students (ages 16 to 21): 30% have computers at home
  Young Professionals (ages 22 to 45): 60% have computers at home or work
  Average: 50%
- Number of Americans with Internet access:
100 million × 50% = 50 million

2. Size of World Wide Web browsing population:
- Number of Americans with Internet access who have visited the Web: assume 1 in 2 = 50 million × 50% = 25 million
- Number of Web visitors who regularly repeat-visit (assume only those people who are very familiar with the Web are willing to make an online book purchase):
  assume 1 in 5 = 25 million × 20% = 5 million

3. Book sales on the Web:
- Percentage of frequent Web users who read books: assume a low 30 percent, since reading and Web browsing are both leisure activities that can consume a great deal of time, and cannot be pursued simultaneously.
- Number of possible online purchasers of books:
  5 million × 30% = 1.5 million
- Percentage of book purchases made online versus through a book store: assume 20 percent, since the primary reasons for purchasing online are either convenience or low price; most book purchasers, however, will prefer to read books immediately on purchase, and will therefore shop book stores more frequently.
- Number of books purchased per year per person: assume 5
- Number of books purchased online:
  1.5 million people × 5 books × 20% = 1.5 million books
- Average price of book: $20.00
- Total online book purchases:
  $20.00 × 1.5 million = $30 million

Elements of an Outstanding Answer

1. If the book distributor were the first to establish an on-line store, then in the absence of competition its annual sales could approach $30 million. Of course, first-year sales will be substantially lower, and will rise slowly year to year thereafter. As the popularity of the Web increases, and people become more accustomed to making online purchases, the $30 million estimate should likewise increase.

Sensitivity analysis:

Market Share	Total Annual Sales
100%	$30 million
75	$22.5
50	$15
25	$7.5

2. Since many of the assumptions in the opportunity assessment were based on either personal experience or conservative attempts to parse populations into smaller subgroupings, the resulting estimated sales number should be checked for reasonableness.

• The distributor should launch the online business only if the economics of the venture are equally or more attractive than those of a retail book store.

• How could we quickly estimate the sales of a retail book store, for comparative purposes? Estimate the costs associated with operating a store, say of the newer big-box variety of 50,000 square feet in a shopping mall:

Cost Item	Amount
Rent ($25 square foot/year)	$1,250,000
Staff (20 people at $40,000/year fully-costed)	800,000
Inventory (assume 50 shelving units, 10 shelves per unit, 20 feet long each, 10 books per foot) $50 \times 10 \times 20 \times 10 = 100,000$ books $\times$ average wholesale price of $15 =	1,500,000
Operations (utilities, maintenance, phone, etc.)	100,000
Allowance for loss: inventory $\times$ 5% =	75,000
Total Cost	$3,725,000

To turn a profit, sales of a large retail book store must exceed $3.725 million, so our estimated sales could be $5 million.

• Compared with $5 million, online sales of $30 million is certainly attractive. Still, the wide disparity may be an indication that our assumptions are somewhat flawed, and as a result our online sales estimate may be slightly exaggerated.

———— • • • ————

Type 9 Pricing

Case 9.1   **Amtrak Rail Ticket**

How does Amtrak price a rail ticket from Boston to Washington, DC?

Elements of a Basic Answer

Framework: Three C's: Customers, Company, Competitors

1. Customers—Amtrak may want to price discriminate among its customers:

   - Amtrak has essentially four customer sets: (1) vacationing travelers, (2) business travelers, (3) students, and (4) commuters. Each of these customers has unique travel patterns. Vacationers will most likely travel during the weekend, often in pairs or families, but may also be present during the week. Business travelers are most common on weekdays, typically during the morning and evening. Students travel most often before and after holidays, and at the beginning and end of semesters. Commuters tend to be most prevalent during the morning and evening hours, riding the train for relatively short distances. For the Boston to Washington route, however, we would only expect to find vacationing, business, and student travelers.

   - Passenger volume is directly correlated to the day of the week, the time of day, the season, and the calendar of holidays. Amtrak may want to consider each of these factors when determining promotional or discounted pricing schemes.

   - Each of the four customer sets is likely to have different price sensitivities: Vacationers may be highly price sensitive and seek family or advance-purchase discounts; business travelers are likely to be less price sensitive, since many of their tickets will be reimbursed by corporations; students and commuters are likely to be the most price sensitive, and may be attracted to age-based or volume discounts.

   - Service expectations also vary for each customer type. Business travelers and commuters are negatively affected by delays and slow service, and as a result may be willing to pay a premium to have guaranteed or faster service. Vacationers and students, on the other hand, may care more about low price than fast service. Still, all four customer sets would surely like to have a seat, a food car, toilets, and maybe even telephones.

- Given such a variety of customer needs and interests, Amtrak could benefit from a pricing strategy that offers different prices to different customers on different days.

2. Company—Amtrak must cover its costs, and still earn a profit:

- Amtrak should price the ticket to at least cover the variable costs and the portion of the fixed costs associated with a one-way trip from Boston to Washington, D.C. Included within the variable costs of the train are labor (1 train conductor, 1 food car agent, 2 ticket collectors), electricity or fuel to operate the locomotive and power the train cabins, drinking water, and miscellaneous toilet items (paper, soap, etc.). Fixed costs include the track, the train locomotive and cars, rail yards, maintenance facilities, corporate offices, customer service facilities, Amtrak information systems and technology, and so on. Only a tiny portion of the total fixed costs, however, should be attributed to operating one train from Boston to Washington. In fact, some of these costs could be considered "sunk" costs (e.g., the track), and therefore should not be attributed to this run at all.

- At a more macro level, a cost-based pricing strategy should also look beyond the simple Boston to Washington route, and consider the cost of operating the total nationwide Amtrak system. It is quite possible that a cost associated with constructing a new rail in California will have to be borne in part by the operation of a train in the Northeast Corridor. Only once these factors are considered can a profitable margin be determined.

3. Competitors—Amtrak must be careful to not price itself out of the market:

- Each customer group mentioned earlier will certainly factor price into their transportation decision. Therefore, the pricing of a one-way Boston to Washington rail ticket must be competitive with alternative transportation methods, such as airplanes (approximately $150 one-way), buses ($45 one-way), rental cars ($50 per day plus gas, tolls and parking), and personal cars (gas, tolls, and parking, plus a portion of insurance, and depreciation of the automobile). To effectively attract each customer group, the basic price of a rail ticket needs to be lower than a flight. But given the greater comfort of a train and perhaps even the faster speed, a rail ticket can cost more than the bus or driving a car.

4. An effective price discriminating strategy would therefore be the following:

Vacationers:	Offer family, group, and senior citizen discounts to attract highly price-sensitive, low time-constrained customers: $50 to $100 one way.
Business Travelers:	Run express trains with reserved seating and special amenities (telephones, laptop plugs, etc.) with higher priced tickets to satisfy time-constrained, price-insensitive travelers: $75 to $125 one way.
Students:	Offer age, multipack ticket, and holiday discounts to satisfy price-sensitive, frequent traveling, seasonal customers: $50 to $100 one way.
Commuters:	(not applicable to the Boston to Washington route)

Elements of an Outstanding Answer

An outstanding answer would graphically argue that the demand curves of the different customer segments are also important drivers of pricing. Take, for example, an illustrative demand curve for business travelers. Although we argued that they had inelastic demand curves, this may hold true for only a certain range of price changes. That is, their demand curve may be a step curve, as seen in Figure AII.2.

Note that raising the price from P_1 to P_2, does not affect the demand for tickets. However, raising the price (only slightly) again to P_3 drastically reduces the demand for tickets. Why? One answer may be that the existence of alternatives creates strong price sensitivities after a certain price range. Another may be corporate policy. Thus, the

Figure AII.2
Step Function Demand Curve for Business Travelers

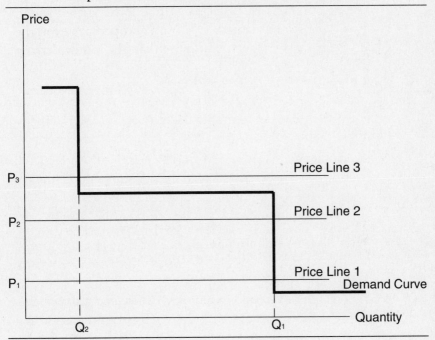

degree of price differentiation depends not only on price elasticity, but also on the nature of the demand function.

● ● ●

TYPE 10   PROFITABILITY LOSS

Case 10.1   Pharmaceutical Drugs

The CEO of a major pharmaceutical company wants to know why the profits of one of its leading over-the-counter drugs declined by 25 percent over the last year.

Elements of a Basic Answer

Framework: Profit = Total revenues − Total costs

Or profit = (Price × Quantity) − (Fixed costs + (Variable costs × Quantity))

1. Total Costs: Understand if the product's costs have changed recently:
   - Total costs can be divided into fixed and variable costs. For this company, examples of fixed costs would include the machinery and equipment used to manufacture the drug, and the building within which the production equipment is housed.

   Q Have the fixed costs increased recently?

   A No, they have remained constant over time. The company has not had to increase the amount of space or the number of machines.

   - Evidently, fixed costs are not responsible for the profit loss. Let's turn to variable costs, which would include the materials used to manufacture the drug, shipping and distribution costs, and marketing and promotion of the product to doctors, hospitals, and the public.

   Q Are the drug's raw materials increasing in price?

   A No, they have remained constant.

   Q How about shipping costs? Do we have difficulty delivering the product to remote destinations?

   A No, we use third-party distributors who purchase the product in bulk from us and then deliver smaller quantities to the end users. We only have to carry the cost of shipping to these centralized distributors, which have not increased substantially over the past year.

   Q Have we changed our marketing efforts?

   A Yes, last year we increased our advertising and promotions budget 5 percent, since we are facing increasing competition.

   - Could this be the reason profits are declining? Only partially, since a 5 percent increase in spending does not necessarily equate to the 25 percent profitability decline. Something else must be responsible for our profit loss.

2. Total Revenues: Understand the sources of revenues for the product:
   - Since total revenues equals price × total quantity, we need to understand if these two inputs have changed.

Q Have you changed the price of the drug, or perhaps offered unusual discounts, in the past year?

A No, the price has remained the same, and we continue to offer the same volume discounts to our most important customers.

Q Then perhaps we have a problem collecting from our customers?

A We've always had approximately 5 percent loss from uncollected bills, but we price our product high enough to cover this loss.

• Next, consider sales volume.

Q Has the total quantity of the drug sold changed recently?

A Yes, it has decreased substantially in the last year.

• Finally, we have identified an element of the profitability equation that has significantly changed. But we cannot stop here—we still have to understand why volume has dropped. Could it be due to declining product quality? Or perhaps due to a declining rate of use among patients? Or even a recent customer preference for substitute products? To answer these questions, we need to better understand the product.

Q Is the drug unique, or are there other products that have the same or similar effects?

A We are currently the only branded product on the market, recognized by doctors, patients, and pharmacists as the leading brand. But dozens of almost identical generic products also exist.

• It would seem that the competition is responsible for our company's declining sales volume, but again we need to understand why. If the generics have always existed, then something else must be causing the sudden volume drop; but if the generics only recently entered the market, then perhaps their arrival has indeed caused the volume decline.

Q How recently have the generics become available?

A Only about a year ago—about the same time our drug patent expired.

• Now we have our answer: The expiration of the company's patent has allowed generics to invade the market, most likely at lower prices, but our company has evidently held the price of its drug constant. As a result, customers have switched to the generics, and our company has had to face lower revenues and hence lower profits.

Elements of an Outstanding Answer

1. Take the case to the next level, by offering recommendations to remedy the situation:
   - The company should reconsider its pricing strategy. Several arguments favor holding the price constant: (a) to maintain an image of a superior, premium product; (b) to continue to extract as much value as possible out of an established brand ("milking" the product); and (c) to avoid the problem that once a price is dropped, it becomes extremely difficult to raise it later.
   - However, a number of different arguments favor a price reduction: (a) to compete with the generics, and perhaps even undercut them; (b) to focus customer attention away from price and toward product reputation when deciding which product to buy; and (c) to increase sales volume and ultimately reap greater revenues and profits despite the lower price.

2. Based on these arguments, a final recommendation could be the following:
   - Lower the price only slightly, to reduce the price disparity with the generics and to restore sales with more price-sensitive customers; continue to lower the price until the share loss is stabilized, but be sure to maintain a slight price premium. As long as the generic products exist, our company is unlikely to restore its original 100 percent market share. The CEO will have to accept some profit loss from a year ago, but by following this strategy, the drug should be able to rely on its brand image to compete.

APPENDIX III

DIRECTORY OF ONE HUNDRED CONSULTING FIRMS

To jump-start your research on consulting firms, we have collected information on one-hundred consulting firms and corporate strategic planning units and presented it in this consolidated resource for you. Although many of the practices listed here are among the largest and best known in the industry, we did not simply select the top one hundred firms.[1] Rather, we deliberately provided a range of practices in terms of size, sector-focus (private, public, and nonprofit), and consulting practice area, to give you a sense of how diverse the opportunities are in the consulting industry. For specific information, contact the firms directly and supplement your research by browsing their Web sites, since recruiting and office information changes frequently and is sometimes specific to factors such as the geographic region or school of the candidate.

In the United States, the recruiting season runs from January to May for undergraduates, from January to May for first-year MBAs seeking summer internships, from September to January (although it may run through May for some firms) for graduating MBAs, and year-round for career-changing professionals.

Abt Associates
55 Wheeler Street
Cambridge, MA 02138
617-492-7100
www.abtassoc.com

Profile
Staff: 1,000
8 offices worldwide

Service Focus
Strategy
Organizational Development
Market Research
Social & Urban Planning

Industry Focus
Government
NGO
Environmental Agencies
Pharmaceuticals/Biotech
Education

Accenture (formerly Andersen Consulting)
33 West Monroe Street
Chicago, IL 60603
312-372-7100
www.ac.com

Profile
Staff: 65,496
115 offices worldwide

Service Focus
Human Resources
Information Technology
Operations Management
Strategy

Industry Focus
Communications
Energy
Financial Services
Pharmaceuticals/Biotech
Manufacturing

Adventis (formerly Renaissance Strategy)
10 Saint James Avenue
    17th Floor
Boston, MA 02116
617-421-9990
www.adventis.com

Profile
Staff: 200+
5 U.S. offices plus London

Service Focus
Strategy

Industry Focus
Communications
Computing
Commerce & Content

The Advisory Board Company
600 New Hampshire Avenue, NW
Washington, DC 20037
202-672-5600
www.advisory.com

Profile
Staff: 400
1 office in Washington, DC

Service Focus
Benchmarking
Research
Strategy
Training
Events

Industry Focus
Healthcare & Life Sciences

American Express Strategic Planning Group

World Financial Center
200 Vesey Street
  38th Floor
New York, NY 10285-3809
212-640-7593
www.americanexpress.com

Profile
Staff: 40
Offices in New York and London

Service Focus
Strategy
New Product Development
New Business Launch
Mergers & Acquisitions
Marketing Strategy

Industry Focus
Financial Services
Travel
Interactive Services

American Management Systems, Inc. (AMS)

4050 Legato Road
Fairfax, VA 22033
703-267-8000
www.amsinc.com

Profile
Staff: 8,031
73 offices worldwide

Service Focus
Human Resources
Information Technology
Operations Management
Strategy

Industry Focus
Government
Communications
Financial Services

Answerthink

1001 Brickwell Bay Drive
  Suite 3000
Miami, FL 33131
877-423-4321
www.answerthink.com

Profile
Staff: 1,400
20 U.S. offices

Service Focus
Information Technology
e-Commerce
Marketing & Branding

Industry Focus
Most industries

Andersen (formerly Arthur Andersen)

69 West Washington Street
Chicago, IL 60602-3002
312-507-0069
www.arthurandersen.com

Profile
Staff: 9,810
385 offices worldwide (including
  tax and audit)

Service Focus
Information Technology
Operations Management
Strategy

Industry Focus
Communications
Government
Financial Services

Aon Consulting
123 North Wacker Drive
  Suite 1100
Chicago, IL 60606
312-701-4800
www.aonconsulting.com

Profile
Staff: 4,300
130 offices worldwide

Service Focus
Human Resources

Industry Focus
Financial Services
Healthcare
Manufacturing

Arthur D. Little
25 Acorn Park
Cambridge, MA 02140
617-498-5000
www.arthurdlittle.com

Profile
Staff: 2,000
45 offices worldwide

Service Focus
Information Technology
Strategy
Operations Management

Industry Focus
Most industries

A.T. Kearney (an EDS company)
222 West Adams Street
Chicago, IL 60606
312-648-0111
www.atkearney.com

Profile
Staff: 2,560
55 offices worldwide

Service Focus
Human Resources
Information Technology
Operations Management
Strategy

Industry Focus
Most industries

Atos Origin
Deccaweg 26
1042 AD Amsterdam
The Netherlands
+31 20 5 653 653
www.origin-it.com

Profile
Staff: 27,000
120 offices worldwide

Service Focus
Information Technology
Operations Management

Industry Focus
Most industries

Avanade
2211 Elliott Avenue
Seattle, WA 98121
206-239-5600

Profile
Staff: NA
17 offices worldwide

Service Focus
Information Technology

Industry Focus
Most industries

Bain & Company, Inc.
Two Copley Place
Boston, MA 02116
617-572-2000
www.bain.com

Profile
Staff: 1,800
26 offices worldwide

Service Focus
Operations Management
Strategy

Industry Focus
Consumer Products
Financial Services
Retail
Technology
Telecommunications
Utilities

Booz•Allen & Hamilton, Inc.
Worldwide Commercial Business
101 Park Avenue
New York, NY 10178
212-551-6000
www.bah.com

Profile
Staff: 7,471
105 offices worldwide

Service Focus
Information Technology
Operations Management
Strategy

Industry Focus
Communications
Energy/Oil & Gas
Government

The Boston Consulting Group, Inc.
Exchange Place
  31st Floor
Boston, MA 02109
617-973-1200
www.bcg.com

Profile
Staff: 2,500
46 offices worldwide

Service Focus
Operations Management
Strategy

Industry Focus
Most industries

Braun Consulting
30 West Monroe
   Suite 300
Chicago, IL 60603
800-68-BRAUN
www.braunconsult.com

Profile
Staff: 250
11 U.S. offices

Service Focus
Strategy
Marketing Strategy
Technology
Product Development & Launch

Industry Focus
Communications
Financial Services
Manufacturing
Packaged Goods
Pharmaceuticals

Breakaway Solutions
Two Seaport Lane
Boston, MA 02210
617-275-3000

Profile
Staff: NA
17 offices worldwide

Service Focus
Information Technology
Marketing
Product Development
Strategy

Industry Focus
Financial Services
Retail
Technology

Buck Consultants, Inc.
One Pennsylvania Plaza
New York, NY 10119-4798
212-330-1000
www.buckconsultants.com

Profile
Staff: 3,100
60 offices worldwide

Service Focus
Human Resources

Industry Focus
Financial Services
Healthcare

**Cambridge Technology
   Partners (CTP)**
8 Cambridge Center
Cambridge, MA 02142
617-374-9800
www.ctp.com

Profile
Staff: 3,732
53 offices worldwide

Service Focus
Information Technology
Operations Management
Strategy

Industry Focus
Business Services
Energy/Oil & Gas
High Technology
Manufacturing

**Cambridge Strategic
   Management Group (CSMG)**
One Boston Place
Boston, MA 02108-4409
617-999-1000
www.csmgusa.com

Profile
Staff: 40
Offices in Boston and London

Service Focus
Strategy
Marketing

Industry Focus
Communications
High-Technology

Cap Gemini Ernst & Young
1114 Avenue of the Americas
   29th Floor
New York, NY 10036
212-944-6464
www.cgey.com

Profile
Staff: 42,685
300+ offices worldwide

Service Focus
Information Technology
Operations Management
Strategy

Industry Focus
Most industries

CBSI
32605 West Twelve Mile Road
   Suite 250
Farmington Hills, MI 48334
248-488-2088
www.cbsiinc.com

Profile
Staff: 4,322
39 offices worldwide

Service Focus
Human Resources
Information Technology
Operations Management
Strategy

Industry Focus
Most industries

Centegy
6539A Dumbarton Circle
Fremont, CA 94555
510-789-1820
www.centegy.com

Profile
Staff: NA
3 U.S. offices

Service Focus
Supply chain solutions

Industry Focus
Most industries

CGI Group
1130 Sherbrooke Street West
   5th Floor
Montreal, Quebec H3 A 2M8
Canada
514-841-3200
www.cgi.ca

Profile
Staff: 8,000
13+ offices worldwide

Service Focus
Information Technology

Industry Focus
Financial Services
Government
Manufacturing
Public Utilities
Telecommunications

CIBER

5251 DTC Parkway
    Suite 1400
Greenwood Village, CO 80111
303-220-0100
www.ciber.com

Profile
Staff: 6,002
45 offices worldwide

Service Focus
Information Technology

Industry Focus
Communications
Financial Services
Government
High Technology
Manufacturing

CMG

Parnell House
25 Wilton Road
London, SW1V ILW
United Kingdom
+44 0-20-7592-4000
www.cmg.com

Profile
Staff: 8,063
82 offices worldwide

Service Focus
Information Technology
Operations Management
Strategy

Industry Focus
Financial Services
Telecommunications
Trade & Industry

Conflict Management Group

9 Waterhouse Street
Cambridge, MA 02138
617-354-5444
www.cmgonline.org

Profile
Staff: NA
Offices worldwide

Service Focus
Negotiation
Conflict Resolution

Industry Focus
Government
NGOs
Nonprofits

Computer Science Corporation (CSC)

2100 East Grand Avenue
El Segundo, CA 90245
310-615-0311
www.csc.com

Profile
Staff: 58,000
40 offices worldwide

Service Focus
Information Technology
Operations Management
Strategy

Industry Focus
Aerospace
Financial Services
Government

Corporate Executive Board

2000 Pennsylvania Avenue, N.W.
Washington, DC 20006
202-777-5000
www.executiveboard.com

Profile
Staff: 250+
2 offices worldwide

Service Focus
Research
Executive Education

Industry Focus
Most industries

debis Systemhaus

D-70771 Leinfelden-Echterdingen
Fasanenweg 9 Germany
+49-711-972-0
www.debis.com

Profile
Staff: 17,200
184 offices worldwide

Service Focus
Information Technology

Industry Focus
Most industries

Deloitte Consulting

1633 Broadway
    35th Floor
New York, NY 10019
212-489-1600
www.dc.com

Profile
Staff: 28,625
95 offices worldwide

Service Focus
Human Resources
Information Technology
Operations Management
Strategy

Industry Focus
Government
Financial Services
Manufacturing

DiamondCluster International

John Hancock Center
875 North Michigan Avenue
    Suite 3000
Chicago, IL 60611
312-255-5000
www.diamondcluster.com

Profile
Staff: 1,100
12 offices worldwide

Service Focus
Information Technology

Industry Focus
Wireless
Financial Services
Consumer Products
Telecommunications
Healthcare
Insurance
Energy

DMR Consulting Group
1000 Sherbrooke Street West
 Suite 1600
Montreal, QC, H3A 3R2
Canada
514-877-3301
www.dmr.com

Profile
Staff: 2,440
65 offices worldwide

Service Focus
Information Technology
Operations Management

Industry Focus
Communications
Financial Services
Government

Dove Consulting
75 Park Plaza
Boston, MA 02116
617-482-2100
www.doveassoc.com

Profile
Staff: 150+
Offices in Boston, Minneapolis, and
 London

Service Focus
Strategy
Organizational Design
Marketing Strategy

Industry Focus
Financial Services
Food & Beverage
Communications

Easton Consultants, Inc.
Four Landmark Square
 Suite 301
Stamford, CT 06901
203-348-8774
www.easton-consult.com

Profile
Staff: 15
1 office in Stamford, CT

Service Focus
Strategy
e-Commerce

Industry Focus
Energy & Utilities
Financial Services
Information Services

Electronic Data Systems
5400 Legacy Drive
Plano, TX 75024-3199
972-604-6000
www.eds.com

Profile
Staff: 121,000
100+ offices worldwide

Service Focus
Information Technology
Outsourcing
Strategy (performed by subsidiary,
    A.T. Kearney)

Industry Focus
Most industries

First Annapolis
900 Elkridge Landing Road
    Suite 400
Linthicum, MD 21090
410-855-8500
www.1st-annapolis.com

Profile
Staff: 20
1 office in Linthicum, MD

Service Focus
Strategy
Risk Analysis
Operations
Marketing

Industry Focus
Financial Services
Utilities
Consumer Goods
Retail

First Consulting Group
111 West Ocean Boulevard
    4th Floor
Long Beach, CA 90802-4632
562-624-5200
www.fcg.com

Profile
Staff: 1,800
22 offices worldwide

Service Focus
Information Technology
Operations Management
Strategy

Industry Focus
Healthcare
Government

First Manhattan Consulting Group
90 Park Avenue
    19th Floor
New York, NY 10016
212-455-9191
www.fmcg.com

Profile
Staff: NA
1 office in New York, NY

Service Focus
Strategy
Operations
Risk Management
Organizational Design
Information Technology
Market Research

Industry Focus
Financial Services
Telecommunications
Insurance

FMI
5151 Glenwood Avenue
    Suite 100
Raleigh, NC 27612
919-785-9320
www.fminet.com

Profile
Staff: 150
Offices in Raleigh, Denver, and
　Tampa

Service Focus
Strategy
Organizational Development
Leadership

Industry Focus
Engineering
Building Construction
Manufacturing
Distribution

The Futures Group International

80 Glastonbury Boulevard
Glastonbury, CT 06033-4409
860-633-3501
www.tfgi.com

Profile
Staff: NA
3 U.S. offices plus Bath, U.K.

Service Focus
Economic Development
Strategy
Marketing

Industry Focus
Government
NGOs
Nonprofits

Gartner Group Consulting Services

56 Top Gallant Road
Stamford, CT 06904-2212
203-964-0096
www.gartner.com

Profile
Staff: 4,000
80 offices worldwide

Service Focus
Market Research
Benchmarking
Training

Industry Focus
Information Technology

Genex

621 North Avenue
　Suite A-150
Atlanta, GA 30308
404-592-3000
www.genex.com

Profile
Staff: NA
Offices in Atlanta and Denver

Service Focus
Information Technology
Marketing

Industry Focus
Automotive
Consumer Products
Financial Services
Media & Entertainment

Gibson Associates

360 W. Butterfield Road
Suite 400
Elmhurst, IL 60126
630-993-0800
www.gibsonconsulting.com

Profile
Staff: 150
3 offices: Chicago, Tampa, and
London

Service Focus
Business Operations

Industry Focus
Most industries

Good Work Associates

85 Willow Street
Building #3
New Haven, CT 06511
888-GWA-TEAM
www.goodworkassociates.com

Profile
Staff: NA
1 office in New Haven, CT

Service Focus
Change Management
Leadership
Organizational Development
Strategy

Industry Focus
Nonprofits
Universities
Government

Grant Thornton

800 One Prudential Plaza
130 East Randolph Street
Chicago, IL 60601
312-856-0001
www.grantthornton.com

Profile
Staff: NA
44 U.S. offices

Service Focus
Information Technology
Performance Management
Strategy

Industry Focus
Construction
Financial Services
Government
Healthcare
Higher Education
Nonprofits

The Hay Group

The Wanamaker Building
100 Penn Square East
Philadelphia, PA 19107-3388
215-861-2000
www.haygroup.com

Profile
Staff: 1,065
73 offices worldwide

Service Focus
Human Resources
Organizational Development

Industry Focus
Most industries

Hewitt Associates, LLC
100 Half Day Road
Lincolnshire, IL 60069
847-295-5000
www.hewitt.com

Profile
Staff: 10,930
75 offices worldwide

Service Focus
Human Resources

Industry Focus
Most industries

Horwath International
415 Madison Avenue
New York, NY 10017
212-838-5566
www.horwath.com

Profile
Staff: 2,299
106 offices worldwide

Service Focus
M&A
Leadership
Financial Advising

Industry Focus
Tax & Accounting
Franchising
Hotel, Travel, & Tourism

**IBM Global Services
Consulting**
Route 9, Town of Mount Pleasant
North Tarrytown, NY 10591
914-332-3000
www.ibm.com/services/consulting

Profile
Staff: NA
165+ offices worldwide

Service Focus
Information Technology
Outsourcing
M&A
Strategy
Marketing

Industry Focus
Most industries

k2 Digital
30 Broad Street
    16th Floor
New York, NY 10004
212-301-8800
www.k2digital.com

Profile
Staff: 40
1 office in New York City

Service Focus
Information Technology
Marketing

Industry Focus
Financial Services
Pharmaceuticals
Publishing
Technology

Keane
Ten City Square
Boston, MA 02129
617-241-9200
www.keane. com

Profile
Staff: 8,335
55 offices worldwide

Service Focus
Human Resources
Information Technology
Operations Management
Strategy

Industry Focus
Financial Services
Government

kpe
860 Broadway
New York, NY 10003
212-652-9600
www.kpe.com

Profile
Staff: NA
Offices in New York, Los Angeles,
    and London

Service Focus
Information Technology
Marketing
Strategy

Industry Focus
Media & Entertainment
Travel & Tourism
Consumer Products

KPMG Consulting
1676 International Drive
Tyson's Tower
McLean, VA 22102
703-747-3000
www.kpmgconsulting.com

Profile
Staff: 17,000
120 offices worldwide

Service Focus
Human Resources
Information Technology
Operations Management
Strategy

Industry Focus
Most industries

Kurt Salmon Associates
628 Green Valley Road
    Suite 206
Greensboro, NC 27408
336-299-0674
www.kurtsalmon.com

Profile
Staff: 600
19 offices worldwide

Service Focus
Information Technology
Strategy
Events
M&A

Industry Focus
Healthcare
Packaged Goods
Retail
Manufacturing

LECG
100 Bush Street
    Suite 1650
San Francisco, CA 94104
415-398-2000
www.lecg.com

313

Profile
Staff: 400
17 offices worldwide

Service Focus
Economics

Industry Focus
Most industries

L.E.K. Consulting
28 State Street
　16th Floor
Boston, MA 02110
617-951-9500
www.lekalcar.com

Profile
Staff: NA
15 offices worldwide

Service Focus
Strategy
M&A

Industry Focus
Aerospace
Pharmaceuticals
Financial Services
Consumer Products
Energy
Telecommunications
Utilities

**Lippincott & Margulies
　(subsidiary of Mercer
　Consulting Group)**
499 Park Avenue
New York, NY 10022
212-521-0000
www.lippincott-margulies.com

Profile
Staff: NA
25 offices worldwide

Service Focus
Branding & Marketing
Events

Industry Focus
Automotive
Financial Services
Healthcare
Publishing
Telecommunications
Travel & Tourism
Utilities

Logica
Stephenson House
75 Hampstead Road
London NW1 2PL
United Kingdom
+44-20-7637-9111
www.logica.com

Profile
Staff: 8,521
100 offices worldwide

Service Focus
Information Technology
Operations Management

Industry Focus
Communications
Financial Services
Government
Automotive

Mainspring

One Main Street
Cambridge, MA 02142
888-588-1066
www.mainspring.com

Profile
Staff: 250
Offices in Cambridge, New York,
    and Chicago

Service Focus
Information Technology
Marketing
Operations
Product Development

Industry Focus
Communications
Financial Services
Retail
Life Sciences
Media

Marakon Associates

300 Atlantic Street
Stamford, CT 06901
800-695-4428
www.marakon.com

Profile
Staff: 200+
Offices in the U.S. and U.K.

Service Focus
Strategy

Industry Focus
Consumer Products
Financial Services
Retail
Chemicals

marchFIRST

South Wacker Drive
    Suite 3500
Chicago, IL 60606
312-922-9200
www.marchfirst.com

Profile
Staff: 8,900
72 offices worldwide

Service Focus
Information Technology
Operations Management
Strategy
Marketing

Industry Focus
Most industries

MarketBridge

4550 Montgomery Avenue
500 North Tower
Bethesda, MD 20814
88-GO-TO-MKT
www.market-bridge.com

Profile
Staff: NA
Offices in Bethesda, MD and
    Boston

Service Focus
Strategy
Sales & Marketing

Industry Focus
Financial Services
Healthcare
Manufacturing
Telecommunications

Mars & Co.
Mars Plaza
124 Mason Street
Greenwich, CT 06830
203-629-9292
www.marsandco.com

Profile
Staff: 200
5 offices worldwide

Service Focus
Strategy

Industry Focus
Most industries

McKinsey & Company, Inc.
55 East 52nd Street
    21st Floor
New York, NY 10022
212-446-7000
www.mckinsey.com

Profile
Staff: 5,670
83 offices worldwide

Service Focus
Information Technology
Operations Management
Strategy

Industry Focus
Most industries

Mercer Management Consulting (subsidiary of Mercer Consulting Group)
1166 Avenue of the Americas
New York, NY 10036
212-345-8000
www.mercermc.com

Profile
Staff: 1,400
23 offices worldwide

Service Focus
Human Resources
Strategy
Marketing
Operations

Industry Focus
Most industries

Mercer Delta (subsidiary of Mercer Consulting Group, formerly Delta Consulting Group)
1177 Avenue of the Americas
New York, NY 10036
212-403-7500
www.mercerdelta.com

Profile
Staff: NA
4 U.S. offices

Service Focus
Organizational Architecture
Leadership

Industry Focus
Most industries

Milliman Global
1301 Fifth Avenue
    Suite 3800
Seattle, WA 98101-2605
206-624-7940
www.woodrowmilliman.com

Profile
Staff: 1,850
100 offices worldwide

Service Focus
Human Resources
Strategy

Industry Focus
Most industries

Monitor Group
Two Canal Park
Cambridge, MA 02141
617-252-2000
www.monitor.com

Profile
Staff: 900
28 offices worldwide

Service Focus
Healthcare
Financial Services
Retail
Media & Entertainment
Strategy

Industry Focus
Financial Services
Healthcare
High Technology
Media & Entertainment
Retail

**National Economic Research
  Association, Inc. (Subsidiary
  of Mercer Consulting Group)**
One Main Street
  Fifth Floor
Cambridge, MA 02142
617-621-0444
www.nera.com

Profile
Staff: 100+
13 offices worldwide

Service Focus
Public Policy
Product Strategy
Risk Management
M&A
Strategy

Industry Focus
Government
Healthcare
Communications
Financial Services
Environment
Pharmaceuticals

Navigant Consulting
615 North Wabash Avenue
Chicago, IL 60611
312-573-5600
www.navigantconsulting.com

Profile
Staff: 1,200
42 offices worldwide

Service Focus
Information Technology
Operations Management
Strategy
M&A

Industry Focus
Communications
Utilities
Telecommunications
Healthcare

PA Consulting Group
123 Buckingham Palace Road
London, United Kingdom SW1W
   9SR
+44-207-730-9000
www.pa-consulting.com

Profile
Staff: 2,000
40 offices worldwide

Service Focus
Information Technology
Operations Management
Strategy

Industry Focus
Energy
Financial Services
Government
Manufacturing
Transportation

Perot Systems
12404 Park Central
Dallas, TX 75251
972-340-5000
www.perotsystems.com

Profile
Staff: 2,300
41 offices worldwide

Service Focus
Information Technology
Strategy

Industry Focus
Healthcare
Communications
Energy
Financial Services
Insurance
Manufacturing
Travel & Transportation
Media

Peterson Consulting
175 W. Jackson Boulevard
   Suite 500
Chicago, IL 60604
312-583-5700
www.petersonworldwide.com

Profile
Staff: 1,700
13 offices worldwide

Service Focus
Information Management
Economic Analysis
Business Outsourcing

Industry Focus
Most industries

Plaut
U.S. Headquarters
1050 Winter Street
Waltham, MA 02451
781-768-0500
www.plaut.com

Profile
Staff: 1,703
25+ offices worldwide

Service Focus
Information Technology
Operations Management
Strategy

Industry Focus
Most industries

PricewaterhouseCoopers
1301 Avenue of the Americas
New York, NY 10019
212-707-6000
www.pwcglobal.com

Profile
Staff: 44,000
200+ offices worldwide

Service Focus
Human Resources
Information Technology
Operations Management
Strategy

Industry Focus
Most industries

razorfish
32 Mercer Street
New York, NY 10013
212-966-5960
www.razorfish.com

Profile
Staff: 1,500
15 offices worldwide

Service Focus
Information Technology
Marketing
Strategy

Industry Focus
Consumer Products
Financial Services
Media & Entertainment
Nonprofits
Telecommunications
Travel & Tourism
Pharmaceuticals
Utilities

Roland Berger & Partner
350 Park Avenue
    27th Floor
New York, NY 10022
212-651-9660
www.rolandberger.com

Profile
Staff: 1,012
30 offices worldwide

Service Focus
Strategy

Industry Focus
Automotive
Financial Services
High Technology
Retail
Transportation

**RSM McGladery (formerly
    McGladery & Pullen)**
1699 Woodfield Road
    Suite 300
Schaumburg, IL 60173-4969
847-517-7070
www.rsmmcgladrey.com

Profile
Staff: 608
300+ offices worldwide

Service Focus
Human Resources
Information Technology
Operations Management
Strategy

Industry Focus
Most industries

Sapient
One Memorial Drive
Cambridge, MA 02142
617–621–0200
www.sapient.com

Profile
Staff: 1,600
19 offices worldwide

Service Focus
Information Technology
Operations Management
Strategy
Marketing

Industry Focus
Energy/Oil & Gas
Financial Services
Media & Publishing
Transportation
Retail

SCA Consulting
633 West 5th Street
    Suite 3300
Los Angeles, CA 90071
213–327–2000
www.scaconsulting.com

Profile
Staff: 100
5 U.S. offices

Service Focus
Human Resources
Organizational Design

Industry Focus
Automotive
Chemicals
Consumer Products
Financial Services
Healthcare

Scient
500 Technology Square
Boston, MA 02139
617–788–2000
www.scient.com

Profile
Staff: NA
11 offices worldwide

Service Focus
Information Technology
Marketing
Strategy

Industry Focus
Financial Services
Healthcare
Media & Publishing
Retail & Consumer Goods
Telecommunications

Sema Group
16 Rue Barbes, 92126 Montrouge
    Cedex
Paris, France
+33–1–40–92–40–92
U.S.: 888–835–7362
www.semagroup.com

Profile
Staff: 21,900
155 offices worldwide

Service Focus
Information Technology

Industry Focus
Financial Services
Manufacturing
Public Sector
Telecommunications

Sibson & Company
600 Alexander Park
   Suite 208
Princeton, NJ 08540
609-520-2700
www.sibson.com

Profile
Staff: NA
10 offices worldwide

Service Focus
Human Resources
Sales & Marketing

Industry Focus
Financial Services
Healthcare

siegelgale
10 Rockefeller Plaza
   3rd Floor
New York, NY 10020
212-707-4000
www.siegelgale.com

Profile
Staff: 400
3 U.S. offices plus London

Service Focus
Marketing & Branding
Product Development
Strategy
Training

Industry Focus
Consumer Products
Financial Services
Media & Entertainment
Retail
Telecommunications

Spherion Technology Architects
823 Commerce Drive
Oak Brook, IL 60523
630-574-3030
www.spherion.com/technology

Profile
Staff: 7,000
66 offices worldwide

Service Focus
Information Technology
Operations Management
Strategy

Industry Focus
Communications
Financial Services
Government

Stax Inc.
359 Green Street
Cambridge, MA 02139
888-654-STAX
www.stax.com

Profile
Staff: 20
4 U.S. offices

Service Focus
Strategy
Marketing
Market Research
M&A
Business Start-up

Industry Focus
Financial Services
Private Equity
Telecommunications
Education
Consumer Goods
Media & Entertainment
Healthcare

Stern Stewart & Co.
1345 Avenue of the Americas
New York, NY 10105
212-261-0600
www.sternstewart.com

Profile
Staff: NA
14 offices worldwide

Service Focus

Industry Focus
Building Materials
Financial Services
Pharmaceuticals
Retail

**Strategic Decisions Group
(SDG)**
2440 Sand Hill Road
Menlo Park, CA 94025
650-854-9000
www.sdg.com

Profile
Staff: NA
6 offices worldwide

Service Focus
Strategy
M&A
Product Development

Industry Focus
Automotive
Electronics
Financial Services
Healthcare
Media & Entertainment
Oil & Gas

Tata Consultancy
3010 LBJ Freeway
  Suite 715
Dallas, TX 75234
972-484-6465
www.tcs.com

Profile
Staff: 10,000
100+ offices worldwide

Service Focus
Information Technology

Industry Focus
Communications
Healthcare
Financial Services
Retail
Telecommunications
Transportation
Utilities

Telcordia Technologies
(formerly Bellcore)
445 South Street
Morristown, NJ 07960
973-829-2000
www.telcordia.com

Profile
Staff: 1,470
37 offices worldwide

Service Focus
Human Resources
Information Technology
Operations Management
Strategy
Training

Industry Focus
Telecommunications

TechPartners International
301 Howard Street
  17th Floor
San Francisco, CA 94105
415-808-9000
www.techpartners.com

Profile
Staff: 600
4 offices worldwide

Service Focus
Information Management

Industry Focus
Most industries

Towers Perrin
335 Madison Avenue
New York, NY 10017-4605
212-309-3400
www.towers.com

Profile
Staff: 8,400
70 offices worldwide

Service Focus
Human Resources
Organizational Development

Industry Focus
Most industries

Viant Corporation
89 South Street
  2nd Floor
Boston, MA 02111
617-531-3700
www.viant.com

Profile
Staff: 400
9 offices worldwide

Service Focus
Information Technology
Marketing
Strategy

Industry Focus
Financial Services
Consumer Products
Retail

VISION Consulting
110 East 42nd Street
New York, NY 10017
212-983-7250
www.vision.com

Profile
Staff: 350
Offices in New York plus London,
   Edinburgh, Belfast, and Dublin

Service Focus
Information Technology

Industry Focus
Financial Services
Transportation
Utilities

Watson Wyatt Worldwide
6707 Democracy Boulevard
   Suite 800
Bethesda, MD 20817
301-581-4600
www.watsonwyatt.com

Profile
Staff: 5,500
85 offices worldwide

Service Focus
Human Resources
Organizational Development
Strategy

Industry Focus
Most industries

William Kent International
2101 Wilson Boulevard
   Suite 1100
Arlington, VA 22201
703-516-7920
www.wkint.com

Profile
Staff: NA
4 offices worldwide

Service Focus
Portfolio Management
Strategy

Industry Focus
Aerospace
Automotive
Building Materials
Chemicals
Consumer Products
Electronics
Food

ZS Associates
1800 Sherman Avenue
   Suite 700
Evanston, IL 60201
847-492-3600
www.zsassociates.com

Profile
Staff: NA
6 offices worldwide

Service Focus
Compensation
Sales & Marketing
Market Research
Product Launch

Industry Focus
Chemicals
Electronics
Financial Services
Insurance
Pharmaceuticals
Telecommunications
Utilities

Notes

Introduction

1. The answers to these case questions and more are provided in Appendix I.

Chapter 1

1. Kennedy Information Research Group.

2. Corporate Decisions, Inc. (CDI) merged with Mercer Management Consulting in 1998.

3. *The Global Management Consulting Marketplace: Key Data, Forecasts & Trends, 2001 Edition,* Kennedy Information Research Group.

4. *The Global Management Consulting Marketplace: Key Data, Forecasts & Trends, 2001 Edition,* Kennedy Information Research Group.

5. Ibid.

6. "A Survey of Management Consultancy," *The Economist,* 1997.

7. *The Global Management Consulting Marketplace: Key Data, Forecasts & Trends, 2001 Edition,* Kennedy Information Research Group.

8. Ibid.

9. "A Survey of Management Consultancy, *The Economist,* 1997.

Chapter 3

1. bainlab Web site, "Welcome" page, February 20, 2001.

2. McKinsey & Company Web site, "Accelerator @ McKinsey" page, February 20, 2001.

NOTES

Chapter 4

1. Donald A. Shön, *The Reflective Practitioner, How Professionals Think in Action,* (New York: Basic Books, 1982).

2. Ibid.

3. Ibid.

4. The added value of cars may be huge, but that does not mean Ford has a large added value. Without Ford, there is still GM, Toyota, and many others.

Chapter 5

1. *Consultant's News,* Kennedy Information Research Group, February 1998; *The Global Management Consulting Marketplace: Key Data, Forecasts & Trends, 2001 Edition,* Kennedy Information Research Group.

Chapter 7

1. Fisher, R., Ury, W., & Patton, B. (1991). *Getting to Yes* (2nd ed.). New York: Penguin Books.

2. Lax, D.A., & Sebenius, J.K. (1986). *The Manager as Negotiator.* New York: The Free Press.

3. *The Global Management Consulting Marketplace: Key Data, Forecasts & Trends, 2001 Edition,* Kennedy Information Research Group.

Appendix I

1. This discussion assumes a basic understanding of accounting. Reference: K.G. Palepu, V.L. Bernard, & P.M. Healy. 1996. *Business Analysis and Valuation: Using Financial Statements,* Cincinnati: South-Western College Publishing.

2. A. Brandenburger and B. Nalebuff. 1996. *Co-opetition.* New York: Doubleday.

Appendix II

1. Boeing corporate information.

Appendix III

1. Information collected from corporate Internet sites, public SEC records, annual reports, and marketing brochures as of May 2001.

Index